Perspectives ON Philosophy OF Science IN Nursing

An Historical and Contemporary Anthology

E. Carol Polifroni is an Associate Professor in the School of Nursing at the University of Connecticut. She earned her bachelor's degree from Saint Anselm College, her master's from New York University, and her doctorate in education from Rutgers University. She teaches classes in leadership and management, administration, contemporary topics, policy, and philosophy of science to undergraduate, graduate, and doctoral students. Carol has had a longtime interest in philosophy of science and is particularly fascinated by its application to patient/family care and health administration.

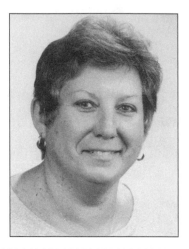

Marylouise Welch is an Associate Professor in the Division of Nursing at Saint Joseph College. She earned her bachelor's degree from the University of Pennsylvania and her master's (nursing) and doctoral degree in anthropology from the University of Connecticut. She teaches nursing theory and care of the patient/family with acute care needs to undergraduate and graduate students and works with an interdisciplinary group on culture. Marylouise is most interested in the relationship between nursing theory, research on trauma survival, and philosophy of science.

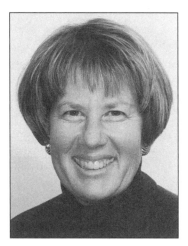

Perspectives on Philosophy of Science in Nursing

An Historical and Contemporary Anthology

EDITED BY:

E. Carol Polifroni, RN, EdD

Associate Professor
University of Connecticut
School of Nursing
Storrs, Connecticut

Marylouise Welch, RN, PhD

Associate Professor of Nursing
Saint Joseph College
West Hartford, Connecticut

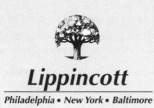

Lippincott

Philadelphia • New York • Baltimore

Acquisitions Editor: Susan M. Glover, RN, MSN
Assistant Editor: Bridget Blatteau
Production Editor: Virginia Barishek
Production Manager: Helen Ewan
Production Service: P.M. Gordon Associates
Compositor: Maryland Composition
Printer/Binder: R.R. Donnelley & Sons/Crawfordsville
Cover Designer: Thomas M. Jackson
Cover Printer: Lehigh Press

Library of Congress Cataloging-in-Publication Data

Perspectives on philosophy of science in nursing: an historical and
   contemporary anthology / edited by E. Carol Polifroni, Marylouise
Welch.
      p.   cm.
   Includes index.
   ISBN 0–7817–1201–7
   1. Nursing—Philosophy.   I. Polifroni, E. Carol.   II. Welch, Marylouise.
   [DNLM: 1. Philosophy, Nursing collected works.   2. Nursing Theory
collected works. WY 86 P4675 1999]
   RT84.5.P475   1999
   610.73′01—dc21
   DNLM/DLC
   for Library of Congress   98–15842
                                                              CIP

Care has been taken to confirm the accuracy of the information presented and to describe generally accepted practices. However, the authors, editors, and publisher are not responsible for errors or omissions or for any consequences from application of the information in this book and make no warranty, express or implied, with respect to the contents of the publication.

The authors, editors and publisher have exerted every effort to ensure that drug selection and dosage set forth in this text are in accordance with current recommendations and practice at the time of publication. However, in view of ongoing research, changes in government regulations, and the constant flow of information relating to drug therapy and drug reactions, the reader is urged to check the package insert for each drug for any change in indications and dosage and for added warnings and precautions. This is particularly important when the recommended agent is a new or infrequently employed drug.

Some drugs and medical devices presented in this publication have Food and Drug Administration (FDA) clearance for limited use in restricted research settings. It is the responsibility of the health care provider to ascertain the FDA status of each drug or device planned for use in their clinical practice.

9 8 7 6 5 4 3 2 1

To the memory of Sheila Packard, RN, PhD (1949–1995) . . . a renegade, a thinker, a fun-loving person . . .

for introducing us to philosophy of science,
for fostering a nontraditional perspective,
for provoking intellectual mischief, and
for being our wonderful friend and colleague.

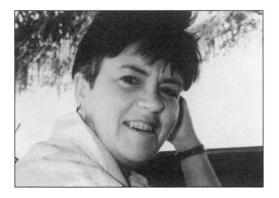

CONTRIBUTORS

Patricia Benner, RN, PhD
Professor
School of Nursing
Department of Physiological Nursing
University of California, San Francisco
San Francisco, California

Sheila Bunting, PhD
Doctoral Student
School of Nursing
Wayne State University
Detroit, Michigan

Jacquelyn C. Campbell, PhD, RN, FAAN
Associate Professor
School of Nursing
Wayne State University
Detroit, Michigan

Barbara A. Carper, RN, EdD
Professor
University of North Carolina
Charlotte, North Carolina

Peggy L. Chinn, RN, PhD, FAAN
Professor
School of Nursing
University of Connecticut
Storrs, Connecticut

William K. Cody, RN, PhD
Associate Professor and Chairperson
Family and Community Nursing
University of North Carolina
Charlotte, North Carolina

Sheila A. Corcoran-Perry, PhD, RN
Associate Professor
University of Minnesota
School of Nursing
Minneapolis, Minnesota

Donald A. Crosby, PhD
Department of Philosophy
Colorado State University
Fort Collins, Colorado

Nancy Drew, RN, PhD
Associate Professor of Nursing
Saint Joseph College
West Hartford, Connecticut

Laura Cox Dzurec, PhD, RN
Oregon State University
Portland, Oregon

Hans-Georg Gadamer, PhD
German philosopher
Faculty at Marburg, Leipzig, Frankfurt, Heidel-
berg, Vanderbilt, Catholic University of Amer-
ica, Boston College, University of Dallas, and
McMaster University

Ruth Ginzberg, PhD
Former Chairperson
Department of Philosophy
Beloit College
Beloit, Wisconsin

Susan R. Gortner, RN, PhD, FAAN

Professor Emeritus of Nursing
Department of Family Health Care Nursing
University of California, San Francisco
San Francisco, California

Jürgen Habermas, PhD

Johann Wolfgang Goethe-Universitat Frankfurt
Frankfurt am Main
Germany

Ian Hacking, PhD

Institute for History and Philosophy of Science
and Technology
University of Toronto
Toronto, Ontario
Canada

Sandra Harding, PhD

Professor
Department of Philosophy
University of California, Los Angeles
Los Angeles, California

Martin Heidegger, PhD*

German philosopher
Studied philosophy under Husserl at the
University of Freiburg
Formerly Rektorat
University of Freiburg

Carl G. Hempel, PhD*

German American philosopher
Formerly faculty at Princeton and Yale

Edmund Husserl, PhD*

German philosopher
Formerly faculty at Universities of Halle,
Gottingen and Freiburg

Evelyn Fox Keller, PhD*

Formerly Visiting Scholar in Science,
Technology and Society
Formerly Professor of Mathematics and
Humanities
Massachusetts Institute of Technology
Northeastern University

Thomas Kuhn, PhD*

Formerly faculty at Harvard, University of California at Berkeley, Princeton, and Massachusetts Institute of Technology

Laurens Laudan, PhD

Fellow
University of Hawaii at Manoa

Victoria Wynn Leonard, RN, PhD

School of Nursing
University of California, San Francisco
San Francisco, California

Marjorie McIntyre, RN, PhD

Assistant Professor
University of Calgary
Faculty of Nursing
Calgary, Alberta
Canada

M. Merleau-Ponty, PhD*

French philosopher
Formerly faculty at Lyons, Sorbonne, and the
College de France

Gail J. Mitchell, RN, PhD

Chief Nursing Officer
Sunnybrook Health Science Centre
Assistant Professor
University of Toronto
Toronto, Ontario
Canada

*Deceased

Margaret A. Newman, PhD, RN, FAAN
Professor
University of Minnesota
School of Nursing
Minneapolis, Minnesota

Sheila A. Packard, RN, PhD*
Formerly faculty at University of Connecticut
Storrs, Connecticut

Marilyn A. Ray, RN, PhD
Professor
Florida Atlantic University
Boca Raton, Florida

Pamela G. Reed, RN, PhD, FAAN
Associate Professor
College of Nursing
University of Arizona
Tucson, Arizona

Moritz Schlick, PhD*
German-Austrian philosopher
Formerly faculty at the Universities of Rostock,
Kiel, and Vienna

Karen L. Schumacher, RN, PhD
University of California, San Francisco
San Francisco, California

A. Marilyn Sime, PhD, RN
Professor
University of Minnesota
School of Nursing
Minneapolis, Minnesota

Janice L. Thompson, RN, PhD
Professor
School of Nursing
University of Southern Maine
Portland, Maine

Bas van Fraassen, PhD
Dutch philosopher of science
Formerly faculty at Yale, University of Toronto,
University of Southern California, and Prince-
ton

Donald Wayne Viney, PhD
Department of Social Science
Pittsburg State University
Pittsburg, Kansas

Jean Watson, RN, PhD, FAAN
University of Colorado
Denver, Colorado

Donna L. Wells, RN, PhD
Assistant Professor
Faculty of Nursing
University of Toronto
Toronto, Ontario
Canada

*Deceased

PREFACE

The genesis of this anthology was the need, identified by the editors, for nursing students to expand their understanding of philosophy and the development of scientific knowledge. It is apparent today that most of us are uninformed and unfamiliar with the historical development of Western knowledge and our philosophical heritage. As teachers we tried to remedy the situation by quick, basic informative sessions on scientific and philosophic concepts and a reliance on secondary sources to give the students summaries of the information. We found this to be an unsatisfactory solution.

We have attempted to identify important currents in philosophy of science that have influenced prominent nurse theorists and knowledge development in nursing. It is clear that nursing science is still on a quest for its philosophical roots and as a discipline has come late to articulating and discussing the important influence of our philosophical origins. It is therefore of paramount importance that subsequent students become more familiar with the original writings of the philosophers of science who are frequently cited in nursing theoretical discussions. A specific philosophical orientation will direct the formulation of the research question, the phenomena selected for study and the choice of technique of inquiry. Nurse scholars need to understand the authors' works unfiltered through the lens of someone else, so that they are better educated to posit research questions that will find answers for future nursing practice.

This anthology, it is hoped, will continue the debate on the need for a plurality and diversity of philosophical perspectives as we strive to define the focus of nursing. This book is intended to further the exploration of the theoretical domain of nursing before we close debate on the actual focus of the discipline.

GUIDE TO THE BOOK

The purpose of this book is to assist the reader in an investigation of philosophy of science in nursing. While the editors and authors have specific views of their own, it is the intent of the book to delve into diversity, origins, and development of thought but not to recommend a specific viewpoint. Each section aims to establish some foundational understanding in the topical area followed by seminal works and manuscripts which illustrate central themes in the topical area. Each section concludes with a series of questions, thoughts, and/or positions to ponder for use in discussions with other readers. Additionally, each section has suggested references that expand upon the viewpoints and schools of thought presented in the section.

This book is designed for use by individuals at varying points in their scholarly inquiry in philosophy of science in nursing. The beginner may use the introductory material in each section as preparatory information to guide them through the original works. The more mature and experienced scholar in philosophy of science may choose to read only the classics we have identified to illustrate the key themes and treatises. In either case, the discussion questions and recommended readings will direct the reader to additional resources to further their understanding of a specific area of thought.

For the novice, it may be helpful to read the discussion questions first, followed by our introduction to each section, and culminating in the reading of the classic works. This may help the reader to grasp the material presented. Upon completion of the readings, the participant may choose to engage in dialogue with another in regard to the questions or attempt to answer them individually. However, the nature of philosophical inquiry is largely dialectic, which involves more than one individual. When the reader is ready to extend their study with readings from the bibliography, they will have accomplished a basic understanding in philosophy of science.

ORGANIZATION OF THE BOOK

The anthology is divided into eight sections. The organization of the book reflects an eclectic approach consistent with the origins of our discipline. The introduction raises the question, what is the focus of the discipline of nursing. That is, what are the phenomena that should be the study of nursing science and what are the problems that nursing science has the potential to answer?

The sections on truth, explanation, and free will versus determinism illustrate topics that have dominated discussions in philosophy of science. The section on free will versus determinism raises questions about individual choice, full and situated freedom, and predetermined sets of circumstances into which one is thrust. How to describe and explain events (phenomena) in the natural world is tackled in the section on explanation. Is there only one truth? Multiple and all competing simultaneously truths are some of the concerns that philosophers of science who write in the section on truth discuss.

The later sections are germane to current discussions on how to develop nursing knowledge and the authors' works contained here are frequently cited in the nursing literature. The central topics (for example, explanation) presented in the first four sections reappear in these later sections. A claim for theories that yield understanding and explanation is the central point of the section on phenomenology and hermeneutics. How to lay bare the effects of power and social relations of dominant groups on knowledge development in subordinate groups is a concern of critical social theorists. This line of critical examination of forces of control has been used by nursing to examine its historically subordinate female role both as practitioners and as theoreticians. The writings in this section reveal the possibilities that critical social theory holds for nursing. In the later part of the twentieth century, as women have begun to achieve graduate degrees, particularly in the natural sciences, the effects of gender on science, that is, who the scientist is, have been examined. The section on gender and science is included because it is a developing domain of inquiry and looks to be fruitful for nursing knowledge development.

The conclusion contains nurse theorists' writings that describe the possibilities that a postmodern view of science has opened up. Postmodernism is an unclear, ambiguous collection of many theoretical viewpoints. It is hoped that this chapter will create many more questions than answers and offer the reader ideas for new creative approaches to theory development in nursing.

E. Carol Polifroni, RN, EdD
Marylouise Welch, RN, PhD

ACKNOWLEDGMENTS

An anthology such as *Perspectives on Philosophy of Science in Nursing* cannot be written without the assistance and guidance of many people. The authors want to first thank the publishers and authors of the works included in this anthology. Without their collective permission, the book would not be. We also want to thank the hundreds of students with whom we have interacted over the past several years. Their insights, difficulties, and perspectives have assisted us in clarifying our thoughts and initiating this work.

The assistance of the individuals from Saint Joseph College, specifically Kathleen Kelley, Catherine Posteraro, and Debbie Ahl, enabled us to proceed from an idea to a product. At the University of Connecticut, David Garnes facilitated our inquiry and gathered data when we were unable to obtain it.

As always, we thank our families for their unyielding support and encouragement. Lastly, we thank each other for enabling ourselves to do our own thing within the context of the larger whole.

Contents

NURSING AND PHILOSOPHY OF SCIENCE: CONNECTIONS AND DISCONNECTIONS

E. Carol Polifroni ● *Marylouise Welch*

PHILOSOPHY OF SCIENCE IN NURSING: AN INTRODUCTION

Science, philosophy and philosophy of science are all topics of great significance to nursing. As the larger society grapples with the meaning and quality of life accompanied by the objectification of the health care world, the need to examine issues of what it means to know, what truth is, how we know and what can be learned from science and philosophy is central to growth in the discipline. Simultaneously, it is imperative that nurse scholars gain an understanding of the diverse scientific and philosophic traditions that have influenced the development of nursing knowledge in order to further develop and enhance our science, our discipline and our profession.

This book examines historical and contemporary thinking in philosophy of science as well as its implications, influences, values and worth for nursing. The intent is to present the historical debates in the development of philosophy of science and relate them to the development of nursing as a science in order to gain a broader and deeper understanding of the philosophical assumptions and underpinnings of much of nursing scientific development.

Crucial questions that pervade the discussions in this text are, "Is nursing a science?" and, if it is, "What do we want or need from nursing science?" Both of these questions have been addressed by nurse scientists (Donaldson & Crowley, 1978; Gortner, 1990; Meleis, 1985; Newman, 1997; Parse, 1987; Watson, 1995), but we can not adequately or even superficially answer either of these questions without an analysis and ultimate understanding of the epistemological and ontological views that define and shape the perspectives of science and nursing.

WHAT IS SCIENCE?

To define science, philosophy and/or philosophy of science would require significantly more than an introductory section to a book. Nonetheless, in order to establish a common ground for discussion, selected views of science are herein addressed. Science can be classified into three major categories: (1) pure versus applied science; (2) law-finding versus fact-finding science; and (3) natural versus social science (Klemke, Hollinger &

Kline, 1988). In the first category, pure sciences are the formal sciences of mathematics and logic, as well as the empirical sciences of both the natural and social sciences: physics, chemistry, biology, psychology, sociology and anthropology. The pure sciences are in contrast to the applied sciences of engineering, aeronautics, agriculture and medicine. In the pure sciences, there is knowledge for knowledge's sake, whereas the applied sciences utilize knowledge for a specific aim beyond knowledge development.

The category of law-finding versus fact-finding science is not without controversy. Law-finding sciences aim to identify universal laws that guide all scientific development and revolutions, and, by their very definition, are applicable everywhere at all times. The essence of law-finding science is the search for universality and maximum generalizability. In contrast, the fact-finding sciences of geography and economics, as two examples, are more concerned and focused on local events and utilization rather than universality. Thus, some argue that fact-finding science is not really scientific or a science when it is individualized and nonuniversal.

The natural sciences versus social sciences category is based on the subject matter and does not search for either universality or facts. Therefore, this category is controversy-ladened as well. Is it a category of science when it does not have a goal but rather only a name? Both natural and social sciences are grounded in the cultural phenomenon of the event as well as the natural phenomenon itself. Is this then a category of science?

Therefore, when the three categories of science are viewed, the first category and distinction between pure and applied science becomes the primary and foremost category of science. The other two categories are seemingly disqualified on the basis of uniqueness, lack of universality, limited articulated differences and an absence of empirical evidence to support the categories as distinctly different items and not merely names of subject matter.

The popular picture is that science is a useful set of theories with practical success in people's lives. It means a public view of verifiable knowledge that focuses on the material or phenomenal world, answering specific questions through investigation. One example is the development of the polio vaccine. A broader view of science is one of the development of certain knowledge domains that contain formal, natural and/or applied elements such as the pure versus applied category discussed above.

AIMS OF SCIENCE

The aims of science differ between the pure and applied categories. In the pure category the aims are two: (1) the pursuit of knowledge and the attainment of truth; and (2) description, explanation, prediction and control of events. The first aim is self-explanatory: knowledge for its own sake is a worthy goal of science, along with the search for truth. In the pure sciences, truth is seen as an absolute, a definite, a singular end wherein only one truth exists. If multiple truths seem possible, it is because the sole, singular truth has not yet been discovered. In the contemporary world, not without controversy and significant disagreement, Horgan (1997) suggests that the end of science is approaching because the single truths (the absolutes) have been found, the goal of science has been met and there is no more purpose to science.

The second aim of science, that of description through control, is an empirical approach to scientific inquiry. The scientist describes an event through an account of the observable and a formulation of propositions. The scientist aims to explain the event by accounting for the facts and the regularities that are observed. An explanation is often the answering of the all-important why question. In prediction, the aim is to derive propositions for events which have not yet occurred, based on the universality of the descriptions and explanations. When description, explanation and prediction are fully actualized, control is reached and the second aim of pure science is met.

For the applied sciences, the aims are different. They are planning, technological progress and the utilization of the forces of nature for practical purposes. In applied sciences, knowledge development for knowledge's sake is not a goal, but rather utilization, the application of the knowledge, is the foremost activity and concern. Planning is identified as a major aim of the applied sciences, in that planning enables society, the science and the people within the science to be prepared for nature's events. Prevention and control permeate the applied scientist's aims and goals through the utilization of knowledge for society's sake. But is taking a theory developed in one discipline and applying it to another the best approach for a practice discipline?

Strasser (1985) expands the discussion of applied science to include a third category, human science. Within human science there are three divisions: practical, theoretical and a combination of both practice and theory. There are three essential characteristics of the human sciences: (1) the scientists communicate with their subjects; (2) the scientists do not objectify their subjects; and (3) the scientists are part of the social world they study.

This framework, with nursing viewed as a practical human science, dictates that from the beginning of theory development the aim is for knowledge specific to an area of praxis. This perspective differs from applied science, in which a theory developed in one discipline is then imported to answer a question in another. Nursing as a practical human science offers potential for future theory development because it integrates the theoretical and practical with the goal of improved patient care.

One must pause here and ponder: Is nursing a science? Is it a pure science or an applied science? What makes it a science? What are the similarities between nursing and the sciences just described? What is truth in nursing and what are our explanations? Do we pursue knowledge for knowledge's sake or do we aim for our science to be applied? Is nursing a science or is it common sense? The reader will be able to both answers these questions and raise additional questions as this material is understood.

CRITERIA FOR SCIENCE

Whether the science, any science, is applied, pure or practical human, there are generally five criteria used to distinguish a science from common sense: intersubjective testability, reliability, definiteness and precision, coherence or systematic character and comprehensiveness and scope (Feigl, 1988). Intersubjective testability is the belief that, in principle, the science can be corroborated by anyone. Intersubjective is a synonym for objective in this case, in that the belief is not based on hallucination or deception and it is not a state of mind but rather truly exists. Furthermore, the belief is neither private nor unique. It can be and must be verified. Embedded in intersubjectivity is the belief that it, the variable, can be empirically tested. The criterion of intersubjective testability then is the premise that the statement, the science, is objective and can be verified if the testing mechanisms are available. The emphasis is not that it has been verified but that it can be tested and ultimately verified.

Reliability is the second criterion distinguishing science from common sense. Reliability is the confirmation of a statement, a set of beliefs, the premises of an argument through repeated tests and the receipt of the same results, the same outcome. Without reliability, there is no ability to either predict or control. Reliability is predicated on repetition and sameness.

The third criterion for a science is definiteness and precision. Exactness and rigidity is a need in a science. Fluidity and accommodation, as well as personalization, are appropriate in common sense but not in science. In other words, "approximately an ounce" is not scientific whereas "30 cubic centimeters" is scientific. "Circular" is common sense whereas "360 degrees" is science. This criterion of definiteness and precision aims to remove ambiguity and vagueness through finite, measurable and clearly identified statements and beliefs.

Coherence or systematic character is the fourth criterion. The notion is the relatedness and wholeness approach to science rather than a series of disjointed and unconnected statements. Within coherence is the belief that the science must be free of contradictions and be universally accepted and uniformly directed.

The last criterion is that of comprehensiveness and scope. The thrust of this criterion is the maximum explanatory power of the science and its related theories. In other words, a science is not a science if it does not explain and address events and related concerns beyond the issue under study at the present time. For instance, Newton's theory of gravity explained falling bodies but it also addressed the revolution of the heavenly bodies and the existence of the tides.

In conclusion, in order for a science, pure, applied or practical human, to earn the traditional distinction of a science it must have the previously addressed five criteria. The reader is now again posed with the question: Is nursing a science? Does nursing possess intersubjective testability, reliability, definiteness and scope, coherence and comprehensiveness? If so, it is likely a science. If not, then what is nursing? Further inquiry and exploration is needed before answering these questions.

WHAT IS PHILOSOPHY?

Despite the achievements and advances of science there still remain questions for which science has no answer. How do philosophy and science help us to understand the complicated and ambiguous relationship between the subjective spirit of the individual and the objective spirit that manifests itself in the physical world? These questions are in the philosophical arena, questions that transcend the material and phenomenal world. Philosophy has as its goal to help humans understand themselves within a world dominated by traditional science. Philosophy is concerned with questions that are more common or abstract and not necessarily amenable to direct investigation. Philosophy of science is an attempt to understand the logical structure of science, to examine the interface of science and other human questions and institutions. It employs logical analysis to examine the methods, goals, outcomes and theories produced by the sciences.

Philosophy originates with the Greek word *philosophia*, which translates as "the love of wisdom." For many, the love of wisdom can be operationalized as critical inquiry and examination of method, experience and meaning. Philosophers, by virtue of both education and intent, hold dialogue on questions human beings are faced with in daily life but rarely talk about. Philosophers are engaged in inquiry concerning the search for truth, the nature of the universe and the meaning of the human experience. The inquiry is thoroughly immersed in the context of the discourse as well as the time and place of the dialogue. Based on the knowledge obtained from the inquiry, a philosopher creates his or her life and lives it within a certain perspective. Philosophy, then, is also a way of life. "Philosophy is a way of life—an essential way—that consists precisely of living according to a certain knowledge; therefore this way of life postulates and requires this certain knowledge. It is thus knowledge which determines the meaning of philosophic life" (Marias, 1967, p. 1). Some argue about this dual approach to philosophy as both knowledge and a way of life in the belief that it is one or the other, but not both. However, the readings and the discussion points which conclude each section will lead the reader to approach philosophy in this dual purpose manner.

Philosophy, as knowledge, is "a fundamental, universal certainty which is also autonomous; that is, philosophy justifies itself; it constantly demonstrates and proves its own validity; it thrives exclusively on evidence. Philosophy is always renewing the reasons for its certainty" (Marias, 1967, p. 2). Philosophy is a quest, a pattern of behavior and inquiry that achieves a perspective on knowledge and meaning. The knowledge and meaning may not be an end but rather the beginning of another quest. The knowledge achieved is continuously assessed and challenged, based on human beings' natural need to know and to learn.

The manner in which the nature of philosophy is approached is based on inquiry and immersion. To engage in a philosophic discussion, the participants must be informed about both the development of the position and knowledgeable of the position itself. Philosophy, then, is heavily indebted to and a part of history. The development of a philosophical position stems from the historical developments of society and learned areas at large. Philosophy draws upon both history and content to create or validate an idea or position. The context of the development as well as the current discourse will, naturally, color the nature of the debate. It is imperative (a word rarely used in philosophy) for the learner of philosophy to engage in a walk through history to provide the needed context for the origin and development of thoughts and associated meanings. This walk is a component of philosophic inquiry.

WHAT IS PHILOSOPHY OF SCIENCE IN NURSING?

Philosophy of science within nursing helps to establish the meaning of science through an understanding and an examination of nursing concepts, theories, laws and aims as they relate to nursing practice. Through such an understanding and deliberate thought, praxis evolves. Philosophy of science in nursing seeks to understand truth, to provide a description of nursing, to propose an understanding of explanation, to examine prediction, causality and law, to critically relate theories, models and scientific systems, and to fully explore determinism and free will. These goals are accomplished through the methods of philosophic inquiry of reflection and dialogue.

HISTORY OF PHILOSOPHY OF SCIENCE AND SCIENCE

The development of a time line, a basis for the reader to contextually ground her- or himself, seems eminently appropriate and helpful. However, it is not without difficulty in that time periods, by their very nature, are specific and exact, whereas the philosophic thought, the patterns of thought and the philosophers themselves transcend the time periods. Nonetheless, this listing of time periods may assist the learner to create a context for the developments addressed throughout the remainder of this book. At the very least, the time line can be used as a basis for discussion and further inquiry.

The following time line, for both the history of science and the history of philosophy of science, was created by blending the tables of contents in both Sahakian's (1968) and Marias's (1967) history of philosophy textbooks, and additions of our own. Those asterisked are more fully described following the complete time line.

Greek Philosophy
    Milesians: the problem of matter
        Thales 624–546 B.C.
    Ionian philosophers: the problem of identity and change
        Pythagoras 580–497 B.C.
    The Sophists: the problem of man
        Socrates 470–399 B.C.
Systematic Philosophy
        Plato 427–347 B.C.
Medieval Philosophy
    Scholasticism
        Thomas Aquinas 1225–1274
Modern Philosophy
    Renaissance Philosophy*
        Francis Bacon 1521–1626
        Thomas Hobbes 1588–1679
        Galileo Galilei 1564–1642
        Johann Kepler 1571–1630
        Isaac Newton 1642–1727
    Continental Rationalists/Seventeenth-Century Idealism*
        René Descartes 1596–1650
        Benedict Spinoza 1632–1677
    British Empiricists
        John Locke 1632–1704
        David Hume 1711–1776
    German Idealists
        Immanuel Kant 1724–1804
        Georg Hegel 1770–1831

British Utilitarianism
    Jeremy Bentham 1748–1832
    John Stuart Mill 1806–1873
Nineteenth-Century Philosophy
    Evolutionary Naturalism
        Charles Darwin 1809–1882
        Herbert Spencer 1820–1903
        Friedrich Nietzsche 1844–1900
    Classical Positivism*
        Auguste Comte 1789–1857
        Ernst Mach 1838–1916
    Marxian Communism
        Karl Marx 1818–1883
        Friedrich Engels 1820–1895
Twentieth-Century Philosophy
    Historicism*
        Wilhelm Dilthey 1833–1911
    Pragmatism*
        Charles Sanders Peirce 1839–1914
        William James 1842–1910
        John Dewey 1859–1952
    Logical Positivism/Vienna School*
        Moritz Schlick 1882–1936
        Rudolf Carnap 1891–1970
        Ludwig Wittgenstein 1889–1951
    Positivism*
        Carl Hempel 1905–1997
        Karl Popper 1902–1994
    Postpositivists*
        Paul Feyerabend 1924–
        Thomas Kuhn 1922–1997
        Bas van Fraassen 1941–
    Phenomenology/Frankfurt School*
        Franz Bretano 1838–1917
        Edmund Husserl 1859–1938
        Maurice Merleau-Ponty 1908–1961
    Existentialism
        Martin Heidegger 1889–1976
        Jean-Paul Sartre 1905–1980
    Postmodernism*
        Richard Rorty 1931–
        Stephen Toulmin 1922–

As one proceeds through this time line, it is important to explain and amplify some of the associated developments with key periods and individuals. Starting with the Renaissance period, the reader can identify that Bacon, Galileo, Newton, and Kepler were all contemporaries. Yet their thinking and patterns of discovery were markedly different.

Kepler advanced the belief in laws of elliptical orbits and that of areas. This was revolutionary thinking for the sixteenth and seventeenth centuries. Galileo developed the art of experimental science, the persistent need for documentation of the science, and the difference between experimental and ideal testing. While Bacon did not support the work of either Galileo or Kepler, he did believe and advance classification of science, envisioned a community of scientists and advanced the belief that a single negative instance refuted a theory. Unlike his contemporaries, Bacon was not interested in the repeated verification of existing theories; he believed that science advanced itself by attempting to refute theories, not by simply asserting that they are true through repetition of like events. Bacon is known as the father of philosophy of science.

Descartes, a rationalist, believed that science and philosophy were united, but also believed that the mind and the body were separate. He believed that all phenomenon in nature can and should be reduced to principles of matter and motion. The Cartesian view of the mind-body disconnection dominated philosophy of science and science for many years after his work.

In the late eighteenth century, Comte advanced his belief in the notion of verification and the importance of empirical verifiability for all science. For Comte, the essence of scientific development was based on empirical verification and mathematics as the basis of all science. He postulated the belief that "society's salvation was to be contingent upon scientific knowledge" (Sahakian, 1968, p. 241). Science is considered positive because of its relationship and underlying value to all of society. He is known as the father of positivism even though the original ideas on which Comte expanded were developed by Saint-Simon.

Dilthey is identified with a philosophy known as historicism. Within this context, the role of history is fundamental. While history has no judgment, the material provides the context, the setting and the resulting understanding (Verstehen) for the philosopher's beliefs and values. Dilthey's work has been recently embraced within the world of nursing science for its contextual grounding and understanding.

Another philosophical movement is that of the pragmatists. Their collective view, while individually operationalized and advanced, was that ideas are largely interpreted and understood through their practical consequences. The notion of application and practicality emerge in all pragmatic philosophical discourse.

From a historical perspective, the term positivism emerges once again, only this time it is called logical positivism. This term is applied to the work of a group of philosophers known as the Vienna circle. The University of Vienna, through its leadership in the philosophy department, led to the development of logical positivism. This movement aimed to "purify" philosophy by addressing only the logical and empirical bases of science. From the logical positivist perspective, there is no room for metaphysics or metaphysical elements, understanding or meaning within the realm of science. Logical positivism, as defined in the Vienna circle, has been largely disputed in the middle to latter half of the twentieth century. The term is often used in a derogatory and pejorative fashion. This interpretation is inconsistent with philosophical inquiry. A view may be rejected but it is not to be denigrated.

Although logical positivism has been rejected, positivism continues to exist. The difference between the two views, as well as the views of classical positivism addressed by Comte, is that positivism is now seen as empiricism. The basis for positivism as a philosophical school of thought is the belief that ideas must be empirically verifiable if the ability to conduct such experiments were developed. In other words, the view need not be verified but rather must have the possibility of verification. Contemporary positivism also addresses the role of understanding within the scientific endeavor as long as it is empirically verifiable.

In the postpositivistic movement, a very broad category which transcends time, it is difficult to identify single thoughts and beliefs. Rather, this category includes a multitude of individuals and perspectives. The most noted individual in the postpositivistic category is Thomas Kuhn. His works have revolutionized scientific discourse, whether it be through acceptance of his perspective or continual dialogue aimed at disputing his beliefs. Kuhn posits that science advances from normal science, the everyday work of the scientist, to revolutions in science which totally discard existing thought. He calls these revolutionary shifts paradigms. Each paradigm is a marked departure from current methods, patterns and beliefs. For Kuhn, he also states that a multitude of paradigms within one discipline is the mark of an immature science. This remark and belief have particular meaning for the world of nursing science, given our current reliance on and utilization of many diverse paradigms.

Phenomenology, as a philosophy, is a twentieth-century development. Phenomenology is explicated in a later section of this book. It is seen as a movement of understanding and the connection between one's experience, one's values and one's perspectives. The phenomenon of concern, the purpose of the investigation, is at the center of the movement as is the perspective of the individual conducting the inquiry. As with positivism, there are many interpretations and operationalizations of phenomenology, all centered around the belief and position that the individual's experience is unique and it is intricately woven to the experiences one has already had and thinks one will have.

The postmodern view is currently developing. For some, it is the antithesis of positivism. The postmodern view discards as irrelevant some standard questions in philosophy of science, such as the search and meaning for truth. For the postmodernist, the perspective is simply that truth may never be achieved and therefore the quest should be simply abandoned. There is every indication it will continue to develop throughout the last decade of this century and on into the next millennium.

In conclusion, the time line provided enables the reader to perceive an historical context for the readings and authors in this book. The time line is meant to be used as a reference without an absolute adherence to the times and period frames, for the works of the individuals go beyond labels and categories.

PURPOSE

The purpose of this book is to explore the concepts of science from a traditional and nontraditional view. Regardless of one's belief about the status of nursing as a science, one cannot be left with anything but questions when faced with the criteria of traditional science as previously discussed. Thus, a major aim of this book is to enable the reader to engage in a discourse to affirm or reject these criteria for nursing as well as other sciences. Are they too rigid, artificial and unilateral? Or can the criteria be applied to the nursing we know? As the readers engage in reflection and dialogue prompted by the readings and questions in this volume, they will be able to explore these questions for themselves and generate new ones as we try to establish a discipline with theoretical formulations useful to nursing practice.

CONCLUSION

The path of this book will take the reader through the journey of philosophy and an understanding of science—philosophy of science. Philosophy of science is a deliberate analysis of the underlying assumptions on which science is based. Philosophy of science engages one in inquiry concerning beliefs about truth, explanation, free will or determinism, gender and science, science as a method or as a philosophy and the notion of action as a result of understanding. Through an examination of the inherent assumptions in each of these views, one is better able to hold true to the methods of the science and to direct inquiry to address the questions raised by science. Without a critical analysis of these assumptions, one is left to engage in scientific endeavors that are neither focused nor philosophically grounded, resulting in theories that may not be substantially adequate for nursing.

DISCUSSION GUIDE

These discussion points are designed to (1) assist the reader in grounding the material, (2) provoke the reader to reflect upon what has been read, and (3) assist the reader to apply the material.

1. What is science?
2. What is philosophy of science?
3. What is the role of culture in the philosophy of science? How is it operationalized?
4. Examine the purpose of tracing the history of the development of science.
5. Is nursing a science? A human science? A cultural science?
6. What are the relationships between science's development and the development of nursing science?
7. Explore the connections between historically significant scientific advancements and the philosophical schools of thought, art and science of nursing in the late 1990s.
8. What is the traditional scientific method? What are the steps? What is its relevance to today's nursing?
9. What is logical positivism? What are the differences between positivism and empiricism? Which scientists support which?
10. What is the relationship between positivism and/or empiricism and empirical knowing?
11. Compare and contrast specific scientists' views on science.
12. How is science classified?
13. Discuss the need for demarcation criteria in nursing science.
14. Nursing is best placed where on the historical development line from positivism to postmodernism?
15. What are the universal laws in nursing?

16. Reflect on the philosophical assumptions of major nurse theorists/paradigms.

17. Where do we go from here in the postmodern era?

REFERENCES

Benner, P. (1989). *The primacy of caring: Stress and coping in health and illness.* Menlo Park: Addison-Wesley.

Donaldson, S. K., & Crowley, D. M. (1978). The discipline of nursing. *Nursing Outlook, 26*(2), 113–120.

Feigl, H. (1988). The scientific outlook: Naturalism and humanism. In E. D. Klemke, R. Hollinger, & A. D. Kline (Eds.), *Philosophy of science* (pp. 427–437). Buffalo, NY: Prometheus Books.

Gortner, S. (1990). Nursing values and science: Toward a philosophy of science. *Image: Journal of Nursing Scholarship, 22*(2), 101–105.

Horgan, J. (1997). *The end of science.* New York: Broadway Books.

Klemke, E. D., Hollinger, R., & Kline, A. D. (1988). *Philosophy of science.* Buffalo, NY: Prometheus Books.

Marias, J. (1967). *History of philosophy.* New York: Dover Publications.

Meleis, A. (1985). *Theoretical nursing.* Philadelphia: Lippincott.

Newman, M. (1997). Experiencing the whole. *Advances in Nursing Science, 20*(1), 34–39.

Parse, R. R. (1987). *Nursing science: Major paradigms, theories and critiques.* Philadelphia: Saunders.

Sahakian, W. (1968). *History of philosophy.* New York: Barnes and Noble.

Strasser, S. (1985). *Understanding and explanation: Basic ideas concerning the humanity of the human sciences.* Pittsburgh: Duquesne University Press.

Watson, J. (1995). Postmodernism and knowledge development in nursing. *Nursing Science Quarterly, 8*(2), 60–64.

Fundamental Patterns of Knowing in Nursing

Barbara A. Carper

It is the general conception of any field of inquiry that ultimately determines the kind of knowledge the field aims to develop as well as the manner in which that knowledge is to be organized, tested and applied. The body of knowledge that serves as the rationale for nursing practice has patterns, forms and structure that serve as horizons of expectations and exemplify characteristic ways of thinking about phenomena. Understanding these patterns is essential for the teaching and learning of nursing. Such an understanding does not extend the range of knowledge, but rather involves critical attention to the question of what it means to know and what kinds of knowledge are held to be of most value in the discipline of nursing.

Identifying Patterns of Knowing

Four fundamental patterns of knowing have been identified from an analysis of the conceptual and syntactical structure of nursing knowledge.[1] The four patterns are distinguished according to logical type of meaning and designated as: (1) empirics, the science of nursing; (2) esthetics, the art of nursing; (3) the component of a personal knowledge in nursing; and

Reprinted with permission from Advances in Nursing Science 1(1): 13–23. © 1978, Aspen Publishers, Inc.

(4) ethics, the component of moral knowledge in nursing.

EMPIRICS: THE SCIENCE OF NURSING

The term nursing science was rarely used in the literature until the late 1950s. However, since that time there has been an increasing emphasis, one might even say a sense of urgency, regarding the development of a body of empirical knowledge specific to nursing. There seems to be general agreement that there is a critical need for knowledge about the empirical world, knowledge that is systematically organized into general laws and theories for the purpose of describing, explaining and predicting phenomena of special concern to the discipline of nursing. Most theory development and research efforts are primarily engaged in seeking and generating explanations which are systematic and controllable by factual evidence and which can be used in the organization and classification of knowledge.

The pattern of knowing which is generally designated as "nursing science" does not presently exhibit the same degree of highly integrated abstract and systematic explanations characteristic of the more mature sciences, although nursing literature reflects this as an ideal form. Clearly there are a number of coexisting, and in a few instances competing, conceptual structures—none of which has achieved the status of what Kuhn calls a scientific paradigm. That is, no single conceptual structure is as yet generally accepted as an example of actual scientific practice "which include[s] law, theory, application, and instrumentation together . . . [and] . . . provide[s] models from which spring particular coherent traditions of scientific research."[2(p10)] It could be argued that some of these conceptual structures seem to have greater potential than others for providing explanations that systematically account for observed phenomena and may ultimately permit more accurate prediction and control of them. However, this is a matter to be determined by research designed to test the validity of such explanatory concepts in the context of relevant empirical reality.

New Perspectives

What seems to be of paramount importance, at least at this stage in the development of nursing science, is that these preparadigm conceptual structures and theoretical models present new perspectives for considering the familiar phenomena of health and illness in relation to the human life process; as such they can and should be legitimately counted as discoveries in the discipline. The representation of health as more than the absence of disease is a crucial change; it permits health to be thought of as a dynamic state or process which changes over a given period of time and varies according to circumstances rather than a static either/or entity. The conceptual change in turn makes it possible to raise questions that previously would have been literally unintelligible.

The discovery that one can usefully conceptualize health as something that normally ranges along a continuum has led to attempts to observe, describe and classify variations in health, or levels of wellness, as expressions of a human being's relationship to the internal and external environments. Related research has sought to identify behavioral responses, both physiological and psychological, that may serve as cues by which one can infer the range of normal variations of health. It has also attempted to identify and categorize significant etiological factors which serve to promote or inhibit changes in health status.

Current Stages

The science of nursing at present exhibits aspects of both the "natural history stage of inquiry" and the "stage of deductively formulated theory." The task of the natural history stage is primarily the description and classification of phenomena which are, generally speaking, ascertainable by direct observation and inspection.[3] But current nursing literature clearly reflects a shift from this descriptive and classification form to increasingly theoretical analysis which is directed toward seeking, or inventing, explanations to account for observed and classified empirical facts. This shift is reflected in the change from a largely observational vocabulary to a new, more theoretical vocabulary whose terms have a distinct meaning and definition only in the context of the corresponding explanatory theory.

Explanations in the several open-system conceptual models tend to take the form commonly labeled functional or teleological.[4] For example, the system models explain a person's level of wellness at any particular point in time as a function of current and accumulated effects of interactions with his or her internal and external environments. The concept of adaptation is central to this type of explanation. Adaptation is seen as crucial in the process of responding to environmental demands (usually classified as stressors), and enables an individual to maintain or reestablish the steady state which is designated as the goal of the system. The developmental models often exhibit a more genetic type of explanation in that certain events, the developmental tasks, are believed to be causally relevant or necessary conditions for the normal development of an individual.

Thus the first fundamental pattern of knowing in nursing is empirical, factual, descriptive and ultimately aimed at developing abstract and theoretical explanations. It is exemplary, discursively formulated and publicly verifiable.

ESTHETICS: THE ART OF NURSING

Few, if indeed any, familiar with the professional literature would deny that primary emphasis is placed on the development of the science of nursing. One is almost led to believe that the only valid and reliable knowledge is that which is empirical, factual, objectively descriptive and generalizable. There seems to be a self-conscious reluctance to extend the term knowledge to include those aspects of knowing in nursing that are not the result of empirical investigation. There is, nonetheless, what might be described as a tacit admission that nursing is, at least in part, an art. Not much effort is made to elaborate or to make explicit this esthetic pattern of knowing in nursing—other than to vaguely associate the "art" with the general category of manual and/or technical skills involved in nursing practice.

Perhaps this reluctance to acknowledge the esthetic component as a fundamental pattern of knowing in nursing originates in the vigorous efforts made in the not-so-distant past to exorcise the image of the apprentice-type educational system. Within the apprentice system, the art of nursing was closely associated with an imitative learning style and the acquisition of knowledge by accumulation of unrationalized experiences. Another likely source of reluctance is that the definition of the term art has been excessively and inappropriately restricted.

Weitz suggests that art is too complex and variable to be reduced to a single definition.[5] To conceive the task of esthetic theory as definition, he says, is logically doomed to failure in that what is called art has no common properties—only recognizable similarities. This fluid and open approach to the understanding and application of the concept of art and esthetic meaning makes possible a wider consideration of conditions, situations and experiences in nursing that may properly be called esthetic, including the creative process of discovery in the empirical pattern of knowing.

ESTHETICS VERSUS SCIENTIFIC MEANING

Despite this open texture of the concept of art, esthetic meanings can be distinguished from those in science in several important aspects. The recognition "that art is expressive rather than merely formal or descriptive," according to Rader, "is about as well established as any fact in the whole field of esthetics."[6(pxvi)] An esthetic experience involves the creation and/or appreciation of a singular, particular, subjective expression of imagined possibilities or equivalent realities which "resists projection into the discursive form of language."[7] Knowledge gained by empirical description is discursively formulated and publicly verifiable. The knowledge gained by subjective acquaintance, the direct feeling of experience, defines discursive formulation. Although an esthetic expression required abstraction, it remains specific and unique rather than exemplary and leads us to acknowledge that "knowledge—genuine knowledge, understanding—is considerably wider than our discourse."[7(p23)]

For Wiedenbach, the art of nursing is made visible through the action taken to provide whatever the patient requires to restore or extend his ability to cope with the demands of his situation.[8] But the action taken, to have an esthetic quality, requires the active transformation of the immediate object—the patient's behavior—into a direct, nonmediated perception of what is significant in it—that is, what need is actually being expressed by the behavior. This perception of the need expressed is not only responsible for the action taken by the nurse but reflected in it.

The esthetic process described by Wiedenbach resembles what Dewey refers to as the difference between recognition and perception.[9] According to Dewey, recognition serves the purpose of identification and is satisfied when a name tag or label is attached according to some stereotype or previously formed scheme of classification. Perception, however, goes beyond recognition in that it includes an active gathering together of details and scattered particulars into an experienced whole for the purpose of seeing what is there. It is perception rather than mere recognition that results in a unity of ends and means which gives the action taken an esthetic quality.

Orem speaks of the art of nursing as being "expressed by the individual nurse through her creativity and style in designing and providing nursing that is effective and satisfying."[10(p155)] The art of nursing is creative in that it requires development of the ability to "envision valid modes of helping in relation to 'results' which are appropriate."[10(p69)] This again invokes Dewey's sense of a perceived unity between an action taken and its result—a perception of the means of the end as an organic whole.[9] The experience of helping must be perceived and designed as an integral component of its desired result rather than conceived separately as an independent action imposed on an independent subject. Perhaps this is what is meant by the concept of nursing the whole patient or total patient care. If so, what are the qualities that enable the creation of a design for nursing care that eliminate or would minimize the fragmentation of means and ends?

Esthetic Pattern of Knowing

Empathy—that is, the capacity for participating in or vicariously experiencing another's feelings—is an important mode in the esthetic pattern of knowing. One gains knowledge of another person's singular, particular, felt experience through empathic acquaintance.[11,12] Empathy is controlled or moderated by psychic distance or detachment in order to apprehend and abstract what we are attending to, and in this sense is objective. The more skilled the nurse becomes in perceiving and empathizing with the lives of others, the more knowledge or understanding will be gained of alternate modes of perceiving reality. The nurse will thereby have available a larger repertoire of choices in design-

ing and providing nursing care that is effective and satisfying. At the same time, increased awareness of the variety of subjective experiences will heighten the complexity and difficulty of the decision making involved.

The design of nursing care must be accompanied by what Langer refers to as sense of form, the sense of "structure, articulation, a whole resulting from the relation of mutually dependent factors, or more precisely, the way the whole is put together."[7(p16)] The design, if it is to be esthetic, must be controlled by the perception of the balance, rhythm, proportion and unity of what is done in relation to the dynamic integration and articulation of the whole. "The doing may be energetic, and the undergoing may be acute and intense," Dewey says, but "unless they are related to each other to form a whole," what is done becomes merely a matter of mechanical routine or of caprice.[9]

The esthetic pattern of knowing in nursing involves the perception of abstracted particulars as distinguished from the recognition of abstracted universals. It is the knowing of a unique particular rather than an exemplary class.

THE COMPONENT OF PERSONAL KNOWLEDGE

Personal knowledge as a fundamental pattern of knowing in nursing is the most problematic, the most difficult to master and to teach. At the same time, it is perhaps the pattern most essential to understanding the meaning of health in terms of individual well-being. Nursing considered as an interpersonal process involves interactions, relationships and transactions between the nurse and the patient-client. Mitchell points out that "there is growing evidence that the quality of interpersonal contacts has an influence on a person's becoming ill, coping with illness and becoming well."[13(p4950)] Certainly the phrase "therapeutic use of self" which has become increasingly prominent in the literature implies that the way in which nurses view their own selves and the client is of primary concern in any therapeutic relationship.

Personal knowledge is concerned with the knowing, encountering and actualizing of the concrete, individual self. One does not know *about* the self; one strives simply to *know* the self. This knowing is a standing in relation to another human being and confronting that human being as a person. This "I-Thou" encounter is unmediated by conceptual categories or particulars abstracted from complex organic wholes.[14] The relation is one of reciprocity, a state of being that cannot be described or even experienced—it can only be actualized. Such personal knowing extends not only to other selves but also to relations with one's own self.

It requires what Buber refers to as the sacrifice of form, i.e., categories or classifications, for a knowing of infinite possibilities, as well as the risk of total commitment.

> Even as a melody is not composed of tones, nor a verse of words, nor a statue of lines—one must pull and tear to turn a unity into a multiplicity— so it is with the human being to whom I say You. . . . I have to do this again and again; but immediately he is no longer You.[14(p59)]

Maslow refers to this sacrifice of form as embodying a more efficient perception of reality in that reality is not generalized nor predetermined by a complex of concepts, expectations, beliefs and stereotypes.[15] This results in a greater willingness to accept ambiguity, vagueness and discrepancy of oneself and others. The risk of commitment involved in personal knowledge is what Polanyi calls the "passionate participation in the act of knowing."[16(p17)]

The nurse in the therapeutic use of self rejects approaching the patient-client as an object and strives instead to actualize an authentic personal relationship between two persons. The individual is considered as an integrated, open system incorporating movement toward growth and fulfillment of human potential. An authentic personal relation requires the acceptance of others in their freedom to create themselves and the recognition that each person is not a fixed entity, but constantly engaged in the process of becoming. How then should the nurse reconcile this with the social and/or professional responsibility to control and manipulate the environmental variables and even the behavior of the person who is a patient in order to maintain or restore a steady state? If a human being is assumed to be free to choose and chooses behavior outside of accepted norms, how will this affect the action taken in the therapeutic use of self by the nurse? What choices must the nurse make in order to know another self in an authentic relation apart from the category of patient, even when categorizing for the purpose of treatment is essential to the process of nursing?

Assumptions regarding human nature, McKay observes, "range from the existentialist to the cybernetic, from the idea of an information processing machine to one of a many splendored being."[17(p399)] Many of these assumptions incorporate in one form or another the notion that there is, for all individuals, a characteristic state which they, by virtue of membership in the species, must strive to assume or achieve. Empirical descriptions and classifications reflect the assumption that being human allows for prediction of basic biological, psychological and social behaviors that will be encountered in any given individual.

Certainly empirical knowledge is essential to the purposes of nursing. But nursing also requires that we be alert to the fact that models of human nature and their abstract and generalized categories refer to and describe behaviors and traits that groups have in common. However, none of these categories can ever encompass or express the uniqueness of the individual encountered as a person, as a "self." These and many other similar considerations are involved in the realm of personal knowledge, which can be broadly characterized as subjective, concrete and existential. It is concerned with the kind of knowing that promotes wholeness and integrity in the personal encounter, the achievement of engagement rather than detachment; and it denies the manipulative, impersonal orientation.

ETHICS: THE MORAL COMPONENT

Teachers and individual practitioners are becoming increasingly sensitive to the difficult personal choices that must be made within the complex context of modern health care. These choices raise fundamental questions about morally right and wrong action in connection with the care and treatment of illness and the promotion of health. Moral dilemmas arise in situations of ambiguity and uncertainty, when the consequences of one's actions are difficult to predict and traditional principles and ethical codes offer no help or seem to result in contradiction. The moral code which guides the ethical conduct of nurses is based on the primary principle of obligation embodied in the concepts of service to people and respect for human life. The discipline of nursing is held to be a valuable and essential social service responsible for conserving life, alleviating suffering and promoting health. But appeal to the ethical "rule book" fails to provide answers in terms of difficult individual moral choices which must be made in the teaching and practice of nursing.

The fundamental pattern of knowing identified here as the ethical component of nursing is focused on matters of obligation or what ought to be done. Knowledge of morality goes beyond simply knowing the norms or ethical codes of the discipline. It includes all voluntary actions that are deliberate and subject to the judgment of right and wrong—including judgments of moral value in relation to motives, intentions and traits of character. Nursing is deliberate action, or a series of actions, planned and implemented to accomplish defined goals. Both goals and actions involve choices made, in part, on the basis of normative judgments, both particular and general. On occasion, the principles and norms by which such choices are made may be in conflict.

According to Berthold, "goals are, of course, value judgments not amenable to scientific inquiry and validation."[18(p196)] Dickoff, James and Wiedenbach also call attention to the need to be aware that the specification of goals serves as "a norm or standard by which to evaluate activity . . . [and] . . . entails taking them as values—that is, signifies conceiving these goal contents as situations worthy to be brought about."[19(p422)]

For example, a common goal of nursing care in relation to the maintenance or restoration of health is to assist patients to achieve a state in which they are independent. Much of the current practice reflects an attitude of value attached to the goal of independence, and indicates nursing actions to assist patients in assuming full responsibility for themselves at the earliest possible moment or to enable them to retain responsibility to the last possible moment. However, valuing independence and attempting to maintain it may be at the expense of the patient's learning how to live with physical or social dependence when necessary—e.g., in instances when prognosis indicates that independence cannot be regained.

Differences in normative judgments may have more to do with disagreements as to what constitutes a "healthy" state of being than lack of empirical evidence or ambiguity in the application of the term. Slote suggests that the persistence of disputes, or lack of uniformity in the application of cluster terms, such as health, is due to "the difficulty of decisively resolving certain sorts of value questions about what is and is not important." This leads him to conclude "that value judgment is far more involved in the making of what are commonly thought to be factual statements than has been imagined."[20(p220)]

The ethical pattern of knowing in nursing requires an understanding of different philosophical positions regarding what is good, what ought to be desired, what is right; of different ethical frameworks devised for dealing with the complexities of moral judgments; and of various orientations to the notion of obligation. Moral choices to be made must then be considered in terms of specific actions to be taken in specific, concrete situations. The examination of the standards, codes and values by which we decide what is morally right should result in a greater awareness of what is involved in making moral choices and being responsible for the choices made. The knowledge of ethical codes will not provide answers to the moral questions involved in nursing, nor will it eliminate the necessity for having to make moral choices. But it can be hoped that:

> The more sensitive teachers and practitioners are to the demands of the process of justification, the more explicit they are about the norms that govern their actions, the more personally engaged they are in assessing surrounding circumstances and potential consequences, the more "ethical" they will be; and we cannot ask much more.[21(p221)]

Using Patterns of Knowing

A philosophical discussion of patterns of knowing may appear to some as a somewhat idle, if not arbitrary and artificial, undertaking having little or no connection with the practical concerns and difficulties encountered in the day-to-day doing and teaching of nursing. But it represents a personal conviction that there is a need to examine the kinds of knowing that provide the discipline with its particular perspectives and significance. Understanding four fundamental patterns of knowing makes possible an increased awareness of the complexity and diversity of nursing knowledge.

Each pattern may be conceived as necessary for achieving mastery in the discipline, but none of them alone should be considered sufficient. Neither are they mutually exclusive. The teaching and learning of one pattern do not require the rejection or neglect of any of the others. Caring for another requires the achievements of nursing science, that is, the knowledge of empirical facts systematically organized into theoretical explanations regarding the phenomena of health and illness. But creative imagination also plays its part in the syntax of discovery in science, as well as in developing the ability to imagine the consequences of alternate moral choices.

Personal knowledge is essential for ethical choices in that moral action presupposes per-sonal maturity and freedom. If the goals of nursing are to be more than conformance to unexamined norms, if the "ought" is not to be determined simply on the basis of what is possible, then the obligation to care for another human being involves becoming a certain kind of person—and not merely doing certain kinds of things. If the design of nursing care is to be more than habitual or mechanical, the capacity to perceive and interpret the subjective experiences of others and to imaginatively project the effects of nursing actions on their lives becomes a necessary skill.

Nursing thus depends on the scientific knowledge of human behavior in health and in illness, the esthetic perception of significant human experiences, a personal understanding of the unique individuality of the self and the capacity to make choices within concrete situations involving particular moral judgments. Each of these separate but interrelated and interdependent fundamental patterns of knowing should be taught and understood according to its distinctive logic, the restricted circumstances in which it is valid, the kinds of data it subsumes and the methods by which each particular kind of truth is distinguished and warranted.

The major significances to the discipline of nursing in distinguishing patterns of knowing are summarized as: (1) the conclusions of the discipline conceived as subject matter cannot be taught or learned without reference to the structure of the discipline—the representative concepts and methods of inquiry that determine the kind of knowledge gained and limit its meaning, scope and validity; (2) each of the fundamental patterns of knowing represents a necessary but not complete approach to the problems and questions in the discipline; and (3) all knowledge is subject to change and revision. Every solution of an existing problem raises new and unsolved questions. These new and as yet unsolved problems require, at times, new methods of inquiry and different conceptual structures; they change the shape and patterns of knowing. With each change in the shape of knowledge, teaching and learning require looking for different points of contact and connection among ideas and things. This clarifies the effect of each new thing known on other things known and the discovery of new patterns by which each connection modifies the whole.

REFERENCES

1. Carper, B. A. "Fundamental Patterns of Knowing in Nursing." PhD dissertation, Teachers College, Columbia University, 1975.
2. Kuhn, T. *The Structure of Scientific Revolutions* (Chicago: University of Chicago Press 1962).
3. Northrop, F. S. C. *The Logic of the Sciences and the Humanities* (New York: The World Publishing Co. 1959).
4. Nagel, E. *The Structure of Science* (New York: Harcourt, Brace and World, Inc. 1961).
5. Weitz, M. "The Role of Theory in Aesthetics" in Rader, M., ed. *A Modern Book of Esthetics* 3rd ed. (New York: Holt, Rinehart and Winston 1960).
6. Rader, M. "Introduction: The Meaning of Art" in Rader, M., ed. *A Modern Book of Esthetics* 3rd ed. (New York: Holt, Rinehart and Winston 1960).
7. Langer, S. K. *Problems of Art* (New York: Charles Scribner and Sons 1957).
8. Wiedenbach, E. *Clinical Nursing: A Helping Art* (New York: Springer Publishing Co., Inc. 1964).
9. Dewey, J. *Art as Experience* (New York: Capricorn Books 1958).
10. Orem, D. E. *Nursing: Concepts of Practice* (New York: McGraw-Hill Book Co. 1971).
11. Lee, V. "Empathy" in Rader, M., ed. *A Modern Book of Esthetics* 3rd ed. (New York: Holt, Rinehart and Winston 1960).
12. Lippo, T. "Empathy, Inner Imitation and Sense-Feeling" in Rader, M., ed. *A Modern Book of Esthetics* 3rd ed. (New York: Holt, Rinehart and Winston 1960).
13. Mitchell, P. H. *Concepts Basic to Nursing* (New York: McGraw-Hill Book Co. 1973).
14. Buber, M. *I and Thou.* Translated by Walter Kaufman (New York: Charles Scribner and Sons 1970).
15. Maslow, A. H. "Self-Actualizing People: A Study of Psychological Health" in Moustakas, C. E., ed. *The Self* (New York: Harper and Row 1956).
16. Polanyi, M. *Personal Knowledge* (New York: Harper and Row 1964).
17. McKay, R. "Theories, Models and Systems for Nursing." *Nurs Res* 18:5 (September–October 1969).
18. Berthold, J. S. "Symposium on Theory Development in Nursing: Prologue." *Nurs Res* 17:3 (May–June 1968).
19. Dickoff, J., James, P., and Wiedenbach, E. "Theory in a Practice Discipline: Part I." *Nurs Res* 17 (September–October 1968).
20. Slote, M. A. "The Theory of Important Criteria." *J Philosophy* 63 (April 14 1966).
21. Greene, M. *Teacher as Stronger* (Belmont, Calif.: Wadsworth Publishing Co., Inc. 1973).

The Focus of the Discipline of Nursing

Margaret A. Newman • *A. Marilyn Sime* • *Sheila A. Corcoran-Perry*

The focus of nursing as a discipline has not been clearly defined but is emergent in the centrality of the concepts of caring and health. The authors propose a focus for nursing as a professional discipline in the form of a statement that identifies a domain of inquiry that reflects the social relevance and nature of its service. Several perspectives from which the focus can be studied are described. The authors assert that a unitary-transformative perspective is essential for the full explication of nursing knowledge.

A discipline is distinguished by a domain of inquiry that represents a shared belief among its members regarding its reason for being. A discipline can be identified by a focus statement in the form of a simple sentence that specifies the area of study. For example, physiology is the study of the function of living systems; sociology is the study of principles and processes governing human society.

A professional discipline, in addition, is defined by social relevance and value orientations.[1,2] The focus is derived from a belief and value system about the profession's social commitment, nature of its service, and area of responsibility for knowledge development. These requisites need expression in the focus state-

ment. For example, medicine is the study of the diagnosis and treatment of human disease. The social relevance and value orientation of medicine as a professional discipline is conveyed by the commitment to alleviate disease.

Knowledge development within a discipline may proceed from several philosophic and scientific perspectives (worldviews). From this standpoint, the focus of a discipline could be considered paradigm free. The purpose of this article is to present a focus for the discipline of nursing and to discuss the implications of differing paradigmatic perspectives for the nature of nursing knowledge.

Concepts Relevant to the Focus of Nursing

The focus of nursing as a professional discipline has emerged most prominently over the past decade. A number of concepts have been identified as central to the study of nursing. An example is the frequently cited tetralogy: person, environment, nursing, and health.[3,4] While identification of these concepts begins to narrow the focus of nursing, there remains the need for more explicit connectedness and social relevance

Discussions in the School of Nursing Curriculum Coordinating Committee stimulated ideas for this article. The authors acknowledge the contributions of other members of the committee: Monica Bossenmaier, Dorothy Fairbanks, Carol Reese, Mariah Snyder, and Patricia Tomlinson. The authors also thank Ellen Egan and Kathleen Sodergren for manuscript critiques.

to describe the field of study that constitutes nursing. Such unconnected concepts do not raise the philosophic issues or scientific questions that stimulate inquiry.

Recently, there has been concentrated emphasis on two concepts as central to nursing: health and caring. Health has been heralded as the centerpiece of nursing knowledge since the days of Florence Nightingale and continues to be discussed by many theorists and researchers.[5-8] The concept of caring also has occupied a prominent position in nursing literature and has been touted as the essence of nursing.[9-11] The accelerated emphasis on health and caring within the past decade has been accentuated by recent Wingspread Conferences[12,13] and the devotion of entire issues of nursing scholarly journals to these concepts.[14,15] These efforts raise questions about nursing's domain of inquiry. Does health or caring represent the focus of the discipline of nursing? Is knowledge gained from research on caring or health specifically identified as nursing knowledge? Although caring and health are indeed central to nursing, no one has developed a unifying focus statement that includes these concepts, and neither concept alone meets the criteria for the focus of a professional discipline. A synthesis of current knowledge development regarding caring and health suggests a focus that meets these criteria.

Caring has generally been linked with the concept of health. In Leininger's historical review of care and caring, she consistently links caring with health and states that "caring is the . . . explanadum for health and well-being."[16(p19)] Watson combines caring and healing in a causal connection and refers repeatedly to "caring-healing."[17] Benner's tenets, as well, specifically link caring with health and well-being.[18]

In a similar fashion, the concept of health is often linked with actions. Pender questions what interventions assist clients in achieving health.[19] Newman submits that the essential question of the discipline of nursing "has something to do with how nurses facilitate the health

of human beings" and poses the question, "What is the quality of relationship that makes it possible for the nurse and patient to connect in a transforming way?"[20(p234)]

Further, in nursing, health means *human* health and, most significantly, human health *experience*. Phillips states that "research should focus on . . . the study of people's *experiencing of their health*, their sense of interconnectedness with others, and specifically how health emerges from a mutual process" (emphasis added).[21(p103)] Pender uses the term "health experience" throughout her recent article on health patterns; she points out that "when illness occurs, it is synthesized as part of the on-going *health experience*" (emphasis added).[19(p116)] Parse has been explicit in her emphasis on human experience as the basis of her theory of man–living–health,[22] which might be rephrased as human health experience.

Considerable evidence exists that caring, health, and health experience are concepts central to the discipline of nursing. These concepts can be related to each other to identify the domain of inquiry for nursing.

A Focus Statement for Nursing

We submit that nursing is the study of *caring in the human health experience*. This focus integrates into a single statement concepts commonly identified with nursing at the metaparadigm level. This focus implies a social mandate and service identity and specifies a domain for knowledge development. The social mandate and service identity are conveyed by a commitment to caring as a moral imperative. It is important to note that at this level, the concepts are not associated with any particular theory.

The domain of inquiry is caring in the human health experience. This focus dictates that nursing's body of knowledge includes caring and human health experience. A body of knowledge that does not include caring and human health experience is not nursing knowledge. For example, knowledge about health without consideration of caring would be knowledge of a discipline of health. Nursing theories would link caring to the human health experience.

The tasks of nursing inquiry will be to examine and explicate the meaning of caring in the human health experience to ascertain the adequacy of this focus for the discipline, and to examine the philosophic and scientific questions provoked by the focus statement.

Differing Paradigmatic Perspectives

What may appear to be confusing and inconsistent meanings of concepts in the proposed focus may actually be a reflection of the use of different paradigms for knowledge explication.[20,23] Nursing research has been conducted from an orientation consistent with at least two, and possibly three, paradigms. Each paradigm specifies a point of view from which the field of study is conceptualized, the assumptions that are inherent in that view, and the basis upon which knowledge claims are accepted. These differing paradigms reflect the shift in focus from physical to social to human science. The three perspectives extant in nursing literature could be described as: particulate-deterministic, interactive-integrative, and unitary-transformative. To explain the effect of a paradigm on the development of nursing knowledge, each perspective will be addressed briefly.

From the particulate-deterministic perspective, phenomena can be viewed as isolatable, reducible entities having definable properties that can be measured. These entities have orderly and predictable connectedness to each other. Change is assumed to be a consequence of antecedent conditions—conditions that, if sufficiently identified and understood, could be used to predict and control change in the phenomena. Relationships within and among entities are viewed as linear and causal. Kinds of knowledge sought include facts and universal laws. Knowledge claims that cannot be refuted are admitted to the body of knowledge. From the perspective of this paradigm, caring in the human health ex-

perience could be studied by examining the concepts that comprise the focus. For example, caring could be isolated for study as a human trait having definable and measurable characteristics. Similarly, health could be reduced and dichotomized in terms of characteristics considered healthy versus those considered unhealthy. Caring also could be studied as a therapeutic intervention affecting patients' health in terms of measurable responses.[23]

From the interactive-integrative perspective (an extension of the particulate-deterministic perspective that takes into account context and experience and legitimized subjective data), phenomena are viewed as having multiple, interrelated parts in relation to a specific context. To explain a phenomenon, the interrelationships of parts and the influence of the context are taken into consideration. Thus, reality is assumed to be multidimensional and contextual. Change in a phenomenon is a function of multiple antecedent factors and probabilistic relationships. Relationships among phenomena may be reciprocal. Knowledge claims may be context dependent and relative. From this perspective, caring in the human health experience would be studied as interactive-integrative phenomena within specific contexts, but still with probabilistic predictability.

The unitary-transformative perspective represents a significant paradigm shift. From this perspective, a phenomenon is viewed as a unitary, self-organizing field embedded in a larger self-organizing field. It is identified by pattern and by interaction with the larger whole. There is interpenetration of fields within fields and diversity within a unified field. Change is unidirectional and unpredictable as systems move through stages of organization and disorganization to more complex organization. Knowledge is personal, involves pattern recognition, and is a function of both viewer and the phenomenon viewed. The subject matter includes thoughts, values, feelings, choices and purpose.[24] Inner reality depicts the reality of the whole. From this perspective, caring in the human health experience would be studied as a unitary-transformative process of mutuality and creative unfolding.

Relationship of Focus to Paradigmatic Perspective

The explication of knowledge relevant to caring in the human health experience is affected by the paradigmatic perspective. As described earlier, concepts in the focus statement could be isolated for study within the first two perspectives, while the unitary-transformative perspective requires the focus to be studied as an indivisible whole. For example, knowledge generated from the particulate-deterministic perspective includes behaviors that characterize caring, physiologic and psychologic aspects of human health, and acontextual rules that relate observable caring behaviors with measurable health outcomes. Examples of knowledge generated from the interactive-integrative perspective include the reciprocal nature of nurse–client interactions, culture-specific caring responses to life process events that are disruptive to health, and rules regarding the influence of specific caring behaviors on the health-related behaviors of particular groups of clients. Knowledge from a unitary-transformative perspective is more difficult to characterize. An example generated from this perspective might be an understanding of the synchrony and mutuality of nurse–client encounters that transcend the time and space limitations of a present situation.

Although multiple perspectives are appropriate for knowledge development in nursing, we are convinced that a unitary-transformative perspective is essential for full explication of the discipline. This position is consistent with a changing world view of the conduct of inquiry into human experience[25–27] and with other nurse scholars who recognize the value of a unitary perspective to nursing inquiry.[22,28–30] Insights from our research and practice reveal a rich and fertile glimpse into caring in the human health experience.

• • • • • • •

The focus of a professional discipline is an area of study defined by the profession's shared social and service commitment. We conclude that the focus of nursing is the study of caring in the human health experience. The explication of nursing knowledge based on this focus takes different forms depending on the perspective of the scientist. We conclude that a unitary perspective is essential for full elaboration of caring in the human health experience. A unified focus derived from the coalescing of theory on caring and health has the potential for claiming the shared vision of nursing.

REFERENCES

1. Johnson DE. Development of theory: A requisite for nursing as a primary health profession. *Nurs Res.* 1974;23(5):372–377.
2. Donaldson SK, Crowley DM. The discipline of nursing. *Nurs Outlook.* 1978;26(2):113–120.
3. Torres G, Yura H. *Today's Conceptual Framework: Its Relationship to the Curriculum Development Process.* New York, NY: National League for Nursing, 1974.
4. Fawcett J. The metaparadigm of nursing: Present status and future refinements. *Image.* 1984;16(3): 84–87.
5. Newman MA. *Health as Expanding Consciousness.* St. Louis, Mo: Mosby, 1986.
6. Meleis AI. Being and becoming healthy: The core of nursing knowledge. *Nurs Sci Q.* 1990;3(3): 107–114.
7. Pender NJ. *Health Promotion in Nursing Practice.* Norwalk, Conn: Appleton & Lange, 1987.
8. Newman MA. Health conceptualizations and related research. *Ann Rev Nurs Res.* 1991;9.
9. Leininger M, ed. *Care: The Essence of Nursing and Health.* Thorofare, N.J.: Slack, 1984.
10. Watson J. *Nursing: The Philosophy and Science of Caring.* Boulder, Col: Colorado Associated University Press, 1985.
11. Benner P, Wrubel J. *The Primacy of Caring.* Menlo Park, Calif: Addison-Wesley, 1989.
12. Stevenson JS, Tripp-Reimer T, eds. *Knowledge About Care and Caring.* Proceedings of a Wingspread Conference, February 1–3, 1989. Kansas City, Mo: American Academy of Nursing, 1990.
13. Duffy ME, Pender NJ, eds. *Conceptual Issues in Health Promotion.* Proceedings of a Wingspread Conference, April 13–15, 1987. Indianapolis, In: Sigma Theta Tau, 1987.

14. *ANS.* 1981:3(2); 1984:6(3); 1988:11(1); 1990: 12(2); 1990:13(1).

15. *Nurs Sci Q.* 1990:3(3).

16. Leininger M. Historic and epistemologic dimensions of care and caring with future directions. In: Stevenson JS, Tripp-Reimer T, eds. *Knowledge About Care and Caring.* Proceedings of a Wingspread Conference, February 1–3, 1989. Kansas City, Mo: American Academy of Nursing, 1990.

17. Watson MJ. New dimensions of human caring theory. *Nurs Sci Q.* 1988;1(4):175–181.

18. Benner P. *Nursing as a caring profession.* Presented at meeting of the American Academy of Nursing; October 16, 1988; Kansas City, MO.

19. Pender NJ. Expressing health through lifestyle patterns. *Nurs Sci Q.* 1990;3(3):115–122.

20. Newman MA. Nursing paradigms and realities. In: Chaska NL, ed. *The Nursing Profession: Turning Points.* St. Louis, Mo: Mosby, 1990.

21. Phillips JR. The different views of health. *Nurs Sci Q.* 1990;3(3):103–104.

22. Parse RR. *Man–Living–Health: A Theory of Nursing.* New York, NY: Wiley, 1981.

23. Morse JM, Solberg SM, Neander WL, Bottorff JL, Johnson JL. Concepts of caring and caring as a concept. *ANS.* 1990;13(1):1–14.

24. Manen MV. *Researching Lived Experience: Human Science for an Action Sensitive Pedagogy.* Albany, NY: State University of New York Press, 1990.

25. Bohm D. *Wholeness and the Implicate Order.* London, England: Routledge & Kegan Paul, 1980.

26. Prigogine I. Order through fluctuation: Self-organization and social system. In: Jantsch E, Waddington CH, eds. *Evolution and Consciousness.* Reading, Mass: Addison-Wesley, 1976.

27. Briggs J, Peat FD. *Turbulent Mirror.* New York, NY: Harper & Row, 1989.

28. Rogers ME. *An Introduction to the Theoretical Basis of Nursing.* Philadelphia, Pa: FA Davis, 1970.

29. Munhall PL. Nursing philosophy and nursing research: In apposition or opposition? *Nurs Res.* 1982;31(3):176–177, 181.

30. Sarter B. Philosophical sources of nursing theory. *Nurs Sci Q.* 1988;1(2):52–59.

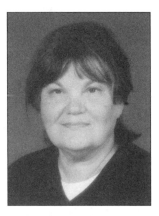

MARGARET A. NEWMAN

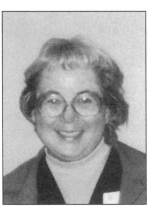

A. MARILYN SIME

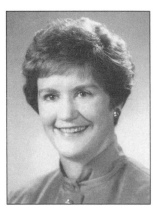

SHEILA A. CORCORAN-PERRY

Nursing Values and Science: Toward a Science Philosophy

Susan R. Gortner

Several premises are proposed for nursing science philosophy in contrast to nursing practice philosophy. These include human understanding, a critical tradition that views science as public knowledge, and use of observation, rationality, explanation, and prediction as a guide to therapy. No argument is made for or against a particular philosophy of science (e.g., positivist, historicist, critical theorist). The debates on the fit of philosophic paradigms with research strategies may soon run their course on the North American continent, as they appear to have done in Scandinavia.

The search for meaning in the universe is the subject matter of philosophy. It is not surprising, therefore, that philosophical discussions now characterize those disciplinary fields examining their purpose, significance, and identity. Nursing in the United States, Canada, Great Britain and elsewhere has publicized formally its purpose and obligation to society through statements on standards for practice (American Nurses' Association [ANA], 1973; Canada Nurses Association [CNA], 1980; Royal College of Nursing [RCN], 1987), codes for practice (ANA, 1976; International Council of Nurses, 1987; RCN, 1987) and social policy statements (ANA, 1980; RCN, 1987). Common themes that might be said to represent nursing philosophy and values commitment are reflected in these statements.

The purpose of this paper is to illustrate how nursing values and philosophy influence thinking about nursing science and research in the United States, Great Britain, and parts of Scandinavia. The position is taken that nursing philosophy represents the belief system of the profession and that it provides perspectives for practice, for scholarship, and for research. This paper will contrast statements of nursing philosophy in the United States and elsewhere and will attempt to show that nursing philosophy can be differentiated from science philosophy. Further, science philosophy can be reframed according to the needs of a discipline for relevant knowledge, empirically and conceptually derived, using a variety of systematic techniques. A philosophic framework for nursing science will be proposed.

Nursing Values

Nursing values portray the concepts of equity, respect for persons and caring (RCN, 1987), health promotion and illness prevention (ANA, 1980; National Center for Nursing Research, 1988), professional competence, and ethical conduct. Fry (1981), who examined the Amer-

Reprinted with permission from IMAGE: Journal of Nursing Scholarship 22(2):101–105. © 1990.

ican standards and codes for practice and research, concluded that the

> concept of nursing embodies the scientific (competence) values of technological skills, scientific inquiry, and knowledge gained by scientific study, as well as humanistic (moral) values of caring and promotion of individual welfare and rights. (p. 5)

Fry suggests that assumptions underlying American statements emphasize (a) the systematic approach to nursing practice (the nursing process) as the means to provide high quality care, (b) the promotion, maintenance and restoration of health as desirable outcomes of nursing action based on the nursing process (i.e., desired goals or ends), and (c) client participation in the health care plan designed to achieve these outcomes.

The British standards have as their underlying assumptions (a) accountability for practice of a high quality, safety, and effectiveness; (b) client participation in the contractual caring relationship; and (c) personalized, warm, understanding *caring* as the core of service. According to the RCN (1987),

> The nursing system must acknowledge the centrality of care in the overall delivery of its service . . . it is the skill and art of caring for another person that transforms the action from a technique to a nursing intervention. (pp. 11–12)

Other statements in this most recent British document emphasize the commitment to a humanistic philosophy and a patient or client advocacy model. Further, there is virtually no mention of obligation to extend knowledge of practice through research as there is in the American statements or of the "phenomena of concern" as in the American social policy statement (ANA, 1980). Stated differently, this most recent British document does not address scientific accountability in practice (Gortner, 1974), nor does it reflect the consensus reached by American nurses in the 1970s that scientific inquiry was the means by which outcomes of nursing action could be identified.

Although the Scandinavian countries are in the process of developing their standards, the publication by the Nordic Nurses Federation (NNF, 1987) of ethical guidelines for nursing research in the Nordic countries acknowledges the nurses' responsibility to "promote health, to prevent illness, to restore health, to prevent death, and to assist to a comfortable death." Further, there is a clear expectation for renewing personal knowledge and skills: "Such an obligation to improve nursing theory and skills implies research in nursing and health care services" (p. 7).

The ICN recently revised its position statement on nursing research. The statement reflects interest in the phenomena of concern stated in the ANA's 1980 social policy statement: individual, family, and group responses to actual and potential health problems. "The future of nursing practice and ultimately the future of health care depends on nursing research designed to constantly generate an up-to-date organized body of nursing knowledge" (p. 1).

It appears that the term "nursing research" in the Nordic and ICN statements is used to describe what in America has come to be called "nursing science" (Gortner, 1980). The United States' usage of nursing science has grown out of a period in our history in which the nature of nursing science was discussed by academic leaders concerned with the preparation of the nurse scientist. In this respect, science, the body of knowledge about the universe, and its manifestations, was distinguished from research, the tool of science (Batey, 1971; Gortner, 1980). This differential terminology now is prevailing in the nursing science institutes at the Universities of Oslo and Bergen as well as at several Finnish universities (Gortner & Lorensen, 1989).

The United States has had an advantage as yet not realized elsewhere in the world of having had government support in the way of grants for nurse scientist training in major universities during the decade 1962 to 1972 (Gortner & Nahm, 1977). The periodic forums that brought together the program directors and faculty members from these grantee institutions produced some of the most thoughtful among early statements on nursing science and the nurse's becoming scientist. Of these was Ellis' essay on values and vicissitudes of the scientist nurse, in which scientific research was viewed as the effective tool of the humanist nurse (Ellis, 1970). Batey's (1972) reflections on values relative to research and to science in nursing, as a result of her own nurse scientist training in sociology, recognized (as did Ellis) the tension between science and humanism but argued for the scientific values of organized skepticism, disinterest, and communality. Fry (1981) gives a foundational place to humanistic values in her analysis, arguing that it is the humanistic value scheme, not the scientific one, that guides humane therapy. A further argument is based on the claim made by Fry that scientific values have no moral content in themselves.

The present author, 15 years ago, urged greater scientific accountability for nursing based on self-reflection and thoughtful analysis of practice but cautioned against a loss of humanistic values while taking on the scientific (Gortner, 1974). That both science and humanism could be accommodated in nursing without loss of purpose and meaning was noted then and is believed to be possible today. What well may be foundational in humanistic philosophy (concern for person and meaning) can remain as philosophy; it need not be translated into scientific strategies (i.e., interpretive designs) and used to the exclusion of other options. Further, the practice of science and the scientific method, the search for explanations, regularities, and predictions about the human state should not be viewed as being incompatible with professional beliefs about practice and societal and personal worth.

Is Science in Nursing Compatible with Humanism?

For the past two decades, nursing scholars have examined the meaning of nursing through philosophical analysis (Ellis, 1983; Gadow,

1980; Lanara, 1982; Patterson & Zderad, 1976; Vaillot, 1962). Lanara recalled the heritage of classical Greek medicine as a healing art, as part of nursing's caring obligation. Nursing as a profession and as a science of caring has been proposed by several American authors (Benner & Wrubel, 1989; Leininger, 1988; Watson, 1985). These proposals have in common a commitment to personhood, holism, and humanistic attention. Further, there is now considerable literature on the need for scientific approaches that will reflect these commitments (Allen, Benner & Diekelmann, 1986; Cull-Wilby & Pepin, 1987; Gortner & Schultz, 1988; Schultz, 1987; Silva & Rothbart, 1984; Stevenson & Woods, 1986; Thompson, 1985).

In all but a few of these essays, science is cast against humanism and hermeneutics, the latter is seen as providing true meaning for all human endeavor including scientific work on humans and by humans. Interestingly, European nurses do not support this dialectic, it appears to be peculiarly American, in part because science does not have the certitude, the *gewissenschaft*, that it has in the United States. In Norway *vitenskap* is the term used for science, it has a broader meaning and tradition beyond that of natural science, incorporating many sources of knowledge not unlike those described by Schultz and Meleis (1988) in a recent account of nursing epistemology. These authors note that valuation of empirical knowledge will require evaluative criteria that are different from either conceptually derived or clinically derived knowledge. Theirs is a refreshing attempt to further understanding values and beliefs about multiple sources of knowledge for a practice field such as nursing.

Changing scientific and philosophical opinions about science in the past two decades have brought about considerable commentary about scientific inquiry and outcome. Science now is viewed as a part of society and not value-free; as such, it is a part of the sociopolitical structure and thus is open to scrutiny. There has been a renewed interest in the history of science, a result of scientists' turning to study their own disciplinary histories as well as philosophy. Kuhn's *Structure of Scientific Revolutions* was first published in the United States in 1962; Winch's *Idea of a Social Science* appeared in Europe about the same time as Kuhn's, according to Phillips (1987). Also influential around this time was Herbert Marcuse's *One-Dimensional Man* (1964). According to Fjelland (personal communication, July 1989), the writings of Marcuse, who emigrated to the United States, as well as others associated with the Frankfurt school of critical social philosophy, particularly Habermas (1971), fit in well with the student reaction against the American and Northern European "establishment," in which science and objectivity were perceived as being overvalued to the detriment of person and humanity. This reaction also was displayed against positivism, or the received view in philosophy of science. In Scandinavian and northern European universities in the 1970s, Marx as humanitarian rather than as political economist was reexamined along with Hegel and other of the German Idealists (Randi Nord & Eli Haugen Bunch, personal communication, February 4, 1988).

Modern version(s) of nineteenth century continental philosophy have emerged to influence the science discussions in some disciplinary fields deeply concerned with the human state. Phenomenology, as articulated by Heidegger (1962), Sartre (1963), and Merleau-Ponty (1962), calls for the appreciation of the human being as supreme being and for self-reflection and understanding as the basis of knowing and acting. Cohen (1987) provided an historical account of the phenomenological movement, differentiating these key leaders. Not addressed in her review is the influence of Heidegger on contemporary interpretative philosophy, namely hermeneutics. Leonard (1989) rectified this situation for nursing readers in a recent essay.

According to Bernstein's (1986) most recent analysis, the issue is less the substitution of hermeneutics for the scientific method as it is acceptance of "the ontological primacy of hermeneutics and its universality" (p. 96).

Hermeneutical understanding can enlighten the human state, a state that has become objectified by scientific advances and technology. Intuition and practical reasoning may well underlie all forms of reasoning including scientific reasoning and the production of scientific knowledge. The foundational nature of hermeneutics for Scandinavian nurse scholars engaged in substantive research programs is a given (Astrid Norberg, personal communication, March 6, 1988). Interestingly, hermeneutics as philosophy has not been transformed there to hermeneutics as method, as it appears to have been transformed in the United States. American scholars might consider this point in reconciling philosophy with modes of inquiry.

The legacy of philosophical positivism continues to guide our beliefs in the scientific method and in careful research strategies and in the conduct of investigations can provide worthwhile and substantial benefits for humankind. The renewed interest in humanism and history has infused us with an appreciation for and sensitivity to the human condition, in the links between objective measures of reality and personal and subjective ones. These links have significant implications for human sciences, among them the health fields.

What seems now to be at stake is whether or not understanding and explanation of the human state can take various forms and whether or not self-understandings and self-theories will be accepted as warranted evidence and thus as measures of "truth." Gergen (1980) suggests that a primary function of such understandings is the capacity to challenge assumptions of the culture, to raise questions about life and to suggest alternative actions: to serve as "generative theory." According to Ziman's (1980) definition, science is public knowledge; if self-defined meanings could be made public and scrutinized, they could be informative, critical, generalizable, and potentially nomothetic. Will such scrutiny distort the faithful interpretation from description that hermeneutical studies aim to present? Probably not, because some excellent public examples now exist in the science literature (Mishel & Murdaugh, 1987). How reproducible and rigorous are the narratives, the data, from such investigations? Herein lies a major debatable question since interpretive studies tend to be idiosyncratic and particularistic, despite cultural and linguistic commonalities. Further, there is no causal requirement for hermeneutical explanation. The explanation is said to lie within the particular history or situation, not in some external human pattern or regularity or "law" that might govern or account for the situation. This lack of causality has serious implications for the human sciences in general and the health sciences in particular. There is loss of generalizability, loss of correspondence with extant theory and diminished power to make "ampliative inferences" that can extend research and therapy. For a practice discipline that needs prescriptive action guides the logic of scientific explanation needs to be coupled with the meaning derived from hermeneutical explanation.

Because hermeneutics can make clear practical wisdom, knowledge, and experience, it has great attraction for the clinician and for the art of clinical diagnosis and treatment. It need not be the sole strategy for inquiry, although it may become a key strategy for practice. This leads to the final question: How should research be conducted in the human enterprise called nursing? More specifically, how might a philosophy of nursing science be framed?

Toward a Nursing Science Philosophy

Human understanding is proposed as a premise of nursing science, in keeping with humanistic traditions in ancient and modern philosophy and in nursing philosophy. If accepted as a basic premise, then nursing research would necessarily incorporate means for determining interpretation of the phenomena of concern from the perspective of the client, patient, or care recipient. These interpretations might be subjected to hermeneutic analysis for their meaning, followed by intersubjective consensual validation by participants. To being the interpretations to intersubjective consensus among scholars requires that they be raised to a level of public information and knowledge, subject to scrutiny, criticism, and further demonstration and empirical testing in other patient-client situations. This strategy might allow for nomothetic explanations as well as idiosyncratic ones.

What is proposed here is what anthropologists would call an emic perspective (Tripp-Reimer, 1984) for most of nursing research. Even if the goal of research is etic, outside the given participant group, one would still argue for consensual validation in the hermeneutic sense (Gortner & Schultz, 1988). But this consensus also has to be brought to the level of public scrutiny, where public this time means other scholar-scientists in addition to the client or subject or informant.

The public nature of human science knowledge, representing rational, informed opinion about the human state, is proposed as a continued premise of nursing science philosophy, in keeping with traditional and modern views of science (Ziman, 1980). Such knowledge generally is obtained through systematic inquiry, with features of theory/observation compatibility, logic, precision, clarity and reproducibility as is characteristic of "good science" (Gortner, 1987). Such knowledge thrives on criticism and attempts to falsify or substantiate its truth claims. Note here that there is no specification of how this knowledge looks: for purposes of nursing science development, it may represent itself in language or numbers or combinations thereof. What is important is that it is publicized, criticized and tried out. Otherwise it becomes ideology.[1]

Observation as a basic, if not foundational, element of knowledge development in nursing science is proposed as another premise. By this is meant the foundational nature of "observables" of the human state; to be observable means that measurement is possible. What if these are feelings, intuitions, preunderstandings? Can these be "observable"? Indeed yes, and in fact this characteristic or capacity may be a unique feature of nursing science as a form of human science. Nursing's skill in capturing the human situation at a given point of time in the health-illness continuum arises from a tradition of intimate, compassionate, caring, and attentive service. Such intimacy promotes sensitivity to cues in the situation that enlarge understanding and guide action. The means is yet to be developed to reframe these feelings and intuitions in a way that they are "observable" and thus believable by others. The American Academy of Nursing's (1986) scientific sessions recommended the use of triangulation (multimethods) and pattern-seeking approaches to capture nursing phenomena; these approaches might accommodate investigators of differing interpretive/analytic philosophies. A "particularistic, pragmatic" plan for holistic nursing inquiry has been detailed by Schultz (1987). Here the whole (meaning and experiences) is assembled with parts (physiological processes or nursing acts) into a single text, in which the investigator reflectively engages with the data, reasons through dialogue, discovers patterns, and uses these dialectically to construct new understandings and meanings. The conclusion or knowledge claims are then assessed for warrantability using Chisholm's (1982) epistemic principles.

Rationality also is a foundational element in nursing science philosophy. Schultz and Meleis (1988) spoke of conceptual knowledge. Nursing conceptual frameworks and theories can be employed deliberately in investigations to determine their empirical relevance. New theories of the generative sort proposed by Gergen (1980) can be inferred from the data coming from personal histories and clinical ethnographies and from the rationality demanded by critical social theory and feminist scholarship. Rational schemes to describe the relationships supposedly seen in the phenomena of interest also might be proposed through the technique now known as causal modeling. Here, data are examined with regard to previously specified models, through

multivariate analytic techniques, and attempts are made to test or generate theories. Here, the "observables," the data, would need transformation from language form to integer form.

Rational philosophies of particular interest to nursing are those employing both critical theory and feminist perspectives. Both are special cases of rationality that apply to situations of social interaction involving authority and power, and both challenge major claims to science based on empirical evidence alone. The arguments for the critical and feminist perspectives have been empirically displayed in research endeavors as well as rationally and ideologically argued by Allen (1985) and Chinn and Wheeler (1985). McLain's (1985) doctoral dissertation and Holter's (1987) theoretical critique are examples of critical theory applications in nursing. An important feminist illustration is Keller's (1985) account of Barbara McClintock's Nobel winning discovery of hybrid corn. The same claims of knowing through intimate attending are made here as have been made by nursing authors in studies of expert caring (Benner & Wrubel, 1989). These claims challenge our contention that scientific knowledge is public knowledge.

Explanatory power is proposed as another premise of philosophy of science in nursing. Human science activities cannot rest only with increased understanding; nor can that understanding be taken as the sole criterion for explanation, as Benner (1985) has proposed. Human patterns and regularities and perhaps even "laws" characterize the human state and undergird the whole enterprise of society and human life. Perhaps concern with the mechanistic philosophy of science has prompted the reaction against explication of patterns. But it is argued here that explication is a necessary requirement of nursing science as a clinical and human science, and that eventually such explanations will guide nursing action as therapy. Even if not brought to the prescriptive level, such explanation enhances knowledge about fundamental processes and thus may inform other disciplinary fields.

To understand aids explanation; certainly understanding informs explanation, but explanation in the sense that is being proposed here must suggest what might occur the next time the event or phenomenon occurs. Thus temporality and predictability are assumed in scientific explanations that are within the definition of explanatory power. Whether control of human phenomena is possible or even desirable are both an ethical and scientific question.

To explain means that some causal process or interaction is involved. Here lies one of the greatest areas of disagreement among nurse scholars including our major theorists. It probably will not be resolved in our lifetimes, just as it has not been resolved through the centuries. Explanation in nursing science philosophy can take a variety of forms, some of which have been illustrated in other essays (Gortner, 1983, 1984). Increasingly, statistical inference and the results of cohort studies and clinical trials can enhance the probability of prediction. To sort out pseudoexplanations, these forms of explanation remain logical rather than intuitive, employing the notion of a contrast class, a causal process, a set of clinically and statistically relevant factors (Salmon, 1978). Although forms of explanation may differ, causal inference must remain a key ingredient.

A final premise of science philosophy is that the knowledge generated must also allow for prescriptions that will guide practice. Whether these are clinically or empirically derived, there is the obligation to act or intervene, in keeping with other helping professions. Basic science has no such mandate for application or therapy.

NOTE

1. A special plea to scholars interested in theory generation and concept discovery is made. Please identify and specify the conditions under which the concept or phenomenon was found. These conditions represent the linkages of the abstraction with reality, increasing the likelihood that the abstraction may be found again. Otherwise who is to know that it is not a fleeting piece of imagination?

REFERENCES

Allen, D. (1985). Nursing research and social control: Alternative modes of science that emphasize understanding and emancipation. **IMAGE: Journal of Nursing Scholarship, 17**(2), 58–64.

Allen, D., Benner, P., & Diekelmann, N. (1986). Three paradigms for nursing research: Methodological considerations. In P. L. Chinn (Ed.), **Nursing research methodology: Issues and explanation** (pp. 23–38). Rockville, MD: Aspen Publications.

American Academy of Nursing. (1986). **Setting the agenda for the year 2000: Knowledge development in nursing.** Kansas City: ANA.

American Nurses' Association. (1973). **Standards of nursing practice.** Kansas City: ANA.

American Nurses' Association (1976). **Code for nurses with interpretive statement.** Kansas City: ANA.

American Nurses' Association (1980). **A social policy statement.** Kansas City: ANA.

Batey, M. (1972). Values relative to research and to science as influenced by a sociological perspective. **Nursing Research, 21,** 504–508.

Benner, P. (1985). Quality of life: A phenomenological perspective on explanation, prediction, and understanding in nursing science. **Advances in Nursing Science, 8**(1), 1–16.

Benner, P., & Wrubel, J. (1989). **The primacy of caring: Stress and coping in health and illness.** Menlo Park: Addison-Wesley.

Bernstein, R. J. (1986). **Philosophical profiles.** Philadelphia: University of Pennsylvania Press.

Canadian Nurses Association. (1980). **Definition of nursing practice and standards of practice.** Ottawa: CNA.

Chinn, P. L., & Wheeler, C. E. (1985). Feminism and nursing. **Nursing Outlook, 33**(2), 74–77.

Chisholm, R. M. (1982). **The foundations of knowing.** Minneapolis: University of Minnesota Press.

Cohen, M. Z. (1987). A historical overview of the phenomenological movement. **IMAGE: Journal of Nursing Scholarship, 19**(1), 31–34.

Cull-Wilby, B., & Pepin, J. (1987). Towards a coexistence of paradigms in nursing knowledge development. **Journal of Advanced Nursing, 12**(4), 515–521.

Ellis, R. (1970). Values and vicissitudes of the scientist nurse. **Nursing Research, 19,** 440–445.

Ellis, R. (1983). Philosophic inquiry. In H. Werley & J. Fitzpatrick (Eds.), **Annual review of nursing research** (Vol. 1) (pp. 211–228). New York: Springer Publishing.

Fry, S. (1981). Accountability in research: The relationship of scientific and humanistic values. **Advances in Nursing Science, 4,** 1–13.

Gadow, S. (1980). Existential advocacy: Philosophical foundations of nursing. In E. Stuart & S. Gadow (Eds.), **Nursing: Images and ideals** (pp. 79–101). New York: Springer Publishing.

Gergen, K. J. (1980). The emerging crisis in life-span developmental theory. In P. Baltes & O. Brien (Eds.), **Life span development and behavior** (Vol. 3), (pp. 31–63). Orlando, FL: Academic Press.

Gortner, S. R. (1974). Scientific accountability in nursing. **Nursing Outlook, 22,** 764–768.

Gortner, S. R. (1980). Nursing science in transition. **Nursing Research, 29**(3), 180–183.

Gortner, S. R. (1983). **Explanation in nursing science: The importance of "why" questions.** Paper presented at the Fifth Annual Graduate Conference: Nursing Knowledge Development, Implementation, and Validation in Practice. Portland, OR: University of Portland.

Gortner, S. R. (1984). Knowledge in a practice discipline: Philosophy and pragmatics. In **Nursing research and policy formation. The case of prospective payment.** Papers of the 1983 Scientific Session of the American Academy of Nursing (pp. 5–17). Kansas City, MO: AAN.

Gortner, S. R. (1987). To build the science. In S. R. Gortner (Ed.), **Nursing science methods: A reader** (pp. 5–15). University of California, San Francisco, 5–16.

Gortner, S. R., & Lorensen, M. (1989). Development of nursing science in Scandinavia. **Nursing Outlook, 37**(3), 123–126.

Gortner, S. R., & Nahm, H. (1977). Overview of nursing research. **Nursing Research, 26,** 10–23.

Gortner, S. R., & Schultz, P. R. (1988). Approaches to nursing science methods. **IMAGE: Journal of Nursing Scholarship, 20**(1), 22–24.

Habermas, J. T. (1971). **Knowledge and human interests** (J. Shapiro, Trans.). Boston: Beacon Press.

Heidegger, M. (1962). **Being and time.** (J. Macquarrie & E. Robinson, Trans.). New York: Harper & Row.

Holter, I. M. (1987). Critical theory. In **Critical theory: An introduction and an exploration of its usefulness as a philosophical foundation for developing nursing theories and for guiding nursing practice and administration** (pp. 8–28). Oslo, Norway: Institutt for Sykepleievitenskap, University of Oslo.

International Council of Nurses. (1987). **Definition: Nursing research.** Geneva: ICN.

Keller, E. F. (1985, October). Contending with a masculine bias in the ideals and values of science. Point of view in the **Chronicle of Higher Education.**

Kuhn, T. (1970). Introduction: II. The route to normal science: III, The nature of normal science. In T. Kuhn (Ed.), **Structure of scientific revolutions.** 2nd ed. enl. (pp. 1–34). Chicago: University of Chicago Press.

Lanara, V. (1982). Development of a scientific foundation for the nursing profession. In K. Lerheim (Ed.), **Proceedings of the Fourth Conference of the Workgroup of European Nurse Researchers** (pp. 98–103). Oslo, Norway: Norwegian Nurses Association.

Leininger, M. (1988). **Care: The essence of nursing and health.** Detroit: Wayne State University Press. (Originally published by Charles Slack, Inc. in 1984).

Leonard, V. W. (1989). A Heideggerian phenomenologic perspective on the concept of person. **Advances in Nursing Science, 11,** 40–55.

Marcuse, H. (1964). **One-dimensional man.** Boston: Beacon Press.

McLain, B. R. (1985). **Patterns of interaction, decision-making, and health care delivery by nurse practitioners and physicians in joint practice.** Unpublished doctoral dissertation. University of San Francisco.

Merleau-Ponty, M. (1962). **Phenomenology of perception.** C. Smith (trans.). London: Routledge and Kegan Paul.

Mishel, M. H., & Murdaugh, C. L. (1987). Family adjustment to heart transplantation: Redesigning the dream. **Nursing Research, 36,** 332–338.

National Center for Nursing Research (1988). **Nursing science: Serving health through research** (Program Announcement). Bethesda, MD: National Institutes of Health.

Nordic Nurses Federation. (1987). **Ethical guidelines for nursing research in the Nordic countries.** Aurskog, Norway: Printing Data Center.

Patterson, J. G., & Zderad, L. T. (Eds.). (1976). **Humanistic nursing.** New York: John Wiley & Sons.

Phillips, D. (1987). The new dynamics of the sciences. In **Philosophy, science, and social inquiry** (pp. 20–36). New York: Pergamon Press.

Royal College of Nursing. (1987). **In pursuit of excellence: A position statement on nursing.** London: Author.

Salmon, W. (1978). Why ask "Why?" An inquiry concerning scientific explanation. **Proceedings and Addresses of the American Philosophical Association, 51,** 683–705.

Sartre, J. P. (1963). **Search for method.** New York: Vintage Books.

Schultz, P. R. (1987). Toward holistic inquiry in nursing: A proposal for synthesis of patterns and methods. **Scholarly Inquiry for Nursing Practice, 1**(2), 135–146.

Schultz, P. R. & Meleis, A. I. (1988). Nursing epistemology: Traditions, insights, questions. **IMAGE: Journal of Nursing Scholarship, 20**(4), 217–221.

Silva, M., & Rothbart, D. (1984). Analysis of changing trends in philosophies of science on nursing theory development and testing. **Advances in Nursing Science, 6**(2), 1–12.

Stevenson, J., & Woods, N. F. (1986). Nursing science and contemporary science: Emerging paradigms. In G. E. Sorensen (Ed.), **Setting the agenda for the year 2000: Knowledge development in nursing** (pp. 6–20). Kansas City: AAN.

Thompson, J. L. (1985). Practical discourse on nursing: Going beyond empiricism and historicism. **Advances in Nursing Science, 7**(4), 59–71.

Tripp-Reimer, T. (1984). Reconceptualizing the construct of health: Integrating emic and etic perspectives. **Research in Nursing and Health, 7,** 101–109.

Vaillot, M. C. (1962). **Commitment to nursing: A philosophical investigation.** Philadelphia: J. B. Lippincott.

Watson, J. (1985). **Nursing: Human science and human caring.** Boulder, CO: Colorado Associated University Press.

Winch, P. (1958). **The idea of a social science and its relation to philosophy.** London: Routledge and Kegan Paul.

Ziman, J. (1980). What is science? In E. D. Klemke, R. Hollinger, & A. D. Kline (Eds.), **Introductory readings in the philosophy of science** (pp. 35–54). Buffalo, NY: Prometheus Books.

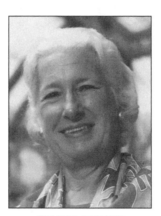

SUSAN R. GORTNER

Objectivity, Value Judgment, and Theory Choice

Thomas Kuhn

In the penultimate chapter of a controversial book first published fifteen years ago, I considered the ways scientists are brought to abandon one time-honored theory or paradigm in favor of another. Such decision problems, I wrote, "cannot be resolved by proof." To discuss their mechanism is, therefore, to talk "about techniques of persuasion, or about argument and counterargument in a situation in which there can be no proof." Under these circumstances, I continued, "lifelong resistance [to a new theory] . . . is not a violation of scientific standards. . . . Though the historian can always find men— Priestley, for instance—who were unreasonable to resist for as long as they did, he will not find a point at which resistance becomes illogical or unscientific."[1] Statements of that sort obviously raise the question of why, in the absence of binding criteria for scientific choice, both the number of solved scientific problems and the precision of individual problem solutions should increase so markedly with the passage of time. Confronting that issue, I sketched in my closing chapter a number of characteristics that scientists share by virtue of the training that licenses their membership in one or another community of specialists. In the absence of criteria able to

dictate the choice of each individual, I argued, we do well to trust the collective judgment of scientists trained in this way. "What better criterion could there be," I asked rhetorically, "than the decision of the scientific group?"[2]

A number of philosophers have greeted remarks like these in a way that continues to surprise me. My views, it is said, make of theory choice "a matter for mob psychology."[3] Kuhn believes, I am told, that "the decision of a scientific group to adopt a new paradigm cannot be based on good reasons of any kind, factual or otherwise."[4] The debates surrounding such choices must, my critics claim, be for me "mere persuasive displays without deliberative substance."[5] Reports of this sort manifest total misunderstanding, and I have occasionally said as much in papers directed primarily to other ends. But those passing protestations have had negligible effect, and the misunderstandings continue to be important. I conclude that it is past time for me to describe, at greater length and with greater precision, what has been on my mind when I have uttered statements like the ones with which I just began. If I have been reluctant to do so in the past, that is largely because I have preferred to devote attention to areas in which my views diverge more sharply from those currently received than they do with respect to theory choice.

What, I ask to begin with, are the characteristics of a good scientific theory? Among a number of quite usual answers I select five, not because they are exhaustive, but because they are individually important and collectively sufficiently varied to indicate what is at stake. First, a theory should be accurate: Within its domain, that is, consequences deducible from a theory should be in demonstrated agreement with the results of existing experiments and observations. Second, a theory should be consistent, not only internally or with itself, but also with other currently accepted theories applicable to related aspects of nature. Third, it should have broad scope: In particular, a theory's consequences should extend far beyond the particular observations, laws, or subtheories it was initially designed to explain. Fourth, and closely related, it should be simple, bringing order to phenomena that in its absence would be individually isolated and, as a set, confused. Fifth—a somewhat less standard item, but one of special importance to actual scientific decisions—a theory should be fruitful of new research findings: It should, that is, disclose new phenomena or previously unnoted relationships among those already known.[6] These five characteristics—accuracy, consistency, scope, simplicity, and fruitfulness— are all standard criteria for evaluating the adequacy of a theory. If they had not been, I would have devoted far more space to them in my book, for I agree entirely with the traditional view that they play a vital role when scientists must choose between an established theory and an upstart competitor. Together with others of much the same sort, they provide *the* shared basis for theory choice.

Nevertheless, two sorts of difficulties are regularly encountered by the men who must use these criteria in choosing, say, between Ptolemy's astronomical theory and Copernicus's, between the oxygen and phlogiston theories of combustion, or between Newtonian mechanics and the quantum theory. Individually the criteria are imprecise: Individuals may legitimately differ about their application to concrete cases. In addition, when deployed together, they repeatedly prove to conflict with one another; accuracy may, for example, dictate the choice of one theory, scope the choice of its competitor. Since these difficulties, especially the first, are also relatively familiar, I shall devote little time to their elaboration. Though my argument does demand that I illustrate them briefly, my views will begin to depart from those long current only after I have done so.

Begin with accuracy, which for present purposes I take to include not only quantitative agreement but qualitative as well. Ultimately it proves the most nearly decisive of all the criteria, partly because it is less equivocal than the others but especially because predictive and explanatory powers, which depend on it, are characteristics that scientists are particularly unwilling to give up. Unfortunately, however, theories cannot always be discriminated in terms of accuracy. Copernicus's system, for example, was not more accurate than Ptolemy's until drastically revised by Kepler more than sixty years after Copernicus's death. If Kepler or someone else had not found other reasons to choose heliocentric astronomy, those improvements in accuracy would never have been made, and Copernicus's work might have been forgotten. More typically, of course, accuracy does permit discriminations, but not the sort that lead regularly to unequivocal choice. The oxygen theory, for example, was universally acknowledged to account for observed weight relations in chemical reactions, something the phlogiston theory had previously scarcely attempted to do. But the phlogiston theory, unlike its rival, could account for the metals' being much more alike than the ores from which they were formed. One theory thus matched experience better in one area, the other in another. To choose between them on the basis of accuracy, a scientist would need to decide the area in which accuracy was more significant. About that matter chemists could and did differ without violating any of the criteria outlined above, or any others yet to be suggested.

However important it may be, therefore, accuracy by itself is seldom or never a sufficient criterion for theory choice. Other criteria must function as well, but they do not eliminate problems. To illustrate I select just two—consistency and simplicity—asking how they functioned in the choice between the heliocentric and geocentric systems. As astronomical theories both Ptolemy's and Copernicus's were internally consistent, but their relation to related theories in other fields was very different. The stationary central earth was an essential ingredient of received physical theory, a tight-knit body of doctrine that explained, among other things, how stones fall, how water pumps function, and why the clouds move slowly across the skies. Heliocentric astronomy, which required the earth's motion, was inconsistent with the existing scientific explanation of these and other terrestrial phenomena. The consistency criterion, by itself, therefore, spoke unequivocally for the geocentric tradition.

Simplicity, however, favored Copernicus, but only when evaluated in a quite special way. If, on the one hand, the two systems were compared in terms of the actual computational labor required to predict the position of a planet at a particular time, then they proved substantially equivalent. Such computations were what astronomers did, and Copernicus's system offered them no labor-saving techniques; in that sense it was not simpler than Ptolemy's. If, on the other hand, one asked about the amount of mathematical apparatus required to explain, not the detailed quantitative motions of the planets, but merely their gross qualitative features—limited elongation, retrograde motion, and the like—then, as every schoolchild knows, Copernicus required only one circle per planet, Ptolemy two. In that sense the Copernican theory was the simpler, a fact vitally important to the choices made by both Kepler and Galileo and thus essential to the ultimate triumph of Copernicanism. But that sense of simplicity was not the only one available, nor even the one most natural to professional astronomers, men whose task was the actual computation of planetary position.

Because time is short and I have multiplied examples elsewhere, I shall here simply assert that these difficulties in applying standard criteria of choice are typical and that they arise no less forcefully in twentieth-century situations than in the earlier and better-known examples I have just sketched. When scientists must choose between competing theories, two men fully committed to the same list of criteria for choice may nevertheless reach different conclusions. Perhaps they interpret simplicity differently or have different convictions about the range of fields within which the consistency criterion must be met. Or perhaps they agree about these matters but differ about the relative weights to be accorded to these or to other criteria when several are deployed together. With respect to divergences of this sort, no set of choice criteria yet proposed is of any use. One can explain, as the historian characteristically does, why particular men made particular choices at particular times. But for that purpose one must go beyond the list of shared criteria to characteristics of the individuals who make the choice. One must, that is, deal with characteristics that vary from one scientist to another without thereby in the least jeopardizing their adherence to the canons that make science scientific. Though such canons do exist and should be discoverable (doubtless the criteria of choice with which I began are among them), they are not by themselves sufficient to determine the decisions of individual scientists. For that purpose the shared canons must be fleshed out in ways that differ from one individual to another.

Some of the differences I have in mind result from the individual's previous experience as a scientist. In what part of the field was he at work when confronted by the need to choose? How long had he worked there; how successful had he been; and how much of his work depended on concepts and techniques challenged by the new theory? Other factors relevant to choice lie outside the sciences. Kepler's early election of Copernicanism was due in part to his immersion in the Neoplatonic and Hermetic movements of his day; German Romanticism predisposed those it affected toward both recognition and acceptance of energy conservation; nineteenth-century British social thought had a similar influence on the availability and acceptability of Darwin's concept of the struggle for existence. Still other significant differences are functions of personality. Some scientists place more premium than others on originality and are correspondingly more willing to take risks; some scientists prefer comprehensive, unified theories to precise and detailed problem solutions of apparently narrower scope. Differentiating factors like these are described by my critics as subjective and are contrasted with the shared or objective criteria from which I began. Though I shall later question that use of terms, let me for the moment accept it. My point is, then, that every individual choice between competing theories depends on a mixture of objective and subjective factors, or of shared and individual criteria. Since the latter have not ordinarily figured in the philosophy of science, my emphasis upon them has made my belief in the former hard for my critics to see.

What I have said so far is primarily simply descriptive of what goes on in the sciences at times of theory choice. As description, furthermore, it has not been challenged by my critics, who reject instead my claim that these facts of scientific life have philosophic import. Taking up that issue, I shall begin to isolate some, though I think not vast, differences of opinion. Let me begin by asking how philosophers of science can for so long have neglected the subjective elements which, they freely grant, enter regularly into the actual theory choices made by individual scientists? Why have these elements seemed to them an index only of human weakness, not at all of the nature of scientific knowledge?

One answer to that question is, of course, that few philosophers, if any, have claimed to possess either a complete or an entirely well-articulated list of criteria. For some time, therefore, they could reasonably expect that further research would eliminate residual imperfections and produce an algorithm able to dictate rational, unanimous choice. Pending that achieve-ment, scientists would have no alternative but to supply subjectively what the best current list of objective criteria still lacked. That some of them might still do so even with a perfected list at hand would then be an index only of the inevitable imperfection of human nature.

That sort of answer may still prove to be correct, but I think no philosopher still expects that it will. The search for algorithmic decision procedures has continued for some time and produced both powerful and illuminating results. But those results all presuppose that individual criteria of choice can be unambiguously stated and also that, if more than one proves relevant, an appropriate weight function is at hand for their joint application. Unfortunately, where the choice at issue is between scientific theories, little progress has been made toward the first of these desiderata and none toward the second. Most philosophers of science would, therefore, I think, now regard the sort of algorithm which has traditionally been sought as a not quite attainable ideal. I entirely agree and shall henceforth take that much for granted.

Even an ideal, however, if it is to remain credible, requires some demonstrated relevance to the situations in which it is supposed to apply. Claiming that such demonstration requires no recourse to subjective factors, my critics seem to appeal, implicitly or explicitly, to the well-known distinction between the contexts of discovery and of justification.[7] They concede, that is, that the subjective factors I invoke play a significant role in the discovery or invention of new theories, but they also insist that that inevitably intuitive process lies outside of the bounds of philosophy of science and is irrelevant to the question of scientific objectivity. Objectivity enters science, they continue, through the processes by which theories are tested, justified, or judged. Those processes do not, or at least need not, involve subjective factors at all. They can be governed by a set of (objective) criteria shared by the entire group competent to judge.

I have already argued that that position does not fit observations of scientific life and shall now assume that that much has been conceded. What is now at issue is a different point: whether or not this invocation of the distinction between contexts of discovery and of justification provides even a plausible and useful idealization. I think it does not and can best make my point by suggesting first a likely source of its apparent cogency. I suspect that my critics have been misled by science pedagogy or what I have elsewhere called textbook science. In science teaching, theories are presented together with exemplary applications, and those applications may be viewed as evidence. But that is not their primary pedagogic function (science students are distressingly willing to receive the word from professors and texts). Doubtless *some* of them were *part* of the evidence at the time actual decisions were being made, but they represent only a fraction of the considerations relevant to the decision process. The context of pedagogy differs almost as much from the context of justification as it does from that of discovery.

Full documentation of that point would require longer argument than is appropriate here, but two aspects of the way in which philosophers ordinarily demonstrate the relevance of choice criteria are worth noting. Like the science textbooks on which they are often modelled, books and articles on the philosophy of science refer again and again to the famous crucial experiments: Foucault's pendulum, which demonstrates the motion of the earth; Cavendish's demonstration of gravitational attraction; or Fizeau's measurement of the relative speed of sound in water and air. These experiments are paradigms of good reason for scientific choice; they illustrate the most effective of all the sorts of argument which could be available to a scientist uncertain which of two theories to follow; they are vehicles for the transmission of criteria of choice. But they also have another characteristic in common. By the time they were performed no scientist still needed to be convinced of the validity of the theory their outcome is now used to demonstrate. Those de-

cisions had long since been made on the basis of significantly more equivocal evidence. The exemplary crucial experiments to which philosophers again and again refer would have been historically relevant to theory choice only if they had yielded unexpected results. Their use as illustrations provides needed economy to science pedagogy, but they scarcely illuminate the character of the choices that scientists are called upon to make.

Standard philosophical illustrations of scientific choice have another troublesome characteristic. The only arguments discussed are, as I have previously indicated, the ones favorable to the theory that, in fact, ultimately triumphed. Oxygen, we read, could explain weight relations, phlogiston could not; but nothing is said about the phlogiston theory's power or about the oxygen theory's limitations. Comparisons of Ptolemy's theory with Copernicus's proceed in the same way. Perhaps these examples should not be given since they contrast a developed theory with one still in its infancy. But philosophers regularly use them nonetheless. If the only result of their doing so were to simplify the decision situation, one could not object. Even historians do not claim to deal with the full factual complexity of the situations they describe. But these simplifications emasculate by making choice totally unproblematic. They eliminate, that is, one essential element of the decision situations that scientists must resolve if their field is to move ahead. In those situations there are always at least some good reasons for each possible choice. Considerations relevant to the context of discovery are then relevant to justification as well; scientists who share the concerns and sensibilities of the individual who discovers a new theory are ipso facto likely to appear disproportionately frequently among that theory's first supporters. That is why it has been difficult to construct algorithms for theory choice, and also why such difficulties have seemed so thoroughly worth resolving. Choices that present problems are the ones philosophers of science need to understand. Philosophically interesting decision procedures must function where, in their absence, the decision might still be in doubt.

That much I have said before, if only briefly. Recently, however, I have recognized another, subtler source for the apparent plausibility of my critics' position. To present it, I shall briefly describe a hypothetical dialogue with one of them. Both of us agree that each scientist chooses between competing theories by deploying some Bayesian algorithm which permits him to compute a value for $p(T,E)$, i.e., for the probability of a theory T on the evidence E available both to him and to the other members of his professional group at a particular period of time. "Evidence," furthermore, we both interpret broadly to include such considerations as simplicity and fruitfulness. My critic asserts, however, that there is only one such value of p, that corresponding to objective choice, and he believes that all rational members of the group must arrive at it. I assert, on the other hand, for reasons previously given, that the factors he calls objective are insufficient to determine in full any algorithm at all. For the sake of the discussion I have conceded that each individual has an algorithm and that all their algorithms have much in common. Nevertheless, I continue to hold that the algorithms of individuals are all ultimately different by virtue of the subjective considerations with which each must complete the objective criteria before any computations can be done. If my hypothetical critic is liberal, he may now grant that these subjective differences do play a role in determining the hypothetical algorithm on which each individual relies during the early stages of the competition between rival theories. But he is also likely to claim that, as evidence increases with the passage of time, the algorithms of different individuals converge to the algorithm of objective choice with which his presentation began. For him the increasing unanimity of individual choices is evidence for their increasing objectivity and thus for the elimination of subjective elements from the decision process.

So much for the dialogue, which I have, of course, contrived to disclose the non sequitur underlying an apparently plausible position. What converges as the evidence changes over time need only be the values of p that individuals compute from their individual algorithms. Conceivably those algorithms themselves also become more alike with time, but the ultimate unanimity of theory choice provides no evidence whatsoever that they do so. If subjective factors are required to account for the decisions that initially divide the profession, they may still be present later when the profession agrees. Though I shall not here argue the point, consideration of the occasions on which a scientific community divides suggests that they actually do so.

My argument has so far been directed to two points. It first provided evidence that the choices scientists make between competing theories depend not only on shared criteria—those my critics call objective—but also on idiosyncratic factors dependent on individual biography and personality. The latter are, in my critics' vocabulary, subjective, and the second part of my argument has attempted to bar some likely ways of denying their philosophic import. Let me now shift to a more positive approach, returning briefly to the list of shared criteria—accuracy, simplicity, and the like—with which I began. The considerable effectiveness of such criteria does not, I now wish to suggest, depend on their being sufficiently articulated to dictate the choice of each individual who subscribes to them. Indeed, if they were articulated to that extent, a behavior mechanism fundamental to scientific advance would cease to function. What the tradition sees as eliminable imperfections in its rules of choice I take to be in part responses to the essential nature of science.

As so often, I begin with the obvious. Criteria that influence decisions without specifying what those decisions must be are familiar in many aspects of human life. Ordinarily, however, they are called, not criteria or rules, but maxims, norms, or values. Consider maxims first. The individual who invokes them when choice is urgent usually finds them frustratingly vague and often also in conflict one with another. Contrast "He who hesitates is lost" with "Look before you leap," or compare "Many hands make light work" with "Too many cooks spoil the broth." Individually maxims dictate different choices, collectively none at all. Yet no one suggests that supplying children with contradictory tags like these is irrelevant to their education. Opposing maxims alter the nature of the decision to be made, highlight the essential issues it presents, and point to those remaining aspects of the decision for which each individual must take responsibility himself. Once invoked, maxims like these alter the nature of the decision process and can thus change its outcome.

Values and norms provide even clearer examples of effective guidance in the presence of conflict and equivocation. Improving the quality of life is a value, and a car in every garage once followed from it as a norm. But quality of life has other aspects, and the old norm has become problematic. Or again, freedom of speech is a value, but so is preservation of life and property. In application, the two often conflict, so that judicial soul-searching, which still continues, has been required to prohibit such behavior as inciting to riot or shouting fire in a crowded theater. Difficulties like these are an appropriate source for frustration, but they rarely result in charges that values have no function or in calls for their abandonment. That response is barred to most of us by an acute consciousness that there are societies with other values and that these value differences result in other ways of life, other decisions about what may and what may not be done.

I am suggesting, of course, that the criteria of choice with which I began function not as rules, which determine choice, but as values, which influence it. Two men deeply committed to the same values may nevertheless, in particular situations, make different choices as, in fact, they do. But that difference in outcome ought not to suggest that the values scientists share are less than critically important either to their decisions or to the development of the enterprise in which they participate. Values like accuracy, consistency, and scope may prove ambiguous in application, both individually and collectively; they may, that is, be an insufficient basis for a *shared* algorithm of choice. But they do specify a great deal: what each scientist must consider in reaching a decision, what he may or may not consider relevant, and what he can legitimately be required to report as the basis for the choice he has made. Change the list, for example by adding social utility as a criterion, and some particular choices will be different, more like those one expects from an engineer. Subtract accuracy of fit to nature from the list, and the enterprise that results may not resemble science at all, but perhaps philosophy instead. Different creative disciplines are characterized, among other things, by different sets of shared values. If philosophy and engineering lie too close to the sciences, think of literature or the plastic arts. Milton's failure to set *Paradise Lost* in a Copernican universe does not indicate that he agreed with Ptolemy but that he had things other than science to do.

Recognizing that criteria of choice can function as values when incomplete as rules has, I think, a number of striking advantages. First, as I have already argued at length, it accounts in detail for aspects of scientific behavior which the tradition has seen as anomalous or even irrational. More important, it allows the standard criteria to function fully in the earliest stages of theory choice, the period when they are most needed but when, on the traditional view, they function badly or not at all. Copernicus was responding to them during the years required to convert heliocentric astronomy from a global conceptual scheme to mathematical machinery for predicting planetary position. Such predictions were what astronomers valued; in their absence, Copernicus would scarcely have been heard, something which had happened to the idea of a moving earth before. That his own version convinced very few is less important than his acknowledgment of the basis on which judgments would have to be reached if heliocentricism were to survive. Though idiosyncrasy must be invoked to explain why Kepler and Galileo were early converts to Copernicus's system, the gaps filled by their efforts to perfect it were specified by shared values alone.

That point has a corollary which may be more important still. Most newly suggested theories do not survive. Usually the difficulties that evoked them are accounted for by more traditional means. Even when this does not occur, much work, both theoretical and experimental, is ordinarily required before the new theory can display sufficient accuracy and scope to generate widespread conviction. In short, before the group accepts it, a new theory has been tested over time by the research of a number of men, some working within it, others within its traditional rival. Such a mode of development, however, *requires* a decision process which permits rational men to disagree, and such disagreement would be barred by the shared algorithm which philosophers have generally sought. If it were at hand, all conforming scientists would make the same decision at the same time. With standards for acceptance set too low, they would move from one attractive global viewpoint to another, never giving traditional theory an opportunity to supply equivalent attractions. With standards set higher, no one satisfying the criterion of rationality would be inclined to try out the new theory, to articulate it in ways which showed its fruitfulness or displayed its accuracy and scope. I doubt that science would survive the change. What from one viewpoint may seem the looseness and imperfection of choice criteria conceived as rules may, when the same criteria are seen as values, appear an indispensable means of spreading the risk which the introduction or support of novelty always entails.

Even those who have followed me this far will want to know how a value-based enterprise of the sort I have described can develop as a science does, repeatedly producing powerful new techniques for prediction and control. To that question, unfortunately, I have no answer at all, but that is only another way of saying that I make no claim to have solved the problem of induction. If science did progress by virtue of some shared and binding algorithm of choice, I would be equally at a loss to explain its success. The lacuna is one I feel acutely, but its presence does not differentiate my position from the tradition.

It is, after all, no accident that my list of the values guiding scientific choice is, as nearly as makes any difference, identical with the tradition's list of rules dictating choice. Given any concrete situation to which the philosopher's rules could be applied, my values would function like his rules, producing the same choice. Any justification of induction, any explanation of why the rules worked, would apply equally to my values. Now consider a situation in which choice by shared rules proves impossible, not because the rules are wrong but because they are, as rules, intrinsically incomplete. Individuals must then still choose and be guided by the rules (now values) when they do so. For that purpose, however, each must first flesh out the rules, and each will do so in a somewhat different way even though the decision dictated by the variously completed rules may prove unanimous. If I now assume, in addition, that the group is large enough so that individual differences distribute on some normal curve, then any argument that justifies the philosopher's choice by rule should be immediately adaptable to my choice by value. A group too small, or a distribution excessively skewed by external historical pressures, would, of course, prevent the argument's transfer.[8] But those are just the circumstances under which scientific progress is itself problematic. The transfer is not then to be expected.

I shall be glad if these references to a normal distribution of individual differences and to the problem of induction make my position appear very close to more traditional views. With respect to theory choice, I have never thought my departures large and have been correspondingly startled by such charges as "mob psychology," quoted at the start. It is worth noting, however, that the positions are not quite identical, and for that purpose an analogy may be helpful. Many properties of liquids and gases can be accounted for on the kinetic theory by supposing that all molecules travel at the same speed. Among such properties are the regularities known as Boyle's and Charles's law. Other characteristics, most obviously evaporation, cannot be explained in so simple a way. To deal with them one must assume that molecular speeds differ, that they are distributed at random, governed by the laws of chance. What I have been suggesting here is that theory choice, too, can be explained only in part by a theory which attributes the same properties to all the scientists who must do the choosing. Essential aspects of the process generally known as verification will be understood only by recourse to the feaures with respect to which men may differ while still remaining scientists. The tradition takes it for granted that such features are vital to the process of discovery, which it at once and for that reason rules out of philosphical bounds. That they may have significant functions also in the philosophically central problem of justifying theory choice is what philosophers of science have to date categorically denied.

What remains to be said can be grouped in a somewhat miscellaneous epilogue. For the sake of clarity and to avoid writing a book, I have throughout this paper utilized some traditional concepts and locutions about the viability of which I have elsewhere expressed serious doubts. For those who know the work in which I have done so, I close by indicating three aspects of what I have said which would better represent my views if cast in other terms, simultaneously indicating the main directions in which such recasting should proceed. The areas I have in mind are: value invariance, subjectivity, and partial communication. If my views of scientific development are novel—a matter about

which there is legitimate room for doubt—it is in areas such as these, rather than theory choice, that my main departures from tradition should be sought.

Throughout this paper I have implicitly assumed that, whatever their initial source, the criteria or values deployed in theory choice are fixed once and for all, unaffected by their participation in transitions from one theory to another. Roughly speaking, but only very roughly, I take that to be the case. If the list of relevant values is kept short (I have mentioned five, not all independent) and if their specification is left vague, then such values as accuracy, scope, and fruitfulness are permanent attributes of science. But little knowledge of history is required to suggest that both the application of these values and, more obviously, the relative weights attached to them have varied markedly with time and also with the field of application. Furthermore, many of these variations in value have been associated with particular changes in scientific theory. Though the experience of scientists provides no philosphical justification for the values they deploy (such justification would solve the problem of induction), those values are in part learned from that experience, and they evolve with it.

The whole subject needs more study (historians have usually taken scientific values, though not scientific methods, for granted), but a few remarks will illustrate the sort of variations I have in mind. Accuracy, as a value, has with time increasingly denoted quantitative or numerical agreement, sometimes at the expense of qualitative. Before early modern times, however, accuracy in that sense was a criterion only for astronomy, the science of the celestial region. Elsewhere it was neither expected nor sought. During the seventeenth century, however, the criterion of numerical agreement was extended to mechanics, during the late eighteenth and early nineteenth centuries to chemistry and such other subjects as electricity and heat, and in this century to many parts of biology. Or think of utility, an item of value not on my initial list. It too has figured significantly in scientific development, but far more strongly and steadily for chemists than for, say, mathematicians and physicists. Or consider scope. It is still an important scientific value, but important scientific advances have repeatedly been achieved at its expense, and the weight attributed to it at times of choice has diminished correspondingly.

What may seem particularly troublesome about changes like these is, of course, that they ordinarily occur in the aftermath of a theory change. One of the objections to Lavoisier's new chemistry was the roadblocks with which it confronted the achievement of what had previously been one of chemistry's traditional goals: the explanation of qualities, such as color and texture, as well as of their changes. With the acceptance of Lavoisier's theory such explanations ceased for some time to be a value for chemists; the ability to explain qualitative variation was no longer a criterion relevant to the evaluation of chemical theory. Clearly, if such value changes had occurred as rapidly or been as complete as the theory changes to which they related, then theory choice would be value choice, and neither could provide justification for the other. But, historically, value change is ordinarily a belated and largely unconscious concomitant of theory choice, and the former's magnitude is regularly smaller than the latter's. For the functions I have here ascribed to values, such relative stability provides a sufficient basis. The existence of a feedback loop through which theory change affects the values which led to that change does not make the decision process circular in any damaging sense.

About a second respect in which my resort to tradition may be misleading, I must be far more tentative. It demands the skills of an ordinary language philosopher, which I do not possess. Still, no very acute ear for language is required to generate discomfort with the ways in which the terms "objectivity" and, more especially, "subjectivity" have functioned in this paper. Let me briefly suggest the respects in which I believe language has gone astray. "Subjective" is a term

with several established uses: In one of these it is opposed to "objective," in another to "judgmental." When my critics describe the idiosyncratic features to which I appeal as subjective, they resort, erroneously I think, to the second of these senses. When they complain that I deprive science of objectivity, they conflate that second sense of subjective with the first.

A standard application of the term "subjective" is to matters of taste, and my critics appear to suppose that that is what I have made of theory choice. But they are missing a distinction standard since Kant when they do so. Like sensation reports, which are also subjective in the sense now at issue, matters of taste are undiscussable. Suppose that, leaving a movie theater with a friend after seeing a western, I exclaim: "How I liked that terrible potboiler!" My friend, if he disliked the film, may tell me I have low tastes, a matter about which, in these circumstances, I would readily agree. But, short of saying that I lied, he cannot disagree with my report that I liked the film or try to persuade me that what I said about my reaction was wrong. What is discussable in my remark is not my characterization of my internal state, my exemplification of taste, but rather my *judgment* that the film was a potboiler. Should my friend disagree on that point, we may argue most of the night, each comparing the film with good or great ones we have seen, each revealing, implicitly or explicitly, something about how he *judges* cinematic merit, about his aesthetic. Though one of us may, before retiring, have persuaded the other, he need not have done so to demonstrate that our difference is one of judgment, not taste.

Evaluations or choices of theory have, I think, exactly this character. Not that scientists never say merely, I like such and such a theory, or I do not. After 1926 Einstein said little more than that about his opposition to the quantum theory. But scientists may always be asked to explain their choices, to exhibit the bases for their judgments. Such judgments are eminently discussable, and the man who refuses to discuss his own cannot expect to be taken seriously. Though there are, very occasionally, leaders of scientific taste, their existence tends to prove to rule. Einstein was one of the few, and his increasing isolation from the scientific community in later life shows how very limited a role taste alone can play in theory choice. Bohr, unlike Einstein, did discuss the bases for his judgment, and he carried the day. If my critics introduce the term "subjective" in a sense that opposes it to judgmental—thus suggesting that I make theory choice undiscussable, a matter of taste—they have seriously mistake my position.

Turn now to the sense in which "subjectivity" is opposed to "objectivity," and note first that it raises issues quite separate from those just discussed. Whether my taste is low or refined, my report that I liked the film is objective unless I have lied. To my judgment that the film was a potboiler, however, the objective–subjective distinction does not apply at all, at least not obviously and directly. When my critics say I deprive theory choice of objectivity, they must, therefore, have recourse to some very different sense of subjective, presumably the one in which bias and personal likes or dislikes function instead of, or in the face of, the actual facts. But that sense of subjective does not fit the process I have been describing any better than the first. Where factors dependent on individual biography or personality must be introduced to make values applicable, no standards of factuality or actuality are being set aside. Conceivably my discussion of theory choice indicates some limitations of objectivity, but not by isolating elements properly called subjective. Nor am I even quite content with the notion that what I have been displaying are limitations. Objectivity ought to be analyzable in terms of criteria like accuracy and consistency. If these criteria do not supply all the guidance that we have customarily expected of them, then it may be the meaning rather than the limits of objectivity that my argument shows.

Turn, in conclusion, to a third respect, or set of respects, in which this paper needs to be recast. I have assumed throughout that the discussions surrounding theory choice are unproblematic, that the facts appealed to in such discussions are independent of theory, and that the discussions' outcome is appropriately called a choice. Elsewhere I have challenged all three of these assumptions, arguing that communication between proponents of different theories is inevitably partial, that what each takes to be facts depends in part on the theory he espouses, and that an individual's transfer of allegiance from theory to theory is often better described as conversion than as choice. Though all these theses are problematic as well as controversial, my commitment to them is undiminished. I shall not now defend them, but must at least attempt to indicate how what I have said here can be adjusted to conform with these more central aspects of my view of scientific development.

For that purpose I resort to an analogy I have developed in other places. Proponents of different theories are, I have claimed, like native speakers of different languages. Communication between them goes on by translation, and it raises all translation's familiar difficulties. That analogy is, of course, incomplete, for the vocabulary of the two theories may be identical, and most words function in the same ways in both. But some words in the basic as well as in the theoretical vocabularies of the two theories—words like "star" and "planet," "mixture" and "compound," or "force" and "matter"—do function differently. Those differences are unexpected and will be discovered and localized, if at all, only by repeated experience of communication breakdown. Without pursuing the matter further, I simply assert the existence of significant limits to what the proponents of different theories can communicate to one another. The same limits make it difficult or, more likely, impossible for an individual to hold both theories in mind together and compare them point by point with each other and with nature. That sort of comparison is, however, the process on which the appropriateness of any word like "choice" depends.

Nevertheless, despite the incompleteness of their communication, proponents of different theories can exhibit to each other, not always easily, the concrete technical results achievable by those who practice within each theory. Little or no translation is required to apply at least some value criteria to those results. (Accuracy and fruitfulness are most immediately applicable, perhaps followed by scope. Consistency and simplicity are far more problematic.) However incomprehensible the new theory may be to the proponents of tradition, the exhibit of impressive concrete results will persuade at least a few of them that they must discover how such results are achieved. For that purpose they must learn to translate, perhaps by treating already published papers as a Rosetta stone or, often more effective, by visiting the innovator, talking with him, watching him and his students at work. Those exposures may not result in the adoption of the theory; some advocates of the tradition may return home and attempt to adjust the old theory to produce equivalent results. But others, if the new theory is to survive, will find that at some point in the language-learning process they have ceased to translate and begun instead to speak the language like a native. No process quite like choice has occurred, but they are practicing the new theory nonetheless. Furthermore, the factors that have led them to risk the conversion they have undergone are just the ones this paper has underscored in discussing a somewhat different process, one which, following the philosophical tradition, it has labeled theory choice.

NOTES

1. *The Structure of Scientific Revolutions,* 2d ed. (Chicago, 1970), pp. 148, 151–152, 159. All the passages from which these fragments are taken appeared in the same form in the first edition, published in 1962.
2. Ibid., p. 170.
3. Imre Lakatos, "Falsification and the Methodology of Scientific Research Programs," in I. Lakatos and A. Musgrave. eds., *Criticism and the Growth of Knowledge* (Cambridge, 1970), pp. 91–195. The quoted phrase, which appears on p. 178, is italicized in the original.
4. Dudley Shapere. "Meaning and Scientific Change," in R. G. Colodny. ed., *Mind and Cosmos: Essays in Contemporary Science and Philosophy.* University of Pittsburgh Series in the Philosophy of Science, vol. 3 (Pittsburgh, 1966), pp. 41–85. The quotation will be found on p. 67.
5. Israel Scheffler, *Science and Subjectivity* (Indianapolis, 1967), p. 81.
6. The last criterion, fruitfulness, deserves more emphasis than it has yet received. A scientist choosing between two theories ordinarily knows that his decision will have a bearing on his subsequent research career. Of course he is especially attracted by a theory that promises the concrete successes for which scientists are ordinarily rewarded.
7. The least equivocal example of this position is probably the one developed in Scheffler, *Science and Subjectivity*, Chap. 4.
8. If the group is small, it is more likely that random fluctuations will result in its members' sharing an atypical set of values and therefore making choices different from those that would be made by a larger and more representative group. External environment—intellectual, ideological, or economic—must systematically affect the value system of much larger groups, and the consequences can include difficulties in introducing the scientific enterprise to societies with inimical values or perhaps even the end of that enterprise within societies where it had once flourished. In this area, however, great caution is required. Changes in the environment where science is practiced can also have fruitful effects on research. Historians often resort, for example, to differences between national environments to explain why particular innovations were initiated and at first disproportionately pursued in particular countries, e.g., Darwinism in Britain, energy conservation in Germany. At present we know substantially nothing about the minimum requisites of the social milieux within which a sciencelike enterprise might flourish.

"The Focus of the Discipline of Nursing": A Critique and Extension

Marjorie McIntyre

Influential writings in nursing tend to align with views held and privileged in the scientific community. By taking this stance nurses resist changes that would advance the discipline and give voice and visibility to marginalized people in society who seek the socially relevant service that nursing purports to offer. The difficulty stems not only from the failure to question the dominance of particular approaches for knowledge generation over others, but also from the failure to recognize that our questions are constructed to support rather than to challenge existing knowledge. Revisioning a pivotal article—"The focus of the discipline of nursing"—enhances its usefulness for nursing curricula.

In the 1991 article "The focus of the discipline of nursing," Newman, Sime, and Corcoran-Perry[1] identified "caring in the human health experience" as the focus statement for the discipline of nursing. Articulating the implications of knowledge generated from different paradigmatic perspectives, the authors effectively supported their stance that the human science perspective is essential for the full explication of nursing knowledge. Although their work clearly accounts for the relationship between the focus statement and a particular perspective, it stops short of addressing the implications of integrating differently generated knowledge into nursing curriculum. Drawing on the experience of using this article in developing and implementing two nursing curricula, the author both critiques and supports ideas Newman et al put forward and describes new possibilities for nursing curricula. Nursing knowledge is inextricable from the assumptions and values underlying its generation. Explicating the assumptions underlying different approaches to knowledge generation in nursing curricula helps nurses avoid unquestioning conformity to existing knowledge and enhances the possibility that they will generate new knowledge and new possibilities.

Review of the Literature

The impetus for Newman and associates' work was to show how the "seemingly disparate work of various members of faculty can indeed relate to a common focus."[2(p10)] First, the authors openly criticized and offered an alternative to the frequently cited metaparadigm concepts of person, health, nursing, and environment as the concepts central to nursing.[3,4] For Newman and associates the unconnected metaparadigm con-

KEY WORDS: caring, critique, focus of nursing, human experience, phenomenology

. . . .

cepts "do not raise the philosophical issues or scientific questions that stimulate inquiry."[1(p2)] Second, these authors concluded that knowledge emanating from the biophysical and biopsychological sciences is relevant, but not sufficient, for the elaboration of nursing science.[2] That is, because they are as valuable as the physical and social sciences, the human sciences are essential for the full generation and conceptualization of nursing knowledge.

Although Newman and associates acknowledged that delineating central concepts has helped to narrow the focus of nursing, they questioned the assumption that the specific concepts identified, and the way they have been traditionally articulated, explicate the "connectedness" and "social relevance" needed to describe the field of study that constitutes nursing.[1(p2)] Central disciplinary concepts, according to the authors, will have different meanings depending on the particular philosophy of science that underlies the generation of such concepts: "Each paradigm specifies a point of view from which the field of study is conceptualized, the assumptions that are inherent in that view, and the basis on which knowledge claims are accepted. These differing paradigms reflect the shift in focus from physical to social to human science."[1(p3)]

Although several authors have suggested that the assumptions and values underlying different worldviews generate different knowledge,[5,6] the strength of Newman et al's position is the inclusion of three perspectives of science (physical, social, and human) that shows a clear distinction between social and human sciences. Presenting three perspectives, as they have done, moves thinking beyond limiting binaries such as positivist and postpositivist, modern and postmodern, and qualitative and quantitative.

The major emphasis of the article—that human science is essential for the full explication of nursing knowledge[1]—is weakened by the authors' inadequate challenge of earlier influential work. For example, in a 1984 article on the metaparadigm, Fawcett[3] gave privilege, albeit

implicitly, to the physical science point of view. In an invited response to Fawcett's classic article on the metaparadigm, Brodie[7] directly challenged several of Fawcett's assumptions, which Newman and associates might have used to support their stance.

The major criticism of Fawcett's work, according to Brodie, is its presentation as a completed final product rather than as "an evolution of a nursing paradigm."[7(p87)] Although she accepted Fawcett's point that congruence of concepts in nursing implies consensus, Brodie argued that "it does not assume common usage and universal acceptance of the meaning of each concept; nor does it establish the validity or testify to the usefulness of the concepts."[7(p88)] Brodie offered the concepts of health and environment as examples of the disagreement shown by the "multiplicity of definitions of health" and the "various conceptualizations of environment."[7(p88)] It is unlikely that many would challenge Brodie's suggestion that health and environment "remain the most ill-defined of all the central concepts."[7(p88)]

Newman and associates indirectly challenge Fawcett's work in claiming that there has been support for considering caring and health as central concepts in the literature since Nightingale. The authors claim that this support is particularly evident in the theoretical and research literature of the past decade. The strength of Newman et al's thesis is not only the concepts identified but also the focus statement itself, which highlights the relationship between the concepts.

The second major point of the article—that the explication of nursing knowledge differs depending on the perspective held—also can be supported by Brodie's[7] criticism of Fawcett's work. The claim that Fawcett "does not articulate a worldvide of science as a way of viewing differing orientations of nursing models"[7(p88)] highlights the importance of and offers support for the stance of Newman and associates. A final aspect enhancing Newman et al's work is the way the authors leave the concept of nursing out of its own definition, an often-cited criticism of the metaparadigm tetralogy.[8]

Since Newman and associates published their research, much has been written about the interface between science and philosophy that adds to an understanding of their work. Although the authors effectively address the interface between science and philosophy, clearer explication might have strengthened the idea that "philosophies of science" is a way of differing between and among orientations within a discipline.

Recently, Kikuchi and Simmons claimed that "in attempting to move beyond traditional scientific methods (objective verifiable knowledge), nurse researchers have not held squarely in view the kind of questions that science is capable of answering and have unwittingly moved into the realm of questions that only philosophy can answer."[9(p6)] These authors claim that understanding science is a philosophic endeavor because the "different views of science are philosophical" views.[9(p23)]

Effects of Paradigm Views on Curricula

My participation in the design and implementation of two different undergraduate nursing curricula, guided by the work of Newman and associates, has provided insight that both supports and suggests extension or revision of their work. What has been most illuminating is the resistance to the curricular changes that provide for the equivalent valuing of the three worldviews. This article discusses the effects of this work on curriculum development and possible sources of the resistance to these effects.

In faculty committee discussions of proposed curriculum themes within the context of existing nursing and educational literature, it became apparent that rather than having one set of assumptions and values (a unified perspective) to guide the curriculum development process, both committees were faced, like Newman and associates, with designing a curriculum that could accommodate two or even three different worldviews. Their work provided a framework for constructively discussing the faculty members' disparate views. Until this point, differences were not always articulated in a way that promoted the cohesion needed for both planning and carrying out a curriculum plan. For curriculum planning, the challenge became how to integrate knowledge generated from various perspectives into one design.

In reviewing the literature and selecting textbooks, both committees encountered considerable confusion in relation to paradigms and worldviews and the language used to articulate them. From this, a commitment evolved not to exclude any worldview from the curriculum. Rather, we deliberately planned the curriculum so that in seeing these differences between worldviews, students might think more critically about what they were learning. The committee members recognized that knowledge of the assumptions and values that underpin a writer's work is an important part of the critique of the work, and the language used to express knowledge can have different meanings depending on the worldview a writer, teacher, or practitioner holds.

To account for the inevitable confusion that arose in considering the different worldviews, the committee adopted the habit of being more inclusive rather than exclusive in our curriculum decision making. Predictably, inclusion was much more difficult to support than exclusion. Inclusion challenged us to generate new ways of thinking and expressing ourselves, whereas exclusion is readily served by existing ideas and language. However, inclusion also involves the risk of adopting an "anything goes" stance, necessitating painstaking accounting for and rethinking of every decision the committees made.

Despite this challenge, committee members have repeatedly been affirmed in their decision to take the more open stance, which we referred to as a "human science philosophy." Critics of this approach often raise the issue that human science is only one worldview, overlooking the point that the major tenet of a human science view is an openness to other worldviews or multiple realities. Such questions arise from another tenet of the human science paradigm; that is, in the study of human phenomena the adoption of reductionist practices—understanding a phenomenon through the limited study of only its elemental parts—is problematic. Tension arises when human phenomena are reduced to smaller elements for teaching or research purposes, raising ethical questions about research and knowledge development that are not sensitive to human phenomena.[10] Polkinghorne discussed the relationship between and among these worldviews: "The subject matter of human science is the human realm. Although the human realm includes physical and biological orders, it is only because of their characteristics as parts of a person that they are included in the subject matter of human science."[10(p259)]

The committee proposed that classroom discussions include a variety of ways of talking about human beings and their experiences, including an emphasis on the importance of the lived life of a person for understanding human experience. That is, teaching strategies were planned to reflect an appreciation of the assumptions and values underpinning a phenomenologic perspective. However, it was intended that students would have many opportunities to appreciate how knowledge generated from a variety of sources, including general or universal knowledge, critically informs our understanding of a particular human experience. The intent of such a stance is not to devalue any particular worldview but to create the opportunity for the voice of the person who lives a particular experience not only to be heard, but to be valued along with other views that inform the human health experience.

DISCIPLINARY CONCEPTS IDENTIFIED BY THE CURRICULUM COMMITTEES

Caring

Caring was identified in the curriculum themes as one of the central concepts for the curriculum, shaping both the study and practice of nursing. Committee discussions within the context of existing educational and nursing literature led to both the planning and the teaching of courses aligned with the assumptions and values sensitive to human beings, human experience, and human health. Our discussions of caring included both caring inquiry and caring practice—not that these were viewed as separate, but rather to emphasize the importance of ethical relating in both the generation and use of nursing knowledge. In situations where knowledge from other disciplines or practices was required, the committees understood that the same ethic of caring would guide the critical consideration of the appropriateness of such knowledge in the enhancement of human health.

CARING INQUIRY

Although the two curriculum committees talked about inquiry differently, in both situations a human science philosophy was understood to underlie the generation and use of knowledge and information. Inquiry was to go beyond a superficial understanding of clients and their individual situations—that is, beyond the application of what is known generally about the specifics of a situation. Rather, inquiry explores theories to help us understand the generalizations that might be made about a health experience, but then goes deeper to see how a particular person's story imparts differences to these general understandings. Caring inquiry is how a nurse learns what matters to a client.

CARING PRACTICE

An ethic of care guides how a professional nurse thinks, feels, and acts in a practice situation. Caring practice is the interface between the personal and professional experience of the nurse and the personal and health experience of the person seeking care.[11]

Human Beings

In the nursing literature human beings have been categorized in the following ways: behavioral systems, human needs, psychosocial beings, biopsychosocial beings, spiritual beings, patient and nursing problems, and nursing and medical diagnoses. In keeping with a more open, nonreductionistic stance that is sensitive to human phenomena, the committee decided to locate what it means to be human with the person who lived a particular experience rather than with the professional. In this way, names and labels used to talk about what it means to be human would be assigned by the person, opening the nurse to many possibilities not yet known or understood by the profession. We intended to locate what it means to be human within a phenomenologic philosophy; that is, what it means to be a human being is located in the world as it is experienced. A phenomenologic philosophy was seen as congruent with the assumptions and values of the human science paradigm that Newman and associates described. The intent was not to have students negate other views but to provide a lens for them to critique knowledge for its sensitivity to human experience.

Human Experience

In nursing, human experience has been talked about as both continuous with and discontinuous with the person. Concepts such as environment and context tend to vary with the assumptions and values about relationships (linear, reciprocal, or interrelational) held by an author. Because of this tendency, clear articulation of what is intended is important in discussion of concepts such as family, community, and culture. Curriculum committee members took the stand that people are continuous with their lived experience and as such cannot be viewed apart from that. Again, the intention is not to dis-

count the other views but to provide nurses with a critical perspective that is sensitive to human phenomena for meaningful participation in discourses on human health experience.

Human Health Experience

Human health is discussed in nursing and related literature in a number of ways. As in the discussion of caring and experience, the assumptions and values (worldview or paradigm) held by the author shape the way health is presented.[1] Health as the absence of disease aligns with the physical science worldview. In this view health is often seen as a goal; the focus is on curing or eradicating disease, and discussions of illness are framed in the language of cause and effect. In this view, health is reduced and dichotomized as healthy or unhealthy.

In contrast, the idea that health is contextually situated aligns with a social science worldview. Changes in health are expressed on a continuum of polarities: wellness and illness. Discussions of health are framed in the language of stress and coping. The environment influences the ability of individuals, families, and communities to cope with illness.

In the human science paradigm, health is constituted within, and inseparable from, the lived experience of a person. As such, health is seen from the perspective of the person who lives it. This accommodates views that include health within illness, disease as a manifestation of health, and possibilities for seeing patterns of health within the lived life of every human being.

Although it is recognized that each of these ways of looking at health is valuable in different ways, committee members generally concurred with the point made by Newman and associates that human science aligns most closely with assumptions sensitive to the human experience of health. This view provides a focus within which students can consider the knowledge generated within other worldviews. Such a view does not negate work on the health of populations but gives the student a perspective to interpret general or universal knowledge in a particular situation.

Health Promotion

Like health, the promotion of health is influenced by the assumptions and values underpinning a particular approach to practice. The intent is to adopt a stance to equalize the power assigned to the knowledge of expert practice with the knowledge of a particular human health experience, privileging neither. The committees recognized that the facts of health and disease, the influence of the context and environment, and the awareness embedded in experience all inform our understanding of a particular human health experience. In the human science paradigm, however, the knowledge arising out of particular experiences such as that of people with acquired immunodeficiency syndrome (AIDS) must be heard. In health promotion and in other matters concerning decision making about matters of health, the curriculum developers saw the interface as being between the personal and professional experience of the nurse and the personal and health experience of a person.

UNDERSTANDING RESISTANCE TO MULTIPLE VIEWS

Although the membership of both curriculum planning committees was faculty directly involved in teaching nursing, and although the input of other faculty and practitioners was solicited throughout the process, when it came to implementation considerable resistance to the idea of teaching different worldviews surfaced. Although it would not be difficult to speculate on the reasons underlying such resistance, it is important to contextualize this resistance beyond the walls of a particular institution and consider the larger society in which the same resistance can be found. My experience of two completely different faculties in different academic communities was very similar.

The decision of both committees was to avoid taking competitive stances and instead to try and understand the resistance. According

to Griffin, an "idealogue has categorical ideas of thought or expression from which she/he will not deviate. She/he dismisses my ideas with labels, epithets, catch phrases. She/he purposely misinterprets me and seizes on small mistakes to humiliate me."[12(p279)] In the words of Smith, the aim of all curriculum members is to present a "relational" not a "divisive" stance, whereby they aim "not for a unified perspective," but rather for a way of "affirming, recognizing, and celebrating the significance of our differences to the growth of the discipline."[13(p46)]

In committee and faculty discussions, the work of Newman and associates was at times seen as divisive in seeming to assume an authoritarian stance in relation to the human science paradigms. Although I did not share this view, I became interested in its frequent occurrence and explored other work in an attempt to make sense of this view. To include the human science view in a curriculum as equally valued and not just other than or inferior to the social and physical sciences raises questions about some of the assumptions within the physical and social science paradigms for nursing. For example, to say that a person who lives an experience is the "authority" challenges the unquestioned authority of the professional. The human science view does not negate the professional's authority, but rather puts it on an equal basis with the authority of recipients of the professional's service. The idea of questioning authority is not only possible but an integral part of the discourses about human health.

Chinn stated that "since myths are based on a particular world view, they function actually to shape and create reality. This view is not necessarily wrong or bad, but it is not universal."[14(p45)] It is possible that the unexamined resistance to multiple realities expressed by some faculty arose from the assumption of universality and thus the authority of a particular view. Frequently committee members were challenged with the questions, "What is the matter with our present approach to nursing curricula?" and "Why question the status quo?" The first question assumes a shared, clearly articulated approach yet to be explicated, and so it is difficult if not impossible to answer. For the answer to the second question, Chinn asked the following: "Why not conceptualize the purposes and goals of our research and theory in terms of the world we want to create? Why not seriously value other ways of knowing? Why not value nursing and health? Why not identify actions, behaviours and assumptions that we know to be consistent with health and behave as scientists in ways that are consistent with our vision?"[14(p49)]

CURRICULUM AS PLANNED AND CURRICULUM AS LIVED

For Aoki[15] the curriculum as planned (that which is prepared in advance) and the curriculum as lived (what everyone in their wisdom actually does) go together to make up any curriculum. As such, curriculum committees must be dynamic groups remaining open to whatever is presented to them for consideration.

Although a number of authors could have been selected to introduce worldviews to beginning students, the work of Newman and associates was introduced as one way that students might begin to appreciate differences in worldviews and understand, albeit at a beginning level, the implications of different worldviews. Parse's[7] totality and simultaneity paradigms or Watson's[16] work on traditional and human sciences could have also been used for this purpose.

LANGUAGE IN NURSING AND OTHER LITERATURE

A final issue that challenged and continues to challenge curriculum committee members and other faculty is what appears to be confusion and contradiction in the literature that can be directly attributed to language. One advantage of the increasing emphasis on work in the human science paradigm is the inevitable realization of language's power to shape human experience.

We have learned to be more thoughtful in how we speak and write human experience as a

way of influencing how and where we locate ourselves as professionals within experience. Curriculum committees and all who have been involved in teaching and planning courses have been faced with the need to rethink their present way of articulating practice, not to change their current thinking, but to clarify it so they can celebrate the inevitable differences that occur between them because they are human.

● ● ● ● ● ●

The work of Newman and associates provides one excellent way to discuss not only different worldviews, but also how people come to hold these views and the implications of such views for both the discipline and practice of nursing. A major implication for integrating differently generated knowledge in nursing curricula is that existing knowledge is challenged, enhancing the possibility that new knowledge and new meanings will be generated within the human health experience.

REFERENCES

1. Newman MA, Sime AM, Corcoran-Perry SA. The focus of the discipline of nursing. *ANS.* 1991;14(1):1–6.
2. Newman MA. Prevailing paradigms in nursing. *Nurs Outlook.* 1992;40(1):10–13.
3. Fawcett J. The metaparadigm of nursing: present status and future refinements. *Image J Nurs Schol.* 1984;16(3):84–87.
4. Flaskerud JH, Halloran EJ. Areas of agreement on nursing theory development. *ANS.* 1980;3(1):1–7.
5. Lincoln YS, Guba EG. Postpositivism and the naturalist paradigm. In: Lincoln YS., Guba EG. *Naturalistic Inquiry.* Beverly Hills, Calif: Sage; 1985.
6. Parse R. *Nursing Science: Major Paradigms. Theories and Critiques.* Philadelphia, Pa: Saunders; 1987.
7. Brodie JN. A response to Dr. J. Fawcett's paper "The metaparadigm of nursing: present status and future refinements." *Image J Nurs Schol.* 1984;16(3):87–89.
8. Conway M. Toward greater specificity of nursing's metaparadigm. *ANS.* 1985;7(4):73–81.
9. Kikuchi J, Simmons H. *Philosophic Inquiry in Nursing.* Beverly Hills, Calif: Sage; 1994.

10. Polkinghorne D. *Methodology for the Human Sciences: Systems of Inquiry.* New York, NY: State University Press; 1983.
11. Bishop A, Scudder J. *Nursing: The Practice of Caring.* New York, NY: National League for Nursing; 1991.
12. Griffin S. The way of all ideology. In: Keohane N, Rosaldo MZ, Gelpi BC, eds. *Feminist Theory: A Critique of Ideology.* Chicago, Ill: University of Chicago Press; 1992.
13. Smith M. Arriving at a philosophy of nursing: discovering? constructing? evolving? In: Kikuchi J, Simmons H, eds. *Developing a Philosophy of Nursing.* Thousand Oaks, Calif: Sage; 1994.
14. Chinn P. Debunking myths in nursing theory and research. *Image J Nurs Schol.* 1985;17(2): 45–49.
15. Aoki T. Legitimating the lived curriculum: The other curriculum that teachers in their practical wisdom know. Presented at the Annual Conference of the Association for Supervision and Curriculum Development, 1992; New Orleans, La.
16. Watson J. *Nursing: Human Science and Human Care.* New York, NY: National League for Nursing; 1988.

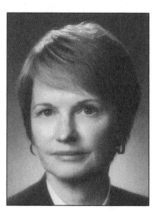

MARJORIE McINTYRE

TRUTH: AN EXPLORATION

E. Carol Polifroni

When faced with the question "What is truth?" one has the option to turn away and dismiss the inquiry as frivolous or meaningless or to begin a journey through the mine fields of philosophical discourse. Given that you are reading this book, the authors believe you have chosen the latter path. The nature of scientific truth is ladened with diverse and divergent beliefs and subsequent premises.

SOURCES OF TRUTH

Our inquiry starts with an examination of the sources of truth. Essentially, truth can be known through five (and perhaps more) major means. Intuition, a flash of insight whose source the receiver can neither fully identify nor explain, is one source of truth. Intuition is often disregarded by those bedded in an empirical world, because neither the source of the intuition nor the reliability and validity of the intuition can be tested or observed. Intuition is an inner belief in the veracity of something or someone. It is a feeling rather than a finding. Intuition may lead to action or not, but in either case the intuitive sense provides one with a defined belief in a specific event or object. However, the intuitive belief can not be validated nor necessarily replicated. But for the receiver, the truth received is no less true.

Authority provides a second source of truth. Authority is of either a sacred nature or a secular stance. In the sacred perspective, one relies on the premise that truth emanates from the supernatural and guidance is received and processed through religious folks. This source of truth is neither challenged nor investigated, but simply accepted as true. Secular sources of authoritative truth, on the other hand, are achieved through the world of science and specialists within a field. For decades, medicine was viewed as the ultimate science wherein treatments were accepted as useful, helpful and truthful. Truthful, in this sense, portrays a positive outcome. In today's world, many accept the medical opinion as a form of gospel, blending the world of scientific authority with the view of supernatural order.

Tradition is another source of truth. The accumulated wisdom of the ages yields definitive beliefs and actions. Tradition, the way we have always done something, is rarely challenged or discussed. The fact that it has been done this way for however long yields a degree of authenticity and, therefore, truthfulness. The absence of verifiable information concerning either the source of the information or the accuracy of the tradition is not of concern for those who accept tradition as a source of truth.

Common sense also serves as a source of truth. The realm of common sense is based on an accumulation of collective guesses, hunches and haphazard trial-and-error learning. When neither the source nor the premises of what we know is known, we tend to call the phenomenon common sense. Common sense differs from intuition in that it is a collective belief rather than an individual insight into the truth of a phenomenon.

Science serves as yet another source of truth. The traditional scientific method, grounded in the act of observation, yields accurate and readily verifiable information known as truth. This type of truth is based on verifiable evidence; ethical neutrality; accurate, precise, systematic, recorded and objective observations; controlled conditions for the observation and trained observers.

For many, science is the ultimate source of truth. For some, science provides little or no truth and other sources prevail. Herein lies the debate within the world of the nature of scientific truth. What is the source of truth? For knowing the source enables one to understand or at least to explore the nature of the truth. Without an appreciation of its source, the mystery continues.

THEORIES OF TRUTH

Truth is *veritas* in Latin and *aletheia* in Greek. The search for truth began with the belief in an objective, absolute truth, but this notion was challenged by the Greeks. Protagoras suggested that truth is relative and not objective, and the debate continues to this day.

To frame the debate, several theories related to truth have been identified; correspondence theory, coherence theory, pragmatic theory, semantic theory and performative theory. The correspondence theory of truth (Aristotle 384–322 B.C. and Aquinas A.D. 1225–1274) suggests that truth is related to and corresponds with reality. Within this theory, there is a connectedness between the issue at hand and the determination of truth. The truth is shaped by the reality which is achieved through perceptions of the world.

Coherence theory, on the other hand, insists upon logical and consistent criteria to evaluate the nature of truth. Truth is true if it is coherent, if it measures up to internal consistency through explanation and affirmation and if it is logical and deductive. Francis Herbert Bradley (1846–1924), an English philosopher, was a strong proponent of the coherence theory for truth.

The pragmatist theory of truth originated with Immanuel Kant (1724–1804) and was elaborated upon by William James (1842–1910). This theory holds that truth is relative and related to the practicality, the utility, the workableness of a solution. In other words, something is not true in and of itself, but rather when it is put to the test of usefulness. That is the origin of truth: does it work? If so, it must be true.

Both the semantic and performative theories of truth have been identified but not widely used. Semantic theory asserts that the nature of truth is within the language and performative theory is the act of agreeing with a statement. The theories of truth, as described within, are more often referred to within the context of realism and anti-realism than in the theoretical context.

REALISM, ANTIREALISM OR IDEALISM

The readings that follow discuss the nature of scientific truth from many perspectives which are summarized as realism, antirealism—or more specifically metaphysical idealism or epistemological idealism—or a phenomenological stance. Realism is the belief that truth is larger than and different from human consciousness. Truth for the realist is an objective reality and the discovery of this reality is the goal of science. Realism rejects both intuition and common sense. Reality embraces the notion of authority, particularly that of the world of the scientist. Realists neither discard nor embrace the element of tradition as a source of truth but rather set out to discover the source of the tradition through observation.

Realism contends that the picture science gives us of the world is true and real, and that the entities postulated do, in fact, exist. The truth of the science is determined by its correspondence with features of the definite world structure. For the realist, real things are not conditioned by being known and they may continue in their unaltered state even when they are not known. For the realist, the world exists either with or without human beings and there is knowledge to be gained which is objective and true and not person-specific. Moritz Schlick (1882–1936), the father of positivism, is a realist and subscribed to the belief that truth exists without dependence on humanity.

As an example, the realist would embrace the notion of an absolute truth which is not conditioned or colored by the nature of man. What is, is, regardless of who the knower is and regardless of what the knower believes. The definitiveness of the realist perspective of truth originates in a central belief on absolute truth and the absence of conditioning or tempering by human beings or any other being for that matter. The search of scientists, from a realist perspective, is to uncover or to discover the single absolute truth.

Bas van Fraassen (1941–) is a North American philosopher who has examined science from both the realist and antirealist perspectives. For him, when science is approached as a realist, the theoretical positions and ideas put forth by the "best and the brightest" within the discipline need to be accepted as true. However, the realist perspective of truth is in sharp contrast to that of the antirealist, and the distinction begins with the antirealist believing in the role of human beings, the knower, in any discussion on truth. Antirealism embraces a variety of philosophical views but all of these embrace the notion that the universe is an embodiment of the mind. All knowable entities are viewed as mental processes in the form of thoughts, ideas, theories, reasoning and/or facts, dependent upon the presence of the knower. In contrast to the realist view, the antirealist subscribes to the belief that human consciousness is at the center of the nature of truth, not independent from it.

For example, the antirealist believes in and values the role of science. However, the antirealist also believes that what science discovers is tempered by human thought and existence. The antirealist does not necessarily believe in an absolute truth but rather believes that truth is personalized within human beings. Thus, for the antirealist, the sources for truth are more varied than for the realist.

Metaphysical idealism emphasizes the analysis of the entire universe as a psychic reality. Subscribers of this view address the belief that if there is a world beyond human consciousness, it must be seen as a consequence of human understanding. Metaphysical idealists believe that truth is conveyed through common acceptance known as consensus. Truth is agreement. Truth for the metaphysical idealist is not based in external world correspondence but rather is bounded by consensual agreement in science. The metaphysical idealist believes that truth changes as paradigms, or worldviews, change.

Another sect of the antirealist perspective is the epistemological idealist. For those holding this view, the identification of reality (truth) is equated to mentally knowable data. Epistemological idealism has strands of premises related to the empirical world in that the meaning of a proposition cannot be known unless it is possible to state the conditions under which the propositions may be verified. Observation serves as the basis for the verification processes.

Constructive empiricism is a contemporary evolution of epistemological idealism. For this view, science aims to give us theories which are empirically adequate and the acceptance of the theory involves a belief only that it is empirically adequate. For the constructive empiricist, the truth is at hand or possibly at hand but the limitation is the science itself. Truth is only that which is observable and science determines the observability of nature. Thus, truth is subjectively determined.

PHENOMENOLOGICAL VIEW OF TRUTH

Lastly, within the nature of scientific truth is the realm of the phenomenological stance. Phenomenology, as philosophy, rejects realism which is entirely objective and idealism wherein truth is subjective. For the phenomenologist, truth lies in the human consciousness. The world may go beyond the bounds of experience but ego is essentially present in the experience. The essence of the experience is the intersubjectivity or the characteristics shared by all persons. The experience itself may be individually tailored to the specific ego or person. Thus, phenomenology is the belief that truth is embedded in the human consciousness and expressed through the essence of universality.

POSTMODERN VIEW OF TRUTH

Rorty (1980) posits that in the postmodern world, which is addressed in greater detail in the concluding section of this book, the discourse on truth should be abandoned. Whether there is a single truth, an absolute truth or multiple truths, for Rorty, is no longer moot. The essence of truth lies within the individual and the individual may change or later alter that view dependent on the context and the circumstances. Thus, the postmodern worldview is that truth is neither singular nor multiple; it is personal and highly individualized and contextually ladened and driven.

CONCLUSION AND READINGS

Each of these diverse perspectives embraces a notion and nature of truth and directs science toward the acquisition of truth within or separate from human consciousness. The following readings illustrate the points addressed above. Hacking lays out the essence of scientific realism as does van Fraassen. Schlick relates material from positivism to that of realism. Laudan presents a different, and perhaps, more inclusive treatise on truth. (See also Kuhn, pp. 34–45 of this volume.) Packard and Polifroni expand upon realism, antirealism and phenomenological stances in regard to truth. Schumacher and Gortner address the same points but tend to embrace a different perspective than that of Packard and Polifroni. Whichever position you accept, the readings will provide rich information which will lead to dialogue and discussion on the essence and relevance of the scientific nature of truth.

DISCUSSION GUIDE

1. Compare and contrast these diverse views of truth:
   a. realism
   b. antirealism
   c. phenomenology
   d. postmodernism
2. What is the role of observables and observation in each of these views?
3. What is the significance of truth for nursing as a profession and as a science?
4. Relate empiricism, positivism, historicism and relativism to the nature of scientific truth. Draw a schema indicating their relationships.
5. How do culture and truth interact?
6. Using clinical examples, illustrate the view of the realist, the antirealist and the phenomenological stances in regard to truth.
7. What is the relationship, if any, between compliance and the views of truth?

REFERENCE

Rorty, R. (1980). *Philosophy and the nature of the mirror.* Princeton: Princeton University Press.

BIBLIOGRAPHY

Boyd, R. (1991). On the current status of scientific realism. In R. Boyd, P. Gasper, & J. D. Trout (Eds.), *The philosophy of science* (pp. 195–222). Cambridge: MIT Press.

Fine, A. (1987). And not anti-realism either. In J. Kourany (Ed.), *Scientific knowledge* (pp. 359–368). Belmont: Wadsworth.

Hacking, I. (1987). Experimentation and scientific realism. In J. Kourany (Ed.), *Scientific knowledge* (pp. 388–399). Belmont: Wadsworth.

Hume, D. (1972). *A treatise of human nature,* Book I. London: Fontana. [Original work published in 1739.]

James, W. (1914). *The meaning of truth.* London: Longmans, Green and Co.

Kikuchi, J. F., Simmons, H., & Romyn, D. (Eds.). (1996). *Truth in nursing inquiry.* Thousand Oaks: Sage.

Laudan, L. (1991). A confrontation of convergent realism. In R. Boyd, P. Gasper, & J. D. Trout (Eds.), *The philosophy of science* (pp. 223–246). Cambridge: MIT Press.

Packard, S., & Polifroni, E. C. (1992). The nature of scientific truth. *Nursing Science Quarterly,* 5(4), 158–163.

Rosaldo, R. (1989). *Culture and truth: The remaking of social analysis.* Boston: Beacon.

Schlick, M. (1979). *Positivism and realism.* Netherlands: Kluwer. (Originally appeared in Erkenntnis III [1932/33].)

Schumacher, K., & Gortner, S. (1992). (Mis)conceptions and reconceptions about traditional science. *Advances in Nursing Science, 14*(4), 1–11.

van Fraassen, B. (1987). Arguments concerning scientific realism. In J. Kourany (Ed.), *Scientific knowledge* (pp. 343–358). Belmont: Wadsworth.

(Mis)conceptions and Reconceptions about Traditional Science

Karen L. Schumacher • Susan R. Gortner

"Traditional" science (ie, scientific work that has evolved from the natural sciences) is still said to rely on theory-neutral facts, quantitative data, and the search for universal laws. This depiction of science is incongruent with much contemporary thinking. This article examines three shifts in recent philosophy that are relevant for nursing science philosophy: the move from foundationalism to an understanding of the fallibility of science, the shift in emphasis from verification to justification of knowledge claims, and the recent examination of explanation by scientific realists. It is suggested that scientific realism may be a fruitful area of inquiry for philosophers of nursing science.

The past decade has witnessed significant commentary on the nature of nursing science and appropriate modes of inquiry, much of which has been published in *Advances in Nursing Science*. Part of the commentary has been directed toward philosophical foundations for nursing science that may be more consonant with the human state than with nature in general[1-7] and has resulted in publication of positions on Heideggerian/phenomenological philosophy,[8,9] critical social theory[10,11] and feminism.[12] In some essays, the approach to science that might be called "traditional" is portrayed as a static and monolithic entity, serving mostly as a foil against which to describe the philosophical position of the author(s).[13,14] As a result, the nursing literature lacks a systematic account of the philosophical underpinnings of the approach to science that evolved from the natural sciences.

This article seeks to balance the discourse about philosophical foundations for nursing science with a description of contemporary or postpositivistic thinking in the philosophy of science. Specifically, it identifies three misconceptions in the nursing critique of traditional science: the purported use of theory-neutral observations, the privilege granted quantitative data in warranting knowledge, and the search for universal laws. It argues that characterizing science in these ways is incongruent with contemporary philosophy of science and suggests some alternative ideas that may provide impetus for philosophical discourse around nursing science.

Before the discussion, however, a clarification of terminology is in order. Numerous terms are used to describe the philosophical basis for what is referred to above as "traditional" science. Empiricism, postempiricism, postpositivism, Cartesianism, objectivism, analytic empiricism, and naturalism are terms used to denote a philosophy of science or an epistemological perspective associated with "scientific method," "empirical research," or simply "science." Even the term "logical positivism" continues to be used as a label[13,14] although logical positivism is generally considered to be dead as a philosophical movement.[6,15,16] While it cannot expect to clear up the terminological confusion, this essay will attempt to avoid falling prey to it. What is referred to as "traditional" science is the epistemological tradition that there is a world "out there" characterized to some extent by patterns and regularities; that it can be known, albeit imperfectly; and that knowing requires the mental discipline imposed by precision, logic, and attention to evidence. In this respect, "traditional" science is distinguished from personal opinion or private experience. This discussion uses the term "science" in the manner in which it is used by Ziman: "Science is public knowledge . . . a consensus of rational opinion over the widest possible field."[17(pp30,31)] In this respect, science is derived from a long intellectual tradition that began with attempts to know about the natural or physical world. However, no analogy is implied here between the physical world and human life. It is the use of disciplined reasoning and observation to discover and explain regularities in the world that makes science what it is. Although the phenomena of interest vary across scientific disciplines and may serve to establish disciplinary boundaries, the nature of scientific thinking has many similarities across disciplines.

Foundationalism in Science

One way in which "traditional" science has been characterized by some nursing scholars is in terms of its reliance on theory-neutral facts.[3,9] For example, Allen, Benner, and Diekelmann assert that "a statement can only be properly regarded as scientific if its truth or falsity can be ascertained by means of theory-neutral observations."[3(p25)] In this statement they implicitly refer to an epistemology that is foundationalist in that observation is seen as an indubitable source of

knowledge. Empiricism in its classical sense was a philosophical doctrine that considered observation to be the foundation of knowledge.[18] Logical positivism was a twentieth-century variant of empiricism that combined an emphasis on observation as the source of knowledge with a logical analysis of the meaning of observation sentences.[19] Knowledge thus secured was considered infallible and led to the belief that certainty in science was possible.

The positivist doctrine that knowledge could be achieved with certainty by basing it on observations has been challenged on a number of fronts by postpositivistic philosophers of science. In nursing, the postpositivist refutation of the claim that there are theory-neutral observations or "brute facts" has been accurately described by Weekes[20] and Thompson.[4] The rejection of the positivistic notion that there are "basic statements" that constitute facts about the "immediately given" rests primarily on the distinction between sensory experience and the cognitive process of perception. As Kuhn put it: "As for a pure observation language, perhaps one will yet be devised. But three centuries after Descartes our hope for such an eventuality still depends exclusively upon a theory of perception and of the mind. And modern psychological experimentation is rapidly proliferating phenomena with which that theory can scarcely deal."[21(p126)] Hanson[22] gives a detailed argument against the notion of theory-neutral observations, showing that what one "observes" depends on perception rather than simply on retinal images. Furthermore, perception, or what stands out as relevant and significant, is a function of one's prior knowledge and experience, which in turn influences how one conceptually organizes sensory experience. If it were not so, we would be bombarded with chaotic, unintelligible sensory data.

Another problem with the idea of theory-neutral observations pertains to the use of instruments to aid the senses.[23–26] Many entities, while unobservable to the unaided human senses, can readily be observed with the aid of instruments. Thus, what must be considered unobservable and therefore theoretical at one point in history may become observable when an appropriate instrument is developed. For example, the cellular constituents of blood, unobservable before the invention of the microscope, are now considered observable. However, such observation presupposes a host of theories about the optics of the microscope as well as the appearance of the cells themselves. Thus, observation with the aid of an instrument can in no way be considered theory-neutral.

The idea that there is no theory-neutral observation language is now widely accepted by philosophers of science as diverse as Popper,[27] Kuhn,[21] Bernstein,[28] and Hanson.[22] The problems identified above have led Newton-Smith to propose that observation and theory, while essentially indistinguishable, may be, for practical purposes, thought of as a continuum ranging from the more observational to the more theoretical. The more observable an entity is, the easier it is to decide with confidence whether or not it applies, the less reliance on instruments is needed, and the easier it is to grasp the nature of the entity without learning a scientific theory.[25]

Two important (and widely accepted) conclusions resulted from the foregoing philosophical work on the nature of observation: there are no theory-neutral facts and there are no absolute knowledge sources. Thus, to claim that science is based on theory-neutral facts is to refer back to a philosophy of science that has been widely discredited. A more contemporary understanding of science is that articulated by Popper.[27] He proposed a fallibilistic conception of knowledge that is nonfoundational in that there are no ultimate sources of knowledge. Instead, science progresses through the elimination of error as successive theories are found to be false and replaced with better theories. Thus, science is a rational endeavor by virtue of its critical attitude, not by the certainty conferred by "brute facts."

The Warrants for Knowledge

In the confusion following the demise of a foundational approach to philosophy of science, there is the risk of going to either of two extremes: radical skepticism or radical subjectivism.[28] However, neither of these extremes is necessary. In the aftermath of positivism, philosophers of science have turned their attention from the origins and foundation of knowledge to concern with the justification of knowledge claims.[18] In other words, a knowledge claim is judged on the merits of the evidence brought to bear on it. This point is essential for understanding contemporary philosophy of science. Its importance is based on the premise that scientific knowledge is public in nature, representing rational, informed, interconsensual opinion.[17,29] It is the justification of knowledge claims or "marshalling good reason in their behalf"[18(p17)] that separates science from private understanding and ideology. The assertion that knowledge claims in science must be warranted is a fundamental assumption in contemporary philosophy of science. However, to say that knowledge claims must be warranted is not to say that there is one privileged way of warranting them that applies equally to all knowledge claims. To establish a scientific knowledge claim, the scientist assembles evidence in its support. But what is the contemporary understanding of evidence?

Certainly observation continues to be an important element in the evidence brought to bear in support of a knowledge claim.[18,27,29,30] However, in the literature pertaining to the warrants for knowledge claims, one can detect a shift in language from the earlier exclusive use of the term "observation" to the more contemporary term "evidence." It is useful to think of support for scientific theories in terms of evidence rather than observation alone, because "evidence" is a more inclusive term; it admits additional types of support for theories such as self-report by the subject, through either questionnaire or interview, as well as the use of reason. Further, it is not as encumbered with philosophical history as is the term "observation." Implied is the assumption that the scientist has considerable latitude in deciding what evidence is needed to evaluate a particular knowledge claim.

Thinking broadly about evidence is important in nursing science, because it allows discourse to shift away from the truism that many phenomena cannot be reduced to sense data or observational terms. More fruitful are discussions about what constitutes "good evidence" for the existence and nature of a phenomenon. For example, family coping processes cannot be reduced to observable terms without losing much of what is inherent in the phenomenon. Such a loss of substantive information is unacceptable. On the other hand, it is not the case that "anything goes" when the scientist is investigating coping processes. The reasonable scientist would want to know what evidence about coping was brought to bear on the research question.

One of the most egregious assumptions about traditional science is that it constitutes a paradigm that disallows the use of qualitative data. This assumption tends to confound method with philosophical perspective and to promote the idea that using both linguistic and numerical data to address a research question violates fundamental philosophical assumptions of one perspective or the other. This assumption supports a "purist" position regarding appropriate data forms and limits the scope of inquiry.[10,31] While it may be the case that qualitative data are the sine qua non of phenomenological research, it is not true that data forms in "traditional" research have to be quantitative. Even though much scientific work within this framework is quantitative and even though some seemingly absurd efforts have been made to reduce mental phenomena to observable physiological parameters, there is no philosophical or historical basis for the supposed identification of traditional science with quantitative methods.[32,33] Research using inductive reasoning based on naturalistic observations and field notes has a respected place

in modern science, going back at least as far as the 19th century biologists. In field work or naturalistic research with persons it is reasonable and necessary to talk with them to elicit their experiences, subjective states, and meanings. The use of such data does not necessarily depart from the canons of traditional science.[34] It simply introduces a uniquely human form of data.

Although traditional science does not require the use of quantitative data, it does require that the scientist examine the evidence brought to bear on a particular question and ask whether it supports the claims of the scientist. One of the considerations in the examination of evidence is whether it is of sufficient scope to adequately address the phenomenon under study. While not identified specifically as such, the scope of scientific evidence has been an implied consideration in the concerns about appropriate data in nursing and other disciplines addressing social phenomena. Specifically, writings about qualitative and quantitative data, multimethod research, and triangulation are implicit efforts to increase the acceptable scope of evidence. Some writers, however, go beyond issues of the nature and scope of evidence and attempt to relate type of evidence to a specific scientific paradigm with the implication that that paradigm determines the type of evidence that is acceptable. Further, qualitative research is sometimes thought to constitute a paradigm rather than a type of evidence.[35]

The type of evidence used by the scientist (ie, numerical or linguistic data) should not be dependent on that paradigm, but rather on the phenomenon under investigation and the specific research question. This position is not novel, but reaffirms what Meleis has called a "passion for substance"[36] rather than philosophy or technique. Some research problems require evidence that is broad in scope in order to draw sound conclusions. In other investigations the need to achieve precision may require evidence that is more narrow in scope. Such decisions have no dogmatic "decision rules" to guide the investigator, nor is there anything in contemporary philosophy of science that requires them. Instead, they are left to the professional judgment of the scientist in the design of studies and to the community of scholars in judgment of investigational findings.

Universality

Traditional science has also been characterized in terms of its search for universal laws that predict and explain phenomena regardless of context.[3,9,37] For example, in describing what they refer to as Paradigm I science, Tinkle and Beaton claim that "this paradigm adopts the view that there is a body of facts and principles to be discovered and understood that are independent of any historical or social context. This search for truth seeks principles that are abstract, general, and universal."[37(p28)]

There are at least two issues inherent in the idea of universal laws. The first is the issue of universality itself, which is often held up as the antithesis of the contextual, historical understanding of human phenomena that nursing seeks. Traditional science is said to isolate phenomena from their contexts for investigation, the results of which are findings then considered "universal" rather than context dependent.

Recent philosophy of science suggests that the reality of universal laws may be as elusive as theory-neutral observations proved to be, even in the physical sciences. Addressing the problem of laws in physics, Cartwright[38] claims that true "laws" are scarce. She goes on to show that statements of lawful relationships usually are qualified by a "ceteris paribus" statement, which says that "all things being equal" such and such a relationship holds. Since all things are often not equal, it is up to the scientist to determine the conditions under which a certain pattern occurs and the conditions under which it changes. Such determinations are required in science in general and are not a special feature of the human sciences. Indeed, Cartwright notes that "I imagine that natural objects are much like people in societies. Their behavior is constrained by some specific laws and by a handful of general principles, but it is not determined in detail, even statistically."[38(p49)]

Even though the belief in universal laws may be misplaced, generalization of findings beyond the particular study sample is clearly valued in traditional approaches to science. If generalization were not allowed it would be difficult for clinicians to use the findings of research not conducted with their own patients. But as noted by Gortner, "all inference is context dependent in some sense."[6] Thus there must be some middle ground of generalization between universal law and the findings in a particular sample. Rather than thinking in terms of universal law, the reasonable scientist asks: To whom can these findings legitimately be generalized?

Although it is a misconception to say that contemporary science is by nature "acontextual," it is probably accurate to say that the way in which "context" is understood varies among investigators. Benner[8] describes person and context as inseparable and mutually constitutive, whereas in traditional science, person and situation variables are frequently isolated for study. While the importance of this distinction should not be discounted, it is an oversimplification to claim that traditional science always seeks universal relationships regardless of the situation. It is more fruitful to ask: What does the incorporation of context into a nursing investigation mean? Is it the inclusion of situational variables? Narrative description of the context from the perspectives of the participants? Both?

The second issue inherent in discussions of universal laws is that of causality and explanation. Statements of law in the classic manner described by Hempel[39,40] and Putnam[41] purport not only to make statements about regularities, but to explain them. In other words, laws deal with the "whys" of phenomena, not simply their occurrence. There is a long and complex tradition in philosophy on causation and explanation, which is beyond the scope of this article. Here we do not argue for a given form of explanation, but simply claim that the idea of causation is necessary in nursing science because of its relevance for clinical practice. Clinicians would be hampered indeed if they did not know the likely consequences of certain events (eg, states, behaviors) under given conditions.

The relevance of explanation for nursing science is based on the argument that causative states or processes are precisely where intervention should be aimed.[23] At the physiological level, the causative relationship between bed rest, diminished ventilation, and postoperative pneumonia has led to the intervention of early ambulation after surgery. At the social level, the lack of social support explains (partially) caregiver depression and has led to the intervention of support groups for caregivers. Illustrative examples like these suggest that causation is simply a matter of a linear relationship, which is not the case. Causation in human science is complex, multifaceted, and possibly multidirectional. However, these difficulties should not deter us from its consideration because it is necessary for clinically relevant science.

A current debate in philosophy of science that has received little attention in nursing may prove useful in thinking about explanation and causation. We refer to the debate between scientific realism and antirealism. The arguments presented shift discourse in philosophy of science away from questions like "How can science be rational if there are no absolute sources of knowledge?" to questions like "What is real?" and "What is the status of theoretical entities in science?"[23(p1)] One of the major distinctions between scientific realism and antirealism is the way in which theoretical entities are understood. (In the language of scientific realism the term "theoretical entity" usually means unobservable entities, states, or processes.) The differing views on theoretical entities have implications for the respective positions on explanation and causality, as shown below.

The antirealists deny the existence of unobservable entities or processes and avoid issues of causality, claiming that scientific theories can describe and predict, but not explain.[23] To take this perspective it is necessary to maintain, to some extent, the distinction between observation and theory because, typically, antirealists assert that the notion of truth or falsity is relevant to observation even though it is not relevant to theory.[25,26,42] One of the most serious consequences of an antirealist construction of theories is that theories cannot explain.[23,25] Because the existence of any explanatory processes "behind" the observable phenomena is denied, science can legitimately only describe and predict observable entities. The logical positivists were antirealists who tried to disallow any discussion of theoretical entities in science, taking instead the extreme empirical position that what is real is observable. Since scientists regularly use theoretical terms ("electron" is the term often used as an example), the logical positivists modified their early position to that of instrumentalism. Instrumentalism is a type of antirealism that claims that theoretical terms are appropriately thought of as instruments, tools, or calculating devices, useful for systematizing and relating observations and for making predictions,[43] but that they do not refer to anything really existent. Since the logical positivists denied the existence of anything "behind" observables, they were opposed to discussions of causes and downplayed explanation.[23] It is the positivists' antirealism that makes their views inappropriate for nursing science. It is not possible in positivism to deal with the subjective aspects of persons, nor with perceived relational processes, nor with explanations without translating them into physiological states or behaviors.

On the other hand, scientific realists claim that unobservable (ie, theoretical) entities or processes have existence; moreover, it is these unobservable processes that often provide explanations for observable phenomena.[23,25,42] Thus, scientific realist discussions of causation focus on unobservable processes. There are three ingredients in scientific realism: ontological, epistemological, and causal.[23,25]

The ontological ingredient of scientific realism makes the claim that the unobservable entities represented by theoretical terms really exist. According to Boyd, the realist thinks of theoretical terms in scientific theories as "putatively referring to expressions; that is, scientific theories should be interpreted 'realistically.' Scientific theories, interpreted realistically, are confirmable and in fact are often confirmed as approximately true. The reality which scientific theories describe is largely independent of our thoughts or theoretical commitments.'[26(pp41–42)] In other words, even though knowledge is always fallible, something like the phenomena postulated by science really exist. Thus, the realist claims that the scientist makes discoveries about the world as it really is.[42]

The epistemological ingredient of scientific realism relates to the notion of verisimilitude or "approximation to the truth."[25,27] Although the "truth" can never be fully established by virtue of the fallibility of all human knowledge, the idea of truth does not need to be abandoned. Rather, the scientist can employ the notion of truth as a regulative ideal, seeking to get closer to the truth by the successive development of better and better theories. In other words, we can, in principle, have warranted belief in theories.[23]

Finally, the causal ingredient of scientific realism relates to the explanatory power of theories. The theoretical or unobservable entities of a theory are causally responsible for, that is, they explain, observable phenomena.[23] If, as the positivists claimed, science can only describe and predict; it does not provide any guidance for intervention if something different from the predicted state is desired. For example, one could predict that mothers who engage actively in a career will be tired and stressed. But if intervention to change this situation for mothers is desired, a deeper understanding is required than prediction allows. The authors agree with Hacking's assertion that the relationship between unobservable theoretical entities and intervention is what makes scientific realism relevant for the practice of science. For the positivist, what is real is simply what can be observed. For the scientific realist, what affects us and what we can affect are also real, whether or not they can be observed.[23] Acknowledging this level of reality leads the scientist to deeper, more probing questions about it.

The interest here is in the causal and epistemological ingredients of scientific realism, because they support the claims that explanations are important in nursing science and practice and that the aim of the scientist is to discover better and better explanations (ie, closer approximations to the truth). However, the reader may well discern metaphysical overtones in the ontological question of whether what is unobservable exists, and a brief comment on these is appropriate. According to Hacking,[23] the current interest in antirealism and scientific realism among philosophers represents a shift in focus away from the rationality of science to consideration of what is "real." This shift raises metaphysical questions that philosophers of science have traditionally been reluctant to address. However, the way in which metaphysical questions are answered has implications for the claims of philosophers about what scientists can attempt to discover. The Enlightenment empiricists, especially Hume and Newton,[23] tried to dispense with the vague idea of "cause" and direct scientific inquiry to description and prediction through observation. The logical positivists were determined to rid science of metaphysics once and for all through their verification principle of meaning,[44] an attempt that failed because the verification principle was unverifiable by its own standards and therefore meaningless. Popper, a realist, argued with the logical positivists, claiming that metaphysical questions are important for science in that they often lead to deeper and more insightful inquiry.[45] The "metaphysical turn" in the philosophy of science of recent decades may be worth pursuing in nursing as we try to reconcile our perspective on human beings and human health with nursing science. Nursing scholars can explore scientific realism for the insights it may provide for a philosophy of nursing science. For now, we propose that scientific realism is relevant to nursing science in the following ways:

1. It supports the full range of nursing theory: descriptive, predictive, and explanatory.
2. It affirms the importance of including subjective client states in nursing theory and refutes the claim of the positivists that if it is not observable, it does not exist.
3. It adds the idea of the *substantive* content of explanations to discussions about *forms* of explanation.
4. It includes the notion of truth as a regulative ideal in science and claims that better theories are theories that are closer to the truth. In other words, some theories are better than others and the task of the scientist is to determine as well as possible which they are.

● ● ● ● ● ●

Traditional science along with its philosophical underpinnings is not the static and monolithic entity that it is sometimes portrayed as. As philosophy of science has become increasingly aligned with the practices of working scientists, its claims for science have become more moderate and qualified. Three significant developments in philosophy of science have occurred in the postpositivist era: the move from foundationalism to an understanding of the fallibility of science, the shift in emphasis from verification to justification of knowledge claims, and the recent examination of explanation by scientific realists. These developments are relevant for nursing science in that they are consonant with such nursing concerns as the appropriate warrants for knowledge, the generalization of research results, and explanation/causation. The issues addressed by scientific realism may be a fruitful area of philosophical inquiry for nurse scholars.

REFERENCES

1. Holmes CA. Alternatives to natural science foundations for nursing. *Int J Nurs Stud.* 1990;27(3): 187–198.
2. Munhall PL. Nursing philosophy and nursing research: In apposition or opposition? *Nurs Res.* 1982;31(3):176–181.
3. Allen D, Benner P, Diekelmann N. Three paradigms for nursing research: Methodological considerations. In: Chinn PL, ed. *Nursing Research Methodology: Issues and Explanation.* Rockville, Md: Aspen Publishers; 1986.
4. Thompson JL. Practical discourse on nursing: Going beyond empiricism and historicism. *ANS.* 1985;7(4):59–71.
5. Silva MC, Rothbart D. An analysis of changing trends in philosophies of science on nursing theory development and testing. *ANS.* 1984;6(2):1–13.
6. Gortner SR. Knowledge in a practice discipline: Philosophy and pragmatics. In: *Nursing Research and Policy Formation: The Case of Prospective Payment.* Papers of the 1983 Scientific Session of the American Academy of Nursing. Kansas City, Mo: American Academy of Nursing; 1983.
7. Watson J. Nursing's scientific quest. *Nurs Outlook.* 1981;29(7):413–416.
8. Benner P. Quality of life: a phenomenological perspective on explanation, prediction, and understanding in nursing science. *ANS.* 1985;8(1):1–14.
9. Leonard VW. A Heideggerian phenomenologic perspective on the concept of person. *ANS.* 1989; 11(4):40–55.
10. Moccia P. A critique of compromise: Beyond the methods debate. *ANS.* 1988;10(4):1–9.
11. Stevens PE. A critical social reconceptualization of environment in nursing: Implications for methodology. *ANS.* 1989;11(4):56–68.
12. Bunting S, Campbell JC. Feminism and nursing: Historical perspectives. *ANS.* 1990;12(4):11–24.
13. Dzurec LC. The necessity for and evolution of multiple paradigms for nursing research: A poststructuralist perspective. *ANS.* 1989;11(4):69–77.
14. Sarnecky MT. Historiography: A legitimate research methodology for nursing. *ANS.* 1990; 12(4):1–10.
15. Phillips DC. After the wake: Postpositivistic educational thought. *Educ Res.* 1983;12(5):4–12.
16. van Fraassen BC. *The Scientific Image.* Oxford, England: Clarendon Press; 1980.
17. Ziman J. What is science? In: Klemke ED, Hollinger R, Kline AD, eds. *Introductory Readings in the Philosophy of Science.* Buffalo, NY: Prometheus Books; 1980.
18. Phillips DC. *Philosophy, Science, and Social Inquiry.* Oxford, England: Pergamon Press; 1987.
19. Ayer AJ. Editor's introduction. In: Ayer AJ, ed. *Logical Positivism.* New York, NY: Free Press, 1959.
20. Weekes DP. Theory-free observation: Fact or fantasy? In: Chinn PL, ed. *Nursing Research Methodol-*

ogy: Issues and Explanation. Rockville, Md: Aspen Publishers; 1986.

21. Kuhn TS. *The Structure of Scientific Revolutions.* 2nd ed. Chicago, Ill: University of Chicago Press; 1970.

22. Hanson NR. *Patterns of Discovery.* Cambridge, England: Cambridge University Press; 1958.

23. Hacking I. *Representing and Intervening.* Cambridge, England: Cambridge University Press; 1983.

24. Maxwell G. The ontological status of theoretical entities. In: Klemke ED, Hollinger R, Kline AD, eds. *Introductory Readings in the Philosophy of Science.* Buffalo, NY: Prometheus Books; 1980.

25. Newton-Smith WH. *The Rationality of Science.* London, England: Routledge & Kegan Paul; 1981.

26. Boyd RN. The current status of scientific realism. In: Leplin J, ed. *Scientific Realism.* Berkeley, Calif: University of California Press; 1984.

27. Popper KR. *Conjectures and Refutations: The Growth of Scientific Knowledge.* New York, NY: Harper & Row; 1963.

28. Bernstein RJ. *Beyond Objectivism and Relativism: Science, Hermeneutics, and Praxis.* Philadelphia, Pa: University of Pennsylvania Press; 1988.

29. Gortner SR. Nursing values and science: Toward a science philosophy. *Image.* 1990;22(2):101–105.

30. Schultz PR, Meleis AI. Nursing epistemology: Traditions, insights, questions. *Image.* 1988;20(4): 217–221.

31. Phillips JR. Research blenders. *Nurs Sci Quart.* 1988;1:4–5.

32. Gortner SR. Nursing's syntax revisited: A critique. *Int J Nurs Stud.* In review.

33. Suppe F. Presented at the first symposium on knowledge development in nursing; September, 1990; Newport, RI.

34. Gortner SR, Schultz PR. Approaches to nursing science methods. *Image.* 1988;20(1):22–24.

35. Guba EC. The alternative paradigm dialog. In: Guba EG, ed. *The Paradigm Dialog.* Newbury Park, Calif: Sage; 1990.

36. Meleis AI. ReVisions in knowledge development: A passion for substance. *Sch Inq Nurs Pract.* 1987;1(1):5–19.

37. Tinkle MB, Beaton JL. Toward a new view of science: Implications for nursing research. *ANS.* 1983; 5(2):27–36.

38. Cartwright N. *How the Laws of Physics Lie.* New York, NY: Oxford University Press; 1983.

39. Hempel C. *Philosophy of Natural Science.* Englewood Cliffs, NJ: Prentice Hall; 1966.

40. Hempel C. *Aspects of Scientific Explanation.* New York; NY: Free Press; 1965.

41. Putnam H. The corroboration of theories. In: Hacking I, ed. *Scientific Revolutions.* New York, NY: Oxford University Press; 1981.

42. McMullin E. A case for scientific realism. In: Leplin J, ed. *Scientific Realism.* Berkeley, Calif: University of California Press; 1984.

43. Hesse M. Laws and theories. In Edwards P, ed. *The Encyclopaedia of Philosophy.* New York, NY: Macmillan; 1967.

44. Carnap R, Pap A, trans. The elimination of metaphysics through logical analysis of language. In: Ayer AJ, ed. *Logical Positivism.* New York, NY: Free Press; 1959.

45. Popper KR. Metaphysics and criticizability. In: Miller D, ed. *Popper Selections.* Princeton, NJ: Princeton University Press; 1985.

Positivism and Realism

Moritz Schlick

I. Preliminary Questions

Every philosophical movement is defined by the principles that it regards as fundamental, and to which it constantly recurs in its arguments. But in the course of historical development, the principles are apt not to remain unaltered, whether it be that they acquire new formulations, and come to be extended or restricted, or that even their meaning gradually undergoes noticeable modifications. At some point the question then arises as to whether we should still speak at all of the development of a single movement, and retain its old name, or whether a new movement has not in fact arisen.

If, alongside the evolved outlook, an 'orthodox' movement still continues to exist, which clings to the first principles in their original form and meaning, then sooner or later some terminological distinction of the old from the new will automatically come about. But where this is not clearly so, and where, on the contrary, the most diverse and perhaps contradictory formulations and interpretations of the principles are bandied about among the various adherents of

a 'movement,' then a hubbub arises, whose result is that supporters and opponents of the view are found talking at cross purposes; everyone seeks out from the principles what he can specifically use for the defense of his own view, and everything ends in hopeless misunderstandings and obscurities. They only disappear when the various principles are separated from each other and tested individually for meaning and truth on their own account, in which process we do best, at first, to disregard entirely the contexts in which they have historically arisen, and the names that have been given to them.

I should like to apply these considerations to the modes of thought grouped under the name of 'positivism.' From the moment when Auguste Comte invented the term, up to the present day, they have undergone a development which provides a good example of what has just been said. I do this, however, not with the historical purpose of establishing, say, a rigorous concept of positivism in its historical manifestation, but rather in order to contribute to a real settlement of the controversy currently carried on about certain principles which rank as positivist axioms. Such a settlement is all the dearer to me, in that I subscribe to some of these principles myself. My only concern here is to make the meaning of these principles as clear as possible; whether, after such clarification, people are still minded to impute them to 'positivism' or not, is a question of wholly subordinate importance.

Originally appeared in *Erkenntnis III* (1932/33); translated by Peter Heath and reprinted in *Moritz Schlick: Philosophical Papers. Volume II* (1925–1936) from *Vienna Circle Collection*, edited by Henk L. Mulder (Kluwer, 1979), pp. 259–284. Reprinted by permission of the Schlick estate and the publisher. Copyright 1979 by Kluwer Academic Publishers.

If every view is to be labelled positivist, which denies the possibility of metaphysics, then nothing can be said against it as a mere definition, and in *this* sense I would have to declare myself a strict positivist. but this, of course, is true only if we presuppose a particular definition of 'metaphysics.' What the definition of metaphysics is, that would have to be made basic here, does not need to interest us at present; but it scarcely accords with the formulations that are mostly current in the literature of philosophy; and closer definitions of positivism that adhere to such formulations lead straight into obscurities and difficulties.

For if, say—as has mostly been done from time immemorial—we assert that metaphysics is the doctrine of 'true being,' of 'reality in itself,' or of 'transcendent being,' this talk of true, real being obviously presupposes that a non-true, lesser or apparent being stands opposed to it, as has indeed been assumed by all metaphysicians since the days of Plato and the Eleatics. This seeming being is said to be the realm of 'appearances,' and while the true transcendent reality is held to be accessible with difficulty only to the efforts of the metaphysician, the special sciences are exclusively concerned with appearances, and the latter are also perfectly accessible to scientific knowledge. The contrast in the knowability of the two 'kinds of being' is then traced to the fact that appearances are 'given' and immediately known to us, whereas metaphysical reality has had to be inferred from them only by a circuitous route. With this we seem to have arrived at a fundamental concept of the positivists, for they, too, are always talking of the 'given,' and state their basic principle mostly by saying that, like the scientist, the philosopher must abide throughout in the given, that an advance beyond it, such as the metaphysician attempts, is impossible or absurd.

It is natural, therefore, to take the given of positivism to be simply identical with the metaphysician's appearances, and to believe that positivism is at bottom a metaphysics from which the transcendent has been omitted or struck out; and such a view may often enough have inspired the arguments of positivists, no less than those of their adversaries. But with this we are already on the road to dangerous errors.

This very term 'the given' is already an occasion for grave misunderstandings. 'To give,' of course, normally signifies a three-termed relation: it presupposes in the first place someone who gives, secondly someone given to, and thirdly something given. For the metaphysician this is quite in order, for the giver is transcendent reality, the receiver is the knowing consciousness, and the latter appropriates what is given to it as its 'content.' But the positivist, from the outset, will obviously have nothing to do with such notions; the given, for him, is to be merely a term for what is simplest and no longer open to question. Whatever term we may choose, indeed, it will be liable to occasion misconceptions; if we talk of 'acquaintance' ['*Erlebnis*'], we seem to presuppose the distinction between he who is acquainted and what he is acquainted with; in employing the term 'content of consciousness,' we appear to burden ourselves with a similar distinction, and also with the complex concept of 'consciousness,' first excogitated, at all events, by philosophical thought.

But even apart from such difficulties, it is possibly still not yet clear what is actually meant by the given. Does it merely include such 'qualities' as 'blue,' 'hot' and 'pain,' or also, for example, relations between them, or the order they are in? Is the similarity of two qualities 'given' in the same sense as the qualities themselves? And if the given is somehow elaborated or interpreted or judged, is this elaboration or judgment not also in turn a given in some sense?

It is not obscurities of this type, however, which give occasion to present-day controversies: it is the question of 'reality' that first tosses among the parties the apple of discord.

If positivism's rejection of metaphysics amounts to a denial of transcendent reality, it seems the most natural thing in the world to conclude that in that case it attributes reality only to non-transcendent being. The main principle of the positivist then seems to run: 'Only the given is real'. Anyone who takes pleasure in plays upon words could even make use of a peculiarity of the German language in order to lend this proposition the air of being a self-evident tautology, by formulating it as: '*Es gibt nur das Gegebene*' [Only the given exists].

What are we to say of this principle?

Many positivists may have stated and upheld it (particularly those, perhaps, who have treated physical objects as 'mere logical constructions' or as 'mere auxiliary concepts'), and others have had it imputed to them by opponents—but we are obliged to say that anyone who asserts this principle thereby attempts to advance a claim that is metaphysical in the same sense, and to the same degree, as the seemingly opposite contention, that 'There is a transcendent reality'.

The problem at issue here is obviously the so-called question as to the reality of the external world, and on this there seem to be two parties: that of 'realism,' which believes in the reality of the external world, and that of 'positivism,' which does not believe in this. I am convinced that in fact it is quite absurd to set two views in contrast to one another in this fashion, since (as with all metaphysical propositions) both parties, at bottom, have not the least notion of what they are trying to say. But before explaining this I should like to show how the most natural interpretations of the proposition 'only the given is real' in fact lead at once to familiar metaphysical views.

As a question about the existence of the 'external' world, the problem can make its appearance only through drawing a distinction of some kind between inner and outer, and this happens inasmuch and insofar as the given is regarded as a 'content' of consciousness, as belonging to a subject (or several) to *whom* it is given. The immediate data are thereby credited with a conscious character, the character of presentations or ideas; and the proposition in question would then assert that *all* reality possesses this character: no being outside consciousness. But this is

nothing else but the basic principle of metaphysical *idealism*. If the philosopher thinks he can speak only of what is given to himself, we are confronted with a solipsistic metaphysics; but if he thinks he may assume that the given is distributed to many subjects, we then have an idealism of the Berkeleyan type.

On this interpretation, positivism would thus be simply identical with the older idealist metaphysics. But since its founders were certainly seeking something quite other than a renewal of that idealism, this view must be rejected as inconsistent with the antimetaphysical purpose of positivism. Idealism and positivism do not go together. The positivist Ernst Laas[1] devoted a work in several volumes to demonstrating the irreconcilable opposition that exists between them in all areas; and if his pupil Hans Vaihinger gave his *Philosophy of As If* the subtitle of an idealist positivism', that is just one of the contradictions that infect this work. Ernst Mach has particularly emphasized that his own positivism has evolved in a direction away from the Berkeleyan metaphysics; he and Avenarius laid much stress on not construing the given as a content of consciousness, and endeavored to keep this notion out of their philosophy altogether.

In view of the uncertainty in the positivists' own camp, it is not surprising if the 'realist' ignores the distinctions we have mentioned and directs his arguments against the thesis that 'there are only contents of consciousness,' or that 'there is only an internal world'. But this proposition belongs to the idealist metaphysics: it has no place in an antimetaphysical positivism, and these counter-arguments do not tell against such a view.

The 'realist' can, indeed, take the line that it is utterly inevitable that the given should be regarded as a content of consciousness, as subjective, or mental—or whatever the term may be; and he would consider the attempts of Avenarius and Mach to construe the given as neutral, and to do away with the inner-outer distinction, as a failure, and would think a theory without metaphysics to be simply impossible. But this line of argument is more rarely encountered. And whatever the position there, we are dealing in any case with a quarrel about nothing, since the 'problem of the reality of the external world' is a meaningless pseudo-problem. It is now time to make this clear.

II. On the Meaning of Statements

It is the proper business of philosophy to seek for and clarify the *meaning* of claims and questions. The chaotic state in which philosophy has found itself throughout the greatest part of its history is traceable to the unlucky fact that firstly it has accepted certain formulations with far too much naivete, as genuine problems, without first carefully testing whether they really possessed a sound meaning; and secondly, that it has believed the answers to certain questions to be discoverable by particular philosophical methods that differ from those of the special sciences. By philosophical analysis we are unable to decide of anything whether it is real; we can only determine what it *means* to claim that it is real; and whether this is then the case or not can only be decided by the ordinary methods of daily life and science, namely by *experience*. So here the task is to get clear whether a meaning can be attached to the question about the reality of the 'external world.'

When are we certain, in general, that the meaning of a question is clear to us? Obviously then, and only then, when we are in a position to state quite accurately the circumstances under which it can be answered in the affirmative—or those under which it would have to receive a negative answer. By these statements, and these alone, is the meaning of the question defined.

It is the first step in every kind of philosophizing, and the basis of all reflection, to realize that it is absolutely impossible to give the meaning of any claim save by describing the state-of-affairs that must obtain if the claim is to be true. If it does not obtain, then the claim is false. The meaning of a proposition obviously consists in this alone, that it expresses a particular state-

of-affairs. This state-of-affairs must actually be pointed out, in order to give the meaning of the proposition. One may say, indeed, that the proposition itself already gives this state-of-affairs; but only, of course, for one who *understands* it. But when do I understand a proposition? When I know the meaning of the words that occur in it? This can be explained by definitions. But in the definitions new words occur, whose meaning I also have to know in turn. The business of defining cannot go on indefinitely, so eventually we come to words whose meaning cannot again be described in a proposition; it has to be pointed out directly; the meaning of the word must ultimately be *shown*, it has to be *given*. This takes place through an act of pointing or showing, and what is shown must be given, since otherwise it cannot be pointed out to me.

In order, therefore, to find the meaning of a proposition, we have to transform it by introduction of successive definitions, until finally only such words appear in it as can no longer be defined, but whose meanings can only be indicated directly. The criterion for the truth or falsity of the proposition then consists in this, that under specific conditions (stated in the definitions) certain data are, or are not, present. Once this is established, I have established everything that the proposition was talking about, and hence I know its meaning. If I am *not* capable, in principle, of verifying a proposition, that is, if I have absolutely no knowledge of how I should go about it, what I would have to do, in order to ascertain its truth or falsity, then I obviously have no idea at all of what the proposition is actually saying; for then I would be in no position to interpret the proposition, in proceeding, by means of the definitions, from its wording to possible data, since insofar as I *am* in a position to do this, I can also, by this very fact, point out the road to verification in principle (even though, for practical reasons, I may often be unable actually to tread it). To state the circumstances under which a proposition is true is *the same* as stating its meaning, and nothing else.

And these 'circumstances,' as we have now seen, have ultimately to be found in the given. Different circumstances imply differences in the given. The *meaning* of every proposition is ultimately determined by the given alone, and by absolutely nothing else.

I do not know if this view should be described as positivistic: though I should like to believe that it has been in the background of all efforts that go under this name in the history of philosophy, whether, indeed, it has been clearly formulated or not. It may well be assumed to constitute the true core and driving force of many quite erroneous formulations that we find among the positivists.

Anyone who has once attained the insight, that the meaning of any statement can be determined only by the given, no longer even grasps the *possibility of another* opinion, for he sees that he has merely discerned the conditions under which opinions can be formulated at all. It would thus be quite erroneous as well to perceive in the foregoing any sort of 'theory of meaning' (in Anglo-Saxon countries the view outlined, that the meaning of a statement is wholly and solely determined by its verification in the given, is commonly called the 'experimental theory of meaning'); that which precedes all formation of theories cannot itself be a theory.

The content of our thesis is in fact entirely trivial (and that is precisely why it can give so much insight); it tells us that a statement only has a specifiable meaning if it makes some testable difference whether it is true or false. A proposition for which the world looks exactly the same when it is true as it does when it is false, in fact says nothing whatever about the world; it is empty, it conveys nothing, I can specify no meaning for it. But a *testable* difference is present only if there is a difference in the given, for to be testable certainly means nothing else but 'demonstrable in the given.'

It is self-evident that the term 'testability' is intended only *in principle*, for the meaning of a proposition does not, of course, depend on whether the circumstances under which we actually find ourselves at a given moment allow of, or prevent, actual verification. The statement that 'there are 10,000 ft mountains on the far side of the moon' is beyond doubt absolutely meaningful, although we lack the technical means for verifying it. And it would remain just as meaningful even if we knew for certain, on scientific grounds of some kind, that no man would ever reach the far side of the moon. Verification always remains *thinkable*, we are always able to say what sort of data we should have to encounter, in order to effect the decision; it is *logically* possible, whatever the situation may be as regards the actual possibility of doing it. And that is all that is at issue here.

But if someone advanced the claim, that within every electron there is a nucleus which is always present, but produces absolutely no effects outside, so that its existence in nature is discernible in no way whatever—then this would be a meaningless claim. For we should at once have to ask the fabricator of this hypothesis: What, then, do you actually *mean* by the presence of this 'nucleus'?, and he could only reply: I mean that something exists there in the electron. We would then go on to ask: What is that supposed to mean? How would it be if this something did not exist? And he would have to reply: In that case, everything else would be exactly as before. For according to his claim, no effects of any kind proceed from this something, and everything observable would remain absolutely unaltered, the realm of the given would not be touched. We would judge that he had not succeeded in conveying to us the meaning of his hypothesis, and that it is therefore vacuous. In this case the impossibility of verification is actually not a factual, but a *logical* impossibility, since the claim that this nucleus is totally without effects rules out, *in principle*, the possibility of deciding by differences in the given.

Nor can it be supposed that the distinction between essential impossibility of verification and a merely factual and empirical impossibility is not sharp, and therefore often hard to draw;

for the 'essential' impossibility is simply a logical one, which differs from the empirical, not by degrees, but absolutely. What is merely empirically impossible still remains *thinkable*; but what is logically impossible is contradictory, and cannot, therefore, be thought at all. We also find, in fact, that with sure instinct, this distinction is always very clearly sensed in the practice of scientific thinking. The physicists would be the first to reject the claim in our example, concerning the eternally hidden nucleus of the electron, with the criticism that this is no hypothesis whatever, but an empty play with words. And on the question of the meaning of their statements, successful students of reality have at all times adopted the standpoint here outlined, in that they acted upon it, even though mostly unawares.

Thus our position does not represent anything strange and peculiar for science, but in a certain sense has always been a self-evident thing. It could not possibly have been otherwise, because only from this standpoint can the truth of a statement be tested at all; since all scientific activity consists in testing the truth of statements, it constantly acknowledges the correctness of our viewpoint by what it does.

If express confirmation be still needed, it is to be found with the utmost clarity at critical points in the development of science, where research is compelled to bring its self-evident presuppositions to consciousness. This situation occurs where difficulties of principle give rise to the suspicion that something may not be in order about these presuppositions. The most celebrated example of this kind, which will forever remain notable, is Einstein's analysis of the concept of time, which consists in nothing else whatever but a statement of the *meaning* of our assertions about the simultaneity of spatially separated events. Einstein told the physicists (and philosophers): you must first say what you *mean* by simultaneity, and this you can only do by showing how the statement 'two events are simultaneous' is verified. But in so doing you have then also established the meaning fully and

without remainder. What is true of the simultaneity concept holds good of every other; every statement has a meaning only insofar as it can be verified; it only *signifies* what is verified and absolutely *nothing* beyond this. Were someone to maintain that it contains more, he would have to be able to say what this more is, and for this he must again say what in the world would be different if he was wrong; but he can say nothing of the kind, for by previous assumption all observable differences have already been utilized in the verification.

In the simultaneity example the analysis of meaning, as is right and proper for the physicist, is carried only so far that the decision about the truth or falsity of a temporal statement resides in the occurrence or non-occurrence of a certain physical event (for example, the coincidence of a pointer with a scale-mark); but it is clear that one may go on to ask: What, then, does it *mean* to claim that the pointer indicates a particular mark on the scale? And the answer to this can be nothing else whatever but a reference to the occurrence of certain data, or, as we are wont to say, of certain 'sensations.' This is also generally admitted, and especially by physicists. "For in the end, positivism will always be right in this", says Planck,[2] "that there is no other source of knowledge but sensations", and this statement obviously means that the truth or falsity of a physical assertion is quite solely dependent on the occurrence of certain sensations (which are a special class of the given).

But now there will always be many inclined to say that this grants only that the truth of a physical statement can be tested in absolutely no other way save by the occurrence of certain sensations, but that this, however, is a different thing from claiming that the very *meaning* of the statement is thereby exhaustively presented. The latter would have to be denied, for a proposition can contain *more* than allows of verification; that the pointer stands at a certain mark on the scale means *more* than the presence of certain sensations (namely, the 'presence of a certain state-of-affairs in the external world').

Of this denial of the identity of meaning and verification the following needs to be said:

1. Such a denial is to be found among physicists only where they leave the proper territory of physical statements and begin to philosophize. (In physics, obviously, we find only statements about the nature or behaviour of things and processes; an express assertion of their 'reality' is needless, since it is always presupposed.) In his own territory the physicist fully acknowledges the correctness of our point of view. We have already mentioned this earlier, and have since elucidated it by the example of the concept of simultaneity. There are, indeed, many philosophers who say: Only relative simultaneity can admittedly be established, but from this it does not follow that there is no such thing as absolute simultaneity, and we continue, as before, to believe in it! There is no way of demonstrating the falsity of this claim; but the great majority of physicists are rightly of the opinion that it is meaningless. It must be emphatically stressed, however, that in both cases we are concerned with exactly the same situation. It makes absolutely no difference, in principle, whether I ask: Does the statement 'two events are simultaneous' mean more than can be verified? Or whether I ask: Does the statement 'the pointer indicates the fifth scale-mark' signify more than can be verified? The physicist who treats the two cases differently is guilty of an inconsistency. He will justify himself by arguing that in the second case, where the 'reality of the external world' is concerned, there is philosophically far more at stake. This argument is too vague for us to be able to assign it any weight, but we shall shortly examine whether anything lies behind it.

2. It is perfectly true that every statement about a physical object or event says more than is verified, say, by the once-and-for-all occurrence of an experience. It is presupposed, rather, that this experience took place under quite specific conditions, whose fulfilment can, of course, be tested in turn only by something given; and it is further presupposed that still other and further verifications (after-tests, confirmations) are

always possible, which themselves of course reduce to manifestations of some kind in the given. In this way we can and must make allowance for sense-deceptions and errors, and it is easy to see how we are classify the cases in which we would say that the observer had merely dreamt that the pointer indicated a certain mark, or that he had not observed carefully, and so on. Blondlot's claims about the N-rays that he thought he had discovered were intended, after all, to say more than that he had had certain visual sensations under certain circumstances, and hence they could also be refuted.[3] Strictly speaking, the meaning of a proposition about physical objects is exhausted only by the provision of indefinitely many possible verifications, and the consequence of this is, that in the last resort such a proposition can never be proved absolutely true. It is generally acknowledged, indeed, that even the most assured propositions of science have always to be regarded merely as hypotheses, which remain open to further definition and improvement. This has certain consequences for the logical nature of such propositions, but they do not concern us here.

Once again: the meaning of a physical statement is never defined by a single isolated verification; it must be conceived, rather, as of the form: If circumstances x are given, data y occur, where indefinitely many circumstances can be substituted for x, and the proposition remains correct on every occasion (this also holds, even if the statement refers to a once-and-for-all occurrence—a historical event—for such an event always has innumerable consequences whose occurrence can be verified). Thus the meaning of every physical statement ultimately lies always in an endless chain of data; the individual datum as such is of no interest in this connection. So if a positivist should ever have said that the individual objects of science are simply the given experiences themselves, he would certainly have been quite wrong; what every scientist seeks, and seeks alone, are rather the rules which govern the connection of experiences, and by which they can be predicted. Nobody denies that the sole verification of natural laws consists in the fact that they provide correct predictions of this type. The oft-heard objection, that the immediately given, which at most can be the object of psychology, is now falsely to be made into an object of physics, is thereby robbed of its force.

3. The most important thing to say, however, is this: If anyone thinks that the meaning of a proposition is not in fact exhausted by what can be verified in the given, but extends far beyond that, then he must at least admit that this surplus of meaning is utterly indescribable, unstatable in any way, and inexpressible by any language. For let him just try to state it! So far as he succeeds in communicating something of the meaning, he will find that the communication consists in the very fact that he has pointed out some circumstances that can serve for verification in the given, and he thereby finds our view confirmed. Or else he may believe, indeed, that he has stated a meaning, but closer examination shows that his words only signify that there is still 'something' there, though nothing whatever is said about its nature. In that case he has really communicated nothing; his claim is meaningless, for one cannot maintain the existence of something without saying *of what* one is claiming the existence. This can be brought out by reference to our example of the essentially indemonstrable 'nucleus of the electron'; but for the sake of clarity we shall analyze yet another example of a very fundamental kind.

I am looking at two pieces of green paper, and establish that they have the same color. The proposition asserting the likeness of color is verified, *inter alia*, by the fact that I twice experience the same color at the same time. The statement 'two patches of the same color are now present' can no longer be reduced to others; it is verified by the fact that it describes the given. It has a good meaning: by virtue of the significance of the words occurring in the statement, this meaning is simply the existence of this similarity of color; by virtue of linguistic usage, the sentence expresses precisely this experi-

ence. I now show one of the two pieces of paper to a second observer, and pose the question: Does he see the green just as I do? Is his color-experience the *same* as mine? This case is *essentially* different from the one just examined. While there the statement was verifiable through the occurrence of an experience of similarity, a brief consideration shows that here such a verification is absolutely impossible. Of course (if he is not color-blind), the second observer also calls the paper *green*; and if I now describe this green to him more closely, by saying that it is more yellowish than this wallpaper, more bluish than this billiard-cloth, darker than this plant, and so on, he will also find it so each time, that is, he will agree with my statements. But even though all his judgments about colors were to agree entirely with mine, I can obviously never conclude from this that he experiences 'the same quality.' It might be that on looking at the green paper he has an experience that I should call 'red'; that conversely, in the cases where I see red, he experiences green, but of course calls it 'red,' and so forth. It might even be, indeed, that my color sensations are matched in him by experiences of sound or data of some other kind; yet it would be impossible in principle ever to discover these differences between his experience and mine. We would agree completely, and could never differ about our surroundings, so long only (and this is absolutely the only precondition that has to be made) as the inner *order* of his experiences agrees with that of mine. Their 'quality' does not come into it at all; all that is required is that they can be brought into a *system* in the same fashion.

All this is doubtless uncontested, and philosophers have pointed out this situation often enough. They have mostly added, however, that such subjective differences are indeed theoretically possible, and that this possibility is in principle very interesting, but that nevertheless it is 'in the highest degree probable' that the observer and I actually experience the *same* green. We, however, must say: The claim that different individuals experience the *same* sensation has this verifiable meaning alone, that all their statements (and of course all their other behavior as well) display certain agreements; hence the claim *means* nothing else whatever but this. It is merely another mode of expression if we say that it is a question of the likeness of two systems of order. The proposition that two experiences of different subjects not only occupy the same place in the order of a system, but *beyond that* are *also* qualitatively like each other, has no meaning for us. It is not false, be it noted, but meaningless: we have no idea at all what it is supposed to signify.

Experience shows that for the majority of people it is very difficult to agree with this. One has to grasp that we are really concerned here with a *logical* impossibility of verification. To speak of the likeness of two data in *the same* consciousness has an acceptable meaning; it can be verified through an immediate experience. But if we wish to talk of the likeness of two data in *different* consciousnesses, that is a new concept; it has to be defined anew, for propositions in which it occurs are no longer verifiable in the old fashion. The new definition is, in fact, the likeness of all reactions of the two individuals; no other can be found. The majority believe, indeed, that no definition is required here; we know straight off what 'like' means, and the meaning is in both cases the same. But in order to recognize this is an error, we have only to recall the concept of simultaneity, where the situation is precisely analogous. To the concept of 'simultaneity at the same place' there corresponds here the concept of 'likeness of experiences in the same individual'; and to 'simultaneity at different places' there corresponds here the 'likeness of experiences in different individuals.' The second is in each case something new in comparison with the first, and must be specially defined. A directly experienceable quality can no more be pointed out for the likeness of two greens in different consciousnesses than for simultaneity at different places; both must be defined by way of a system of relations.

Many philosophers have tried to overcome the difficulty that seemed to confront them here by all sorts of speculations and thought-experiments, in that they have spoken, say, of a universal consciousness (God) embracing all individuals, or have imagined that perhaps by an artificial linkage of the nerve-systems of two people the sensations of the one might be made accessible to the other and could be compared—but all this is useless, of course, since even by such fantastical methods it is in the end only contents of one and the same consciousness that are directly compared; but the question is precisely whether a comparison is possible between qualities insofar as they belong to different consciousnesses, and *not* the same one.

It must be admitted, therefore, that a proposition about the likeness of the experiences of two different persons has no other *stateable* meaning save that of a certain agreement in their reactions. Now it is open to anyone to believe that such a proposition also possesses another, more direct meaning; but it is certain that this meaning is not verifiable, and that there can be no way at all of starting or pointing out what this meaning is supposed to be. From this it follows, however, that there is absolutely no way at all in which such a meaning could be made a topic of discussion; there could be absolutely no talk about it, and it can in no way enter into any language whereby we communicate with each other.

And what has, we hope, become clear from this example, is of quite general application. All we can understand in a proposition is what it conveys; but a meaning can be communicated only if it is verifiable. Since propositions are nothing else but a vehicle of communication, we can assign to their meaning only what can be communicated. For this reason I should insist that 'meaning' can never signify anything but 'stateable meaning.'

But even if someone insisted that there was a nonverifiable meaning, this would actually be of no consequence whatever; for in everything he says and asks, and in everything that we ask him and reply to him, *such* a meaning can never in any way come to light. In other words, if such a thing were to exist, all our utterances and arguments and modes of behavior would still remain totally untouched by it, whether it was a question of daily life, of ethical or aesthetic attitude, of science of any kind, or of philosophy. Everything would be exactly as though there were no unverifiable meaning, for insofar as anything was different, it would in fact be verifiable through this very difference.

That is a serious situation, and we must absolutely demand that it be taken seriously. One must guard above all things against confusing the present logical impossibility with an empirical incapacity, just as though some technical difficulties and human imperfection were to blame for the fact that only the verifiable can be expressed, and as though there were still some little backdoor through which an unstateable meaning could slip into the daylight and make itself noticeable in our speech and behavior! No! The incommunicability is an absolute one; anyone who believes in a nonverifiable meaning (or more accurately, we shall have to say, imagines he believes in this) must still confess that only *one* attitude remains in regard to it: absolute silence. It would be of no use either to him or us, however, often he asserted: 'but there is a nonverifiable meaning,' for this statement is itself devoid of meaning, and says nothing.

III. What Does 'Reality' Mean? What Does 'External World' Mean?

We are now prepared to make application of the foregoing to the so-called problem of the reality of the external world.

Let us ask: What meaning has it, if the 'realist' says 'there is an external world'? or even: What meaning attaches to the claim (which the realist attributes to the positivist) 'there is no external world'?

To answer the question, it is necessary, of course, to clarify the significance of the words 'there is' and external world.' Let us begin with

the first. 'There is x' amounts to saying 'x is real' or 'x is actual'. So what does it mean if we attribute actuality (or reality) to an object? It is an ancient and very important insight of logic or philosophy, that the proposition 'x is actual' is totally different in kind from a proposition that attributes any sort of *property* to x (such as 'x is hard'). In other words, actuality, reality or existence is not a property. The statement 'the dollar in my pocket is round' has a totally different logical form from the statement 'the dollar in my pocket is actual.' In modern logic this distinction is expressed by an altogether different symbolism, but it had already been very sharply emphasized by Kant, who, as we know, in his critique of the so-called ontological proof of God's existence had correctly found the error of this proof in the fact that existence was treated like a property there.

In daily life we very often have to speak of actuality or existence, and for that very reason it cannot be hard to discover the meaning of this talk. In a legal battle it often has to be established whether some document really exists, or whether this has merely been falsely claimed, say, by one of the parties; nor is it wholly unimportant to me, whether the dollar in my pocket is merely imaginary or actually real. Now everybody knows in what way such a reality-claim is verified, nor can there be the least doubt about it; the reality of the dollar is proved by this, and this alone, that by suitable manipulations I furnish myself certain tactual or visual sensations, on whose occurrence I am accustomed to say: this is a dollar. The same holds of the document, only there we should be content, on occasion, with certain statements by others claiming to have seen the document, that is, to have had perceptions of a quite specific kind. And the 'statements of others' again consist in certain acoustic, or—if they were written utterances— visual perceptions. There is need of no special controversy about the fact that the occurrence of certain sense-perceptions among the data *always* constitutes the sole criterion for propositions about the reality of a 'physical' object or event, in daily life no less than in the most refined assertions of science. That there are okapis in Africa can be established only by observing such animals. But it is not necessary that the object or event 'itself' should have to be perceived. We can imagine, for example, that the existence of a trans-Neptunian planet might be inferred by observation of perturbations with just as much certainty as by direct perception of a speck of light in the telescope. The reality of the atom provides another example, as does the back side of the moon.

It is of great importance to state that the occurrence of some one particular experience in verifying a reality-statement is often not recognized as such a verification, but that it is throughout a question of regularities, of law-like connections; in this way true verifications are distinguished from illusions and hallucinations. If we say of some event or object—which must be marked out by a description—that it is *real*, this means, then, that there is a quite specific connection between perceptions or other experiences, that under given circumstances certain data are presented. By this alone is it verified, and hence this is also its only stateable meaning.

This, too, was already formulated, in principle, by Kant, whom nobody will accuse of 'positivism.' Reality, for him, is a category, and if we apply it anywhere, and claim of an object that it is real, then all this asserts, in Kant's opinion, is that it belongs to a law-governed connection of perceptions.

It will be seen that for us (as for Kant; and the same must apply to any philosopher who is aware of his task) it is merely a matter of saying what is meant when we ascribe real existence to a thing in life or in science; it is in no sense a matter of correcting the claims of ordinary life or of research. I must confess that I should charge with folly and reject *a limine* every philosophical system that involved the claim that clouds and stars, mountains and the sea, were not actually real, that the 'physical world' did not exist, and that the chair against the wall

ceases to be every time I turn my back on it. Nor do I seriously impute such a claim to any thinker. It would, for example, be undoubtedly a quite mistaken account of Berkeley's philosophy if his system were to be understood in this fashion. He, too, in no way denied the reality of the physical world, but merely sought to explain what we mean when we attribute reality to it. Anyone who says here that unperceived things are ideas in the mind of God is not in fact denying their existence, but is seeking, rather, to understand it. Even John Stuart Mill was not wanting to deny the reality of physical objects, but rather to explain it, when he declared them to be 'permanent possibilities of sensation,' although I do consider his mode of expression to have been very unsuitably chosen.

So if 'positivism' is understood to mean a view that denies reality to bodies, I should simply have to declare it absurd; but I do not believe that such an interpretation of positivist opinions, at least as regards their competent exponents, would be historically just. Yet, however that may be, we are concerned only with the issue itself. And on this we have established as follows: our principle, that the question about the meaning of a proposition is identical with the question about its verification, leads us to recognize that the claim that a thing is real is a statement about lawful connections of experiences; it does *not*, however, imply this claim to be false. (There is therefore no denial of reality to physical objects in favor of sensations.)

But opponents of the view presented profess themselves by no means satisfied with this assertion. So far as I can see, they would answer as follows: 'You do, indeed, acknowledge completely the reality of the physical world, but—as we see it—only in words. You simply *call* real what we should describe as mere conceptual constructions. When *we* use the word "reality," we mean by it something quite different from you. Your definition of the real reduces it to experiences; but we mean something quite independent of all experiences. We mean something that possesses the same independence that you obviously concede only to the data, in that you reduce everything else to them, as the not-further-reducible.'

Although it would be a sufficient rebuttal to request our opponents to reflect once more upon how reality-statements are verified, and how verification is connected with *meaning*, I do in fact recognize the need to take account of the psychological attitude from which this argument springs, and therefore beg attention to the following considerations, whereby a modification of this attitude may yet, perhaps, be effected.

Let us first enquire whether, on our view, a 'content of consciousness' is credited with a reality that is denied to a physical object. We ask, therefore: does the claim that a feeling or sensation is real have a meaning different from the claim that a physical object is real? For us, this can mean only: are different types of verification involved in the two cases? The answer is: no!

To clarify this, we need to enter a little into the logical form of reality-statements. The general logical recognition that an existence-statement can be made about a datum only if it is marked out by a description, but not if it is given by an immediate indication, is also valid, of course, for the 'data of consciousness.' In the language of symbolic logic, this is expressed by the fact that an existence-claim must contain an 'operator.' In Russell's notation, for example, a reality-statement has the form $(\exists x)fx$, or in words, 'there is an x that has the property f.' The form of words 'there is a,' where 'a' is supposed to be the individual name of a directly indicated object, therefore means no more than 'this here'; this form of words is meaningless, and in Russell's symbolism it cannot even be written down. We have to grasp the idea that Descartes's proposition 'I am'—or, to put it better, 'contents of consciousness exist'—is absolutely meaningless; it expresses nothing, and contains no knowledge. This is due to the fact that 'contents of consciousness' occurs in this

connection as a mere *name* for the given; no characteristic is asserted, whose presence could be tested. A proposition has meaning, and is verifiable, only if I can state under what circumstances it would be true, and under what circumstances it would be false. But how am I to describe the circumstances under which the proposition 'My contents of consciousness exist' would be false? Every attempt would lead to ridiculous absurdities, to such propositions, say, as 'It is the case that nothing is the case,' or the like. Hence I am self-evidently unable to describe the circumstances that make the proposition true (just try it!). Nor is there any doubt whatever that Descartes, with his proposition, had really obtained no knowledge, and was actually no wiser than before.

No, the question about the reality of an experience has meaning only where this reality can also be meaningfully *doubted*. I can ask, for example: Is it really true that I felt joy on hearing that news? This can be verified or falsified exactly as when we ask, say: Is it true that Sirius has a companion (that this companion is real)? That I felt joy on a particular occasion can be verified, for example, by examination of other people's statements about my behaviour at the time, by my finding of a letter that I then wrote, or simply by the return to me of an exact memory of the emotion I experienced. Here, therefore, there is not the slightest difference of principle: to be real always means to stand in a definite connection with the given. Nor is it otherwise, say, with an experience that is present at this very moment. I can quite meaningfully ask, for example (in the course, say, of a physiological experiment): Do I now actually feel a pain or not? (Notice that 'pain,' here, does not function as an individual name for a 'this here,' but represents a conceptual term for a describable class of experiences.) Here, too, the question is answered by establishing that in conjunction with certain circumstances (experimental conditions, concentration of attention, etc.) an experience with certain describable properties occurs. Such describable properties would be, for example: similarity to an experience that has occurred under certain other circumstances; tendency to evoke certain reactions; and so on.

However we may twist and turn, it is impossible to interpret a reality-statement otherwise than as fitting into a perceptual context. It is absolutely the *same* kind of reality that we have to attribute to the data of consciousness and to physical events. Scarcely anything in the history of philosophy has created more confusion than the attempt to pick out one of the two as true 'being.' Wherever the term 'real' is intelligibly used, it has one and the same meaning.

Our opponent, perhaps, will still feel his position unshaken by what we have said, having the impression, rather, that the arguments here presented presuppose a starting-point at which he cannot, from the outset, station himself. He has to concede that the decision about the reality or unreality of anything in experience takes place, in every case, in the manner outlined, but he claims that in this way we only arrive at what Kant called *empirical* reality. It designates the area governed by the observations of daily life and of science, but beyond this boundary there lies something else, *transcendent* reality, which cannot be inferred by strict logic, and is thus no postulate of the understanding, though it is a postulate of sound *reason*. It is the only true *external world*, and this alone is at issue in the philosophical problem of the existence of the external world. The discussion thereupon abandons the question about the meaning of the term 'reality,' and turns to that about the meaning of the term 'external world.'

The term 'external world' is obviously used in two different ways: firstly in the usage of daily life, and secondly as a technical term in philosophy.

Where it occurs in everyday life, it has, like the majority of expressions employed in practical affairs, an intelligibly stateable meaning. In contrast to the 'internal world,' which covers memories, thoughts, dreams, wishes and feel-

ings, the 'external world' means nothing else, here, but the world of mountains and trees, houses, animals and men. What it means to maintain the existence of a certain object in this world, is known to every child; and it was necessary to point out that it really means absolutely nothing *more* than what the child knows. We all know how to verify the proposition, say, that 'There is a castle in the park before the town.' We perform certain acts, and if certain exactly specifiable states-of-affairs come about, then we say: 'Yes, there really is a castle there'; otherwise we say: 'That statement was an error or a lie.' And if somebody now asks us: 'But was the castle there in the night as well, when nobody saw it?' we answer: 'Undoubtedly! for it would have been impossible to build it in the period from early this morning till now, and besides, the state of the building shows that it was not only already *in situ* yesterday, but has been there for a hundred years, and hence since before we were born.' We are thus in possession of quite specific empirical criteria for whether houses and trees were also there when we were not seeing them, and whether they already existed before our birth, and will exist after our death. That is to say, the claim that these things 'exist independently of us' has a perfectly clear, testable meaning, and is obviously to be answered in the affirmative. We are very well able to distinguish such things in a stateable way from those that only occur 'subjectively,' 'in dependence upon ourselves.' If, owing to an eye defect, I see, for example, a dark speck when I look at the wall opposite me, I say of it that it is there only when I look, whereas I say of the wall that it is also there when I am not looking. The verification of this difference is in fact very easy, and both claims assert precisely what is contained in these verifications and nothing more.

So if the term 'external world' is taken in the everyday sense, the question about its existence simply means: Are there, in addition to memories, wishes and ideas, also stars, clouds, plants and animals, and my own body? We have just affirmed once more that it would be utterly absurd to say no to this question. There are obviously houses and clouds and animals existing independently of us, and I have already said earlier that a thinker who denied the existence of the external world in this sense would have no claim to our attention. Instead of telling us what we mean when we speak of mountains and plants, he wishes to persuade us that there are no such things at all!

But now how about science? When it speaks of the external world, does it, unlike daily life, mean something other than things such as houses and trees? It seems to me that this is by no means the case. For atoms and electric fields, or whatever else the physicist may speak of, are precisely what houses and trees consist of, according to his teaching; the one must therefore be real in the same sense as the other. The objectivity of mountains and clouds is just exactly the same as that of protons and energies; the latter stand in no greater contrast to the 'subjectivity' of feelings, say, or hallucinations, than do the former. We have long since convinced ourselves, in fact, that the existence of even the most subtle of the 'invisible' things postulated by the scientist is verified, in principle, in exactly the same way as the reality of a tree or a star.

In order to settle the dispute about realism, it is of the greatest importance to alert the physicist to the fact that his external world is nothing else but the *nature* which also surrounds us in daily life, and is not the 'transcendent world' of the metaphysicians. The difference between the two is again quite particularly evident in the philosophy of Kant. Nature, and everything of which the physicist can and must speak, belongs, in Kant's view, to empirical reality, and the meaning of this (as already mentioned) is explained by him exactly as we have also had to do. Atoms, in Kant's system, have no transcendent reality—they are not 'things-in-themselves.' Thus the physicist cannot appeal to the Kantian philosophy; his arguments lead only to the empirical external world that we all acknowledge,

not to a transcendent one; his electrons are not metaphysical entities.

Many scientists speak, nonetheless, of the necessity of having to postulate the existence of an external world as a *metaphysical* hypothesis. They never do this, indeed, within their own science (although all the necessary hypotheses of a science ought to occur *within* it), but only at the point where they leave this territory and begin to philosophize. The transcendent external world is actually something that is referred to exclusively in philosophy, never in a science or in daily life. It is simply a technical term, whose meaning we now have to inquire into.

How does the transcendent or metaphysical external world differ from the empirical one? In philosophical systems it is thought of as subsisting somehow behind the empirical world, where the word 'behind' is also supposed to indicate that this world is not *knowable* in the same sense as the empirical, that it lies beyond a boundary that divides the accessible from the inaccessible.

This distinction originally has its ground in the view formerly shared by the majority of philosophers, that to know an object requires that it be immediately given, directly experienced; knowledge is a kind of intuition, and is perfect only if the known is directly present to the knower, like a sensation or a feeling. So what cannot be immediately experienced or intuited remains, on this view, unknowable, ungraspable, transcendent, and belongs to the realm of things-in-themselves. Here, as I have elsewhere had to state on numerous occasions, we simply have a confusion of knowing with mere acquaintance or experiencing. But such a confusion is certainly not committed by modern scientists; I do not believe that any physicist considers knowledge of the electron to consist in its entering bodily, by an act of intuition, into the scientist's consciousness; he will take the view, rather, that for complete knowledge the only thing needed is for the regularity of an electron's behaviour to be so exhaustively stated that all formulae in which its properties occur in any way are totally confirmed by experience. In other words, the electron, and all physical realities likewise, are *not* unknowable things-in-themselves, and do not belong to a transcendent, metaphysical reality, if this is characterized by the fact that it embraces the unknowable.

Thus we again return to the conclusion that all the physicist's hypotheses can relate only to *empirical* reality, if by this we mean the knowable. It would in fact be a self-contradiction to wish to assume something unknowable as a hypothesis. For there must always be specific *reasons* for setting up a hypothesis, since it is, after all, supposed to fulfil a specific purpose. What is assumed in the hypothesis must therefore have the property of fulfilling this purpose, and of being precisely so constituted as to be justified by these reasons. But in virtue of this very fact certain statements are made of it, and these contain *knowledge* of it. And they contain, indeed, *complete* knowledge of it, since *only* that can be hypothetically assumed for which there are reasons in experience.

Or does the scientific 'realist' wish to characterize the talk of not immediately experienced objects as a metaphysical hypothesis for some reason other than the nonexistent one of its unknowability? To this, perhaps, he will answer 'yes.' In fact it can be seen from numerous statements in the literature, that the physicist by no means couples his claim of a transcendent world with the claim that it is unknowable; on the contrary, he (quite rightly) takes the view that the nature of extra-mental things is reflected with perfect correctness in his equations. Hence the external world of the physical realist is not that of traditional metaphysics. He employs the technical term of the philosophers, but what he designates by means of it has seemed to us to be merely the external world of everyday life, whose existence is doubted by nobody, not even the 'positivist.'

So what is this other reason that leads the 'realist' to regard his external world as a metaphysical assumption? Why does he want to distinguish it from the empirical external world that

we have described? The answer to this question leads us back again to an earlier point in our argument. For the 'realistic' physicist is perfectly content with our description of the external world, except on one point: he thinks that we have not lent it enough *reality*. It is not by its unknowability or any other feature that he takes his 'external world' to differ from the empirical one; it is simply and solely by the fact that another, higher reality attaches to it. This often finds expression even in the terminology; the word 'real' is often reserved for this external world, in contrast to the merely 'ideal', 'subjective' content of consciousness, and the mere 'logical constructions' into which 'positivism' is accused of dissolving reality.

But now even the physical realist has a dim feeling that, as we know, reality is not a 'property'; hence he cannot simply pass from our empirical external world to his transcendent one by attributing to it the feature of 'reality' over and above the features that we, too, ascribe to all physical objects; yet that is how he talks, and this illegitimate leap, whereby he leaves the realm of the meaningful, would in fact be 'metaphysical,' and is also felt to be such by himself.

We now have a clear view of the situation, and can judge it on the basis of the preceding considerations.

Our principle, that the truth and falsity of all statements, including those about the reality of a physical object, can be tested only in the 'given', and that *therefore* the meaning of all statements can likewise be formulated and understood only by means of the given—this principle has been wrongly construed as if it claimed or presupposed that only the given is real. Hence the 'realist' feels compelled to contradict the principle, and to set up the counterclaim, that the meaning of a reality-statement is by no means exhausted in mere assertions of the form 'Under these particular circumstances this particular experience will occur' (where these assertions, on our view, are in any case an infinite multitude); the meaning, he says, in fact lies *beyond this* in something else, which must be referred to, say, as 'independent existence', 'transcendent being' or the like, and of which our principle provides no account.

To this we ask: Well, then, *how* does one give an account of it? What do these words 'independent existence' and 'transcendent being' mean? In other words, what testable difference does it make in the world, whether an object has transcendent being or not?

Two answers are given here. The first runs: It makes a quite enormous difference. For a scientist who believes in a 'real external world' will feel and work quite differently from one who merely aims at 'describing sensations.' The former will regard the starry heaven, whose aspect recalls to him the inconceivable sublimity and size of the universe, and his own human smallness, with feelings of awe and devotion quite different from those of the latter, to whom the most distant galactic systems are but 'complexes of his own sensations.' The first will be devoted to his task with an enthusiasm, and will feel in his knowing of the objective world a satisfaction, that are denied to the second, since he takes himself to be concerned only with constructions of his own.

To this first answer we have this to say: If, in the behaviour of two thinkers, there should anywhere occur a difference such as has here been described—and it would in fact involve an observable state-of-affairs—and were we to insist upon so expressing this difference as to say that the first believes in a real external world, and the other not—well, even so, the *meaning* of our assertion still consists solely in what we observe in the behavior of the two. That is to say, the words 'absolute reality,' or 'transcendent being,' or whatever other terms we may use for it, now *signify* absolutely nothing else but certain states of feeling which arise in the two whenever they contemplate the universe, or make reality-statements, or philosophize. The fact of the matter is, that employment of the words 'independent existence,' 'transcendent reality' and so on, is simply and solely the expression of a feeling, a psychological attitude of the speaker (which

may in the end, moreover, apply to all metaphysical propositions). If someone assures us that there is a real external world in the supra-empirical sense of the term, he thinks, no doubt, that he has thereby conveyed a truth about the world; but in actuality his words express a quite different state-of-affairs, namely the mere presence of certain feelings, which provoke him to specific reactions of a verbal or other nature.

If the self-evident still needs to be specially dwelt on, I should like to underline—but in that case with maximum emphasis, and with stress upon the *seriousness* of what I am saying—that the nonmetaphysician does not differ from the metaphysician by the fact, say, that he lacks those feelings to which the other gives expression by way of the propositions of a 'realistic' philosophy, but only by the fact that he has recognized that these propositions by no means have the meaning that they seem to have, and are therefore to be avoided. He will give expression to the same feelings in a *different* way. In other words, this confrontation of the two types of thinker, set up in the 'realist's' first answer, was misleading and erroneous. If anyone is so unfortunate as not to feel the sublimity of the starry heaven, then the blame lies on something other than a logical analysis of the concepts of reality and the external world. To suppose that the opponent of metaphysics is incapable, say, of justly estimating the greatness of Copernicus, because in a certain sense the Ptolemaic view reflects the empirical situation just as well as the Copernican, seems to me no less strange than to believe that the 'positivist' cannot be a good father to his family, because according to his theory his children are merely complexes of his own sensations, and it is therefore senseless to make provision for their welfare after his death. No, the world of the non-metaphysician is the same world as that of everybody else; it lacks nothing that is needed in order to make meaningful all the statements of science and all the actions of daily life. He merely refuses to add meaningless statements to his description of the world.

We come to the *second* answer that can be

given to the question about the meaning of the claim that there is a transcendent reality. It simply consists in admitting that it makes absolutely no difference for experience whether we postulate something else existing behind the empirical world or not; metaphysical realism cannot therefore be actually tested or verified. Thus it cannot be further stated what is meant by this claim; yet something *is* meant thereby, and the meaning can also be understood without verification.

This is nothing else but the view criticized in the previous Section, that the meaning of a proposition has nothing to do with its verification, and it only remains for us to repeat once more our earlier general criticism, as applied to this particular Case. We must reply, therefore: Well now! You are giving the name 'existence' or 'reality' here to something that is utterly inexpressible and cannot be explained or stated in any fashion. You think, nonetheless, that these words have a meaning. As to that, we shall not quarrel with you. But this much is certain: by the admission just made, this meaning cannot in any way become manifest, cannot be expressed by any oral or written communication, or by any gesture or act. For if this were possible, a testable empirical situation would exist; there would be something *different* in the world, if the proposition 'There is a transcendent world' were true, from if it were false. This differentness would then signify the meaning of the words 'real external world,' and hence it would be an empirical meaning—that is, this real external world would again be merely the empirical world which we, too, acknowledge, like everyone else. Even to speak, merely, of another world, is logically impossible. There can be no discussion about it, for a nonverifiable existence cannot enter as meaning into any possible proposition. Anyone who still believes in such a thing—or imagines he believes—can only do so in silence. There are arguments only for something that can be said.

The results of our discussion can be summarized as follows:

1. The principle, that the meaning of every proposition is exhaustively determined by its verification in the given, seems to me a legitimate, unassailable core of the 'positivist' schools of thought.

   But within these schools it has seldom come clearly to light, and has often been mingled with so many untenable principles, that a logical clean-up is necessary. If we want to call the result of this clean-up 'positivism,' which might well be justified on historical grounds, we should have, perhaps, to affix a differentiating adjective: the term[4] 'logical' or 'logistic positivism' is often used; otherwise the expression 'consistent empiricism' has seemed to me appropriate.

2. This principle does not mean, nor does it follow from it, that only the given is real; such a claim would actually be meaningless.

3. Consistent empiricism, therefore, does *not* deny, either, the existence of an external world; it merely points out the empirical meaning of this existence-claim.

4. It is not an 'as if theory.' It does not say, for example, that everything behaves as if there were physical independent bodies; on the contrary, for it, too, everything is real that the nonphilosophizing scientist declares to be real. The subject matter of physics does not consist of sensations, but of laws. The formulation employed by some positivists, that bodies 'are mere complexes of sensations' is therefore to be rejected. The only correct view is that propositions about bodies can be transformed into propositions of like meaning about the regularity of occurrence of sensations.[5]

5. Logical positivism and realism are therefore not opposed; anyone who acknowledges our principle must actually be an empirical realist.

6. There is opposition only between consistent empiricism and the metaphysician,

and it is directed as much against the realist as the idealist (the former is designated in our discussion as a 'realist,' in quotation-marks).

7. The denial of the existence of a transcendent external world would be just as much a metaphysical proposition as its assertion; the consistent empiricist does not therefore deny the transcendent, but declares both its denial and its affirmation to be equally devoid of meaning.

This last distinction is of the greatest importance. I am convinced that the main resistances to our viewpoint stem from the fact that the difference between the falsity and the meaninglessness of a proposition is not heeded. The proposition 'Talk of a metaphysical external world is meaningless' does *not* say 'There is no metaphysical external world,' but something *toto coelo* different. The empiricist does not say to the metaphysician: 'Your words assert something false,' but 'Your words assert nothing at all!' He does not contradict the metaphysician, but says: 'I do not understand you.'

NOTES

1. E. Laas, *Idealismus und Positivismus. Eine kritische Auseinandersetzung,* Berlin 1879–1881.
2. M. Planck, *Positivismus und reale Aussenwelt,* Leipzig 1931, p. 14.
3. Cf. ibid. p. 11.
4. Cf. the article by A. E. Blumberg and H. Feigl ["Logical Positivism"] in *The Journal of Philosophy* 28 (1931); see also E. Kaila ['Der logistische Neupositinsmus. Eine kritische Studie'] in *Annaies Universitatis Aboensis* 13 (1930), and A. Petzäll ["Logistischer Positivismus"] in *Göreborgs Högskolas Arsskrift* 37 (1931).
5. On this, as on the content of the whole essay, cf. the article by H. Cornelius ['Zur Kritik der wissenschaftlichen Grundbegriffe'] in *Erkenntnis* 2 (1931). The formulations there are admittedly not free from objection. Cf. also the outstanding discussion by Philipp Frank in chapter X of his book *Das Kausalgesetz und seine Grenzen,* Wien 1932, and Rudolf Carnap, *Scheinprobleme in der Philosophie,* Leipzig and Berlin 1928.

Arguments Concerning Scientific Realism

Bas van Fraassen

The rigor of science requires that we distinguish well the undraped figure of nature itself from the gay-colored vesture with which we clothe it at our pleasure.

> —*Heinrich Hertz, quoted by Ludwig Boltzmann,*
> *letter to* Nature, *28 February 1895*

In our century, the first dominant philosophy of science was developed as part of logical positivism. Even today, such an expression as "the received view of theories" refers to the views developed by the logical positivists, although their heyday preceded the Second World War.

. . . I shall examine and criticize the main arguments that have been offered for scientific realism. These arguments occurred frequently as part of a critique of logical positivism. But it is surely fair to discuss them in isolation, for even if scientific realism is most easily understood as a reaction against positivism, it should be able to stand alone. The alternative view which I advocate—for lack of a traditional name I shall call it *constructive empiricism*—is equally at odds with positivist doctrine.

Scientific Realism and Constructive Empiricism

In philosophy of science, the term "scientific realism" denotes a precise position on the question of how a scientific theory is to be under-

stood, and what scientific activity really is. I shall attempt to define this position, and to canvass its possible alternatives. Then I shall indicate, roughly and briefly, the specific alternative which I shall advocate. . . .

STATEMENT OF SCIENTIFIC REALISM

What exactly is scientific realism? A naive statement of the position would be this: The picture which science gives us of the world is a true one, faithful in its details, and the entities postulated in science really exist—the advances of science are discoveries, not inventions. That statement is too naive; it attributes to the scientific realist the belief that today's theories are correct. It would mean that the philosophical position of an earlier scientific realist such as C. S. Peirce had been refuted by empirical findings. I do not suppose that scientific realists wish to be committed, as such, even to the claim that science will arrive in due time at theories true in all respects—for the growth of science might be an endless self-correction; or worse, Armageddon might occur too soon.

But the naive statement has the right flavor. It answers two main questions: It characterizes a scientific theory as a story about what there really is, and scientific activity as an enterprise of discovery, as opposed to invention. The two questions of what a scientific theory is, and what a scientific theory does, must be answered by any philosophy of science. The task we have at this point is to find a statement of scientific realism that shares these features with the naive statement, but does not saddle the realists with unacceptably strong consequences. It is especially important to make the statement as weak as possible if we wish to argue against it, so as not to charge at windmills.

As clues I shall cite some passages, most of which will also be examined below in the contexts of the authors' arguments. A statement of Wilfrid Sellars is this:

> to have good reason for holding a theory is *ipso facto* to have good reason for holding that the entities postulated by the theory exist.[1]

This addresses a question of epistemology, but also throws some indirect light on what it is, in Sellars's opinion, to hold a theory. Brian Ellis, who calls himself a scientific entity realist rather than a scientific realist, appears to agree with that statement of Sellars, but gives the following formulation of a stronger view:

> I understand scientific realism to be the view that the theoretical statements of science are, or purport to be, true generalized descriptions of reality.[2]

This formulation has two advantages: It focuses on the understanding of the theories without reference to reasons for belief, and it avoids the suggestion that to be a realist you must believe current scientific theories to be true. But it gains the latter advantage by use of the word *purport*, which may generate its own puzzles.

Hilary Putnam, in a passage which I shall cite again [later], gives a formulation which he says he learned from Michael Dummett:

> A realist (with respect to a given theory or discourse) holds that (1) the sentences of that theory are true or false; and (2) that what makes them true or false is something external—that is to say, it is not (in general) our sense data, actual or potential, or the structure of our minds, or our language, etc.[3]

He follows this soon afterwards with a further formulation which he credits to Richard Boyd:

> That terms in mature scientific theories typically refer (this formulation is due to Richard Boyd),

that the theories accepted in a mature science are typically approximately true, that the same term can refer to the same thing even when it occurs in different theories—these statements are viewed by the scientific realist . . . as part of any adequate scientific description of science and its relations to its objects.[4]

None of these were intended as definitions. But they show I think that truth must play an important role in the formulation of the basic realist position. They also show that the formulation must incorporate an answer to the question what it is to *accept* or *hold* a theory. I shall now propose such a formulation, which seems to me to make sense of the above remarks, and also renders intelligible the reasoning by realists which I shall examine below—without burdening them with more than the minimum required for this.

Science aims to give us, in its theories, a literally true story of what the world is like; and acceptance of a scientific theory involves the belief that it is true. This is the correct statement of scientific realism.

Let me defend this formulation by showing that it is quite minimal, and can be agreed to by anyone who considers himself a scientific realist. The naive statement said that science tells a true story; the correct statement says only that it is the aim of science to do so. The aim of science is of course not to be identified with individual scientists' motives. The aim of the game of chess is to checkmate your opponent; but the motive for playing may be fame, gold, and glory. What the aim is determines what counts as success in the enterprise as such; and this aim may be pursued for any number of reasons. Also, in calling something *the* aim, I do not deny that there are other subsidiary aims which may or may not be means to that end: Everyone will readily agree that simplicity, informativeness, predictive power, explanation are (also) virtues. Perhaps my formulation can even be accepted by any philosopher who considers the most important aim of science to be something which only *requires* the finding of true theories—given that I wish to give the weakest formulation of the doctrine that is generally acceptable.

I have added "literally" to rule out as realist such positions as imply that science is true if "properly understood" but literally false or meaningless. For that would be consistent with conventionalism, logical positivism, and instrumentalism. I will say more about this below; and also on pp. 356–357, where I shall consider Dummett's views further.

The second part of the statement touches on epistemology. But it only equates acceptance of a theory with belief in its truth.[5] It does not imply that anyone is ever rationally warranted in forming such a belief. We have to make room for the epistemological position, today the subject of considerable debate, that a rational person never assigns personal probability 1 to any proposition except a tautology. It would, I think, be rare for a scientific realist to take this stand in epistemology, but it is certainly possible.[6]

To understand qualified acceptance we must first understand acceptance *tout court*. If acceptance of a theory involves the belief that it is true, then tentative acceptance involves the tentative adoption of the belief that it is true. If belief comes in degrees, so does acceptance, and we may then speak of a degree of acceptance involving a certain degree of belief that the theory is true. This must of course be distinguished from belief that the theory is approximately true, which seems to mean belief that some member of a class centering on the mentioned theory is (exactly) true. In this way the proposed formulation of realism can be used regardless of one's epistemological persuasion.

ALTERNATIVES TO REALISM

Scientific realism is the position that scientific theory construction aims to give us a literally true story of what the world is like, and that acceptance of a scientific theory involves the belief that it is true. Accordingly, anti-realism is a position according to which the aim of science can

well be served without giving such a literally true story, and acceptance of a theory may properly involve something less (or other) than belief that it is true.

What does a scientist do then, according to these different positions? According to the realist, when someone proposes a theory, he is asserting it to be true. But according to the anti-realist, the proposer does not assert the theory; *he displays it*, and claims certain virtues for it. These virtues may fall short of truth: empirical adequacy, perhaps; comprehensiveness, acceptability for various purposes. This will have to be spelled out, for the details here are not determined by the denial of realism. For now we must concentrate on the key notions that allow the generic division.

The idea of a literally true account has two aspects: The language is to be literally construed; and so construed, the account is true. This divides the anti-realists into two sorts. The first sort holds that science is or aims to be true, properly (but not literally) construed. The second holds that the language of science should be literally construed, but its theories need not be true to be good. The anti-realism I shall advocate belongs to the second sort.

It is not so easy to say what is meant by a literal construal. The idea comes perhaps from theology, where fundamentalists construe the Bible literally, and liberals have a variety of allegorical, metaphorical, and analogical interpretations, which "demythologize." The problem of explicating "literal construal" belongs to the philosophy of language. . . . [B]elow, where I briefly examine some of Michael Dummett's views, I shall emphasize that "literal" does not mean "truth-valued." The term "literal" is well enough understood for general philosophical use, but if we try to explicate it we find ourselves in the midst of the problem of giving an adequate account of natural language. It would be bad tactics to link an inquiry into science to a commitment to some solution to that problem. The following remarks, and those on pp.

356–357, should fix the usage of "literal" sufficiently for present purposes.

The decision to rule out all but literal construals of the language of science rules out those forms of anti-realism known as *positivism* and *instrumentalism*. First, on a literal construal, the apparent statements of science really are statements, *capable of* being true or false. Secondly, although a literal construal can elaborate, it cannot change logical relationships. (It is possible to elaborate, for instance, by identifying what the terms designate. The "reduction" of the language of phenomenological thermodynamics to that of statistical mechanics is like that: Bodies of gas are identified as aggregates of molecules, temperature as mean kinetic energy, and so on.) On the positivists' interpretation of science, theoretical terms have meaning only through their connection with the observable. Hence they hold that two theories may in fact *say the same thing* although in form they contradict each other. (Perhaps the one says that all matter consists of atoms, while the other postulates instead a universal continuous medium; they will say the same thing nevertheless if they agree in their observable consequences, according to the positivists.) But two theories which contradict each other in such a way can "really" be saying the same thing only if they are not literally construed. Most specifically, if a theory says that something exists, then a literal construal may elaborate on what that something is, but will not remove the implication of existence.

There have been many critiques of positivist interpretations of science, and there is no need to repeat them. . . .

CONSTRUCTIVE EMPIRICISM

To insist on a literal construal of the language of science is to rule out the construal of a theory as a metaphor or simile, or as intelligible only after it is "demythologized" or subjected to some other sort of "translation" that does not preserve logical form. If the theory's statements include "There are electrons," then the theory says that there are electrons. If in addition they include "Electrons are not planets," then the theory says, in part, that there are entities other than planets.

But this does not settle very much. It is often not at all obvious whether a theoretical term refers to a concrete entity or a mathematical entity. Perhaps one tenable interpretation of classical physics is that there are no concrete entities which are forces—that "there are forces such that. . ." can always be understood as a mathematical statement asserting the existence of certain functions. That is debatable.

Not every philosophical position concerning science which insists on a literal construal of the language of science is a realist position. For this insistence relates not at all to our epistemic attitudes toward theories, nor to the aim we pursue in constructing theories, but only to the correct understanding of *what a theory says*. (The fundamentalist theist, the agnostic, and the atheist presumably agree with each other [though not with liberal theologians] in their understanding of the statement that God, or gods, or angels exist.) After deciding that the language of science must be literally understood, we can still say that there is no need to believe good theories to be true, nor to believe *ipso facto* that the entities they postulate are real.

Science aims to give us theories which are empirically adequate; and acceptance of a theory involves as belief only that it is empirically adequate. This is the statement of the anti-realist position I advocate; I shall call it *constructive empiricism*.

This formulation is subject to the same qualifying remarks as that of scientific realism on pp. 343–345 above. In addition it requires an explication of "empirically adequate." For now, I shall leave that with the preliminary explication that a theory is empirically adequate exactly if what it says about the observable things and events in this world is true—exactly if it "saves the phenomena." A little more precisely: Such a theory has at least one model that all the actual phenomena fit inside. I must emphasize that this refers to *all* the phenomena; these are not exhausted by those actually observed, nor even by those observed at some time, whether past, present, or future. . . .

The distinction I have drawn between realism and anti-realism, insofar as it pertains to acceptance, concerns only how much belief is involved therein. Acceptance of theories (whether full, tentative, to a degree, etc.) is a phenomenon of scientific activity which clearly involves more than belief. One main reason for this is that we are never confronted with a complete theory. So if a scientist accepts a theory, he thereby involves himself in a certain sort of research programme. That programme could well be different from the one acceptance of another theory would have given him, even if those two (very incomplete) theories are equivalent to each other with respect to everything that is observable—insofar as they go.

Thus acceptance involves not only belief but a certain commitment. Even for those of us who are not working scientists, the acceptance involves a commitment to confront any future phenomena by means of the conceptual resources of this theory. It determines the terms in which we shall seek explanations. If the acceptance is at all strong, it is exhibited in the person's assumption of the role of explainer, in his willingness to answer questions *ex cathedra*. Even if you do not accept a theory, you can engage in discourse in a context in which language use is guided by that theory—but acceptance produces such contexts. There are similarities in all of this to ideological commitment. A commitment is of course not true or false: The confidence exhibited is that it will be *vindicated*.

This is a preliminary sketch of the *pragmatic* dimension of theory acceptance. Unlike the epistemic dimension, it does not figure overtly in the disagreement between realist and anti-realist. But because the amount of belief involved in acceptance is typically less according to anti-realists, they will tend to make more of the pragmatic aspects. It is as well to note here the important difference. Belief that a theory is true, or that it is empirically adequate, does not imply, and is not implied by, belief that full acceptance of the theory will be vindicated. To see this, you need only consider here a person who has quite definite beliefs about the future of the human race, or about the scientific community and the influences thereon and practical limitations we have. It might well be, for instance, that a theory which is empirically adequate will not combine easily with some other theories which we have accepted in fact, or that Armageddon will occur before we succeed. Whether belief that a theory is true, or that it is empirically adequate, can be equated with belief that acceptance of it would, under ideal research conditions, be vindicated in the long run, is another question. It seems to me an irrelevant question within philosophy of science, because an affirmative answer would not obliterate the distinction we have already established by the preceding remarks. (The question may also assume that counterfactual statements are objectively true or false, which I would deny.)

Although it seems to me that realists and anti-realists need not disagree about the pragmatic aspects of theory acceptance, I have mentioned it here because I think that typically they do. We shall find ourselves returning time and again, for example, to requests for explanation to which realists typically attach an objective validity which anti-realists cannot grant.

The Theory/Observation "Dichotomy"

For good reasons, logical positivism dominated the philosophy of science for thirty years. In 1960, the first volume of *Minnesota Studies in the Philosophy of Science* published Rudolf Carnap's "The Methodological Status of Theoretical Concepts," which is, in many ways, the culmination of the positivist programme. It interprets science by relating it to an observation language (a postulated part of natural language which is devoid of theoretical terms).

Two years later this article was followed in the same series by Grover Maxwell's "The Ontological Status of Theoretical Entities," in title and theme a direct counter to Carnap's. This is the *locus classicus* for the new realists' contention that the theory observation distinction cannot be drawn.

I shall examine some of Maxwell's points directly, but first a general remark about the issue. Such expressions as "theoretical entity" and "observable—theoretical dichotomy" are, on the face of it, examples of category mistakes. Terms or concepts are theoretical (introduced or adapted for the purposes of theory construction); entities are observable or unobservable. This may seem a little point, but it separates the discussion into two issues. Can we divide our language into a theoretical and non-theoretical part? On the other hand, can we classify objects and events into observable and unobservable ones?

Maxwell answers both questions in the negative, while not distinguishing them too carefully. On the first, where he can draw on well-known supportive essays by Wilfrid Sellars and Paul Feyerabend, I am in total agreement. All our language is thoroughly theory-infected. If we could cleanse our language of theory-laden terms, beginning with the recently introduced ones like "VHF receiver," continuing through "mass" and "impulse" to "element" and so on into the prehistory of language formation, we would end up with nothing useful. The way we talk, and scientists talk, is guided by the pictures provided by previously accepted theories. This is true also, as Duhem already emphasized, of experimental reports. Hygienic reconstructions of language such as the positivists envisaged are simply not on. . . .

But does this mean that we must be scientific realists? We surely have more tolerance of ambiguity than that. The fact that we let our language be guided by a given picture, at some point, does not show how much we believe about that picture. When we speak of the sun coming up in the morning and setting at night, we are guided by a picture now explicitly disavowed. When Milton wrote *Paradise Lost* he deliberately let the old geocentric astronomy guide his poem, although various remarks in passing clearly reveal his interest in the new astronomical discoveries and speculations of his time. These are extreme examples, but show that no immediate conclusions can be drawn from the theory-ladenness of our language.

However, Maxwell's main arguments are directed against the observable-unobservable distinction. Let us first be clear on what this distinction was supposed to be. The term "observable" classifies putative entities (entities which may or may not exist). A flying horse is observable—that is why we are so sure that there aren't any—and the number seventeen is not. There is supposed to be a correlate classification of human acts: An unaided act of perception, for instance, is an observation. A calculation of the mass of a particle from the deflection of its trajectory in a known force field is not an observation of that mass.

It is also important here not to confuse *observing* (an entity, such as a thing, event, or process) and *observing that* (something or other is the case). Suppose one of the Stone Age people recently found in the Philippines is shown a tennis ball or a car crash. From his behavior, we see that he has noticed them; for example, he picks up the ball and throws it. But he has not seen *that* it is a tennis ball, or *that* some event is a car crash, for he does not even have those concepts. He cannot get that information through perception; he would first have to learn a great deal. To say that he does not see the same things and events as we do, however, is just silly; it is a pun which trades on the ambiguity between seeing and seeing that. (The truth-conditions for our statement "x observes *that A*" must be such that what concepts x has, presumably related to the language x speaks if he is human, enter as a variable into the correct truth definition, in some way. To say that x observed the tennis ball, therefore, does not imply at all that *x* observed that it was a tennis ball; that would require some conceptual awareness of the game of tennis.)

The arguments Maxwell gives about observability are of two sorts: one directed against the possibility of drawing such distinctions, the other against the importance that could attach to distinctions that can be drawn.

The first argument is from the continuum of cases that lie between direct observation and inference:

> there is, in principle, a continuous series beginning with looking through a vacuum and containing these as members: looking through a window-pane, looking through glasses, looking through binoculars, looking through a low-power microscope, looking through a high-power microscope, etc., in the order given. The important consequence is that, so far, we are left without criteria which would enable us to draw a non-arbitrary line between "observation" and "theory".[7]

This continuous series of supposed acts of observation does not correspond directly to a continuum in what is supposed observable. For if something can be seen through a window, it can also be seen with the window raised. Similarly, the moons of Jupiter can be seen through a telescope; but they can also be seen without a telescope if you are close enough. That something is observable does not automatically imply that the conditions are right for observing it now. The principle is:

> X is observable if there are circumstances which are such that, if X is present to us under those circumstances, then we observe it.

This is not meant as a definition, but only as a rough guide to the avoidance of fallacies.

We may still be able to find a continuum in what is supposed detectable: Perhaps some things can only be detected with the aid of an optical microscope, at least: perhaps some require an electron microscope, and so on. Maxwell's problem is: Where shall we draw the line between what is observable and what is only detectable in some more roundabout way?

Granted that we cannot answer this question without arbitrariness, what follows? That "observable" is a *vague predicate*. There are many puzzles about vague predicates, and many sophisms designed to show that, in the presence of vagueness, no distinction can be drawn at all. In Sextus Empiricus, we find the argument that incest is not immoral, for touching your mother's big toe with your little finger is not immoral, and all the rest differs only by degree. But predicates in natural language are almost all vague, and there is no problem in their use; only in formulating the logic that governs them.[8] A vague predicate is usable provided it has clear cases and clear countercases. Seeing with the unaided eye is a clear case of observation. Is Maxwell then perhaps challenging us to present a clear counter-case? Perhaps so, for he says "I have been trying to support the thesis that any (non-logical) term is a *possible* candidate for an observation term."

A look through a telescope at the moons of Jupiter seems to me a clear case of observation, since astronauts will no doubt be able to see them as well from close up. But the purported observation of micro-particles in a cloud chamber seems to me a clearly different case—if our theory about what happens there is right. The theory says that if a charged particle traverses a chamber filled with saturated vapor, some atoms in the neighborhood of its path are ionized. If this vapor is decompressed, and hence becomes supersaturated, it condenses in droplets on the ions, thus marking the path of the particle. The resulting silver-grey line is similar (physically as well as in appearance) to the vapor trail left in the sky when a jet passes. Suppose I point to such a trail and say: "Look, there is a jet!"; might you not say: "I see the vapor trail, but where is the jet?" Then I would answer: "Look just a bit ahead of the trail . . . there! Do you see it?" Now, in the case of the cloud chamber this response is not possible. So while the particle is detected by means of the cloud chamber, and the detection is based on observation, it is clearly not a case of the article's being observed.

As second argument, Maxwell directs our attention to the "can" in "what is observable is what can be observed." An object might of course be temporarily unobservable—in a rather different sense: It cannot be observed in the circumstances in which it actually is at the moment, but could be observed if the circumstances were more favorable. In just the same way, I might be temporarily invulnerable or invisible. So we should concentrate on "observable" *tout court*, or on (as he prefers to say) "unobservable in principle." This Maxwell explains as meaning that the relevant scientific theory *entails* that the entities cannot be observed in any circumstances. But this never happens, he says, because the different circumstances could be ones in which we have different sense organs—electron-microscope eyes, for instance.

This strikes me as a trick, a change in the subject of discussion. I have a mortar and pestle made of copper and weighing about a kilo. Should I call it breakable because a giant could break it? Should I call the Empire State Building portable? Is there no distinction between a portable and a console record player? The human organism is, from the point of view of physics, a certain kind of measuring apparatus. As such it has certain inherent limitations—which will be described in detail in the final physics and biology. It is these limitations to which the "able" in "observable" refers—our limitations, *qua* human beings.

As I mentioned, however, Maxwell's article also contains a different sort of argument: Even if there is a feasible observable/unobservable distinction, this distinction has no importance. The point at issue for the realist is, after all, the reality of the entities postulated in science. Suppose that these entities could be classified into observable and others; what relevance should that have to the question of their existence?

Logically, none. For the term "observable" classifies putative entities and has logically nothing to do with existence. But Maxwell must have more in mind when he says: "I conclude that the drawing of the observational–theoreti-

cal line at any given point is an accident and a function of our physiological make-up, . . . and, therefore, that it has no ontological significance whatever."[9] No ontological significance if the question is only whether "observable" and "exists" imply each other—for they do not; but significance for the question of scientific realism?

Recall I defined scientific realism in terms of the aim of science and epistemic attitudes. The question is what aim scientific activity has, and how much we shall believe when we accept a scientific theory. What is the proper form of acceptance: belief that the theory, as a whole, is true; or something else? To this question, what is observable by us seems eminently relevant. Indeed, we may attempt an answer at this point: To accept a theory is (for us) to believe that it is empirically adequate—that what the theory says *about what is observable* (by us) is true.

It will be objected at once that, on this proposal, what the anti-realist decides to believe about the world will depend in part on what he believes to be his, or rather the epistemic community's, accessible range of evidence. At present, we count the human race as the epistemic community to which we belong; but this race may mutate, or that community may be increased by adding other animals (terrestrial or extra-terrestrial) through relevant ideological or moral decisions ("to count them as persons"). Hence the anti-realist would, on my proposal, have to accept conditions of the form

> If the epistemic community changes in fashion Υ, then my beliefs about the world will change in manner Z.

To see this as an objection to anti-realism is to voice the requirement that our epistemic policies should give the same results independent of our beliefs about the range of evidence accessible to us. That requirement seems to me in no way rationally compelling; it could be honored, I should think, only through a thoroughgoing scepticism or through a commitment to wholesale leaps of faith. But we cannot settle the major questions of epistemology *en passant* in philosophy of science; so I shall just conclude that it is, on the face of it, not irrational to commit oneself only to a search for theories that are empirically adequate, ones whose models fit the observable phenomena, while recognizing that what counts as an observable phenomenon is a function of what the epistemic community is (that *observable* is *observable-to-us*).

The notion of empirical adequacy in this answer will have to be spelled out very carefully if it is not to bite the dust among hackneyed objections. . . . But the point stands: Even if observability has nothing to do with existence (is, indeed, too anthropocentric for that), it may still have much to do with the proper epistemic attitude to science.

Inference to the Best Explanation

A view advanced in different ways by Wilfrid Sellars, J.J.C. Smart, and Gilbert Harman is that the canons of rational inference require scientific realism. If we are to follow the same patterns of inference with respect to this issue as we do in science itself, we shall find ourselves irrational unless we assert the truth of the scientific theories we accept. Thus Sellars says: "As I see it, to have good reason for holding a theory is *ipso facto* to have good reason for holding that the entities postulated by the theory exist."[10]

The main rule of inference invoked in arguments of this sort is the rule of *inference to the best explanation*. The idea is perhaps to be credited to C. S. Peirce,[11] but the main recent attempts to explain this rule and its uses have been made by Gilbert Harman.[12] I shall only present a simplified version. Let us suppose that we have evidence *E,* and are considering several hypotheses, say *H* and *H'*. The rule then says that we should infer *H* rather than *H'* exactly if *H* is a better explanation of *E* than *H'* is. (Various qualifications are necessary to avoid inconsistency: We should always try to move to the best overall explanation of all available evidence.)

It is argued that we follow this rule in all "ordinary" cases; and that if we follow it consistently everywhere, we shall be led to scientific realism, in the way Sellars's dictum suggests. And surely there are many telling "ordinary" cases: I hear scratching in the wall, the patter of little feet at midnight, my cheese disappears— and I infer that a mouse has come to live with me. Not merely that these apparent signs of mousely presence will continue, not merely that all the observable phenomena will be as if there is a mouse, but that there really is a mouse.

Will this pattern of inference also lead us to belief in unobservable entities? Is the scientific realist simply someone who consistently follows the rules of inference that we all follow in more mundane contexts? I have two objections to the idea that this is so.

First of all, what is meant by saying that we all *follow* a certain rule of inference? One meaning might be that we deliberately and consciously "apply" the rule, like a student doing a logic exercise. That meaning is much too literalistic and restrictive; surely all of mankind follows the rules of logic much of the time, while only a fraction can even formulate them. A second meaning is that we act in accordance with the rules in a sense that does not require conscious deliberation. That is not so easy to make precise, since each logical rule is a rule of permission (*modus ponens* allows you to infer *B* from *A* and (if *A* then *B*), but does not forbid you to infer (*B or A*) instead). However, we might say that a person behaved in accordance with a set of rules in that sense if every conclusion he drew could be reached from his premises via those rules. But this meaning is much too loose; in this sense we always behave in accordance with the rule that any conclusion may be inferred from any premise. So it seems that to be following a rule, I must be willing to believe all conclusions it allows, while definitely unwilling to believe conclusions at variance with the ones it allows—or else, change my willingness to believe the premises in question.

Therefore the statement that we all follow a certain rule in certain cases is a *psychological hypothesis* about what we are willing and unwilling to do. It is an empirical hypothesis, to be confronted with data, and with rival hypotheses. Here is a rival hypothesis: We are always willing to believe that the theory which best explains the evidence is empirically adequate (that all the observable phenomena are as the theory says they are).

In this way I can certainly account for the many instances in which a scientist appears to argue for the acceptance of a theory or hypothesis on the basis of its explanatory success. (A number of such instances are related by Thagard.[13]) For, remember: I equate the acceptance of a scientific theory with the belief that it is empirically adequate. We have therefore two rival hypotheses concerning these instances of scientific inference, and the one is apt in a realist account, the other in an anti-realist account.

Cases like the mouse in the wainscoting cannot provide telling evidence between those rival hypotheses. For the mouse *is* an observable thing; therefore "there is a mouse in the wainscoting" and "All observable phenomena are as if there is a mouse in the wainscoting" are totally equivalent; each implies the other (given what we know about mice).

It will be countered that it is less interesting to know whether people do follow a rule of inference than whether they ought to follow it. Granted; but the premise that we all follow the rule of inference to the best explanation when it comes to mice and other mundane matters—that premise is shown wanting. It is not warranted by the evidence, because that evidence is not telling *for* the premise *as against* the alternative hypothesis I proposed, which is a relevant one in this context.

My second objection is that even if we were to grant the correctness (or worthiness) of the rule of inference to the best explanation, the realist needs some further premise for his argument. For this rule is only one that dictates a choice when given a set of rival hypotheses. In other words, we need to be committed to belief in one of a range of hypotheses before the rule can be applied. Then, under favorable circum-

stances, it will tell us which of the hypotheses in that range to choose. The realist asks us to choose between different hypotheses that explain the regularities in certain ways; but his opponent always wishes to choose among hypotheses of the form "theory *T* is empirically adequate." So the realist will need his special extra premise that every universal regularity in nature needs an explanation before the rule will make realists of us all. And that is just the premise that distinguishes the realist from his opponents (and which I shall examine in more detail . . . below). . . .

I have kept this discussion quite abstract; but more concrete arguments by Sellars, Smart, and Putnam will be examined below. It should at least be clear that there is no open-and-shut argument from common sense to the unobservable. Merely following the ordinary patterns of inference in science does not obviously and automatically make realists of us all.

Limits of the Demand for Explanation

In this section and the next . . . , I shall examine arguments for realism that point to explanatory power as a criterion for theory choice. That this is indeed a criterion I do not deny. But these arguments for realism succeed only if the demand for explanation is supreme—if the task of science is unfinished, *ipso facto*, as long as any pervasive regularity is left unexplained. I shall object to this line of argument, as found in the writings of Smart, Reichenbach, Salmon, and Sellars, by arguing that such an unlimited demand for explanation leads to a demand for hidden variables, which runs contrary to at least one major school of thought in twentieth-century physics. I do not think that even these philosophers themselves wish to saddle realism with logical links to such consequences; but realist yearnings were born among the mistaken ideals of traditional metaphysics.

In his book *Between Science and Philosophy*, Smart gives two main arguments for realism. One is that only realism can respect the important distinction between *correct* and *merely useful* theories. He calls "instrumentalist" any view that locates the importance of theories in their use, which requires only empirical adequacy and not truth. But how can the instrumentalist explain the usefulness of his theories?

> Consider a man (in the sixteenth century) who is a realist about the Copernican hypothesis but instrumentalist about the Ptolemaic one. He can explain the instrumental usefulness of the Ptolemaic system of epicycles because he can prove that the Ptolemaic system can produce almost the same predictions about the apparent motions of the planets as does the Copernican hypothesis. Hence the assumption of the realist truth of the Copernican hypothesis explains the instrumental usefulness of the Ptolemaic one. Such an explanation of the instrumental usefulness of certain theories would not be possible if *all* theories were regarded as merely instrumental.[14]

What exactly is meant by "such an explanation" in the last sentence? If no theory is assumed to be true, then no theory has its usefulness explained as following from the truth of another one—granted. But would we have less of an explanation of the usefulness of the Ptolemaic hypothesis if we began instead with the premise that the Copernican gives implicitly a very accurate description of the motions of the planets as observed from earth? This would not assume the truth of Copernicus's heliocentric hypothesis, but would still entail that Ptolemy's simpler description was also a close approximation of those motions.

However, Smart would no doubt retort that such a response pushes the question only one step back: What explains the accuracy of predictions based on Copernicus's theory? If I say, the empirical adequacy of that theory, I have merely given a verbal explanation. For of course Smart does not mean to limit his question to actual predictions—it really concerns all actual and possible predictions and retrodictions. To put it quite concretely: What explains the fact that all observable planetary phenomena fit Copernicus's theory (if they do)? From the medieval de-

bates, we recall the nominalist response that the basic regularities are merely brute regularities and have no explanation. So here the anti-realist must similarly say: That the observable phenomena exhibit these regularities, because of which they fit the theory, is merely a brute fact, and may or may not have an explanation in terms of unobservable facts "behind the phenomena"—it really does not matter to the goodness of the theory, nor to our understanding of the world.

Smart's main line of argument is addressed to exactly this point. In the same chapter he argues as follows. Suppose that we have a theory T which postulates micro-structure directly, and macrostructure indirectly. The statistical and approximate laws about macroscopic phenomena are only partially spelled out perhaps, and in any case derive from the precise (deterministic or statistical) laws about the basic entities. We now consider theory T', which is part of T, and says only what T says about the macroscopic phenomena. (How T' should be characterized I shall leave open, for that does not affect the argument here.) Then he continues:

> I would suggest that the realist could (say) . . . that the success of T' is explained by the fact that the original theory T is true of the things that it is ostensibly about; in other words by the fact that there really are electrons or whatever is postulated by the theory T. If there were no such things, and if T were not true in a realist way, would not the success of T' be quite inexplicable? One would have to suppose that there were innumerable lucky accidents about the behavior mentioned in the observational vocabulary, so that they behaved miraculously as *if* they were brought about by the nonexistent things ostensibly talked about in the theoretical vocabulary.[15]

In other passages, Smart speaks similarly of "cosmic coincidences." The regularities in the observable phenomena must be explained in terms of deeper structure, for otherwise we are left with a belief in lucky accidents and coincidences on a cosmic scale.

I submit that if the demand for explanation

implicit in these passages were precisely formulated, it would at once lead to absurdity. For if the mere fact of postulating regularities, without explanation, makes T' a poor theory, T will do no better. If, on the other hand, there is some precise limitation on what sorts of regularities can be postulated as basic, the context of the argument provides no reason to think that T' must automatically fare worse than T.

In any case, it seems to me that it is illegitimate to equate being a lucky accident, or a coincidence, with having no explanation. It was by coincidence that I met my friend in the market—but I can explain why I was there, and he can explain why he came, so together we can explain how this meeting happened. We call it a coincidence, not because the occurrence was inexplicable, but because we did not severally go to the market in order to meet.[16] There cannot be a requirement upon science to provide a theoretical elimination of coincidences, or accidental correlations in general, for that does not even make sense. There is nothing here to motivate the demand for explanation, only a restatement in persuasive terms. . . .

Limits to Explanation: A Thought Experiment

Wilfrid Sellars was one of the leaders of the return to realism in philosophy of science and has, in his writings of the past three decades, developed a systematic and coherent scientific realism. I have discussed a number of his views and arguments elsewhere; but will here concentrate on some aspects that are closely related to the arguments of Smart, Reichenbach, and Salmon just examined.[17] Let me begin by setting the stage in the way Sellars does.

There is a certain oversimplified picture of science, the "levels picture," which pervades positivist writings and which Sellars successfully demolished.[18] In that picture, singular observable facts ("this crow is black") are scientifically explained by general observable regularities ("all crows are black"), which in turn are explained by highly theoretical hypotheses not restricted in what they say to the observable. The three levels are commonly called those of *fact*, of *empirical law*, and of *theory*. But, as Sellars points out, theories do not explain, or even entail such empirical laws—they only show why observable things obey these so-called laws to the extent they do.[19] Indeed, perhaps we have no such empirical laws at all: All crows are black—except albinos; water boils at 100°C—provided atmospheric pressure is normal; a falling body accelerates—provided it is not intercepted, or attached to an aeroplane by a static line; and so forth. On the level of the observable we are liable to find only putative laws heavily subject to unwritten *ceteris paribus* qualifications.

This is, so far, only a methodological point. We do not really expect theories to "save" our common everyday generalizations, for we ourselves have no confidence in their strict universality. But a theory which says that the microstructure of things is subject to *some* exact, universal regularities must imply the same for those things themselves. This, at least, is my reaction to the points so far. Sellars, however, sees an inherent inferiority in the description of the observable alone, an incompleteness which requires (*sub specie* the aims of science) an introduction of an unobservable reality behind the phenomena. This is brought out by an interesting "thought-experiment."

Imagine that at some early stage of chemistry it had been found that different samples of gold dissolve in *aqua regia* at different rates, although "as far as can be observationally determined, the specimens and circumstances are identical."[20] Imagine further that the response of chemistry to this problem was to postulate two distinct micro-structures for the different samples of gold. Observationally unpredictable variation in the rate of dissolution is explained by saying that the samples are mixtures (not compounds) of these two (observationally identical) substances, each of which has a fixed rate of dissolution.

In this case we have explanation through laws

which have no observational counterparts that can play the same role. Indeed, no explanation seems possible unless we agree to find our physical variables outside the observable. But science aims to explain, must try to explain, and so must require a belief in this unobservable micro-structure. So Sellars contends.

There are at least three questions before us. Did this postulation of micro-structure really have no new consequences for the observable phenomena? Is there really such a demand upon science that it must explain—even if the means of explanation bring no gain in empirical predictions? And thirdly, could a *different* rationale exist for the use of a micro-structure picture in the development of a scientific theory in a case like this?

First, it seems to me that these hypothetical chemists did postulate new observable regularities as well. Suppose the two substances are A and B, with dissolving rates x and $x + y$ and that every gold sample is a mixture of these substances. Then it follows that every gold sample dissolves at a rate no lower than x and no higher than $x + y$; *and* that between these two any value may be found—to within the limits of accuracy of gold mixing. None of this is implied by the data that different samples of gold have dissolved at various rates between x and $x + y$. So Sellars's first contention is false.

We may assume, for the sake of Sellars's example, that there is still no way of predicting dissolving rates any further. Is there then a categorical demand upon science to explain this variation which does not depend on other observable factors? . . . [A] precise version of such a demand (Reichenbach's principle of the common cause) could result automatically in a demand for hidden variables, providing a "classical" underpinning for indeterministic theories. Sellars recognized very well that a demand for hidden variables would run counter to the main opinions current in quantum physics. Accordingly he mentions ". . . the familiar point that the irreducibly and lawfully statistical ensembles

of quantum-mechanical theory are mathematically inconsistent with the assumption of hidden variables."[21] Thus, he restricts the demand for explanation, in effect, to just those cases where it is *consistent* to add hidden variables to the theory. And consistency is surely a logical stopping point.

This restriction unfortunately does not prevent the disaster. For while there are a number of proofs that hidden variables cannot be supplied so as to turn quantum mechanics into a classical sort of deterministic theory, those proofs are based on requirements much stronger than consistency. To give an example, one such assumption is that two distinct physical variables cannot have the same statistical distributions in measurement on all possible states.[22] Thus it is assumed that, if we cannot point to some possible difference in empirical predictions, then there is no real difference at all. If such requirements were lifted, and consistency alone were the criterion, hidden variables could indeed be introduced. I think we must conclude that science, in contrast to scientific realism, does not place an overriding value on explanation in the absence of any gain for empirical results.

Thirdly, then, let us consider how an anti-realist could make sense of those hypothetical chemists' procedure. After pointing to the new empirical implications which I mentioned two paragraphs ago, he would point to methodological reasons. By imagining a certain sort of micro-structure for gold and other metals, say, we might arrive at a theory governing many observationally disparate substances; and this might then have implications for new, wider empirical regularities when such substances interact. This would only be a hope, of course; no hypothesis is guaranteed to be fruitful—but the point is that the true demand on science is not for explanation *as such*, but for imaginative pictures which have a hope of suggesting new statements of observable regularities and of correcting old ones. . . .

. . . The Ultimate Argument

. . . In . . . "What is Mathematical Truth," Putnam . . . gives what I shall call the *Ultimate Argument*. He begins with a formulation of realism which he says he learned from Michael Dummett:

> A realist (with respect to a given theory or discourse) holds that (1) the sentences of that theory are true or false; and (2) that what makes them true or false is something external—that is to say, it is not (in general) our sense data, actual or potential, or the structure of our minds, or our language, etc.[23]

This formulation is quite different from the one I have given even if we instantiate it to the case in which that theory or discourse is science or scientific discourse. Because the wide discussion of Dummett's views has given some currency to his usage of these terms, and because Putnam begins his discussion in this way, we need to look carefully at this formulation.

In my view, Dummett's usage is quite idiosyncratic. Putnam's statement, though very brief, is essentially accurate. In his "Realism," Dummett begins by describing various sorts of realism in the traditional fashion, as disputes over whether there really exist entities of a particular type. But he says that in some cases he wishes to discuss, such as the reality of the past and intuitionism in mathematics, the central issues seem to him to be about other questions. For this reason he proposes a new usage: He will take such disputes

> as relating, not to a class of entities or a class of terms, but to a class of *statements* . . . . Realism I characterize as the belief that statements of the disputed class possess an objective truth-value, independently of our means of knowing it: They are true or false in virtue of a reality existing independently of us. The anti-realist opposes to this the view that statements of the disputed class are to be understood only by reference to the sort of thing which we count as evidence for a statement of that class.[24]

Dummett himself notes at once that nominalists are realists in this sense.[25] If, for example, you say that abstract entities do not exist, and sets are abstract entities, hence sets do not exist, then you will certainly accord a truth-value to all statements of set theory. It might be objected that if you take this position then you have a decision procedure for determining the truth-values of these statements (*false* for existentially quantified ones, *true* for universal ones, apply truth tables for the rest). Does that not mean that, on your view, the truth-values are not independent of our knowledge? Not at all; for you clearly believe that if we had not existed, and a *fortiori* had had no knowledge, the state of affairs with respect to abstract entities would be the same.

Has Dummett perhaps only laid down a necessary condition for realism, in his definition, for the sake of generality? I do not think so. In discussions of quantum mechanics we come across the view that the particles of microphysics are real and obey the principles of the theory, but at any time t when "particle x has exact momentum p" is true then "particle x has position q" is neither true nor false. In any traditional sense, this is a realist position with respect to quantum mechanics.

We note also that Dummett has, at least in this passage, taken no care to exclude non-literal construals of the theory, as long as they are truth-valued. The two are not the same; when Strawson construed "The king of France in 1905 is bald" as neither true nor false, he was not giving a nonliteral construal of our language. On the other hand, people tend to fall back on non-literal construals typically in order to be able to say, "properly construed, the theory is true."

Perhaps Dummett is right in his assertion that what is really at stake, in realist disputes of various sorts, is questions about language—or, if not really at stake, at least the only serious philosophical problems in those neighborhoods. Certainly the arguments in which he engages are profound, serious, and worthy of our attention. But it seems to me that his terminology ill accords with the traditional one. Certainly I wish to define scientific realism so that it need not imply that all statements in the theoretical language are true or false (only that they are all capable of being true or false, that is, there are conditions for each under which it has a truth-value); to imply also that the aim at least is that the theories should be true. And the contrary position of constructive empiricism is not anti-realist in Dummett's sense, since it also assumes scientific statements to have truth-conditions entirely independent of human activity or knowledge. But then, I do not conceive the dispute as being about language at all.

In any case Putnam himself does not stick with this weak formulation of Dummett's. A little later in the paper he directs himself to scientific realism *per se*, and formulates it in terms borrowed, he says, from Richard Boyd. The new formulation comes in the course of a new argument for scientific realism, which I shall call the Ultimate Argument:

> the positive argument for realism is that it is the only philosophy that doesn't make the success of science a miracle. That terms in mature scientific theories typically refer (this formulation is due to Richard Boyd), that the theories accepted in a mature science are typically approximately true, that the same term can refer to the same thing even when it occurs in different theories—these statements are viewed by the scientific realist not as necessary truths but as part of the only scientific explanation of the success of science, and hence as part of any adequate scientific description of science and its relations to its objects.[26]

Science, apparently, is required to explain its own success. There is this regularity in the world, that scientific predictions are regularly fulfilled; and this regularity, too, needs an explanation. Once *that* is supplied we may perhaps hope to have reached the *terminus de jure*?

The explanation provided is a very traditional one—*adequatio ad rem*, the "adequacy" of the theory to its objects, a kind of mirroring of the structure of things by the structure of ideas—Aquinas would have felt quite at home with it.

Well, let us accept for now this demand for a scientific explanation of the success of science. Let us also resist construing it as merely a restatement of Smart's "cosmic coincidence" argument, and view it instead as the question why we have successful scientific theories at all. Will this realist explanation with the Scholastic look be a scientifically acceptable answer? I would like to point out that science is a biological phenomenon, an activity by one kind of organism which facilitates its interaction with the environment. And this makes me think that a very different kind of scientific explanation is required.

I can best make the point by contrasting two accounts of the mouse who runs from its enemy, the cat. St. Augustine already remarked on this phenomenon, and provided an intensional explanation: The mouse *perceives that* the cat is its enemy, hence the mouse runs. What is postulated here is the "adequacy" of the mouse's thought to the order of nature: The relation of enmity is correctly reflected in his mind. But the Darwinist says: Do not ask why the *mouse* runs from its enemy. Species which did not cope with their natural enemies no longer exist. That is why there are only ones who do.

In just the same way, I claim that the success of current scientific theories is no miracle. It is not even surprising to the scientific (Darwinist) mind. For any scientific theory is born into a life of fierce competition, a jungle red in tooth and claw. Only the successful theories survive—the ones which *in fact* latched on to actual regularities in nature.[27]

NOTES

1. *Science, Perception and Reality* (New York: Humanities Press, 1962); cf. the footnote on p. 97. See also my review of his *Studies in Philosophy and its History*, in *Annals of Science*, January 1977.
2. Brian Ellis, *Rational Belief Systems* (Oxford: Blackwell, 1979), p. 28.
3. Hilary Putnam, *Mathematics, Matter and Method* (Cambridge: Cambridge University Press, 1975), Vol. 1, pp. 69f.

4. Putnam, op. cit., p. 73, n. 29. The argument is reportedly developed at greater length in Boyd's forthcoming book *Realism and Scientific Epistemology* (Cambridge University Press).

5. Hartry Field has suggested that "acceptance of a scientific theory involves the belief that it is true" be replaced by "any reason to think that any part of a theory is not, or might not be, true, is reason not to accept it." The drawback of this alternative is that it leaves open what epistemic attitude acceptance of a theory does involve. This question must also be answered, and as long as we are talking about full acceptance—as opposed to tentative or partial or otherwise qualified acceptance—I cannot see how a realist could do other than equate that attitude with full belief. (That theories believed to be false are used for practical problems, for example, classical mechanics for orbiting satellites, is of course a commonplace.) For if the aim is truth, and acceptance requires belief that the aim is served . . . I should also mention the statement of realism at the beginning of Richard Boyd, "Realism, Underdetermination, and a Causal Theory of Evidence," *Noûs*, 7 (1973), 1–12. Except for some doubts about his use of the terms *explanation* and *causal relation* I intend my statement of realism to be entirely in accordance with his. Finally, see C. A. Hooker, "Systematic Realism," *Synthese*, **26** (1974), 409–97; esp. pp. 409 and 426.

6. More typical of realism, it seems to me, is the sort of epistemology found in Clark Glymour's book, *Theory and Evidence* (Princeton: Princeton University Press, 1980), except of course that there it is fully and carefully developed in one specific fashion. (See esp. his chapter "Why I Am Not a Bayesian" for the present issue.) But I see no reason why a realist, as such, could not be a Bayesian of the type of Richard Jeffrey, even if the Bayesian position has in the past been linked with anti-realist and even instrumentalist views in philosophy of science.

7. G. Maxwell, "The Ontological Status of Theoretical Entities." *Minnesota Studies in Philosophy of Science*, III (1962), p. 7.

8. There is a great deal of recent work on the logic of vague predicates: especially important, to my mind, is that of Kit Fine ("Vagueness, Truth, and Logic." *Synthese*, **30** [1975] 265–300) and Hans Kamp. The latter is currently working on a new theory of vagueness that does justice to the "vagueness of vagueness" and the context-dependence of standards of applicability for predicates.

9. Op. cit., p. 15. . . . At this point . . . I may be suspected of relying on modal distinctions which I criticize elsewhere. After all, I am making a distinction between human limitations and accidental factors. A certain apple was dropped into the sea in a bag of refuse, which sank; relative to that information it is necessary that no one ever observed the apple's core. That information, however, concerns an accident of history, and so it is not human limitations that rule out observation of the apple core. But unless I assert that some facts humans are essential, or physically necessary, and others accidental, how can I make sense of this distinction? This question raises the difficulty of a philosophical retrenchment for modal language. This I believe to be possible through an ascent to pragmatics. In the present case, the answer would be, to speak very roughly, that the scientific theories we accept are a determining factor for the set of features of the human organism counted among the limitations to which we refer in using the term "observable."

10. See n. 1 above.

11. Cf. P. Thagard, doctoral dissertation, University of Toronto, 1977, and "The Best Explanation: Criteria for Theory Choice." *Journal of Philosophy*, **75** (1978), 76–92.

12. "The Inference to the Best Explanation." *Philosophical Review*, **74** (1965), 88–95 and "Knowledge, Inference, and Explanation." *American Philosophical Quarterly*, **5** (1968), 164–73. Harman's views were further developed in subsequent publications (*Nous*, 1967; *Journal of Philosophy*, 1968; in M. Swain (ed.), *Induction*, 1970; in H.-N. Castañeda (ed.), *Action, Thought, and Reality*, 1975; and in his book *Thought*, Ch. 10). I shall not consider these further developments here.

13. See n. 11 above.

14. J. J. C. Smart, *Between Science and Philosophy* (New York: Random House, 1968), p. 151.

15. Ibid., pp. 150f.

16. This point is clearly made by Aristotle, *Physics*, II, Chs. 4–6 (see esp. 196^a 1–20; 196^b 20–197^a 12).

17. See my "Wilfrid Sellars on Scientific Realism," *Dialogue*, **14** (1975). 606–16; W. Sellars, "Is Scientific Realism Tenable?" pp. 307–34 in F. Suppe and P. Asquith (eds.), *PSA 1976* (East Lansing, Mich.: Philosophy of Science Association, 1977), vol. II, 307–34; and my "On the Radical Incompleteness of the Manifest Image," ibid., 335–43; and see n. 1 above.

18. W. Sellars. "The Language of Theories," in his *Science, Perception and Reality* (London: Routledge and Regan Paul, 1963).

19. Op. cit., p. 121.

20. Ibid., p. 121.

21. Ibid., p. 123.

22. See my "Semantic Analysis of Quantum Logic," in C. A. Hooker (ed.), *Contemporary Research in the Foundations and Philosophy of Quantum Theory*

(Dordrecht: Reidel, 1973), Part III, Sects. 5 and 6.

23. See n. 3 above.

24. Michael Dummett, *Truth and Other Enigmas* (Cambridge, Mass., Harvard University Press, 1978), p. 146 (see also pp. 358–61).

25. Dummett adds to the cited passage that he realizes that his characterization does not include all the disputes he had mentioned, and specifically excepts nominalism about abstract entities. However, he includes scientific realism as an example (op cit., pp. 146f.).

26. See n. 4 above.

27. Of course, we can ask specifically why the *mouse* is one of the surviving species. How *it* survives, and answer this, on the basis of whatever scientific theory we accept, in terms of its brain and environment. The analogous question for theories would be why, say, Balmer's formula for the line spectrum of hydrogen survives as a successful hypothesis. In that case too we explain, on the basis of the physics we accept now, why the spacing of those lines satisfies the formula. Both the question and the answer are very different from the global question of the success of science, and the global answer of realism. The realist may now make the *further* objection that the anti-realist cannot answer the question about the mouse specifically, nor the one about Balmer's formula, in this fashion, since the answer is in part an assertion that the scientific theory, used as basis of the explanation, is true. This is a quite different argument, which I . . . take up in Ch. 4, Sect. 4, and Ch. 5 [of *The Scientific Image*].

In his most recent publications and lectures Hilary Putnam has drawn a distinction between two doctrines, metaphysical realism and internal realism. He denies the former and identifies his preceding scientific realism as the latter. While I have at present no commitment to either side of the metaphysical dispute, I am very much in sympathy with the critique of Platonism in philosophy of mathematics, which forms part of Putnam's arguments. Our disagreement about scientific (internal) realism would remain, of course, whenever we came down to earth after deciding to agree or disagree about metaphysical realism, or even about whether this distinction makes sense at all.

Dissecting the Holist Picture of Scientific Change

Larry Laudan

It is now more than twenty years since the appearance of Thomas Kuhn's *The Structure of Scientific Revolutions*. For many of us entering the field two decades ago, that book made a powerful difference. Not because we fully understood it; still less because we became converts to it. It mattered, rather, because it posed in a particularly vivid form some direct challenges to the empiricism we were learning from the likes of Hempel, Nagel, Popper, and Carnap.

Philosophers of science of that era had no doubts about whom and what the book was attacking. If Kuhn was right, all the then-reigning methodological orthodoxies were simply wrong. It was a good deal less clear what Kuhn's positive message amounted to, and not entirely because many of Kuhn's philosophical readers were too shocked to read him carefully. Was he saying that theories were really and always incommensurable so that rival scientists invariably misunderstood one another, or did he mean it when he said that the problem-solving abilities of rival theories could be objectively compared? Did he really believe that accepting a new theory was a "conversion experience," subject only to the Gestalt-like exigencies of the religious

life? In the first wave of reaction to Kuhn's bombshell, answers to such questions were not easy to find.

Since 1962 most of Kuhn's philosophical writings have been devoted to clearing up some of the ambiguities and confusions generated by the language of the first edition of *The Structure of Scientific Revolutions*. By and large, Kuhn's message has been an ameliorative and conciliatory one, to such an extent that some passages in his later writings make him sound like a closet positivist. More than one commentator has accused the later Kuhn of taking back much of what made his message interesting and provocative in the first place.[1]

But that is not entirely fair, for if many of Kuhn's clarifications have indeed taken the sting out of what we once thought Kuhn's position was, there are several issues about which the later Kuhn is both clear *and* controversial. Significantly, several of those are central to the themes of this essay . . . .

Kuhn, then, will be my immediate target, but I would be less than candid if I did not quickly add that the views I discuss here have spread considerably beyond the Kuhnian corpus. To some degree, almost all of us who wrote about scientific change in the 1970s (present company included) fell prey to some of the confusions I describe. In trying to characterize the mechanisms of theory change, we have tended to lapse into sloppy language for describing change. However, because Kuhn's is the best-known ac-

From Chapter 4 of *Science and Values: An Essay on the Aims of Science and Their Role in Scientific Debate* by Larry Laudan (1984), pp. 67–102, 141–144. Reprinted by permission of the Regents of the University of California and the University of California Press. © 1984, The Regents of the University of California.

count of scientific change, and because Kuhn most overtly makes several of the mistakes I want to discuss, this chapter focuses chiefly on his views. Similar criticisms can be raised with varying degrees of severity against authors as diverse as Foucault, Lakatos, Toulmin, Holton, and Laudan.

Kuhn on the Units of Scientific Change

It is notorious that the key Kuhnian concept of a paradigm is multiply ambiguous. Among its most central meanings are the following three: First and foremost, a paradigm offers a conceptual framework for classifying and explaining natural objects. That is, it specifies in a generic way the sorts of entities that are thought to populate a certain domain of experience and it sketches out how those entities generally interact. In short, every paradigm will make certain claims about what populates the world. Such ontological claims mark that paradigm off from others, since each paradigm is thought to postulate entities and modes of interaction which differentiate it from other paradigms. Second, a paradigm will specify the appropriate methods, techniques, and tools of inquiry for studying the objects in the relevant domain of application. Just as different paradigms have different ontologies, so they involve substantially different methodologies. (Consider, for instance, the very different methods of research and theory evaluation associated with behaviorism and cognitive psychology respectively.) These methodological commitments are persistent ones, and they characterize the paradigm throughout its history. Finally, the proponents of different paradigms will, according to Kuhn, espouse different sets of cognitive goals or ideals. Although the partisans of two paradigms may (and usually do) share some aims in common, Kuhn insists that the goals are not fully overlapping between followers of rival paradigms. Indeed, to accept a paradigm is, for Kuhn, to subscribe to a complex of cognitive values which the proponents of no other paradigm accept fully.

Paradigm change, on this account, clearly represents a break of great magnitude. To trade in one paradigm for another is to involve oneself in changes at each of . . . three levels . . . : We give up one ontology for another, one methodology for another, and one set of cognitive goals for another. Moreover, according to Kuhn, this change is *simultaneous* rather than *sequential*. . . .

. . . Kuhn portrays paradigm changes in ways that make them seem to be abrupt and global ruptures in the life of a scientific community. So great is this supposed transition that several of Kuhn's critics have charged that, despite Kuhn's proclaimed intentions to the contrary, his analysis inevitably turns scientific change into a nonrational or irrational process. In part, but only in part, it is Kuhn's infelicitous terminology that produces this impression. Notoriously, he speaks of the acceptance of a new paradigm as a "conversion experience,"[2] conjuring up a picture of the scientific revolutionary as a born-again Christian, long on zeal and short on argument. At other times he likens paradigm change to an "irreversible Gestalt-shift."[3] Less metaphorically, he claims that there is never a point at which it is "unreasonable" to hold onto an old paradigm rather than to accept a new one.[4] Such language does not encourage one to imagine that paradigm change is exactly the result of a careful and deliberate weighing-up of the respective strengths of rival contenders. But impressions based on some of Kuhn's more lurid language can probably be rectified by cleaning up some of the vocabulary of *The Structure of Scientific Revolutions*, a task on which Kuhn has been embarked more or less since the book first appeared.[5] No changes of terminology, however, will alter the fact that some central features of Kuhn's model of science raise serious roadblocks to a rational analysis of scientific change. The bulk of this chapter is devoted to examining some of those impediments. Before we turn to that examination, however, I want to stress early on that my complaint with Kuhn is not merely that he has failed to give any normatively robust or rational account of theory change, serious as that failing is. As I show below, he has failed even at the descriptive or narrative task of offering an accurate story about the manner in which large-scale changes of scientific allegiance occur.

But there is a yet more fundamental respect in which Kuhn's approach presents obstacles to an understanding of the dynamics of theory change. Specifically, by insisting that individual paradigms have an integral and static character—that changes take place only between, rather than within, paradigms—Kuhn has missed the single feature of science which promises to mediate and rationalize the transition from one world view or paradigm to another. Kuhn's various writings on this subject leave the reader in no doubt that he thinks the parts of a paradigm go together as an inseparable package. As he puts it in *The Structure of Scientific Revolutions*, "In learning a paradigm the scientist acquires theory, methods, and standards together, usually in an *inextricable* mix."[6] This theme of the inextricable and inseparable ingredients of a paradigm is a persistent one in Kuhn's work. One key aim of this chapter is to show how drastically we need to alter Kuhn's views about how tightly the pieces of a paradigm's puzzle fit together before we can expect to understand how paradigmlike change occurs.

LOOSENING UP THE FIT

Without too heavy an element of caricature, we can describe world-view models such as Kuhn's along the following lines: One group or faction in the scientific community accepts a particular "big picture." That requires acquiescence in a certain ontology of nature, acceptance of a specific set of rules about how to investigate nature, and adherence to a set of cognitive values about the teleology of natural inquiry (i.e., about the goals that science seeks). On this analysis, large-scale scientific change involves the replacement of one such world view by another, a process that entails the simultaneous repudiation of the key elements of the old picture and the adoption

of corresponding (but of course different) elements of the new. In short, scientific change looks something like Figure 9-1.

When scientific change is construed so globally, it is no small challenge to see how it could be other than a conversion experience. If different scientists not only espouse different theories but also subscribe to different standards of appraisal and ground those standards in different and conflicting systems of cognitive goals, then it is difficult indeed to imagine that scientific change could be other than a whimsical change of style or taste. There could apparently never be compelling grounds for saying that one paradigm is better than another, for one has to ask: Better relative to which standards and whose goals? To make matters worse—much worse—Kuhn often suggested that each paradigm is more or less automatically guaranteed to satisfy its own standards and to fail the standards of rival paradigms, thus producing a kind of self-reinforcing solipsism in science. As he once put it, "To the extent, as significant as it is incomplete, that two scientific schools disagree about what is a problem and what is a solution, they will inevitably talk through each other when debating the merits of their respective paradigms. In the partially circular arguments that regularly result, *each* paradigm will be shown to satisfy more or less the criteria that it dictates for itself and to fall short of those dictated by its opponent."[7] Anyone who writes prose of this sort must think that scientific decision-making is fundamentally capricious. Or at least so many of us thought in the mid- and late 1960s, as philosophers began to digest Kuhn's ideas. In fact, if one looks at several discussions of Kuhn's work dating from that period, one sees this theme repeatedly. Paradigm change, it was said, could not possibly be

WV1 (ontology 1, methodology 1, values 1)

$\downarrow$

WV2 (ontology 2, methodology 2, values 2)

FIGURE 9-1. Kuhn's Picture of Theory Change

a reasoned or rational process. Kuhn, we thought, has made science into an irrational "monster."

Kuhn's text added fuel to the fire by seeming to endorse such a construal of his own work. In a notorious discussion of the shift from the chemistry of Priestley to that of Lavoisier and Dalton, for instance, Kuhn asserted that it was perfectly reasonable for Priestley to hold onto phlogiston theory, just as it was fully rational for most of his contemporaries to be converting to the oxygen theory of Lavoisier. According to Kuhn, Priestley's continued adherence to phlogiston was reasonable because—given Priestley's cognitive aims and the methods he regarded as appropriate—his own theory continued to look good. Priestley lost the battle with Lavoisier, not because Priestley's paradigm was objectively inferior to its rivals, but rather because most of the chemists of the day came to share Lavoisier's and Dalton's views about what was important and how it should be investigated.

The clear implication of such passages in Kuhn's writings is that interparadigmatic debate is necessarily inconclusive and thus can never be brought to rational closure. When closure does occur, it must therefore be imposed on the situation by such external factors as the demise of some of the participants or the manipulation of the levers of power and reward within the institutional structure of the scientific community. Philosophers of science, almost without exception, have found such implications troubling, for they directly confute what philosophers have been at pains for two millennia to establish: to wit, that scientific disputes, and more generally all disagreements about matters of fact, are in principle open to rational clarification and resolution. It is on the strength of passages such as those I have mentioned that Kuhn has been charged with relativism, subjectivism, irrationalism, and a host of other sins high on the philosopher's hit list.

There is some justice in these criticisms of Kuhn's work, for . . . Kuhn has failed over the past twenty years to elaborate any coherent ac-count of consensus formation, that is, of the manner in which scientists could ever agree to support one world view rather than another. But that flaw, serious though it is, can probably be remedied. . . . [W]e solve the problem of consensus once we realize that *the various components of a world view are individually negotiable and individually replaceable in a piecemeal fashion* (that is, in such a manner that replacement of one element need not require wholesale repudiation of all the other components). Kuhn himself grants, of course, that some components of a world view can be revised; that is what "paradigm articulation" is all about. But for Kuhn, as for such other world view theorists as Lakatos and Foucault, the central commitments of a world view, its "hard core" (to use Lakatos's marvelous phrase), are not revisable—short of rejecting the entire world view. The core ontology of a world view or paradigm, along with its methodology and axiology, comes on a take-it-or-leave-it basis. Where these levels of commitment are concerned, Kuhn (along with such critics of his as Lakatos) is an uncompromising holist. Consider, for instance, his remark: "Just because it is a transition between incommensurables, the transition between competing paradigms cannot be made a step at a time . . . like the Gestalt-switch, it must occur all at once or not at all."[8] Kuhn could hardly be less ambiguous on this point.

But paradigms or research programs need not be so rigidly conceived, and typically they are not so conceived by scientists; nor, if we reflect on it a moment, should they be so conceived. . . . [T]here are complex justificatory interconnections among a scientist's ontology, his methodology, and his axiology. If a scientist's methodology fails to justify his ontology; if his methodology fails to promote his cognitive aims; if his cognitive aims prove to be utopian—in all these cases the scientist will have compelling reasons for replacing one component or other of his world view with an element that does the job better. Yet he need not modify everything else.

To be more precise, the choice confronting a scientist whose world view is under strain in this manner need be nothing like as stark as the choice sketched in Figure 9-1 (where it is a matter of sticking with what he knows best unchanged or throwing that over for something completely different), but rather a choice where the modification of one core element—while retaining the others—may bring a decided improvement. Schematically, the choice may be one between

$$O^1 \ \& \ M^1 \ \& \ A^1 \qquad (1)$$

and

$$O^2 \ \& \ M^1 \ \& \ A^1 \qquad (2)$$

Or, between (1) and

$$O^1 \ \& \ M^2 \ \& \ A^1 \qquad (3)$$

Or, to exhaust the simple cases, it may be between (1) and

$$O^1 \ \& \ M^1 \ \& \ A^2 \qquad (4)$$

. . . [C]hoices like those between (1) and (2), or between (1) and (3), are subject to strong normative constraints. And . . . choices of the sort represented between (1) and (4) are also, under certain circumstances, equally amenable to rational analysis.

In all these examples there is enough common ground between the rivals to engender hope of finding an "Archimedean standpoint" which can rationally mediate the choice. When such commonality exists, there is no reason to regard the choice as just a matter of taste or whim; nor is there any reason to say of such choices, as Kuhn does (recall his characterization of the Priestley–Lavoisier exchange), that there can be no compelling grounds for one preference over another. Provided theory change occurs one level at a time, there is ample scope for regarding it as a thoroughly reasoned process.

But the crucial question is whether change actually does occur in this manner. If one thinks quickly of the great transitions in the history of science, they *seem* to preclude such a stepwise analysis. The shift from (say) an Aristotelian to a Newtonian world view clearly involved changes on all three levels. So, too, did the emergence of psychoanalysis from nineteenth-century mechanistic psychology. But before we accept this wholesale picture of scientific change too quickly, we should ask whether it might not acquire what plausibility it enjoys only because our characterizations of such historical revolutions make us compress or telescope a number of gradual changes (one level at a time, as it were) into what, at our distance in time, can easily appear as an abrupt and monumental shift.

By way of laying out the core features of a more gradualist (and, I argue, historically more faithful) picture of scientific change, I will sketch a highly idealized version of theory change. Once it is in front of us, I will show in detail how it makes sense of some real cases of scientific change. Eventually, we will want a model that can show how one might move from an initial state of disagreement between rival traditions or paradigms to consensus about which one is better. But, for purposes of exposition, I want to begin with a rather simpler situation, namely, one in which consensus in favor of one world view or tradition gives way eventually to consensus in favor of another, without scientists ever being faced with a choice as stark as that between two well-developed, and totally divergent, rival paradigms. My "tall tale," represented schematically in Figure 9-2, might go like this: At any given time, there will be at least one set of values, methods, and theories which one can identify as operating in any field or subfield of science. Let us call this collective C_1, and its components T_1, M_1, and A_1. These components typically stand in . . . complex justificatory relationships to one another . . . ; that is, A_1 will justify M_1 and harmonize with T_1; M_1 will justify T_1 and exhibit the realizability of A_1; and T_1 will constrain M_1 and exemplify A_1. Let us suppose that someone then proposes a new theory, T_2, to replace T_1. The rules M_1 will be consulted and they may well indicate grounds for preferring T_2

Changing element   Adjudicating factors

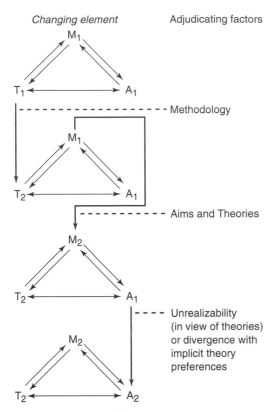

FIGURE 9-2. Unitraditional Change

to T_1. Suppose that they do, and that we thereby replace T_1 with T_2. As time goes by, certain scientists may develop reservations about M_1 and propose a new and arguably superior methodology, M_2. Now a choice must be made between M_1 and M_2. As we have seen, that requires determining whether M_1 or M_2 offers more promise of realizing our aims. Since that determination will typically be an empirical matter, both A_1 and the then-prevailing theory, T_2, will have to be consulted to ascertain whether M_1 or M_2 is optimal for securing A_1. Suppose that, in comparing the relative efficacy of achieving the shared values, A_1, cogent arguments can be made to show that M_2 is superior to M_1. Under the circumstances, assuming scientists behave rationally, M_2 will replace M_1. This means that as new theories, T_3, T_4, . . . , T_n, emerge later, they

will be assessed by rules M_2 rather than M_1. Suppose, still further along in this fairy tale, we imagine a challenge to the basic values themselves. Someone may, for instance, point to new evidence suggesting that some element or other of A_1 is unrealizable. Someone else may point out that virtually none of the theories accepted by the scientific community as instances of good science exemplify the values expressed in A_1 (Or, it may be shown that A_1 is an inconsistent set in that its component aspirations are fundamentally at odds with one another.) Under such circumstances, scientists may rationally decide to abandon A_1 and to take up an alternative, consistent set of values, A_2, should it be available . . .

Now that we have this hypothetical sequence before us, let us imagine a historian called Tom, who decides many years later to study this episode. He will doubtless be struck by the fact that a group of scientists who once accepted values A_1, rules M_1, and theory T_1 came over the course of, say, a decade or two to abandon the whole lot and to accept a new complex, C_2, consisting of A_2, M_2, and T_2. Tom will probably note, and rightly too, that the partisans of C_2 have precious little in common with the devotees of C_1. Surely, Tom may well surmise, here was a scientific revolution if ever there was one, for there was dramatic change at every level. If Tom decides to call the view that scientists eventually came to hold "Paradigm 2," and the view from which they began "Paradigm 1," then he will be able to document the existence of a massive paradigm shift between what (at our remoteness in time) appear to be conceptually distant and virtually incommensurable paradigms.

The point, of course, is that a sequence of belief changes which, described at the microlevel, appears to be a perfectly reasonable and rational sequence of events may appear, when represented in broad brushstrokes that drastically compress the temporal dimension, as a fundamental and unintelligible change of world view. This kind of tunnel vision, in which a sequence of gradual shifts is telescoped into one abrupt and mighty transformation, is a folly which every historian is taught to avoid. Yet knowing that one should avoid it and actually doing so are two different things. Once we recognize this fallacy for what it is, we should probably hesitate to accept too quickly the models of the holists and big-picture builders. For, if our fairy story has anything of the truth about it (that is, if change is, or more weakly even if it could be, more piecemeal than the holistic accounts imply), there may yet be room for incorporating changes of methods and of cognitive values into a rational account of scientific activity. My object in the rest of this chapter is to offer some reasons to believe that the fairy tale is a good deal closer to the mark than its holistic rivals.

But before I present the evidence needed for demythologizing my story, we have to add a new twist to it. As I pointed out above, this story concerns what I call a "unitraditional paradigm shift." It reveals how it might be possible for scientists, originally advocates of one tradition or paradigm, to come around eventually to accept what appears to be a very different view of the world, not to say a very different view of what science is. I call such a change unitraditional because it is not prompted or provoked by the availability of a well-articulated rival world view. If you like, the unitraditional picture explains how one could get paradigm change by developments entirely internal to the dynamic of a particular paradigm. More interesting, and more challenging, is the problem of multitraditional paradigm shifts, that is, basic changes of world view which arise from competition between rival paradigms. To deal with such cases, we need to complicate our fairy story a bit.

Here, we need to imagine two of our complexes already well developed, and radically divergent (i.e., with different ontologies, different methodologies, and different axiologies). If we ask under what circumstances it would be reasonable for the partisans of C_1 to abandon it and accept C_2, some answers come immediately to mind. Suppose, for instance, it can be shown that the central theories of C_1 look worse than the theories of C_2, even by the standards of C_1. . . . Kuhn denies that this is possible, since he says that the theories associated with a particular paradigm will always look better by its standards than will the theories of rival paradigms. . . . But as we have already seen, there is no way of guaranteeing in advance that the methods and standards of C_1 will always give the epistemic nod to theories associated with C_1, since it is always possible (and has sometimes happened) that rival paradigms to C_1 will develop theories that do a better job of satisfying the methodological demands of C_1 than do the theories developed within C_1 itself. Alternatively, suppose someone shows that there is a set of methods M_3 which is more nearly optimal than M_1 for achieving the aims of C_1, and that those methods give the epistemic nod to the theories of C_2 rather than those of C_1. Or, suppose that someone shows that the goals of C_1 are deeply at odds with the attributes of some of the major theories of science—theories that the partisans of C_1 themselves endorse—and that, by contrast, the cognitive values of C_2 are typified by those same theories. Again, new evidence might emerge that indicates the nonrealizability of some of the central cognitive aims of C_1 and the achievability of the aims of C_2. In all these circumstances (and several obvious ones which I shall not enumerate), the only reasonable thing for a scientist to do would be to give up C_1 and to embrace C_2.

. . . [W]e see that the transition from one paradigm or world view to another can itself be a step-wise process, requiring none of the wholesale shifts in allegiance at every level required by Kuhn's analysis. The advocates of C_1 might, for instance, decide initially to accept many of the substantive theories of C_2, while still retaining for a time the methodology and axiology of C_1. At a later stage they might be led by a different chain of arguments and evidence to accept the methodology of C_2 while retaining C_1's axiology. Finally, they might eventually come to share the values of C_2. As William Whewell showed more than a century ago, precisely some such series of shifts occurred in the gradual capitulation of Cartesian physicists to the natural philosophy of Newton.[9]

In effect, I am claiming the solution of the problem of consensus formation in the multi-paradigm situation to be nothing more than a special or degenerate instance of unitraditional change. It follows that, if we can show that the unitraditional fairy tale has something going for it, then we will solve both forms of the consensus-formation problem simultaneously. The core question is whether the gradualist myth, which I have just sketched out, is better supported by the historical record than the holistic picture associated with Kuhn.

One striking way of formulating the contrast between the piecemeal and the holistic models, and thus designing a test to choose between them, is to ask a fairly straightforward question about the historical record: Is it true that the major historical shifts in the methodological rules of science and in the cognitive values of scientists have invariably been contemporaneous with one another *and* with shifts in substantive theories and ontologies? The holistic account is clearly committed to an affirmative answer to the question. Indeed, it is a straightforward corollary of Kuhn's analysis that changes in rules or values, when they occur, will occur only when a scientific revolution takes place, that is, only when there is a concomitant shift in theories, methods, and values. A change in values without an associated change in basic ontology is not a permissible variation countenanced in the Kuhnian scheme.[10] Nor is a change in methods possible for Kuhn without a paradigm change. Kuhn's analysis flatly denies that the values and norms of a "mature" science can shift in the absence of a revolution. Yet there are plenty of examples one may cite to justify the assertion made here that changes at the three levels do not always go together. I shall mention two such examples.

Consider, first, a well-known shift at the level of methodological rules. From the time of Bacon until the early nineteenth century most scientists subscribed to variants of the rules of inductive inference associated with Bacon, Hume, and Newton. The methods of agreement, difference, and concomitant variations were a standard part of the repertoire of most working scientists for two hundred years. These rules, at least as then understood, foreclosed the postulation of any theoretical or hypothetical entities, since observable bodies were the only sort of objects and properties to which one could apply traditional inductive methods. More generally . . . , thinkers of the Enlightenment believed it important to develop rules of inquiry which would exclude unobservable entities and bring to heel the tendency of scientists to indulge their *l'esprit de système*. Newton's famous third rule of reasoning in philosophy, the notorious "hypotheses non fingo," was but a particularly succinct and influential formulation of this trenchant empiricism.

It is now common knowledge that by the late nineteenth century this methodological orientation had largely vanished from the writings of major scientists and methodologists. Whewell, Peirce, Helmholtz, Mach, Darwin, Hertz, and a host of other luminaries had, by the 1860s and 1870s, come to believe that it was quite legitimate for science to postulate unobservable entities, and that most of the traditional rules of inductive reasoning had been superseded by the logic of hypothetico-deduction. Elsewhere I have described this shift in detail.[11] What is important for our purposes is both that it occurred and when it occurred. That it took place would be denied, I think, by no one who studies the record; determining precisely when it occurred is more problematic, although probably no scholar would quarrel with the claim that it comes in the period from 1800 to 1860. And a dating as fuzzy as that is sufficient to make out my argument.

For here we have a shift in the history of the explicit methodology of the scientific community as significant as one can imagine—from methods of enumerative and eliminative induction to the method of hypothesis—occurring across the spectrum of the theoretical sciences, from celestial mechanics to chemistry and biology. . . . Yet where is the larger and more global scientific revolution of which this methodological shift was the concomitant? There were of course revolutions, and important ones, in this period. Yet this change in methodology cannot be specifically linked to any of the familiar revolutions of the period. The method of hypothesis did not become the orthodoxy in science of the late nineteenth century because it rode on the coattails of any specific change in ontology or scientific values. So far as I can see, this methodological revolution was independent of any particular program of research in any one of the sciences, which is not to say that it did not reflect some very general tendencies appearing across the board in scientific research. The holist model, which would have us believe that changes in methodological orientation are invariably linked to changes in values and ontology, is patently mistaken here. Nor, if one reflects on the nature of methodological discussion, should we have expected otherwise. . . . [M]ethodological rules can reasonably be criticized and altered if one discovers that they fail optimally to promote our cognitive aims. If our aims shift, as they would in a Kuhnian paradigm shift, we would of course expect a reappraisal of our methods of inquiry in light of their suitability for promoting the new goals. But, even when our goals shift not at all, we sometimes discover arguments and evidence which indicate that the methods we have been using all along are not really suitable for our purposes. Such readjustments of methodological orientation, in the absence of a paradigm shift . . . pose a serious anomaly for Kuhn's analysis.

What about changes in aims, as opposed to rules? Is it not perhaps more plausible to imagine, with Kuhn, that changes of cognitive values are always part of broader shifts of paradigm or world view? Here again, the historical record speaks out convincingly against this account.

Consider, very briefly, one example: the abandonment of "infallible knowledge" as an epistemic aim for science. As before, my historical account will have to be "potted" for purposes of brevity; but there is ample serious scholarship to back up the claims I shall be making.[12]

That scholarship has established quite convincingly that, during the course of the nineteenth century, the view of science as aiming at certainty gave way among most scientists to a more modest program of producing theories that were plausible, probable, or well tested. As Peirce and Dewey have argued, this shift represents one of the great watersheds in the history of scientific philosophy: the abandonment of the quest for certainty. More or less from the time of Aristotle onward, scientists had sought theories that were demonstrable and apodictically certain. Although empiricists and rationalists disagreed about precisely how to certify knowledge as certain and incorrigible, all agreed that science was aiming exclusively at the production of such knowledge. This same view of science largely prevailed at the beginning of the nineteenth century. But by the end of that century this demonstrative and infallibilist ideal was well and truly dead. Scientists of almost every persuasion were insistent that science could, at most, aspire to the status of highly probable knowledge. Certainty, incorrigibility, and indefeasibility ceased to figure among the central aims of most twentieth-century scientists.

The full story surrounding the replacement of the quest for certainty by a thoroughgoing fallibilism is long and complicated; I have attempted to sketch out parts of that story elsewhere.[13] What matters for our purposes here is not so much the details of this epistemic revolution, but the fact that this profound transformation was not specifically associated with the emergence of any new scientific paradigms or research programs. The question of timing is crucial, for it is important to see that this deep shift in axiological sensibilities was independent of any specific change in scientific world view or paradigm. No new scientific tradition or paradigm in the nineteenth century was associated with a specifically fallibilist axiology. Quite the reverse, fallibilism came to be associated with virtually every major program of scientific research by the mid- to late nineteenth century. Atomists and antiatomists, wave theorists and particle theorists, Darwinians and Lamarckians, uniformitarians and catastrophists—all subscribed to the new consensus about the corrigibility and indemonstrability of scientific theories. A similar story could be told about other cognitive values which have gone the way of all flesh. The abandonment of intelligibility, of the requirement of picturable or mechanically constructible models of natural processes, of the insistence on "complete" descriptions of nature— all reveal a similar pattern. The abandonment of each of these cognitive ideals was largely independent of shifts in basic theories about nature.

Once again, the holistic approach leads to expectations that are confounded by the historical record. Changes in values and changes in substantive ontologies or methodologies show no neat isomorphism. Change certainly occurs at all levels, and sometimes changes are concurrent, but there is no striking covariance between the timing of changes at one level and the timing of those at any other. I conclude from such examples that scientific change is substantially more piecemeal than the holistic model would suggest. Value changes do not always accompany, nor are they always accompanied by, changes in scientific paradigm. Shifts in methodological rules may, but need not, be associated with shifts in either values or ontologies. The three levels, although unquestionably interrelated, do not come as an inseparable package on a take-it-or-leave-it basis.

This result is of absolutely decisive importance for understanding the processes of scientific change. Because these changes are not always concomitant, we are often in a position to hold one or two of the three levels fixed while we decide whether to make modifications at the disputed level. The existence of these (temporarily) fixed and thus shared points of perspective provides a crucial form of triangulation. Since theories, methodologies, and axiologies stand together in a kind of justificatory triad, we can use those doctrines about which there is agreement to resolve the remaining areas where we disagree. The uncontested levels will not always resolve the controversy, for underdetermination is an ever present possibility. But the fact that the levels of agreement are sometimes insufficient to terminate the controversy provides no comfort for Kuhn's subjectivist thesis that those levels of agreement are never sufficient to resolve the debate. As logicians say, we need to be very careful about our quantifiers here. Some writers have not always exercised the care they should. Kuhn, for instance, confusedly slides from (*a*) the correct claim that the shared values of scientists are, in certain situations, incapable of yielding unambiguously a preference between two rival theories to (*b*) the surely mistaken claim that the shared values of scientists are never sufficient to warrant a preference between rival paradigms. Manifestly in some instances, the shared rules and standards of methodology are unavailing. But neither Kuhn nor anyone else has established that the rules, evaluative criteria, and values to which scientists subscribe are generally so ambiguous in application that virtually any theory or paradigm can be shown to satisfy them. And we must constantly bear in mind the point that, even when theories are underdetermined by a set of rules or standards, many theories will typically be ruled out by the relevant rules; and if one party to a scientific debate happens to be pushing for a theory that can be shown to violate those rules, then the rules will eliminate that theory from contention.

What has led holistic theorists to misdescribe so badly the relations among these various sorts of changes? As one who was himself once an advocate of such an account, I can explain specifically what led me into thinking that change on the various levels was virtually simultaneous. If one focuses, as most philosophers of science have, on the processes of justification in science, one begins to see systemic linkages among what

I earlier called factual, methodological, and axiological ideas. One notices further that beliefs at all three levels shift through time. Under the circumstances it is quite natural to conjecture that these various changes may be interconnected. Specifically, one can imagine that the changes might well be simultaneous, or at least closely dependent on one another. The suggestion is further borne out—at least to a first approximation—by an analysis of some familiar scientific episodes. It is clear, for instance, that the scientific revolution of the seventeenth century brought with it changes in theories, ontologies, rules, and values. Equally, the twentieth-century revolution in relativity theory and quantum mechanics brought in its wake a shift in both methodological and axiological orientations among theoretical physicists. But as I have already suggested, these changes came seriatim, not simultaneously. More to the point, it is my impression that the overwhelming majority of theory transitions in the history of science (including shifts as profound as that from creationist biology to evolution, from energeticist to atomistic views on the nature of matter, from catastrophism to uniformitarianism in geology, from particle to wave theories of light) have not taken place by means of Gestalt-like shifts at all levels concurrently. Often, change occurs on a single level only (e.g., the Darwinian revolution or the triumph of atomism, where it was chiefly theory or ontology that changed); sometimes it occurs on two levels simultaneously; rarely do we find an abrupt and wholesale shift of doctrines at all three levels.

This fact about scientific change has a range of important implications for our understanding of scientific debate and scientific controversy. Leaving aside the atypical case of simultaneous shifts at all three levels . . ., it means that most instances of scientific change—including most of the events we call scientific revolutions—occur amid a significant degree of consensus at a variety of levels among the contending parties. Scientists may, for instance, disagree about specific theories yet agree about the appropriate rules for theory appraisal. They may even disagree about both theories and rules but accept the same cognitive values. Alternatively, they may accept the same theories and rules yet disagree about the cognitive values they espouse. In all these cases there is no reason to speak (with Kuhn) of "incommensurable choices" or "conversion experiences," or (with Foucault) about abrupt "ruptures of thought," for there is in each instance the possibility of bringing the disagreement to rational closure. Of course, it may happen in specific cases that the mechanisms of rational adjudication are of no avail, for the parties may be contending about matters that are underdetermined by the beliefs and standards the contending parties share in common. But, even here, we can still say that there are rational rules governing the game being played, and that the moves being made (i.e., the beliefs being debated and the arguments being arrayed for and against them) are in full compliance with the rules of the game.

Above all, we must bear in mind that it has never been established that such instances of holistic change constitute more than a tiny fraction of scientific disagreements. Because such cases are arguably so atypical, it follows that sociologists and philosophers of science who predicate their theories of scientific change and cognition on the presumed ubiquity of irresolvable standoffs between monolithic world views (of the sort that Kuhn describes in *Structure of Scientific Revolutions*) run the clear risk of failing to recognize the complex ways in which rival theories typically share important background assumptions in common. To put it differently, global claims about the immunity of interparadigmatic disputes to rational adjudication (and such claims are central in the work of both Kuhn and Lakatos) depend for their plausibility on systematically ignoring the piecemeal character of most forms of scientific change and on a gross exaggeration of the impotence of rational considerations to bring such disagreements to closure. Beyond that, I have argued that, even if interparadigmatic clashes had the character Kuhn says they do (namely, of involving little or no overlap at any of the three levels), it still would not follow that there are no rational grounds for a critical and comparative assessment of the rival paradigms. In sum, no adequate support has been provided for the claim that clashes between rival scientific camps can never, or rarely ever, be resolved in an objective fashion. The problem of consensus formation, which I earlier suggested was the great Kuhnian enigma, . . . can be resolved, but only if we realize that science has adjudicatory mechanisms whose existence has gone unnoticed by Kuhn and the other holists.

But it would be misleading to conclude this treatment of Kuhn and the holist theory of theory change on such a triumphal note, for we have yet to confront directly and explicitly another relevant side of Kuhn's work: specifically, his claim, elaborated through a variety of arguments, that methodological rules and shared cognitive values (on which I have laid so much stress as instruments of closure and consensus formation) are impotent to resolve large-scale scientific disagreement. We must now turn to that task directly.

Kuhn's Critique of Methodology

Several writers (e.g., Quine, Hesse, Goodman) have asserted that the rules or principles of scientific appraisal underdetermine theory choice. For reasons I have tried to spell out elsewhere,[14] such a view is badly flawed. Some authors, for instance, tend to confuse the logical underdetermination of theories by data with the underdetermination of theory choice by methodological rules. Others (e.g., Hesse and Bloor) have mistakenly taken the logical underdetermination of theories to be a license for asserting the causal underdetermination of our theoretical beliefs by the sensory evidence to which we are exposed.[15] But there is a weaker, and much more interesting, version of the thesis of underdetermination, which has been developed most fully in Kuhn's recent writings. Indeed, it is one of the strengths

of Kuhn's challenge to traditional philosophy of science that he has "localized" and given flesh to the case for underdetermination, in ways that make it prima facie much more telling. In brief, Kuhn's view is this: If we examine situations where scientists are required to make a choice among the handful of paradigms that confront them at any time, we discover that the relevant evidence and appropriate methodological standards fail to pick out one contender as unequivocally superior to its extant rivals. I call such situations cases of "local" underdetermination, by way of contrasting them with the more global forms of underdetermination (which say, in effect, that the rules are insufficient to pick out any theory as being uniquely supported by the data). Kuhn offers four distinct arguments for local underdetermination. Each is designed to show that, although methodological rules and standards do constrain and delimit a scientist's choices or options, those rules and standards are never sufficient to compel or unequivocally to warrant the choice of one paradigm over another.

1. THE "AMBIGUITY OF SHARED STANDARDS" ARGUMENT

Kuhn's first argument for methodological underdetermination rests on the purported ambiguity of the methodological rules or standards that are shared by advocates of rival paradigms. The argument first appeared in *The Structure of Scientific Revolutions* (1962) and has been extended considerably in his later *The Essential Tension* (1977). As he put it in the earlier work, "lifelong resistance [to a new theory] . . . is not a violation of scientific standards . . . though the historian can always find men—Priestley, for instance—who were unreasonable to resist for as long as they did, he will not find a point at which resistance becomes illogical or unscientific."[16] Many of Kuhn's readers were perplexed by the juxtaposition of claims in such passages as these. On the one hand, we are told that Priestley's continued refusal to accept the theory of Lavoisier was "unreasonable"; but we are also told that Priestley's refusal was neither "illogical" nor "unscientific." To those inclined to think that being "scientific" (at least in the usual sense of that term) required one to be "reasonable" about shaping one's beliefs, Kuhn seemed to be talking gibberish. On a more sympathetic construal, Kuhn seemed to be saying that a scientist could always interpret the applicable standards of appraisal, whatever they might be, so as to "rationalize" his own paradigmatic preferences, whatever they might be. This amounts to claiming that the methodological rules or standards of science never make a real or decisive difference to the outcome of a process of theory choice; if any set of rules can be used to justify any theory whatever, then methodology would seem to amount to just so much window dressing. But that construal, it turns out, is a far cry from what Kuhn intended. As he has made clear in later writings, he wants to bestow a positive, if (compared with the traditional view) much curtailed, role on methodological standards in scientific choice.

What Kuhn apparently has in mind is that the shared criteria, standards, and rules to which scientists explicitly and publicly refer in justifying their choices of theory and paradigm are typically "ambiguous" and "imprecise," so much so that "individuals [who share the same standards] may legitimately differ about their application to concrete cases."[17] Kuhn holds that, although scientists share certain cognitive values "and must do so if science is to survive, they do not all apply them in the same way. Simplicity, scope, fruitfulness, and even accuracy can be judged differently (which is not to say they may be judged arbitrarily) by different people."[18] Because, then, the shared standards are ambiguous, two scientists may subscribe to "exactly the same standard" (say, the rule of simplicity) and yet endorse opposing viewpoints.

Kuhn draws some quite large inferences from the presumed ambiguity of the shared standards or criteria. Specifically, he concludes that every case of theory choice must involve an admixture of objective and subjective factors, since (in

Kuhn's view) the shared, and presumably objective, criteria are too amorphous and ambiguous to warrant a particular preference. He puts the point this way: "I continue to hold that the algorithms of individuals are all ultimately different by virtue of the subjective considerations with which each [scientist] must complete the objective criteria before any computations can be done."[19] As this passage makes clear, Kuhn believes that, because the shared criteria are too imprecise to justify a choice, and because—despite that imprecision—scientists do manage to make choices, those choices *must* be grounded in individual and subjective preferences different from those of his fellow scientists. As he says, "every individual choice between competing theories depends on a mixture of objective and subjective factors, or of shared and individual criteria."[20] And, the shared criteria "are not by themselves sufficient to determine the decisions of individual scientists."[21]

This very ambitious claim, if true, would force us to drastically rethink our views of scientific rationality. Among other things, it would drive us to the conclusion that every scientist has different reasons for his theory preferences from those of his fellow scientists. The view entails, among other things, that it is a category mistake to ask (say) why physicists think Einstein's theories are better than Newton's; for, on Kuhn's analysis, there must be as many different answers as there are physicists. We might note in passing that this is quite an ironic conclusion for Kuhn to reach. Far more than most writers on these subjects, he has tended to stress the importance of community and socialization processes in understanding the scientific enterprise. Yet the logic of his own analysis drives him to the radically individualistic position that every scientist has his own set of reasons for theory preferences and that there is no real consensus whatever with respect to the grounds for theory preference, not even among the advocates of the same paradigm. Seen from this perspective, Kuhn tackles what I earlier called the problem of consensus by a maneuver that trivializes the problem; for if we must give a separate and discrete explanation for the theory preferences of each member of the scientific community—which is what Kuhn's view entails—then we are confronted with a gigantic mystery at the collective level, to wit, why the scientists in a given discipline—each supposedly operating with his own individualistic and idiosyncratic criteria, each giving a different "gloss" to the criteria that are shared—are so often able to agree about which theories to bet on. But we can leave it to Kuhn to sort out how he reconciles his commitment to the social psychology of science with his views about the individual vagaries of theory preference. What must concern us is the question whether Kuhn has made a plausible case for thinking that the shared or collective criteria must be supplemented by individual and subjective criteria.

The first point to stress is that Kuhn's thesis purports to apply to all scientific rules or values that are shared by the partisans of rival paradigms, not just to a selected few, notoriously ambiguous ones. We can grant straightaway that some of the rules, standards, and values used by scientists ("simplicity" would be an obvious candidate) exhibit precisely that high degree of ambiguity which Kuhn ascribes to them. But Kuhn's general argument for the impotence of shared rules to settle disagreements between scientists working in different paradigms cannot be established by citing the occasional example. Kuhn must show us, for he claims as much, that there is something in the very nature of those methodological rules that come to be shared among scientists which makes the application of those rules or standards invariably inconclusive. He has not established this result, and there is a good reason why he has not: It is false. To see that it is, one need only produce a methodological rule widely accepted by scientists which can be applied to concrete cases without substantial imprecision or ambiguity. Consider, for instance, one of Kuhn's own examples of a widely shared scientific standard, namely, the requirement that an acceptable theory must be inter-

nally consistent and logically consistent with accepted theories in other fields. (One may or may not favor this methodological rule. I refer to it here only because it is commonly regarded, including by Kuhn, as a methodological rule that frequently plays a role in theory evaluation.)

I submit that we have a very clear notion of what it is for a theory to be internally consistent, just as we understand perfectly well what it means for a theory to be consistent with accepted beliefs. Moreover, on at least some occasions we can tell whether a particular theory has violated the standard of (internal or external) consistency. Kuhn himself, in a revealing passage, grants as much; for instance, when comparing the relative merits of geocentric and heliocentric astronomy, Kuhn says that "the consistency criterion, by itself, therefore, spoke unequivocally for the geocentric tradition."[22] (What he has in mind is the fact that heliocentric astronomy, when introduced, was inconsistent with the then-reigning terrestrial physics, whereas the assumptions of geocentric astronomy were consistent with that physics.) Note that in this case we have a scientific rule or criterion "speaking unequivocally" in favor of one theory and against its rival. Where are the inevitable imprecision and ambiguity which are supposed by Kuhn to afflict all the shared values of the scientific community? What is ambiguous about the notion of consistency? The point of these rhetorical questions is to drive home the fact that, even by Kuhn's lights, some of the rules or criteria widely accepted in the scientific community do not exhibit that multiplicity of meanings which Kuhn has described as being entirely characteristic of methodological standards.

One could, incidentally, cite several other examples of reasonably clear and unambiguous methodological rules. For instance, the requirements that theories should be deductively closed or that theories should be subjected to controlled experiments have not generated a great deal of confusion or disagreement among scientists about what does and does not constitute closure or a control. Or, consider the rule that theories should lead successfully to the prediction of results unknown to their discoverer; so far as I am aware, scientists have not differed widely in their construal of the meaning of this rule. The significance of the nonambiguity of many methodological concepts and rules is to be found in the fact that such nonambiguity refutes one of Kuhn's central arguments for the incomparability of paradigms and for its corollary, the impotence of methodology as a guide to scientific rationality. There are at least some rules that are sufficiently determinate that one can show that many theories clearly fail to satisfy them. We need not supplement the shared content of these objective concepts with any private notions of our own in order to decide whether a theory satisfies them.

2. THE "COLLECTIVE INCONSISTENCY OF RULES" ARGUMENT

As if the ambiguity of standards was not bad enough, Kuhn goes on to argue that the shared rules and standards, when taken as a collective, "repeatedly prove to conflict with one another."[23] For instance, two scientists may each believe that empirical accuracy and generality are desirable traits in a theory. But, when confronted with a pair of rival (and thus incompatible) theories, one of which is more accurate and the other more general, the judgments of those scientists may well differ about which theory to accept. One scientist may opt for the more general theory; the other, for the more accurate. They evidently share the same standards, says Kuhn, but they end up with conflicting appraisals. Kuhn puts it this way: ". . . in many concrete situations, different values, though all constitutive of good reasons, dictate different conclusions, different choices. In such cases of value-conflict (e.g., one theory is simpler but the other is more accurate) the relative weight placed on different values by different individuals can play a decisive role in individual choice."[24]

Because many methodological standards do pull in different directions, Kuhn thinks that the scientist can pretty well go whichever way he likes. Well, not quite any direction he likes, since—even by Kuhn's very liberal rules—it would be unreasonable for a scientist to prefer a theory (or paradigm) which failed to satisfy any of the constraints. In Kuhn's view, we should expect scientific disagreements or dissensus to emerge specifically in those cases where (a) no available theory satisfied all the constraints and (b) every extant theory satisfied some constraints not satisfied by its rivals. That scientists sometimes find themselves subscribing to contrary standards, I would be the first to grant. . . . But Kuhn is not merely saying that this happens occasionally; he is asserting that such is the nature of any set of rules or standards that any group of reasonable scientists might accept. As before, our verdict has to be that Kuhn's highly ambitious claim is just that; he never shows us why families of methodological rules should always or even usually be internally inconsistent. He apparently expects us to take his word for it that he is just telling it as it is.[25] I see no reason why we should follow Kuhn in his global extrapolations from the tiny handful of cases he describes. On the contrary, there are good grounds for resisting, since there are plenty of sets of consistent methodological standards. Consider, for instance, one of the most influential documents of nineteenth-century scientific methodology, John Stuart Mill's *System of Logic*. Mill offered there a set of rules or canons for assessing the soundness of causal hypotheses. Nowadays those rules are still called "Mill's methods," and much research in the natural and social sciences utilizes them, often referring to them as the methods of agreement, difference, and concomitant variations. To the best of my knowledge, no one has ever shown that Mill's methods exhibit a latent tendency toward contradiction or conflict of the sort that Kuhn regards as typical of systems of methodological rules. To go back further in history, no one has ever shown that Bacon's or Descartes's or Newton's or Herschel's famous canons of reasoning are internally inconsistent. The fact that numerous methodologies of science may be cited which have never been shown to be inconsistent casts serious doubts on Kuhn's claim that any methodological standards apt to be shared by rival scientists will tend to exhibit mutual inconsistencies.

Kuhn could have strengthened his argument considerably if, instead of focusing on the purported tensions in sets of methodological rules, he had noted, rather, that whenever one has more than one standard in operation, it is conceivable that we will be torn in several directions. And this claim is true, regardless of whether the standards are strictly inconsistent with one another or not (just so long as there is not a complete covariance between their instances). If two scientists agree to judge theories by two standards, then it is trivially true that, depending upon how much weight each gives to the two standards, their judgments about theories may differ. Before we can make sense of how to work with several concurrent standards, we have to ask (as Kuhn never did) about the way in which these standards do (or should) control the selection of a preferred theory. Until we know the answer to that question, we will inevitably find that the standards are of little use in explaining scientific preferences. Kuhn simply assumes that all possible preference structures (i.e., all possible differential weightings of the applicable standards) are equally viable or equally likely to be exemplified in a working scientist's selection procedures. . . .

To sum up the argument to this point: I have shown that Kuhn is wrong in claiming that all methodological rules are inevitably ambiguous and in claiming that scientific methodologies consisting of whole groups of rules always or even usually exhibit a high degree of internal "tension." Since these two claims were the linchpins in Kuhn's argument to the effect that shared criteria "are not by themselves sufficient to determine the decisions of individual scientists,"[26] we are entitled to say that Kuhn's effort to establish a general form of local underdetermination falls flat.

3. THE SHIFTING STANDARDS ARGUMENT

Equally important to Kuhn's critique of methodology is a set of arguments having to do with the manner in which standards are supposed to vary from one scientist to another. In treating Kuhn's views on this matter, I follow Gerald Doppelt's excellent and sympathetic explication of Kuhn's position.[27] In general, Kuhn's model of science envisages two quite distinct ways in which disagreements about standards might render scientific debate indeterminate or inconclusive. In the first place, the advocates of different paradigms may subscribe to different methodological rules or evaluative criteria. Indeed, *may* is too weak a term here, for, as we have seen, Kuhn evidently believes that associated with each paradigm is a set of methodological orientations that are (at least partly) at odds with the methodologies of all rival paradigms. Thus, he insists that whenever a "paradigm shift" occurs, this process produces "changes in the standards governing permissible problems, concepts and explanations."[28] This is quite a strong claim. It implies, among other things, that the advocates of different paradigms invariably have different views about what constitutes a scientific explanation and even about what constitutes the relevant facts to be explained (viz., the "permissible problems"). If Kuhn is right about these matters, then debate between the proponents of two rival paradigms will involve appeal to different sets of rules and standards associated respectively with the two paradigms. One party to the dispute may be able to show that his theory is best by his standards, while his opponent may be able to claim superiority by his.

As I have shown in detail earlier in this chapter, Kuhn is right to say that scientists sometimes subscribe to different methodologies (including different standards for explanation and facticity). But he has never shown, and I believe him to be chronically wrong in claiming, that disagreements about matters of standards and rules neatly coincide with disagreements about substantive matters of scientific ontology. Rival scientists advocating fundamentally different theories or paradigms often have the same standards of assessment (and interpret them identically); on the other hand, adherents to the same paradigm will frequently espouse different standards. In short, methodological disagreements and factual disagreements about basic theories show no striking covariances of the kind required to sustain Kuhn's argument about the intrinsic irresolvability of interparadigmatic debate. It was the thrust of my earlier account of "piecemeal change" to show why Kuhn's claims about irresolvability will not work.

But, of course, a serious issue raised by Kuhn still remains before us. If different scientists sometimes subscribe to different standards of appraisal (and that much is surely correct), then how is it possible for us to speak of the resolution of such disagreements as anything other than an arbitrary closure? . . . Provided there are mechanisms for rationally resolving disagreements about methodological rules and cognitive values . . . the fact that scientists often disagree about such rules and values need not, indeed should not, be taken to show that there must be anything arbitrary about the resolution of such disagreements.

4. THE PROBLEM-WEIGHTING ARGUMENT

As I have said earlier, Kuhn has another argument up his sleeve which he and others think is germane to the issue of the rationality of comparative theory assessment. Specifically, he insists that the advocates of rival paradigms assign differential degrees of importance to the solution of different sorts of problems. Because they do, he says that they will often disagree about which theory is better supported, since one side will argue that it is most important to solve a certain problem, while the other will insist on the centrality of solving a different problem. Kuhn poses the difficulty in these terms: "If there were but one set of scientific problems, one world within which to work on them, and one set of standards for their solution, paradigm competition might be settled more or less rou-

tinely by some process like counting the number of problems solved by each. But, in fact, these conditions are never met completely. The proponents of competing paradigms are always at least slightly at cross purposes . . . the proponents will often disagree about the list of problems that any candidate for paradigm must resolve."[29]

In this passage Kuhn runs together two issues which it is well to separate: One concerns the question (just addressed in the preceding section) about whether scientists have different standards of explanation or solution; the other (and the one that concerns us here) is the claim that scientists working in different paradigms want to solve different problems and that, because they do, their appraisals of the merits of theories will typically differ. So we must here deal with the case where scientists have the same standards for what counts as solving a problem but where they disagree about which problems are the most important to solve. As Kuhn puts it, "scientific controversies between the advocates of rival paradigms involve the question: which problems is it more significant to have solved? Like the issue of competing standards, that question of values can be answered only in terms of criteria that lie outside of normal science altogether."[30] Kuhn is surely right to insist that partisans of different global theories or paradigms often disagree about which problems it is most important to solve. But the existence of such disagreement does not establish that interparadigmatic debate about the epistemic support of rival paradigms is inevitably inconclusive or that it must be resolved by factors that lie outside the normal resources of scientific inquiry.

At first glance, Kuhn's argument seems very plausible: The differing weights assigned to the solution of specific problems by the advocates of rival paradigms may apparently lead to a situation in which the advocates of rival paradigms can each assert that their respective paradigms are the best because they solve precisely those problems they respectively believe to be the most important. No form of reasoning, insists Kuhn, could convince either side of the merits of the opposition or of the weakness of its own approach in such circumstances.

To see where Kuhn's argument goes astray in this particular instance, we need to dissect it at a more basic level. Specifically, we need to distinguish two quite distinct senses in which solving a problem may be said to be important. A problem may be important to a scientist just in the sense that he is particularly curious about it. Equally, it may be important because there is some urgent social or economic reason for solving it. Both sorts of considerations may explain why a scientist regards it as urgent to solve the problem. Such concerns are clearly relevant to explaining the motivation of scientists. But these senses of problem importance have no particular epistemic or probative significance. When we are assessing the evidential support for a theory, when we are asking how well supported or well tested that theory is by the available data, we are not asking whether the theory solves problems that are socially or personally important. Importance, in the sense chiefly relevant to this discussion, is what we might call epistemic or probative importance. One problem is of greater epistemic or probative significance than another if the former constitutes a more telling test of our theories than does the latter.

So, if Kuhn's point is to be of any significance for the epistemology of science (or, what amounts to the same thing, if we are asking how beliefworthy a theory is), then we must imagine a situation in which the advocates of different paradigms assign conflicting degrees of epistemic import to the solution of certain problems. Kuhn's thesis about such situations would be, I presume, that there is no rational machinery for deciding who is right about the assignment of epistemic weight to such problems. But that seems wrong-headed, or at least unargued, for philosophers of science have long and plausibly maintained that the primary function of scientific epistemology is precisely to ascertain the (epistemic) importance of any piece of con-

firming or disconfirming evidence. It is not open to a scientist simply to say that solving an arbitrarily selected problem (however great its subjective significance) is of high probative value. Indeed, it is often true that the epistemically most salient problems are ones with little or no prior practical or even heuristic significance. (Consider that Brownian motion was of decisive epistemic significance in discrediting classical thermodynamics, even though such motion had little intrinsic interest prior to Einstein's showing that such motion was anomalous for thermodynamics.) The whole point of the theory of evidence is to desubjectify the assignment of evidential significance by indicating the kinds of reasons that can legitimately be given for attaching a particular degree of epistemic importance to a confirming or refuting instance. Thus, if one maintains that the ability of a theory to solve a certain problem is much more significant epistemically than its ability to solve another, one must be able to give reasons for that epistemic preference. Put differently, one has to show that the probative significance of the one problem for testing theories of a certain sort is indeed greater than that of the other. He might do so by showing that the former outcome was much more surprising than or more general than the latter. One may thus be able to motivate a claim for the greater importance of the first problem over the second by invoking relevant epistemic and methodological criteria. But if none of these options is open to him, if he can answer the question, "Why is solving this problem more important probatively than solving that one?" only by replying, in effect, "because I am interested in solving this rather than that," then he has surrendered any claim to be shaping his beliefs rationally in light of the available evidence.

We can put the point more generally: The rational assignment of any particular degree of probative significance to a problem must rest on one's being able to show that there are viable methodological and epistemic grounds for assigning that degree of importance rather than

READING 9 / DISSECTING THE HOLIST PICTURE OF SCIENTIFIC CHANGE **123**

another. Once we see this, it becomes clear that the degree of empirical support which a solved problem confers on a paradigm is not simply a matter of how keenly the proponents of that paradigm want to solve the problem.

Let me expand on this point by using an example cited extensively by both Kuhn and Doppelt: the Daltonian "revolution" in chemistry. As Doppelt summarizes the Kuhnian position, ". . . the pre-Daltonian chemistry of the phlogiston theory and the theory of elective affinity achieved reasonable answers to a whole set of questions effectively abandoned by Dalton's new chemistry."[31] Because Dalton's chemistry failed to address many of the questions answered by the older chemical paradigm, Kuhn thinks that the acceptance of Dalton's approach deprived "chemistry of some actual and much potential explanatory power."[32] Indeed, Kuhn is right in holding that, during most of the nineteenth century, Daltonian chemists were unable to explain many things that the older chemical traditions could make sense of. On the other hand, as Kuhn stresses, Daltonian chemistry could explain a great deal that had eluded earlier chemical theories. In short, "the two paradigms seek to explain different kinds of observational data, in response to different agendas of problems."[33] This "loss" of solved problems during transitions from one major theory to another is an important insight of Kuhn's . . . . But this loss of problem-solving ability through paradigm change, although real enough, does not entail, as Kuhn claims, that proponents of old and new paradigms will necessarily be unable to make congruent assessments of how well tested or well supported their respective paradigms are.

What leads Kuhn and Doppelt to think otherwise is their assumption that the centrality of a problem on one's explanatory agenda necessarily entails one's assigning a high degree of epistemic or probative weight to that problem when it comes to determining how well supported a certain theory or paradigm is. But that assumption is usually false. In general, the observations to which a reasonable scientist attaches the most probative or epistemic weight are those instances that test a theory especially "severely" (to use Popper's splendid term). The instances of greatest probative weight in the history of science (e.g., the oblate shape of the "spherical" earth, the Arago disk experiment, the bending of light near the sun, the recession of Mercury's perihelion, the reconstitution of white light from the spectrum) have generally not been instances high on the list of problems that scientists developed their theories to solve. A test instance acquires high probative weight when, for example, it involves testing one of a theory's surprising or counterintuitive predictions, or when it represents a kind of crucial experiment between rival theories. The point is that a problem or instance does not generally acquire great probative strength in testing a theory simply because the advocates of that theory would like to be able to solve the problem. Quite the reverse, many scientists and philosophers would say. After all, it is conventional wisdom that a theory is not very acutely tested if its primary empirical support is drawn from the very sort of situations it was designed to explain. Most theories of experimental design urge—in sharp contrast with Kuhn—that theories should not be given high marks simply because they can solve the problems they were invented to solve. In arguing that the explanatory agenda a scientist sets for himself automatically dictates that scientist's reasoned judgments about well-testedness, Kuhn and Doppelt seem to have profoundly misconstrued the logic of theory appraisal.

Let us return for a moment to Kuhn's Dalton example. If I am right, Dalton might readily have conceded that pre-Daltonian chemistry solved a number of problems that his theory failed to address. Judged as theories about the qualitative properties of chemical reagents, those theories could even be acknowledged as well supported *of their type*. But Dalton's primary interests lie elsewhere, for he presumably regarded those earlier theories as failing to address what he considered to be the central problems of chemistry. But this is not an epistemic judgment; it is a pragmatic one. It amounts to saying: "These older theories are well-tested and reliable theories for explaining certain features of chemical change; but those features happen not to interest me very much." In sum, Kuhn and Doppelt have failed to offer us any grounds for thinking that a scientist's judgment about the degree of evidential support for a paradigm should or does reflect his personal views about the problems he finds most interesting. That, in turn, means that one need not share an enthusiasm for a certain paradigm's explanatory agenda in order to decide whether the theories that make up that paradigm are well tested or ill tested. It appears to me that what the Kuhn-Doppelt point really amounts to is the truism that scientists tend to invest their efforts exploring paradigms that address problems those scientists find interesting. That is a subjective and pragmatic matter which can, and should, be sharply distinguished from the question whether one paradigm or theory is better tested or better supported than its rivals. Neither Kuhn nor Doppelt has made plausible the claim that, because two scientists have different degrees of interest in solving different sorts of problems, it follows that their epistemic judgments of which theories are well tested and which are not will necessarily differ.

We are thus in a position to conclude that the existence of conflicting views among scientists about which problems are interesting apparently entails nothing about the *incompatibility* or *incommensurability* of the epistemic appraisals those scientists will make. That in turn means that these real differences of problem-solving emphasis between advocates of rival paradigms do nothing to undermine the viability of a methodology of comparative theory assessment, insofar as such a methodology is epistemically rather than pragmatically oriented. It seems likely that Kuhn and Doppelt have fallen into this confusion because of their failure to see that acknowledged differences in the motivational appeal of various problems to various scientists constitutes no rationale for asserting the existence of correlative differences in the probative weights properly assigned to those problems by those same scientists.

The appropriate conclusion to draw from the features of scientific life to which Kuhn and Doppelt properly direct our attention is that the pursuit of (and doubtless the recruitment of scientists into) rival paradigms is influenced by pragmatic as well as by epistemic considerations. That is an interesting thesis, and probably a sound one, but it does nothing to undermine the core premise of scientific epistemology: that there are principles of empirical or evidential support which are neither paradigm-specific, hopelessly vague, nor individually idiosyncratic. More important, these principles are sometimes sufficient to guide our preferences unambiguously.[34]

NOTES

1. Alan Musgrave spoke for many of Kuhn's readers when he noted, apropos of the second edition of *The Structure of Scientific Revolutions*, that in "his recent writings, then, Kuhn disowns most of the challenging ideas ascribed to him by his critics . . . the new, more real Kuhn who emerges . . . [is] but a pale reflection of the old, revolutionary Kuhn" (Musgrave, 1980, p. 51).
2. Kuhn, 1962.
3. Ibid.
4. Ibid., p. 159.
5. As Kuhn himself remarks, he has been attempting "to eliminate misunderstandings for which my own past rhetoric is doubtless partially responsible" (1970, pp. 259–260).
6. Kuhn, 1962, p. 108; my italics.
7. Ibid., pp. 108–109.
8. Ibid., p. 149.
9. See Whewell's remarkably insightful essay of 1851, where he remarks, apropos the transition from one global theory to another: "the change . . . is effected by a transformation, or series of transformations, of the earlier hypothesis, by means of which it is brought nearer and nearer to the second [i.e., later]" (1851, p. 139).
10. Some amplification of this point is required. Kuhn evidently believes that there are some values that transcend specific paradigms. He mentions such examples as the demand for accuracy, consistency, and

simplicity. The fortunes of these values are not linked to specific paradigms. Thus, if they were to change, such change would presumably be independent of shifts in paradigms. In Kuhn's view, however, these values have persisted unchanged since the seventeenth century. Or, rather, scientists have invoked these values persistently since that time; strictly speaking, on Kuhn's analysis, these values are changing constantly, since each scientist interprets them slightly differently. For a detailed discussion of Kuhn's handling of these quasi-shared values, see the final section of this chapter.

11. See Laudan, 1981.
12. For an extensive bibliography on this issue, see Laudan, 1968.
13. See Laudan, 1981.
14. See Laudan, forthcoming.
15. See ibid. for a lengthy treatment of some issues surrounding underdetermination of theories.
16. Kuhn, 1962, p. 159.
17. Kuhn, 1977, p. 322.
18. Ibid., p. 262.
19. Ibid., p. 329.
20. Ibid., p. 325; see also p. 324.
21. Ibid., p. 325.
22. Ibid., p. 323.
23. Ibid., p. 322.
24. Kuhn, 1970, p. 262.
25. "What I have said so far is primarily simply descriptive of what goes on in the sciences at times of theory choice" (Kuhn, 1977, p. 325).
26. Kuhn, 1977, p. 325.
27. Doppelt, 1978. Whereas Kuhn's own discussion of these questions in *The Structure of Scientific Revolutions* rambles considerably, Doppelt offers a succinct and perspicacious formulation of what is, or at least what should have been, Kuhn's argument. Although I quarrel with Doppelt's analysis at several important points, my own thoughts about these issues owe a great deal to his writings.
28. Kuhn, 1962, p. 104.
29. Ibid., pp. 147–148.
30. Ibid., p. 110.
31. Doppelt, 1978, p. 42.
32. Kuhn, 1962, p. 107.
33. Ibid., p. 43.
34. Even on the pragmatic level, however, it is not clear that the Doppeltian version of Kuhn's relativistic picture of scientific change will stand up, for Doppelt is at pains to deny that there can be any short-term resolution between the advocates of rival axiologies. If the arguments of the preceding chapter have any cogency, it seems entirely possible that pragmatic relativism, every bit as much as its epistemic counterpart, is question begging.

REFERENCES

Doppelt, Gerald (1978). "Kuhn's Epistemological Relativism: An Interpretation and Defense," *Inquiry* 21: 33–86.

Gutting, Gary, ed. (1980). *Paradigms and Revolutions*. Notre Dame: University of Notre Dame Press.

Kuhn, Thomas (1962). *The Structure of Scientific Revolutions*. Chicago: University of Chicago Press.

——— (1970). "Reflections on My Critics." In I. Lakatos and A. Musgrave, *Criticism and the Growth of Knowledge*. Cambridge: Cambridge University Press.

——— (1977). *The Essential Tension*. Chicago: University of Chicago Press.

Laudan, Larry (1968). "Theories of Scientific Method from Plato to Mach," *History of Science* 7:1–63.

——— (1981). *Science and Hypothesis*. Dordrecht: Reidel.

——— (forthcoming). *Science and Method*.

Musgrave, Alan (1980). "Kuhn's Second Thoughts." In Gutting, 1980.

Whewell, William (1851). "Of the Transformation of Hypotheses in the History of Science," *Transactions of the Cambridge Philosophical Society* 9:139–147.

The Nature of Scientific Truth

Sheila A. Packard ● *E. Carol Polifroni*

The purpose of this article is to share with the readers the authors' views on the need for a philosophical foundation in nursing scholarship. The philosophical premises of realism, idealism, and empiricism are discussed. In addition, the research methods most appropriately used with each philosophical stance are identified and discussed. The authors strongly suggest that nursing epistemology will not advance along the lines of good science until all nursing theorists, thinkers, and philosophers identify their under-pinning philosophical positions prior to the discovery of theory, through research and other scientific endeavors. A nursing science fiction account of discovery and theory is used to illustrate the points made within the article.

Nursing literature in recent years has increasingly turned toward an examination of issues related to the development of a unique epistemology. Theoretical constructs have been analyzed and dissected, the worthiness of particular theories being determined to some extent by their "fit" with the real world and their concomitant applicability to practice, education, and research (Packard & Polifroni, 1991; Sarter, 1988; Schultz & Meleis, 1988; Smith, 1988; Visintainer, 1986). Methodologies as well as the generalized premises of induction versus deduction are currently under debate (Clarke & Yaros, 1988; Duffy, 1987; Gortner & Schultz, 1988; Moccia, 1988; Norbeck, 1987; Phillips, 1988). The proliferation of nursing science has quite naturally led to these analyses. It seems that a new era has been entered where critical appraisal of both common knowledge and new contributions to the field must be carefully scrutinized.

It is the purpose of this article to add to the self-appraisal taking place in nursing science. The fundamental issues emanating from the philosophy of science must be fully addressed in the critique and analysis of the emerging body of knowledge. Diverse philosophical views regarding the nature of scientific truth and the question of observability will be offered as a basis for a more profound examination of nursing epistemology.

The issues pertaining to truth and its availability are not mutually exclusive. Perhaps the best way to approach explanation in this arena is to enter into a bit of nursing science fiction upon which a discussion may be based.

Dayincalm Theory

In the days before the invention of the quark-perceptograph there lived a pensive nurse scientist named Marion Dayincalm. Dr. Dayincalm, through her own practice, began to reflect on a particular phenomenon concerning nursing care. It seemed as though certain nurses had more success in relieving pain than others. She

· ·
Reprinted by permission of Chestnut House Publications from Nursing Science Quarterly 5:4. © 1992, Chestnut Hill Publications.

noted further that this appeared to have something to do with how much tactile contact the nurse had with the patient and how often the nurse smiled. Dayincalm began to speculate about the mechanism of this occurrence. On a common sense level, it could be said that smiling and touching are observable behaviors and human beings tend to respond to these behaviors positively. Being a thinker, though, Dayincalm wondered if there wasn't an underlying explanation. She postulated that pain, which was at least some form of field disturbance, might be affected by smile (a symptom of positive force) and touching (the channeling of that force). However, no tool existed at the time which could measure such a force.

Dayincalm recognized her difficulties. However, she felt that she was onto something. She proceeded to develop a theory and to examine it by testing it to determine the consequences. Her theory held great promise for the alleviation of suffering. While only speculating as to the nature of the "force," Dayincalm described the aspects of the force that were apparent and constructed a model pertaining to the phenomenon of concern. Interestingly enough, when her postulates were used as a guide to practice, a patient's pain often diminished.

The SAT (smile and touch) theory aroused severe criticism in the world of nursing science. This criticism often took the form of, "In order to account for the facts, Dayincalm must assume a force exists. The qualities of this force can't be measured. Thus, the very postulates of her theory preclude their being observed; they are unobservable in principle." This general remark was then followed by various interpretations and analyses of Dayincalm's SAT theory. According to one of these analyses, the force was merely convenient fiction useful for facilitating the thinking of scientists but not to be taken seriously in the sphere of knowledge. A closely related view held that the SAT theory was just a tool, useful for organizing observational statements and producing, perhaps, desired results, and it made no more sense to question the

essence of the force than to ask about the nature of a hammer or any other tool.

In actuality, most scientists agreed that theories such as Dayincalm's played a useful role in scientific enterprise. However, some were concerned with the problems that could arise when metaphysical entities were pondered. Others maintained that while Dayincalm's force might exist in reality, it should not be the concern of nursing. They asserted that if she had used the correct methodology, she would have discovered sooner, and with less effort, all of the propositions relating to SAT without the superfluous link (the force) in the causal chain. Yet another group held that understanding must be directed toward the lived experience of individuals, not toward transcendent data.

Fortunately, Dayincalm lived to see the invention of the quarkperceptograph. Her force was identified through readings taken by the new instrument, and, in fact, specific patterns of force were determined that coincided with the assertions of SAT theory. In reaction to this validation of Dayincalm's claims, some critics were compelled to modify their views. One group of scientists stated that Dayincalm's force never had been unobservable in principle because the SAT theory did not imply the impossibility of finding a means (the quarkperceptograph) of observing it. A more radical cadre contended that the force was in fact not observed at all; it was argued that what was detected by means of the quarkperceptograph was merely an image rather than reality itself.

The problems confronted by the scientists in this fictional account are, coincidentally, those facing nursing as it moves into the 21st century.

The Nature of Scientific Truth

Perhaps the most fundamental question pertaining to the development of nursing epistemology concerns the essence of scientific truth. The fundamental premises about truth must be confronted by all of those intent upon producing knowledge, in that it governs the aim of science.

Indeed, ideas about the nature of truth are not new; they predate Socrates, when scattered groups of Greek philosophers attempted to describe the way the world really is beyond everyday appearances (Solomon, 1985). Today, the question "What is truth?" divides philosophers of science. It is beyond the scope of this article to trace currently held perspectives from antiquity. However, several important positions on the nature of scientific truth can be briefly described.

Realism is one philosophical stance regarding the nature of truth. Essentially, the realist perspective maintains that a definite world structure exists. It is possible to obtain a substantial amount of reliable and relatively observer-independent information concerning this world structure. Its features may not be restricted to that which is observable. This view culminates in the idea that science aims at (and may achieve) access to the definite world structure at some future time. The "truth" of nursing science is therefore determined by its correspondence with features of the definite world structure (Fine, 1984). Realism, succinctly stated, contends that the picture science gives of the world is true, is real, and that the entities postulated do, in fact, exist (van Fraassen, 1976). In addition, real things are in no sense conditioned by their being known. They may continue to exist unaltered when they are not known (Sahakian, 1968).

In contrast to the realist perspective, idealism or anti-realism incorporates a wide variety of philosophical views pertaining to truth (Sahakian, 1968). Its diverse adherents, however, agree on the fundamental hypothesis that the universe is the embodiment of the mind. Ultimate reality transcends phenomena. And all knowable things are viewed as mental entities (in the form of thought, theory, reasoning, ideas, and facts) dependent upon the presence of a knower (Aiken, 1956; Sahakian, 1968; Solomon, 1985). A distinction can be drawn between two of the more commonly espoused brands of idealism.

Metaphysical idealism emphasizes the analysis of the entire universe as a psychic reality (Sahakian, 1968). If there is a world reality beyond human consciousness, it must be seen as a consequence of human understanding (Aiken, 1956). Metaphysical idealism contends that science indeed aims to be true but may not be literally construed; truth is conveyed by common acceptance. This type of idealism encompasses a paradigm-relative concept of truth as discussed by Kuhn (1970). Where realism orients the scientist to face out to an unknown world structure, these idealists counter with a notion of truth which reflects external world correspondence and is bounded by consensual agreement in scientific dialogue. Behaviorism, which fixes the limits of truth at what is accepted by the scientific community, is an example of this brand of anti-realism (Fine, 1984). Truth is grounded in consensus, and the metaphysical aspects of realism may be cast aside.

Epistemological idealism emphasizes the identification of reality with mentally knowable data (Sahakian, 1968). This position is commonly known as empiricism and may be traced to the positive philosophy of Comte (1853). For this brand of idealism, the meaning of proposition cannot be known unless it is possible to state the conditions under which the proposition may be verified (verification principle). Sense observation or information ultimately derived by means of sense observation is necessary for this verification (Aiken, 1956).

The more contemporary version of this perspective (constructive empiricism) contends that science aims only to provide theories that are empirically adequate and that acceptance of a theory necessitates *only* that it is empirically adequate (van Fraassen, 1976). The only truth to be imagined is that which is at our fingertips. It avoids the pitfalls of earlier brands of empiricism (the conception of theory as a deductively closed logical system in the vocabulary of which there is imposed an epistemologically significant distinction between observables and unobservables) by allowing science itself to dictate that which is empirically verifiable. Again, truth is not as elusive as in realism. To the empiricist, only that which is observable exists, and science decides what is observable (Fine, 1984).

The opposing views of scientific truth, where truth is seen as either entirely objective (realism) or utterly subjective (idealism), were rejected by Husserl (1956) in his phenomenological philosophy. Although disputed by Paci (1972), Merleau-Ponty (1945) considered phenomenology the mediation between the two polarities. The phenomenological stance asserts that truth dwells within the consciousness. The world may be beyond the bounds of the experience, but ego is always present in experience. Reality is disclosed only through individual consciousness (Paci, 1972). Pure phenomenon possesses a subjectivity to the particular ego which experiences it, but essence possesses an intersubjectivity, a characteristic shared by all persons. The experience of sound as a pure phenomenon is the private subjective state of the person experiencing it, but the essence of sound, its universal characteristics (comparable to mathematical principles), is common to all persons (intersubjectivity). Experience is therefore of two types: ordinary (or individual) and essential (or universal) (Sahakian, 1968; Solomon, 1985). Phenomenology is an attempt to study consciousness in order to determine the essences or universals.

The philosophical notions of truth may be stated simply as: (a) a stance based on realism wherein truth is larger than and different from human consciousness, an objective reality, the discovery of which may be seen as the goal of all science; (b) a metaphysical idealist stance which holds that truth is delineated by a consensus of scientists, allowing for the rise and fall of competing paradigms; (c) an epistemologic idealist stance whereby truth is no more and no less than that which may be reached through empirical means; and, (d) a phenomenological stance where truth may be identified through the study of essential experience (Aiken, 1956; Carnap, 1970; Churchland, 1982; Fine, 1984; Gurwitsch, 1974; Maxwell, 1962; Paci, 1972; Sahakian, 1968; Solomon, 1985; van Fraassen, 1976). Each of these philosophical positions has something to say about the aims of the scientific enterprise. That is, each position directs science toward the acquisition of a particular sort of truth (be it within or separate from the realm of human consciousness).

Dayincalm's SAT Theory and Truth

The hypothetical situation of Dayincalm's work may be used to further illustrate the philosophical positions regarding scientific truth. The question which is fundamental to evaluating the worthiness of the SAT theory is posited within the philosophy of science. To wit, does the theory represent truth?

From the perspective of realism, there is an objective world structure which may or may not include Dayincalm's force. Truth, from this stance, is often elusive and perhaps just beyond the grasp of the working scientist. However, the possibility exists that the mysteries of the universe may be eventually unmasked. When Dayincalm first set forth her assertions, those scientists espousing realism acknowledged that her work played a useful role in scientific speculation. They were willing to accept that the force might exist, and, that in some way, this entity was part of a larger world reality. Truth is not dependent upon human abilities. Therefore, Dayincalm might be given the benefit of the doubt until proven otherwise. As it happened, the quarkperceptograph was invented, which gave credence to the propositions of the SAT theory. The realists took satisfaction in stating that the theory now stood up to more fully developed scrutiny, the force never having been considered unobservable in principle. However, recognizing the limitations inherent in human endeavors, the realists continued to anticipate modifications to theory.

The positions of the idealists, who link truth to human consciousness, contrasted with some of the realists' appraisals. Some idealists (those of the truth-as-acceptance ilk) were generally accepting of Dayincalm's theory. Whether her thesis was a convenient fiction or a tool, it was generally thought to be useful in organizing observations and in producing results in the areas of practice and education. It also had its applications in research. However, these idealists believed that the true value in the SAT theory had little to do with the postulated force. Pragmatically, the smile and touch behaviors were enough to support the theory without any reference to a supra-empirical entity such as the force. The theory as it was originally designed was deemed acceptable to the nursing science community, and, therefore, it could be viewed as truth. Smile and touch seemed to work. Why complicate a nice simple assertion? The nature of the force was not the concern of nursing science. The subsequent discovery of the quark-perceptograph had little impact upon this group of thinkers. Since the theory had already gained credence, it had been established as truth and would remain so until a competing theory took its place.

The other group of idealists (empiricists) initially viewed Dayincalm's ideas with skepticism. They stated that her theory was based upon assumptions which could not be verified. The force as proposed was unobservable and, therefore, could not be measured. This being the case, the SAT theory, while in some instances useful, did not pass the test of scientific rigor. Metaphysical phenomena were irrelevant in the proliferation of nursing epistemology. The advent of the quarkperceptograph did much to change the view of some empiricists. The con-

structive empiricists were satisfied that the force had been proven to exist based on the findings of the new instrument. Yet a cadre of skeptics (the more traditional logical empiricists) pondered the nature of the quarkperceptograph. Since it was an extension of the human sensory apparatus, perhaps its findings were not to be trusted.

Lastly, the phenomenologists received Dayincalm's theory in yet a different way. This cadre of scientists centered their attention on the lived experience of those persons being smiled at and touched. Since human consciousness is the only object which may be studied, it was the essential experience of patients that mattered. They held that attention should be restricted to the absolute data of pure consciousness. The content of consciousness is the only indisputable and authentic data. This content stands prior to all scientific explanation, interpretation and theorizing. Phenomenological analysis excludes everything which transcends the bounds of experience, as well as cause and effect relationships. The phenomenologists, therefore, contended that nothing about smile and touch in itself may be known directly. It is only the experience reported by patients that constitutes any evidence of this phenomenon. The nurse's act of smiling or touching is irrelevant to an understanding of the essential experience of pain relief. Dayincalm's theory per se was of little interest to the phenomenologists. SAT theory was yet another scientific explanation which was off the beam.

Observables and Unobservables

The controversy over scientific truth has directed attention toward the concept of observability. A problem facing all science, including nursing science, is the determination of what is meant by the term "observable." This becomes particularly salient when it may be noted that authors of research textbooks commonly state that "observation" is the basic unifying principle across all methodologies (Polit & Hungler, 1988; Wilson, 1985; Woods & Catanzaro, 1988).

On the surface, observability would seem to be a characteristic of an entity that is rather straightforward. Either something may or may not be seen, touched, heard, and so forth. The problem arises when the scientist attempts to draw a line between what is observable and what is not observable by ordinary means. If an entity may be seen or heard only through some extension of the human sensory apparatus, is it empirically available or does it pass into the realm of being present theoretically? In this regard Maxwell (1962) states,

> It really does seem awkward to say that when people who wear glasses describe what they see they are talking about shadows, while those who employ unaided vision talk about physical things—or that when we look through a windowpane we can only infer it is raining while if we raise the window we may "observe directly" that it is. The point I am making is there is, in principle, a continuous series beginning with looking through a vacuum and containing these as members: looking through a window pane, looking through glasses, looking through binoculars, looking through a low-power microscope, looking through a high-power microscope, etc. The important consequence is that so far, we are left without criteria which would enable us to draw a nonarbitrary line between "observation" and "theory." (p. 22)

Scientists through their work and through their acceptance of certain theories cannot avoid the defining of observability and its implications. A range exists from the most conservative view (only entities immediately available to human senses) to the most liberal view (anything that is even remotely able to be observed if and when instrumentation exists). These views overlap with the philosophical notions of realism and idealism.

The more conservative perspectives are held by idealists. This is logical since truth to these scientists, as previously mentioned, is contingent upon human consciousness. What is unavailable and cannot be observed concretely and at present is not true. In this way the logical empiricist position ultimately speaks to the need for the grounding of data in observational terms. Carnap (1970) asserts that there are different levels of abstraction among the concepts of empirical science. In order to find out whether the more abstract concepts hold in a certain case, one must carry out a more complex procedure which also rests finally on observations. A slightly more moderate perspective is held by the constructive empiricists. Van Fraassen (1976) contends that descriptive excellence in theory is the ultimate measure of truth and ontology at all levels of cognition, even at the observational level. Constructive empiricists are willing to allow for not only direct observables but also detectables (entities which can be indirectly examined, as, for example, through a high-power telescope or sonar apparatus). In essence, empiricists have a generally narrow view of observation. Other idealists in a somewhat middle-of-the-road approach emphasize the need for observability in the establishment of theory but are willing to allow the scientific community to determine the constitution of observation. Thus there is a bit more latitude (as perhaps beyond immediate sensory information) given to observation and therefore theory development. Science collectively decides on appropriate instrumentation.

The most liberal stance is taken by scientists who espouse realism. Churchland (1982) asserts that observational concepts are just as theory-laden as any others, since the integrity of those concepts is contingent on the integrity of the theories in which they are embedded. Therefore observational ontology is rendered exactly as dubious as nonobservational ontology. There is, from the realist's view, no reason for resisting commitment to unobservable ontologies while allowing commitment to observable ontologies. The line between observable and non-observable or theoretical entities is blurred.

By its very nature, phenomenology disregards the use of instrumentation in arriving at truth. While intersubjectivity is acknowledged (meaning that others are known to exist), it is the patterns found in individual human experiences (essential experience) that are sought in scientific enterprise (Paci, 1972; Sahakian, 1968). The acquisition of data relevant to universal experience does not follow along the lines of traditional scientific methodology where measurement becomes a salient issue.

Epistemological Considerations in Nursing

The foregoing discussion has centered on ideas of truth and how truth may be achieved in science. These fundamental philosophical notions must also be considered in the development of nursing epistemology. Views of scientific truth provide a platform for appraisal of nursing theories and a way to better understand the various research methods.

THEORY

A more profound critique of nursing theory is possible only when the philosophical perspective of the theorist is examined. Indeed, a particular theorist may not have set out to formulate a framework which defines truth, but this is what theory accomplishes. Each thinker in nursing holds a position on the nature of scientific truth, whether explicitly stated or implicitly inferred. Every theory is based upon an idea of what truth might be and where it might be found. The evaluator of theory may agree or disagree with the theorist's position. It would be very difficult for a critic to value any theory that is based upon a view of truth inconsistent with or in opposition to his or her own view. In some

respects, this explains much about the appeal of certain theories to specific individuals.

Competing ideas about the nature of truth are more fundamental than the discussion of wholes or parts, let alone the applicability, simplicity, and generality of a theory. It may be contended that such discussions must begin with a determination of a theorist's assumptions about the nature of scientific truth. Without this knowledge, the value of a theory cannot be fully appraised.

RESEARCH METHODS

Recent literature is replete with discussions of appropriate methodologies for the acquisition of scientific knowledge in nursing. Most scholars are only too familiar with the qualitative/quantitative debate and its offspring of blended methods. The occurrence of such dialogue and controversy is not only to be expected but perhaps also necessary as nursing experiences the growing pains of maturing as a science. However, the essential issue which must be understood is that methodology of any sort is simply a means to an end. It is absurd to argue the value of one approach over another without this end in mind. The philosophical positions held on the nature of truth and notions of observability again become of paramount importance. The acceptance or rejection of a method must be fundamentally based upon a perspective regarding scientific truth. It may be asserted that the research question determines the method, but it must also be recognized that philosophical notions about scientific truth determine the research question.

Nursing's newfound attraction for blended research is that it ostensibly offers the best of all worlds: adherence to stringent scientific quantification while at the same time seeking a richer more qualifiable truth. Herein, however, lies the fatal flaw. It is not possible to simultaneously contend that truth is any combination of the projection of human consciousness and independent of this same consciousness. That is to say, either one believes that scientific truth is in the form of a separate and definite world structure, or that scientific truth consists only of what is accessible and measurable by human beings, or that truth is found in the lived experience of individuals. Thus, blended research is possible only when the methods used are noncontradictory. The notion of scientific truth is not altered by virtue of methodology for the working scientist. Quantitative research may be blended only with certain sorts of qualitative approaches such as the Dickoff and James (1968) version of factor isolating. In most cases, quantification cannot be triangulated or combined with interpretative methodologies simply because they do not aim at the same scientific truth. No scientist can blend that which is fundamentally inconsistent. "Good science" cannot be a sophisticated sort of cognitive dissonance. Good science emanates from a solid philosophical base wherein the ends determine the means, rather than the other way around.

Conclusion

As nursing moves into the 21st century, it may be expected that dialogue and debate centering on epistemological concerns will proliferate. This article has attempted to draw the reader's attention to some foundational issues relevant to any discussion of the means and ends of nursing science. Addressing the philosophical basis of knowledge development is an essential component of nursing scholarship.

REFERENCES

Aiken, H. (1956). *The age of ideology*. New York: New American Library of World Literature.

Carnap, R. (1970). *Foundations of logic and mathematics*. Chicago: University of Chicago Press.

Churchland, P. M. (1982). The anti-realist epistemology of van Fraassen's scientific image. *Pacific Philosophical Quarterly, 66*(2).

Clarke, P., & Yaros, P. (1988). Commentary: Transitions to new methodologies in nursing science. *Nursing Science Quarterly, 3,* 147–151.

Comte, A. (1853). *The positive philosophy of Auguste Comte* (H. Martineau, Trans.). London: Trubner. (free translation of Comte's *Cours de Philosophia Positive*, 1840–1842).

Dickoff, J., & James, P. (1968). A theory of theories: A position paper. *Nursing Research, 17*(3), 197–203.

Duffy, M. (1987). Methodological triangulation: A vehicle for merging quantitative and qualitative research methods. *IMAGE: Journal of Nursing Scholarship, 19*(3), 130–133.

Fine, A. (1984). Is scientific realism compatible with quantum physics? *Nous, 18,* 51–66.

Gortner, S., & Schultz, P. (1988). Approaches to nursing science methods. *IMAGE: Journal of Nursing Scholarship, 20*(1), 22–24.

Gurwitsch, A. (1974). *Phenomenology and the theory of science*. Evanston: Northwestern University Press.

Husserl, E. (1956). Philosophy as a rigorous science. *Cross Currents, 6,* 227–246, 325–344.

Kuhn, T. (1970). *The structure of scientific revolutions* (2nd ed.). Chicago: University of Chicago Press.

Maxwell, G. (1962). The ontological status of theoretical entities. *Minnesota Studies in Philosophy of Science, 3,* 3–14.

Merleau-Ponty, M. (1945). *Phenomenologic de la perception* (C. Smith, Trans.). Paris: Gallimard.

Moccia, P. (1988). A critique of compromise: Beyond the methods debate. *Advances in Nursing Science, 10*(4), 1–9.

Norbeck, J. (1987). In defense of empiricism. *IMAGE: Journal of Nursing Scholarship, 19*(1), 28–30.

Paci, E. (1972). *The function of the sciences and the meaning of man*. Evanston: Northwestern University Press.

Packard, S., & Polifroni, E. C. (1991). Dilemmas in nursing science. *Nursing Science Quarterly, 4,* 7–13.

Phillips, J. (1988). Research blenders. *Nursing Science Quarterly, 1,* 4–5.

Polit, D., & Hungler, B. P. (1988). *Nursing research: Principles and methods* (2nd ed.). Philadelphia: Lippincott.

Sahakian, W. (1968). *History of philosophy*. New York: Harper & Row.

Sarter, B. (1988). Philosophical sources of nursing theory. *Nursing Science Quarterly, 1,* 52–59.

Schultz, P., & Meleis, A. (1988). Nursing epistemology: Tradition, insights, questions. *IMAGE: Journal of Nursing Scholarship, 20*(4), 217–222.

Smith, M. J. (1988). Perspectives on nursing science. *Nursing Science Quarterly, 1,* 80–85.

Solomon, R. (1985). *Introducing philosophy.* San Diego: Harcourt Brace & Jovonovich.

van Fraassen, B. B. (1976). To save the phenomena. *The Journal of Philosophy, 73*(18), 633–637.

Visintainer, M. (1986). The nature of nursing knowledge and theory in nursing. *IMAGE: Journal of Nursing Scholarship, 18*(2), 32–38.

Wilson, H. S. (1985). *Research in nursing.* Menlo Park: Addison Wesley.

Woods, N., & Catanzaro, M. (1988). *Nursing research: Theory and practices.* St. Louis: Mosby.

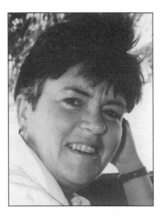 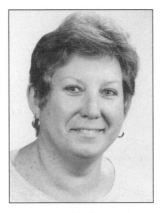

SHEILA A. PACKARD   E. CAROL POLIFRONI

Experimentation and Scientific Realism

Ian Hacking

Experimental physics provides the strongest evidence for scientific realism. Entities that in principle cannot be observed are regularly manipulated to produce new phenomena and to investigate other aspects of nature. They are tools, instruments not for thinking but for doing.

The philosopher's standard "theoretical entity" is the electron. I will illustrate how electrons have become experimental entities, or experimenter's entities. In the early stages of our discovery of an entity, we may test hypotheses about it. Then it is merely a hypothetical entity. Much later, if we come to understand some of its causal powers and use it to build devices that achieve well-understood effects in other parts of nature, then it assumes quite a different status.

Discussions about scientific realism or antirealism usually talk about theories, explanation, and prediction. Debates at that level are necessarily inconclusive. Only at the level of experimental practice is scientific realism unavoidable—but this realism is not about theories and truth. The experimentalist need only be a realist about the entities used as tools.

A Plea for Experiments

No field in the philosophy of science is more systematically neglected than experiment. Our grade school teachers may have told us that sci-

entific method is experimental method, but histories of science have become histories of theory. Experiments, the philosophers say, are of value only when they test theory. Experimental work, they imply, has no life of its own. So we lack even a terminology to describe the many varied roles of experiment. Nor has this one-sidedness done theory any good, for radically different types of theory are used to think about the same physical phenomenon (e.g., the magneto-optical effect). The philosophers of theory have not noticed this and so misreport even theoretical enquiry.

Different sciences at different times exhibit different relationships between "theory" and "experiment." One chief role of experiment is the creation of phenomena. Experimenters bring into being phenomena that do not naturally exist in a pure state. These phenomena are the touchstones of physics, the keys to nature, and the source of much modern technology. Many are what physicists after the 1870s began to call "effects": the photoelectric effect, the Compton effect, and so forth.[1] A recent high-energy extension of the creation of phenomena is the creation of "events," to use the jargon of the trade. Most of the phenomena, effects, and events created by the experimenter are like plutonium: They do not exist in nature except possibly on vanishingly rare occasions.[2]

In this paper I leave aside questions of methodology, history, taxonomy, and the purpose of experiment in natural science. I turn to the purely philosophical issue of scientific real-

Reprinted by permission from Philosophical Topics 13(1):71–87. © 1983.

ism. Simply call it "realism" for short. There are two basic kinds: realism about entities and realism about theories. There is no agreement on the precise definition of either. Realism about theories says that we try to form true theories about the world, about the inner constitution of matter and about the outer reaches of space. This realism gets its bite from optimism: We think we can do well in this project and have already had partial success. Realism about entities—and I include processes, states, waves, currents, interactions, fields, black holes, and the like among entities—asserts the existence of at least some of the entities that are the stock in trade of physics.[3]

The two realisms may seem identical. If you believe a theory, do you not believe in the existence of the entities it speaks about? If you believe in some entities, must you not describe them in some theoretical way that you accept? This seeming identity is illusory. *The vast majority of experimental physicists are realists about entities but not about theories.* Some are, no doubt, realists about theories too, but that is less central to their concerns.

Experimenters are often realists about the entities that they investigate, but they do not have to be so. R. A. Millikan probably had few qualms about the reality of electrons when he set out to measure their charge. But he could have been skeptical about what he would find until he found it. He could even have remained skeptical. Perhaps there is a least unit of electric charge, but there is no particle or object with exactly that unit of charge. Experimenting on an entity does not commit you to believing that it exists. Only manipulating an entity, in order to experiment on something else, need do that.

Moreover, it is not even that you use electrons to experiment on something else that makes it impossible to doubt electrons. Understanding some causal properties of electrons, you guess how to build a very ingenious, complex device that enables you to line up the electrons the way you want, in order to see what will happen to something else. Once you have the right experimental idea, you know in advance roughly how to try to build the device, because you know that this is the way to get the electrons to behave in such and such a way. Electrons are no longer ways of organizing our thoughts or saving the phenomena that have been observed. They are now ways of creating phenomena in some other domain of nature. Electrons are tools.

There is an important experimental contrast between realism about entities and realism about theories. Suppose we say that the latter is belief that science aims at true theories. Few experimenters will deny that. Only philosophers doubt it. Aiming at the truth is, however, something about the indefinite future. Aiming a beam of electrons is using present electrons. Aiming a finely tuned laser at a particular atom in order to knock off a certain electron to produce an ion is aiming at present electrons. There is, in contrast, no present set of theories that one has to believe in. If realism about theories is a doctrine about the aims of science, it is a doctrine laden with certain kinds of values. If realism about entities is a matter of aiming electrons next week or aiming at other electrons the week after, it is a doctrine much more neutral between values. The way in which experimenters are scientific realists about entities is entirely different from ways in which they might be realists about theories.

This shows up when we turn from ideal theories to present ones. Various properties are confidently ascribed to electrons, but most of the confident properties are expressed in numerous different theories or models about which an experimenter can be rather agnostic. Even people in a team, who work on different parts of the same large experiment, may hold different and mutually incompatible accounts of electrons. That is because different parts of the experiment will make different uses of electrons. Models good for calculations on one aspect of electrons will be poor for others. Occasionally, a team actually has to select a member with a quite different theoretical perspective simply to get someone who can solve those experimental problems. You may choose someone with a foreign training, and whose talk is well-nigh incommensurable with yours, just to get people who can produce the effects you want.

But might there not be a common core of theory, the intersection of everybody in the group, which is the theory of the electron to which all the experimenters are realistically committed? I would say common lore, *not* common core. There are a lot of theories, models, approximations, pictures, formalisms, methods, and so forth involving electrons, but there is no reason to suppose that the intersection of these is a theory at all. Nor is there any reason to think that there is such a thing as "the most powerful nontrivial *theory* contained in the intersection of all the theories in which this or that member of a team has been trained to believe." Even if there are a lot of shared beliefs, there is no reason to suppose they form anything worth calling a theory. Naturally, teams tend to be formed from like-minded people at the same institute, so there is usually some real shared theoretical basis to their work. That is a sociological fact, not a foundation for scientific realism.

I recognize that many a scientific realism concerning theories is a doctrine not about the present but about what we might achieve, or possibly an ideal at which we aim. So to say that there is no present theory does not count against the optimistic aim. The point is that such scientific realism about theories has to adopt the Peircean principles of faith, hope, and charity. Scientific realism about entities needs no such virtues. It arises from what we can do at present. To understand this, we must look in some detail at what it is like to build a device that makes the electrons sit up and behave.

Our Debt to Hilary Putnam

It was once the accepted wisdom that a word such as "electron" gets its meaning from its place in a network of sentences that state theoretical laws. Hence arose the infamous problems of incommensurability and theory change. For if a theory is modified, how could a word such as "electron" go on meaning the same? How could different theories about electrons be compared, since the very word "electron" would differ in meaning from theory to theory?

Putnam saved us from such questions by inventing a referential model of meaning. He says that meaning is a vector, refreshingly like a dictionary entry. First comes the syntactic marker (part of speech); next the semantic marker (general category of thing signified by the word); then the stereotype (clichés about the natural kind, standard examples of its use, and present-day associations. The stereotype is subject to change as opinions about the kind are modified). Finally, there is the actual referent of the word, the very stuff, or thing, it denotes if it denotes anything. (Evidently dictionaries cannot include this in their entry, but pictorial dictionaries do their best by inserting illustrations whenever possible.)[4]

Putnam thought we can often guess at entities that we do not literally point to. Our initial guesses may be jejune or inept, and not every naming of an invisible thing or stuff pans out. But when it does, and we frame better and better ideas, then Putnam says that, although the stereotype changes, we refer to the same kind of thing or stuff all along. We and Dalton alike spoke about the same stuff when we spoke of (inorganic) acids. J. J. Thomson, H. A. Lorentz, Bohr, and Millikan were, with their different theories and observations, speculating about the same kind of thing, the electron.

There is plenty of unimportant vagueness about when an entity has been successfully "dubbed," as Putnam puts it. "Electron" is the name suggested by G. Johnstone Stoney in 1891 as the name for a natural unit of electricity. He had drawn attention to this unit in 1874. The name was then applied to the subatomic particles of negative charge, which J. J. Thomson, in 1897, showed cathode rays consist of. Was Johnstone Stoney referring to the electron?

Putnam's account does not require an unequivocal answer. Standard physics books say that Thomson discovered the electron. For once I might back theory and say that Lorentz beat him to it. Thomson called his electrons "corpuscles," the subatomic particles of electric charge. Evidently, the name does not matter much. Thomson's most notable achievement was to measure the mass of the electron. He did this by a rough (though quite good) guess at e, and by making an excellent determination of e/m, showing that m is about $1/1800$ the mass of the hydrogen atom. Hence it is natural to say that Lorentz merely postulated the existence of a particle of negative charge, while Thomson, determining its mass, showed that there is some such real stuff beaming off a hot cathode.

The stereotype of the electron has regularly changed, and we have at least two largely incompatible stereotypes, the electron as cloud and the electron as particle. One fundamental enrichment of the idea came in the 1920s. Electrons, it was found, have angular momentum, or "spin." Experimental work by O. Stern and W. Gerlach first indicated this, and then S. Goudsmit and G. E. Uhlenbeck provided the theoretical understanding of it in 1925. Whatever we think, Johnstone Stoney, Lorentz, Bohr, Thomson, and Goudsmit were all finding out more about the same kind of thing, the electron.

We need not accept the fine points of Putnam's account of reference in order to thank him for giving us a new way to talk about meaning. Serious discussion of inferred entities need no longer lock us into pseudo-problems of incommensurability and theory change. Twenty-five years ago the experimenter who believed that electrons exist, without giving much credence to any set of laws about electrons, would have been dismissed as philosophically incoherent. Now we realize it was the philosophy that was wrong, not the experimenter. My own relationship to Putnam's account of meaning is like the experimenter's relationship to a theory. I do not literally believe Putnam, but I am happy to employ his account as an alternative to the unpalatable account in fashion some time ago.

Putnam's philosophy is always in flux. His account of reference was intended to bolster scientific realism. But now, at the time of this writing (July 1981), he rejects any "metaphysical realism" but allows "internal realism."[5] The internal realist acts, in practical affairs, as if the entities occurring in his working theories did in fact exist. However, the direction of Putnam's metaphysical anti-realism is no longer scientific. It is not peculiarly about natural science. It is about chairs and livers too. He thinks that the world does not naturally break up into our classifications. He calls himself a transcendental idealist. I call him a transcendental nominalist. I use the word "nominalist" in the old-fashioned way, not meaning opposition to "abstract entities" like sets, but meaning the doctrine that there is no nonmental classification in nature that exists over and above our own human system of naming.

There might be two kinds of internal realist, the instrumentalist about science and the scientific realist. The former is, in practical affairs where he uses his present scheme of concepts, a realist about livers and chairs but thinks that electrons are only mental constructs. The latter thinks that livers, chairs, and electrons are probably all in the same boat, that is, real at least within the present system of classification. I take Putnam to be an internal scientific realist rather than an internal instrumentalist. The fact that either doctrine is compatible with transcendental nominalism and internal realism shows that our question of scientific realism is almost entirely independent of Putnam's internal realism.

Interfering

Francis Bacon, the first and almost last philosopher of experiments, knew it well: The experimenter sets out "to twist the lion's tail." Experimentation is interference in the course of nature; "nature under constraint and vexed; that is to say, when by art and the hand of man she is forced out of her natural state, and squeezed and molded."[6] The experimenter is convinced of the reality of entities, some of whose causal properties are sufficiently well understood that they can be used to interfere *elsewhere* in nature. One is impressed by entities that one can use to test conjectures about other, more hypothetical entities. In my example, one is sure of the electrons that are used to investigate weak neutral currents and neutral bosons. This should not be news, for why else are we (nonskeptics) sure of the reality of even macroscopic objects, but because of what we do with them, what we do to them, and what they do to us?

Interference and interaction are the stuff of reality. This is true, for example, at the borderline of observability. Too often philosophers imagine that microscopes carry conviction because they help us see better. But that is only part of the story. On the contrary, what counts is what we can do to a specimen under a microscope, and what we can see ourselves doing. We stain the specimen, slice it, inject it, irradiate it, fix it. We examine it using different kinds of microscopes that employ optical systems that rely on almost totally unrelated facts about light. Microscopes carry conviction because of the great array of interactions and interferences that are possible. When we see something that turns out to be unstable under such play, we call it an artifact and say it is not real.[7]

Likewise, as we move down in scale to the truly unseeable, it is our power to use unobservable entities that makes us believe they are there. Yet, I blush over these words "see" and "observe." Philosophers and physicists often use these words in different ways. Philosophers tend to treat opacity to visible light as the touchstone of reality, so that anything that cannot be touched or seen with the naked eye is called a theoretical or inferred entity. Physicists, in contrast, cheerfully talk of observing the very entities that philosophers say are not observable. For example, the fermions are those fundamental constituents of matter such as electron neutrinos and deuterons and, perhaps, the notorious quarks. All are standard philosophers' "unobservable" entities. C. Y. Prescott, the initiator of the experiment described below, said in a recent lecture, that "of these fermions, only the t quark is yet unseen. The failure to observe $t\bar{t}$ states in e^+e^- annihilation at PETRA remains a puzzle."[8] Thus, the physicist distinguishes among the philosophers' "unobservable" entities, noting which have been observed and which not. Dudley Shapere has just published a valuable study of this fact.[9] In his example, neutrinos are used to see the interior of a star. He has ample quotations such as "neutrinos present the only way of directly observing" the very hot core of a star.

John Dewey would have said that fascination with seeing-with-the-naked-eye is part of the spectator theory of knowledge that has bedeviled philosophy from earliest times. But I do not think Plato or Locke or anyone before the nineteenth century was as obsessed with the sheer opacity of objects as we have been since. My own obsession with a technology that manipulates objects is, of course, a twentieth-century counterpart to positivism and phenomenology. Its proper rebuttal is not a restriction to a narrower domain of reality, namely, to what can be positivistically seen with the eye, but an extension to other modes by which people can extend their consciousness.

Making

Even if experimenters are realists about entities, it does not follow that they are right. Perhaps it is a matter of psychology: Maybe the very skills that make for a great experimenter go with a certain cast of mind which objectifies whatever it thinks about. Yet this will not do. The experimenter cheerfully regards neutral bosons as merely hypothetical entities, while electrons are real. What is the difference?

There are an enormous number of ways in which to make instruments that rely on the causal properties of electrons in order to produce desired effects of unsurpassed precision. I shall illustrate this. The argument—it could be called the "experimental argument for realism"—is not that we infer the reality of electrons from our success. We do not make the instruments and then infer the reality of the electrons, as when we test a hypothesis, and then believe it because it passed the test. That gets the time order wrong. By now we design apparatus relying on a modest number of home truths about electrons, in order to produce some other phenomenon that we wish to investigate.

That may sound as if we believe in the electrons because we predict how our apparatus will behave. That too is misleading. We have a number of general ideas about how to prepare polarized electrons, say. We spend a lot of time building prototypes that do not work. We get rid of innumerable bugs. Often we have to give up and try another approach. Debugging is not a matter of theoretically explaining or predicting what is going wrong. It is partly a matter of getting rid of "noise" in the apparatus. "Noise" often means all the events that are not understood by any theory. The instrument must be able to isolate, physically, the properties of the entities that we wish to use, and damp down all the other effects that might get in our way. *We are completely convinced of the reality of electrons when we regularly set to build—and often enough succeed in building—new kinds of device that use various well understood causal properties of electrons to interfere in other more hypothetical parts of nature.*

It is not possible to grasp this without an example. Familiar historical examples have usually become encrusted by false theory-oriented philosophy or history, so I will take something new. This is a polarizing electron gun whose acronym is PEGGY II. In 1978, it was used in a fundamental experiment that attracted attention even in *The New York Times*. In the next section I describe the point of making PEGGY II. To do that, I have to tell some new physics. You may omit reading this and read only the engineering section that follows. Yet it must be of interest to know the rather easy-to-understand significance

of the main experimental results, namely, that parity is not conserved in scattering of polarized electrons from deuterium, and that, more generally, parity is violated in weak neutral-current interactions.[10]

Parity and Weak Neutral Currents

There are four fundamental forces in nature, not necessarily distinct. Gravity and electromagnetism are familiar. Then there are the strong and weak forces (the fulfillment of Newton's program, in the *Optics*, which taught that all nature would be understood by the interaction of particles with various forces that were effective in attraction or repulsion over various different distances, i.e., with different rates of extinction).

Strong forces are 100 times stronger than electromagnetism but act only over a minuscule distance, at most the diameter of a proton. Strong forces act on "hadrons," which include protons, neutrons, and more recent particles, but not electrons or any other members of the class of particles called "leptons."

The weak forces are only 1/10,000 times as strong as electromagnetism, and act over a distance 100 times greater than strong forces. But they act on both hadrons and leptons, including electrons. The most familiar example of a weak force may be radioactivity.

The theory that motivates such speculation is quantum electrodynamics. It is incredibly successful, yielding many predictions better than one part in a million, truly a miracle in experimental physics. It applies over distances ranging from diameters of the earth to 1/100 the diameter of the proton. This theory supposes that all the forces are "carried" by some sort of particle: Photons do the job in electromagnetism. We hypothesize "gravitons" for gravity.

In the case of interactions involving weak forces, there are charged currents. We postulate that particles called "bosons" carry these weak forces.[11] For charged currents, the bosons may be either positive or negative. In the 1970s, there arose the possibility that there could be weak "neutral" currents in which no charge is carried or exchanged. By sheer analogy with the vindicated parts of quantum electrodynamics, neutral bosons were postulated as the carriers in weak neutral interactions.

The most famous discovery of recent high-energy physics is the failure of the conservation of parity. Contrary to the expectations of many physicists and philosophers, including Kant,[12] nature makes an absolute distinction between right-hand-edness and left-handedness. Apparently, this happens only in weak interactions.

What we mean by right- or left-handed in nature has an element of convention. I remarked that electrons have spin. Imagine your right hand wrapped around a spinning particle with the fingers pointing in the direction of spin. Then your thumb is said to point in the direction of the spin vector. If such particles are traveling in a beam, consider the relation between the spin vector and the beam. If all the particles have their spin vector in the same direction as the beam, they have right-handed (linear) polarization, while if the spin vector is opposite to the beam direction, they have left-handed (linear) polarization.

The original discovery of parity violation showed that one kind of product of a particle decay, a so-called muon neutrino, exists only in left-handed polarization and never in right-handed polarization.

Parity violations have been found for weak *charged* interactions. What about weak *neutral* currents? The remarkable Weinberg-Salam model for the four kinds of force was proposed independently by Stephen Weinberg in 1967 and A. Salam in 1968. It implies a minute violation of parity in weak neutral interactions. Given that the model is sheer speculation, its success has been amazing, even awe-inspiring. So it seemed worthwhile to try out the predicted failure of parity for weak neutral interactions. That would teach us more about those weak forces that act over so minute a distance.

The prediction is: Slightly more left-handed polarized electrons hitting certain targets will scatter than right-handed electrons. Slightly more! The difference in relative frequency of the two kinds of scattering is 1 part in 10,000, comparable to a difference in probability between 0.50005 and 0.49995. Suppose one used the standard equipment available at the Stanford Linear Accelerator Center in the early 1970s, generating 120 pulses per second, each pulse providing one electron event. Then you would have to run the entire SLAC beam for twenty-seven years in order to detect so small a difference in relative frequency. Considering that one uses the same beam for lots of experiments simultaneously, by letting different experiments use different pulses, and considering that no equipment remains stable for even a month, let alone twenty-seven years, such an experiment is impossible. You need enormously more electrons coming off in each pulse—between 1000 and 10,000 more electrons per pulse than was once possible. The first attempt used an instrument now called PEGGY I. It had, in essence, a high-class version of J. J. Thomson's hot cathode. Some lithium was heated and electrons were boiled off. PEGGY II uses quite different principles.

Peggy II

The basic idea began when C. Y. Prescott noticed (by chance!) an article in an optics magazine about a crystalline substance called gallium arsenide. GaAs has a curious property; when it is struck by circularly polarized light of the right frequencies, it emits lots of linearly polarized electrons. There is a good, rough and ready quantum understanding of why this happens, and why half the emitted electrons will be polarized, three-fourths of these polarized in one direction and one-fourth polarized in the other.

PEGGY II uses this fact, plus the fact that GaAs emits lots of electrons owing to features of its crystal structure. Then comes some engineering—it takes work to liberate an electron from a surface. We know that painting a surface with the right stuff helps. In this case, a thin layer of cesium and oxygen is applied to the crystal. Moreover, the less air pressure around the crystal, the more electrons will escape for a given amount of work. So the bombardment takes place in a good vacuum at the temperature of liquid nitrogen.

We need the right source of light. A laser with bursts of red light (7100 Ångstroms) is trained on the crystal. The light first goes through an ordinary polarizer, a very old-fashioned prism of calcite, or Iceland spar[13]—this gives linearly polarized light. We want circularly polarized light to hit the crystal, so the polarized laser beam now goes through a cunning device called a Pockel's cell, which electrically turns linearly polarized photons into circularly polarized ones. Being electric, it acts as a very fast switch. The direction of circular polarization depends on the direction of current in the cell. Hence, the direction of polarization can be varied randomly. This is important, for we are trying to detect a minute asymmetry between right- and left-handed polarization. Randomizing helps us guard against any systematic "drift" in the equipment.[14] The randomization is generated by a radioactive decay device, and a computer records the direction of polarization for each pulse.

A circularly polarized pulse hits the GaAs crystal, resulting in a pulse of linearly polarized electrons. A beam of such pulses is maneuvered by magnets into the accelerator for the next bit of the experiment. It passes through a device that checks on a proportion of polarization along the way. The remainder of the experiment requires other devices and detectors of comparable ingenuity, but let us stop at PEGGY II.

Bugs

Short descriptions make it all sound too easy; therefore, let us pause to reflect on debugging. Many of the bugs are never understood. They are eliminated by trial and error. Let me illustrate three different kinds of bugs: (1) the essential technical limitations that, in the end, have to be factored into the analysis of error; (2) simpler mechanical defects you never think of until they are forced on you; and (3) hunches about what might go wrong.

Here are three examples of bugs:

(1) Laser beams are not as constant as science fiction teaches, and there is always an irremediable amount of "jitter" in the beam over any stretch of time.

(2) At a more humdrum level, the electrons from the GaAs crystal are back-scattered and go back along the same channel as the laser beam used to hit the crystal. Most of them are then deflected magnetically. But some get reflected from the laser apparatus and get back into the system. So you have to eliminate these new ambient electrons. This is done by crude mechanical means, making them focus just off the crystal and, thus, wander away.

(3) Good experimenters guard against the absurd. Suppose that dust particles on an experimental surface lie down flat when a polarized pulse hits it, and then stand on their heads when hit by a pulse polarized in the opposite direction. Might that have a systematic effect, given that we are detecting a minute asymmetry? One of the team thought of this in the middle of the night and came down next morning frantically using antidust spray. They kept that up for a month, just in case.[15]

Results

Some 10^{11} events were needed to obtain a result that could be recognized above systematic and statistical error. Although the idea of systematic error presents interesting conceptual problems, it seems to be unknown to philosophers. There were systematic uncertainties in the detection of right- and left-handed polarization, there was some jitter, and there were other problems about the parameters of the two kinds of beam.

These errors were analyzed and linearly added to the statistical error. To a student of statistical inference, this is real seat-of-the-pants analysis with no rationale whatsoever. Be that as it may, thanks to PEGGY II the number of events was big enough to give a result that convinced the entire physics community.[16] Left-handed polarized electrons were scattered from deuterium slightly more frequently than right-handed electrons. This was the first convincing example of parity-violation in a weak neutral current interaction.

Comment

The making of PEGGY II was fairly nontheoretical. Nobody worked out in advance the polarizing properties of GaAs—that was found by a chance encounter with an unrelated experimental investigation. Although elementary quantum theory of crystals explains the polarization effect, it does not explain the properties of the actual crystal used. No one has got a real crystal to polarize more than 37 percent of the electrons, although in principle 50 percent should be polarized.

Likewise, although we have a general picture of why layers of cesium and oxygen will "produce negative electron affinity," that is, make it easier for electrons to escape, we have no quantitative understanding of why this increases efficiency to a score of 37 percent.

Nor was there any guarantee that the bits and pieces would fit together. To give an even more current illustration, future experimental work, briefly described later in this paper, makes us want even more electrons per pulse than PEGGY II can give. When the aforementioned parity experiment was reported in *The New York Times*, a group at Bell Laboratories read the newspaper and saw what was going on. They had been constructing a crystal lattice for totally unrelated purposes. It uses layers of GaAs and a related aluminum compound. The structure of this lattice leads one to expect that virtually all the electrons emitted would be polarized. As a

consequence, we might be able to double the efficiency of PEGGY II. But, at present, that nice idea has problems. The new lattice should also be coated in work-reducing paint. The cesium-oxygen compound is applied at high temperature. Hence the aluminum tends to ooze into the neighboring layer of GaAs, and the pretty artificial lattice becomes a bit uneven, limiting its fine polarized-electron-emitting properties.[17] So perhaps this will never work. Prescott is simultaneously reviving a souped-up new thermionic cathode to try to get more electrons. Theory would not have told us that PEGGY II would beat out thermionic PEGGY I. Nor can it tell if some thermionic PEGGY III will beat out PEGGY II.

Note also that the Bell people did not need to know a lot of weak neutral current theory to send along their sample lattice. They just read *The New York Times*.

Moral

Once upon a time, it made good sense to doubt that there were electrons. Even after Thomson had measured the mass of his corpuscles, and Millikan their charge, doubt could have made sense. We needed to be sure that Millikan was measuring the same entity as Thomson. Thus, more theoretical elaboration was needed, and the idea had to be fed into many other phenomena. Solid state physics, the atom, and superconductivity all had to play their part.

Once upon a time, the best reason for thinking that there are electrons might have been success in explanation. Lorentz explained the Faraday effect with his electron theory. But the ability to explain carries little warrant of truth. Even from the time of J. J. Thomson, it was the measurements that weighed in, more than the explanations. Explanations, however, did help. Some people might have had to believe in electrons because the postulation of their existence could explain a wide variety of phenomena. Luckily, we no longer have to pretend to infer from explanatory success (i.e., from what makes our minds feel good). Prescott and the team from the SLAC do not explain phenomena with electrons. They know how to use them. Nobody in his right mind thinks that electrons "really" are just little spinning orbs about which you could, with a small enough hand, wrap your fingers and find the direction of spin along your thumb. There is, instead, a family of causal properties in terms of which gifted experimenters describe and deploy electrons in order to investigate something else, for example, weak neutral currents and neutral bosons. We know an enormous amount about the behavior of electrons. It is equally important to know what does *not* matter to electrons. Thus, we know that bending a polarized electron beam in magnetic coils does not affect polarization in any significant way. We have hunches, too strong to ignore although too trivial to test independently: For example, dust might dance under changes of directions of polarization. Those hunches are based on a hard-won sense of the kinds of things electrons are. (It does not matter at all to this hunch whether electrons are clouds or waves or particles.)

When Hypothetical Entities Become Real

Note the complete contrast between electrons and neutral bosons. Nobody can yet manipulate a bunch of neutral bosons, if there are any. Even weak neutral currents are only just emerging from the mists of hypothesis. By 1980, a sufficient range of convincing experiments had made them the object of investigation. When might they lose their hypothetical status and become commonplace reality like electrons?—when we use them to investigate something else.

I mentioned the desire to make a better electron gun than PEGGY II. Why? Because we now "know" that parity is violated in weak neutral interactions. Perhaps by an even more grotesque statistical analysis than that involved in the parity experiment, we can isolate just the weak interactions. For example, we have a lot of interactions, including electromagnetic ones,

which we can censor in various ways. If we could also statistically pick out a class of weak interactions, as precisely those where parity is not conserved, then we would possibly be on the road to quite deep investigations of matter and antimatter. To do the statistics, however, one needs even more electrons per pulse than PEGGY II could hope to generate. If such a project were to succeed, we should then be beginning to use weak neutral currents as a manipulable tool for looking at something else. The next step toward a realism about such currents would have been made.

The message is general and could be extracted from almost any branch of physics. I mentioned earlier how Dudley Shapere has recently used "observation" of the sun's hot core to illustrate how physicists employ the concept of observation. They collect neutrinos from the sun in an enormous disused underground mine that has been filled with old cleaning fluid (i.e., carbon tetrachloride). We would know a lot about the inside of the sun if we knew how many solar neutrinos arrive on the earth. So these are captured in the cleaning fluid. A few neutrinos will form a new radioactive nucleus (the number that do this can be counted). Although, in this study, the extent of neutrino manipulation is much less than electron manipulation in the PEGGY II experiment, we are nevertheless plainly using neutrinos to investigate something else. Yet not many years ago, neutrinos were about as hypothetical as an entity could get. After 1946 it was realized that when mesons disintegrate giving off, among other things, highly energized electrons, one needed an extra nonionizing particle to conserve momentum and energy. At that time this postulated "neutrino" was thoroughly hypothetical, but now it is routinely used to examine other things.

Changing Times

Although realisms and anti-realisms are part of the philosophy of science well back into Greek pre-history, our present versions mostly descend from debates at the end of the nineteenth century about atomism. Anti-realism about atoms was partly a matter of physics; the energeticists thought energy was at the bottom of everything, not tiny bits of matter. It also was connected with the positivism of Comte, Mach, K. Pearson, and even J. S. Mill. Mill's young associate Alexander Bain states the point in a characteristic way, apt for 1870:

> Some hypotheses consist of assumptions as to the minute structure and operation of bodies. From the nature of the case these assumptions can never be proved by direct means. Their merit is their suitability to express phenomena. They are Representative Fictions.[18]

"All assertions as to the ultimate structure of the particles of matter," continues Bain, "are and ever must be hypothetical. . . . The kinetic theory of heat serves an important intellectual function." But we cannot hold it to be a true description of the world. It is a representative fiction.

Bain was surely right a century ago, when assumptions about the minute structure of matter could not be proved. The only proof could be indirect, namely, that hypotheses seemed to provide some explanation and helped make good predictions. Such inferences, however, need never produce conviction in the philosopher inclined to instrumentalism or some other brand of idealism.

Indeed, the situation is quite similar to seventeenth-century epistemology. At that time, knowledge was thought of as correct representation. But then one could never get outside the representations to be sure that they corresponded to the world. Every test of a representation is just another representation. "Nothing is so much like an idea as an idea," said Bishop Berkeley. To attempt to argue to scientific realism at the level of theory, testing, explanation, predictive success, convergence of theories, and so forth is to be locked into a world of representations. No wonder that scientific anti-realism is so permanently in the race. It is a variant on "the spectator theory of knowledge."

Scientists, as opposed to philosophers, did, in general, become realists about atoms by 1910. Despite the changing climate, some anti-realist variety of instrumentalism or fictionalism remained a strong philosophical alternative in 1910 and in 1930. That is what the history of philosophy teaches us. The lesson is: Think about practice, not theory. Anti-realism about atoms was very sensible when Bain wrote a century ago. Anti-realism about *any* submicroscopic entities was a sound doctrine in those days. Things are different now. The "direct" proof of electrons and the like is our ability to manipulate them using well-understood low-level causal properties. Of course, I do not claim that reality is constituted by human manipulability. Millikan's ability to determine the charge of the electron did something of great importance for the idea of electrons—more, I think, than the Lorentz theory of the electron. Determining the charge of something makes one believe in it far more than postulating it to explain something else. Millikan got the charge on the electron; but better still, Uhlenbeck and Goudsmit in 1925 assigned angular momentum to electrons, brilliantly solving a lot of problems. Electrons have spin, ever after. The clincher is when we can put a spin on the electrons, and thereby get them to scatter in slightly different proportions.

Surely, there are innumerable entities and processes that humans will never know about. Perhaps there are many in principle we can never know about, since reality is bigger than us. The best kinds of evidence for the reality of a postulated or inferred entity is that we can begin to measure it or otherwise understand its causal powers. The best evidence, in turn, that we have this kind of understanding is that we can set out, from scratch, to build machines that will work fairly reliably, taking advantage of this or that causal nexus. Hence, engineering, not theorizing, is the best proof of scientific realism about entities. My attack on scientific anti-realism is analogous to Marx's onslaught on the idealism of his day. Both say that the point is not to understand the world but to change it. Perhaps there are some entities which in theory we can know about only through theory (black holes). Then our evidence is like that furnished by Lorentz. Perhaps there are entities which we shall only measure and never use. The experimental argument for realism does not say that only experimenter's objects exist.

I must now confess a certain skepticism, about, say, black holes. I suspect there might be another representation of the universe, equally consistent with phenomena, in which black holes are precluded. I inherit from Leibniz a certain distaste for occult powers. Recall how he inveighed against Newtonian gravity as occult. It took two centuries to show he was right. Newton's ether was also excellently occult—it taught us lots: Maxwell did his electromagnetic waves in ether, H. Hertz confirmed the ether by demonstrating the existence of radio waves. Albert A. Michelson figured out a way to interact with the ether. He thought his experiment confirmed G. G. Stoke's ether drag theory, but, in the end, it was one of the many things that made ether give up the ghost. A skeptic such as myself has a slender induction: Long-lived theoretical entities which do not end up being manipulated commonly turn out to have been wonderful mistakes.

NOTES

1. C.W.F. Everitt suggests that the first time the word "effect" is used this way in English is in connection with the Peltier effect, in James Clerk Maxwell's 1873 *Electricity and Magnetism*, par. 249, p. 301. My interest in experiment was kindled by conversation with Everitt some years ago, and I have learned much in working with him on our joint (unpublished) paper. "Theory or Experiment, Which Comes First?"
2. Ian Hacking, "Spekulation, Berechnung und die Erschaffnung der Phanomenen." In *Versuchungen: Aufsätze zur Philosophie. Paul Feverabends*, no. 2, ed. P. Duerr (Frankfort, 1981), 126–158.
3. Nancy Cartwright makes a similar distinction in her book, *How the Laws of Physics Lie* (Oxford: Oxford University Press, 1983). She approaches realism from the top, distinguishing theoretical laws (which

do not state the facts) from phenomenological laws (which do). She believes in some "theoretical" entities and rejects much theory on the basis of a subtle analysis of modeling in physics. I proceed in the opposite direction, from experimental practice. Both approaches share an interest in real life physics as opposed to philosophical fantasy science. My own approach owes an enormous amount to Cartwright's parallel developments, which have often preceded my own. My use of the two kinds of realism is a case in point.

4. Hilary Putnam, "How Not to Talk About Meaning," "The Meaning of 'Meaning,'" and other papers in *Mind, Language and Reality*, Philosophical Papers. Vol. 2 (Cambridge: Cambridge University Press, 1975).
5. These terms occur in, e.g., Hilary Putnam, *Meaning and the Moral Sciences* (London: Routledge and Kegan Paul, 1978), 123–130.
6. Francis Bacon, *The Great Instauration*, in *The Philosophical Works of Francis Bacon*, trans. Ellis and Spedding, ed. J. M. Robertson (London, 1905), 252.
7. Ian Hacking, "Do We See Through a Microscope?" *Pacific Philosophical Quarterly* 62 (1981): 305–322.
8. C. Y. Prescott, "Prospects for Polarized Electrons at High Energies." SLAC-PUB-2630, Stanford Linear Accelerator, October 1980, p. 5.
9. "The Concept of Observation in Science and Philosophy," *Philosophy of Science* 49 (1982): 485–526. See also K. S. Shrader-Frechette, "Quark Quantum Numbers and the Problem of Microphysical Observation," *Synthese* 50 (1982), 125–146, and ensuing discussion in that issue of the journal.
10. I thank Melissa Franklin, of the Stanford Linear Accelerator, for introducing me to PEGGY II and telling me how it works. She also arranged discussion with members of the PEGGY II group, some of whom are mentioned below. The report of experiment E-122 described here is "Parity Non-conservation in Inelastic Electron Scattering," C. Y. Prescott et al., in *Physics Letters*. I have relied heavily on the in-house journal, the *SLAC Beam Line*, report no. 8, October 1978. "Parity Violation in Polarized Electron Scattering." This was prepared by the in-house science writer Bill Kirk.
11. The odd-sounding bosons are named after the Indian physicist, S. N. Bose (1894–1974), also remembered in the name "Bose-Einstein statistics" (which bosons satisfy).
12. But excluding Leibniz, who "knew" there had to be some real, natural difference between right- and left-handedness.
13. Iceland spar is an elegant example of how experimental phenomena persist even while theories about

them undergo revolutions. Mariners brought calcite from Iceland to Scandinavia. Erasmus Bartholinus experimented with it and wrote it up in 1609. When you look through these beautiful crystals you see double, thanks to the so-called ordinary and extra-ordinary rays. Calcite is a natural polarizer. It was our entry to polarized light, which for three hundred years was the chief route to improved theoretical and experimental understanding of light and then electromagnetism. The use of calcite in PEGGY II is a happy reminder of a great tradition.

14. It also turns GaAs, a 3/4 to 1/4 left-hand/right-hand polarizer, into a 50-50 polarizer.
15. I owe these examples to conversation with Roger Miller of SLAC.
16. The concept of a "convincing experiment" is fundamental. Peter Gallison has done important work on this idea, studying European and American experiments on weak neutral currents conducted during the 1970s.
17. I owe this information to Charles Sinclair of SLAC.
18. Alexander Bain, *Logic, Deductive and Inductive* (London and New York, 1870), 362.

EXPLANATION IN SCIENCE

E. Carol Polifroni

Why does something happen? Why do we bathe everyone the same way when people have different preferences? Why do we incorporate industrial economics into health care when one is empirically driven and the other is not? Some (Gortner, 1992; Hempel, 1965; Polifroni & Packard, 1995) suggest that a why question seeks an answer that provides a scientific explanation. In contrast, some why questions ask not for an answer or explanation per se, but rather a reason or an *epistemic* (Hempel, 1965, p. 335). These latter types of questions seek support of an assertion rather than a scientific explanation of the phenomenon.

In the profession of nursing, we answer questions with regularity, but do we pose questions aiming for an explanation? Are the questions posed simply to seek an empirical answer, or is there a greater goal in mind? As one explores the clinical world of nursing practice, we are faced with too few explanation-seeking questions. All too often we simply repeat what we did yesterday because it was done the day before. Rarely do we ponder the reason why we are doing something. As patient days shorten in the acute care world, the time and opportunity for why questions lessens while the need for why questions increases disproportionately. The reason-seeking or epistemic questions are a component of human nature. Explanation-driven questions are within the world of science.

CRITERIA FOR SCIENTIFIC EXPLANATIONS

An explanation is a statement or set of statements. It is more than a yes or a no. It is more than a few-word response. It is not, on the other hand, a treatise. The premises on which the explanation are based are called the explanans. The premises are statements which account for the phenomenon which is expressed in the explanandum or conclusion. The phenomenon of concern is the event one is attempting to explain.

Carl Hempel (1905–1997), a German-American philosopher, is the individual who fully defined and articulated the meaning of explanation in science. According to Hempel (1965), a proposed explanation is deemed solid if it meets the conditions of logical and empirical adequacy. Logical adequacy is met in each of three ways:

1. The explanans contains at least one law of nature.
2. The explanandum is a logical consequence of the explanans.
3. The explanans must be empirically based and testable by empirical means.

Laws of nature are general laws which apply universally. These laws will be discussed later in this introductory section. The explanans must be composed of at least one general law in order for them to meet the condition of logical adequacy. Furthermore, the explanandum, the conclusion, must be deductively surmised from the empirically verifiable general law and explanans. In other words, the premises provide the foundation for the conclusion, the answer in the form of an explanation.

The premises within the explanans must include empirical content (measurable, observable and therefore testable) and be capable of empirical verification. The issue of whether they have been tested or not is not a concern; it is the possibility of testing which is important. When these three criteria are met, the condition of logical adequacy has been fulfilled.

Empirical adequacy is met when the sentences constituting the explanans are true. Thus, the premises must have undergone some type of empirical verification in order for this condition of empirical adequacy to have been met.

Given that an explanation is an answer to a why question, scientific explanations must be deductively valid. Thus, it is impossible for the premises to be true and the conclusion to be false. If the premises have met the conditions of logical and empirical adequacy, including the general laws and empirical veracity, then the deductive answer, the explanation, must also be true. However, if the premises (explanans) are either deleted or false, the explanadum will necessarily be false.

Hempel believed that antecedent conditions and a full exposure of them are also necessary for an adequate explanation to take place. While the antecedent conditions are not a formal part of the previously stated conditions for logical and empirical adequacy, they can be included for our discussion purposes. Antecedent conditions are those conditions, states or status realized prior to or at the same time as the phenomenon of concern. Hempel believed that an explanation was valid only when the antecedent conditions were understood and accepted as part of the premises, the explanans.

PREDICTION AND EXPLANATION

Within the world of nursing, we predict what events will occur based on our experience and the data available to us at the time of the prediction. Hempel (1965) believes that in order for a prediction to be valid, it must meet the same criteria as an explanation: logical and empirical adequacy. Thus, if an event or phenomenon has already occurred, then an explanation may be provided. If an account of the phenomenon is attempted prior to the actual presentation or occurrence, then it is a prediction. Regardless of when the conclusion or answer is made, the conditions of logical and empirical adequacy must be met.

The nursing clinical practice arena is replete with premises and statements labeled as answers or explanations. However, we must explore the notion of general laws prior to concluding that nursing has explanations which meet the criteria of logical and empirical adequacy. A general law is "a statement of universal conditional form which is capable of being confirmed or disconfirmed by suitable empirical findings" (Hempel, 1965, p. 231). General laws serve the purpose of connecting events into patterns which form the basis for both prediction and explanation (p. 232).

COVERING LAWS

A covering law is a general law which applies to all experiences and explains all phenomena. Hempel, in his book *Aspects of Scientific Explanation* (1965), using a seminal work of Dray (1957), identifies and illustrates four types of covering laws: deductive nomological, causal explanation, inductive statistical and deductive statistical covering laws. Deductive nomological covering laws dominate most scientific explanations and are based on the criteria of logical and empirical adequacy. Deductive nomological covering laws are universalities which have been logically deduced, flow from the premises (general laws) and have been empirically verified. Deductive nomological covering laws (laws of nature) form the basis for deductive nomological explanations, which are the type previously described as answers to why questions.

Causal explanations as a second type of covering law are based on deterministic laws. As discussed in Section 4 on determinism, absolutes are considered givens within the deterministic worldview. Thus, a causal explanation asserts a general or specified connection between characteristics of events based on the absolute givens within the scientific world. In a causal explanation, as a covering law, if *a* and *b*, then *c* is a given, an automatic, an absolute. *C* is caused by *a* and *b* in combination and nothing can be done to alter the conclusion of *c* when *a* and *b* are present. *C* is an absolute when *a* and *b* are present.

Statistical covering laws are divided into two types and are very briefly defined here. A statistical law is either inductive or deductive. The difference for these covering laws from either deductive nomological or causal explanation is the reliance on statistical laws or principles of statistical form. In simple terms, statistical explanations as covering laws are used to provide an answer to a why question using probability as a base rather than empirical verifiability.

CONCLUSIONS AND READINGS

In exploring the world of nursing science, the reader is urged to explore the realm of covering laws and general laws within nursing practice. Are there sufficient covering and general laws to explain nursing treatments, procedures and diagnoses? Nancy Cartwright, a noted English economist and philosopher (1981), posits that the problem with the covering law principle as a basis for explanation is that there are simply too few. Where are the laws of nature and the general laws which govern or control or explain or predict nursing science? Do we ask enough explanation-seeking questions—why questions—or are we simply content with epistemic questions which are not based on either general laws or subject to the conditions of logical and empirical adequacy?

As the latter question is pondered, another dimension must be added. Is explanation in the physical and natural sciences, as we have just addressed, the same as explanation in practice-based sciences such as nursing? Furthermore, some posit that nursing is a human science (Mitchell & Cody, 1992; Parse, 1987; Watson, 1995) and, as such, is not bound by the explanatory nature of the physical sciences. What is a human science? Is the aim of a human science explanation based on logical and empirical conditions of adequacy? Is a human science based on general laws and covering law models? Whether nursing is a human science or a practice-based science using physical and natural sciences as well as its own scientific base, is the aim of nursing inquiry explanation or something else? Several philosophers and researchers suggest that nursing's aim is understanding and interpretation of meaning and the human condition rather than seemingly endless answers to why questions. These ideas are more fully explored in Section 5 on hermeneutics and phenomenology.

The selections for the present section ask the reader to explore the views of explanation in greater depth. Hempel and van Fraassen address explanation within the physical sciences and other sciences, respectively. Gortner, an American nurse-philosopher and physiologist, lays out the debate and offers her insight to the discourse. Polifroni and Packard examine two polar opposite views of explanation and suggest a middle position originally posited by Miller (1983). In totality, the readings provide a diverse and comprehensive exploration of explanation in science.

Discussion Guide

1. What is scientific explanation?
2. What is the difference between a scientific explanation and a nonscientific explanation?
3. What is a covering law?
4. What are the covering laws, if any, in nursing science?
5. What is the relationship between the type of question and the type of explanation?
6. What is the role of explanation in nursing science? Nursing theory? Nursing practice?
7. What is the goal of nursing science: explanation or interpretation or . . .?
8. What is the relationship between explanation in the physical sciences and explanation in human science?
9. Describe the role/significance/value of causality in nursing science?
10. What methods of inquiry stem from explanation in the physical sciences?
11. What are Dilthey's, Heidegger's, and Mitchell and Cody's view of the nature of human science?
12. Compare and contrast the goals of explanation in natural science and human science?
13. Discuss 'Is nursing a human science?'
14. Should nursing's epistemology be based on a search for explanation, understanding or . . .?
15. Reflect on understanding, Understanding, Dasein.
16. What is the relationship between explanation in human science and hermeneutics?
17. What methods of inquiry stem from human science explanation?

References

Cartwright, N. (1981). The reality of causes in a world of instrumental laws. *PSA 1980*. Michigan: Philosophy of Science Association, pp. 38–48.
Dray, W. (1957). *Laws and explanation in history*. Oxford: Oxford University Press.

Gortner, S. (1992). Nursing's syntax revisited: A critique of philosophies said to influence nursing theories. *International Journal of Nursing Studies, 30*(6), 422–433.

Hempel, C. (1965). *Aspects of scientific explanation.* New York: Macmillan.

Miller, R. (1983). Fact and method in the social sciences. In R. Boyd, P. Gasper, & J. D. Trout (Eds.), *The philosophy of science* (pp. 743–762). Cambridge: MIT Press.

Mitchell, G., & Cody, W. (1992). Nursing knowledge and human science: Ontological and epistemological considerations. *Nursing Science Quarterly, 5*(2), 54–61.

Parse, R. R. (1987). *Nursing science: Major paradigms, theories and critiques.* Philadelphia: Saunders.

Polifroni, E. C., & Packard, S. (1995). Explanation in nursing science. *Canadian Journal of Nursing Research 27*(2):45–58.

Watson, J. (1995). Postmodernism and knowledge development in nursing. *Nursing Science Quarterly, 8*(2), 60–64.

BIBLIOGRAPHY

Boyd, R. (1991). On the current status of scientific realism. In R. Boyd, P. Gasper, & J. D. Trout (Eds.), *The philosophy of science* (pp. 195–222). Cambridge: MIT Press.

Cartwright, N. (1991). The reality of causes in a world of instrumental laws. In R. Boyd, P. Gasper, & J. D. Trout (Eds.), *The philosophy of science* (pp. 379–386). Cambridge: MIT Press.

Fine, A. (1987). And not anti-realism either. In J. Kourany (Ed.), *Scientific knowledge* (pp. 359–368). Belmont: Wadsworth.

Gortner, S. (1990). Nursing values and science: Toward a science of philosophy. *IMAGE: Journal of Nursing Scholarship, 22,* 101–105.

Hacking, I. (1987). Experimentation and scientific realism. In J. Kourany (Ed.), *Scientific knowledge* (pp. 388–399). Belmont: Wadsworth.

———. (1990). *Representing and intervening: Introductory topics in the philosophy of natural science.* Cambridge: Cambridge University Press.

Hempel, C. (1991). Laws and their roles in scientific explanation. In R. Boyd, P. Gasper, & J. D. Trout (Eds.), *The philosophy of science* (pp. 299–316). Cambridge: MIT Press.

Hiley, D., Bohman, J., & Shusterman, R. (Eds.). (1991). *The interpretative turn.* Ithaca: Cornell University Press.

James, W. (1914). *The meaning of truth.* London: Longmans, Green and Co.

Kikuchi, J. F., Simmons, H., & Romyn, D. (Eds.). (1996). *Truth in nursing inquiry.* Thousand Oaks: Sage.

Laudan, L. (1991). A confrontation of convergent realism. In R. Boyd, P. Gasper, & J. D. Trout (Eds.), *The philosophy of science* (pp. 223–246). Cambridge: MIT Press.

Putnam, H. (1991). Explanation and reference. In R. Boyd, P. Gasper, & J. D. Trout (Eds.), *The philosophy of science* (pp. 171–186). Cambridge: MIT Press.

Ruben, D.-H. (Ed.). (1993). *Explanation.* Oxford: Oxford University Press.

van Fraassen, B. (1987). Arguments concerning scientific realism. In J. Kourany (Ed.), *Scientific knowledge* (pp. 343–358). Belmont: Wadsworth.

———. (1991). The pragmatics of explanation. In R. Boyd, P. Gasper, & J. D. Trout (Eds.), *The philosophy of science* (pp. 317–328). Cambridge: MIT Press.

Whitehead, A. N. (1925). *Science and the modern world.* New York: The Free Press.

Nursing's Syntax Revisited: A Critique of Philosophies Said to Influence Nursing Theories*

Susan R. Gortner

Lodged within the syntax of a discipline are the value systems and research constraints that influence theory development and research strategies. Humanism and postmodern philosophy have challenged natural science philosophical influences on nursing's syntax. This paper examines the construction of nursing's syntax from empiricist, hermeneuticist, feminist, and critical social theory views. In this critique, two requirements are placed on the world views: (1) they must accommodate theoretical (realist) terms important to nursing; and (2) they should provide explanatory power for these terms within nursing's disciplinary substance. Arguments are continued for a "within-the-discipline" structure, a substantive and syntactical structure for the discipline of nursing that recognizes the centrality of biobehavioral processes in the practice of nursing [Gortner, *IMAGE: J. Nurs. Scholarship* **22,** 101–105 (1990)].

Introduction

Over a decade ago Donaldson and Crowley (1978) presented a landmark paper before the Western Society for Nursing Research, on the structural and syntactical features of nursing as a discipline, following characterizations developed by Schwab (1964). They identified the "substantive structure" as those conceptualizations, borrowed or invented, which are consonant with the perspective of the discipline; in contrast, the "syntax" of the discipline refers to "the research methodologies and criteria used to justify the acceptance of the statements as true within the discipline" (p. 119). Lodged within the syntax are the value systems and research constraints that influence theory generation and research designs; these "function to ensure that enquiry will result in conclusions and statements that are appropriate, valid, and reliable for the purpose of the discipline" (p. 119). Theories are both descriptive and prescriptive in this scheme, as shown in Fig. 12-1, and intercept the substance and the syntax in Donaldson and Crowley's representation.

Both the substance and syntax, as the structural elements of the discipline, can reflect the nursing perspective of humanism and concern with the whole person. Yet this perspective can

* Based on an invited paper presented at the First Symposium on Knowledge Development sponsored by the College of Nursing, University of Rhode Island, Newport Beach, U.S.A., 7 September 1990 and revised during a sabbatical as professeure invitee, faculte des science infirmieres, Universite de Montreal, Canada, Spring 1991.

Reprinted by permission from the International Journal of Nursing Studies 30(6):477–488, 1993, Elsevier Science, Ltd, Oxford, England. © 1993, Elsevier Science, Ltd.

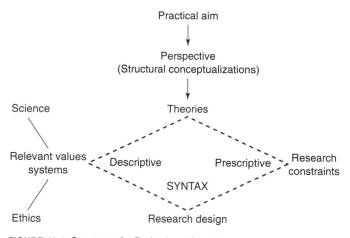

FIGURE 12-1. Structure of a Professional Discipline.
Source: Donaldson, S., & Crowley, D. (1978). The structure of the discipline.
Nursing Outlook 26, 119.

be problematic for the development of the discipline, since holism stands in direct opposition to objectivism and its associated reductionism. Accordingly social philosophy has become increasingly popular as a conceptual base for contemporary nursing. Natural science philosophy, including the philosophy of biology, appears now to have little conceptual value for nursing so that the associated view of humans as living organisms or entities is being supplanted by the view of humans as social beings. Hermeneutics has been proposed as an alternative syntax for the discipline, along with feminism and/or critical social theory and other non-naturalistic world views (Allen, 1985; Moccia, 1988; Benner and Wrubel, 1989; Holden, 1990; Holmes, 1990). What will these modifications of syntax accomplish for nursing as an emerging disciplinary field? How will the questions of substance be formulated and pursued? This is an issue first identified by Donaldson and Crowley in the conclusion of their 1978 paper and subsequently emphasized by Meleis (1987) nearly a decade later. Should particular phenomenological social philosophies continue their ascendancy in nursing, there will be ontological as well as epistemological consequences. The belief sys-

tems or ontologies may disallow reality outside of the human, the existence of biobehavioral patterns and regularities, and even theories. The belief systems or ontologies will determine the nature of explanations about phenomena, and whether explanations can become generalizations or not (Collin, 1992).

The purpose of this paper is to re-examine construction of the syntax (the value systems and research constraints), from empiricist, hermeneutic, feminist and critical social theory views. In this examination two requirements will be placed on the world views, in keeping with the author's scientific orientation. The requirements are that world views should accommodate theoretical (realist) terms important to nursing, and they should provide explanatory power for these terms within nursing's disciplinary substance.[1] Scientific realism maintains that theoretical terms and abstractions arising from scientific work exist, refer to the real world, and may or may not be true (Boyd, 1984). Explanatory power is the capacity of a set of propositions not only to account for a given event but to generalize to other events of the same set. Explanations therefore need to be nomothetic (that is law-like or general) as well as idiosyncratic (specific to the case, the particular, the singular). Explanations must cover the phenomena ["save the phenomena" in the van Fraassen (1980) terminology] and also predict what might happen the next time the same set of circumstances occurs (a traditional feature of scientific explanations). In the critique offered in this paper, arguments will continue for a "within-the-discipline" structure, a substantive and syntactical structure for the discipline of nursing that recognizes the centrality of biobehavioral processes in the practice of nursing (Gortner, 1990).

Origins of the Critique

Identification of supposed positivistic influences on nursing's syntax (i.e. theory and research) appears to have arisen from the Suppe and Jacox (1985) critique of nursing theories, in which the requirement of operationalization is said to be posivitistic. Jacox subsequently has acknowledged that her earlier writings on theory development (Jacox, 1974) were unduly influenced by positivism. Interestingly, neither Whall (1989) or Meleis (1991) could find direct evidence of positivistic influence on nursing practice (Whall) or theory (Meleis), although Whall (personal communication, 1991) has observed that the "truth criteria" (i.e. are the relationships empirically verifiable) proposed for evaluation of nursing theories had positivistic overtones. Other critiques of natural science and positivistic science orientations have come from critical social theorists in nursing (Thompson, 1985, 1987; Allen, 1985; Moccia, 1988), from proponents of phenomenological and interpretive views (Benner, 1985; Benner and Wrubel, 1989; Leonard, 1989) and from some nursing philosophers who advocate caring as the leitmotif of nursing (Gadow, 1980; Eriksson, 1990; Newman *et al.*, 1991).

These criticisms contain a central theme that positivism is antithetical to nursing's disciplinary orientation, an orientation or perspective that is framed by humanistic concepts, values and practices. Because of these humanistic intentions, it is argued that the research needs to be humanistic. The position that philosophical viewpoints necessarily should guide and direct research strategy may be termed the "purist" position. The "nonpurist" position has argued for theoretical and methodological pluralism, and toward a consensus regarding nursing philosophy of science (Gortner, 1990; Nagle and Mitchell, 1991). Still another position, "the radical separationist thesis", has been offered by Suppe at a knowledge development symposium (Suppe, 1990). This position argues that a discipline's theory and research are distinct and not necessarily congruent in philosophy (humanistic) and strategy (empiricist or phenomenological). Epistemology provides "no evidential role" for knowledge claims; rather philosophy can play a role in credentialing knowledge claims, a process of legitimatizing the claim into the shared body of information the discipline accepts and uses.[2] This position would allow humanism to be the dominant nursing perspective while allowing scientists to engage other themes and inquiry forms at various levels of analysis (Suppe, 1990).[3]

The stakes are high, for the arguments strike at the very belief systems of nursing scholarship and how we credential, accept as legitimate, the discoveries arising from scholarly work. How will we decide which is the more important question: "How is it that we know?", "What do we know?" or "What does it mean to be a person?" (patient or nurse). The first two questions have been the heart of Ph.D. training in the discipline. The third is raised by those advocating moral, social and political foundations for nursing's epistemology. How we respond will determine whether our conceptualizations can be microanalytic (e.g. cellular, biological) as well as microanalytic (e.g. social or cultural), whether the syntax can be objective and logical as well as interpretive and reflective, and whether we can model the human system/state at various levels (e.g. cell, organ, system) or rest with meanings and motives within the context of culture and society.[4]

Positivism/Empiricism

Suppe and Jacox's (1985) essay on philosophic influences on nursing theory development appears to be the major source for contentions that nursing theory has been influenced by positivism. Whether this contention of influence is accurate, despite assertions in our literature that it is, would depend on evidence that we don't have and preferably would have to be garnered from the theorists themselves. At the conference where this paper was originally presented, both Hesook Suzie Kim and Callista Roy were present; neither acknowledged the supposed influence of positivism on their own writings. Kim believes (personal communication, 1991) that the logical positivist influence on early theoretical works in nursing was selective and circumspective rather than dogmatic. Indeed, the reference by theoreticians to propositions and terms that are capable of empirical demonstration and testability might better reflect a (scientific) realist position rather than a logical positivistic or antirealist position. This skepticism about supposed positivistic influences prompted Whall to examine American nursing practice guides for the period 1950–1970; she failed to find evidence of positivistic influence and commented that it was strange, indeed, to have purported influence in one sector (theory) and not in the other (practice) (Whall, 1989).

In portrayals of philosophical positions, it is important to bear in mind that old distinctions no longer suffice. Much of the critique of positivism has been rendered against the form known as logical positivism, and the Vienna Circle. That form of positivism is no longer extant, and to continue to reference it (e.g. Sarnecky, 1990) is to ignore its demise in the late '60s (Glymour, 1980; Hacking, 1981; Schumacher and Gortner, 1992). Even in Benner and Wrubel's recent portrayal, positivism is equated with empiricism and illustrated through a mechanistic, reductionist principle: "the complex can be best understood in terms of its basic atomic components, components that bear no intrinsic relation to one another" (Benner and Wrubel, 1989, p. 32). This statement about contemporary empiricist views regarding the process of science continues fallacious equivocations of empiricism with reductionism, atomism, and quantification. There is no historical basis for the association of positivism with quantification; statistical theory and practices arose not from philosophy but from agricultural science.

Rather there is a postpositivistic view, a contemporary empiricist view (Schumacher and Gortner, 1992; Gortner and Schultz, 1988; Norbeck, 1986) that continues belief in observables, in careful scientific strategies that bear results that can be corroborated if not confirmed. This modern view has arisen in part through the historicist criticism of Kuhn (1970), Lakatos (1970), Laudan (1977) and others, including the positivists themselves. Contemporary empiricism recognizes the fallacies of the principle of verification, the impossibility of separating fact from theory and thus of making scientific endeavors antirealist (as the logical positivists attempted), acknowledges the theoryladeness of observation and experience, and does not differentiate the context of discovery from justification in scientific work. Modern empiricists, along with clinical scientists, are concerned with complex phenomena, some of which can be reduced and partitioned for study and some of which cannot. What guides a research program is a significant problem area, as for example pain or recovery or caregiving strain or postpartal depression, for which explanation and understanding are sought. Extant theory is used generally, hence the hypothetico-deductive terminology. Yet generative theory is not ruled out; in fact Roy's experience with brain damaged adults during her Robert Wood Johnson Clinical Nurse Scholar's program is credited with the revisions and adjustments made subsequently in her theoretical position. Her work reflects clearly the thinking of an empiricist scholar (Roy, 1989).

In the following features are reflected the strengths of empiricist scholarship: (1) specification of factors assumed to be key to understanding and explanation of the phenomenon under study and (2) the expectation for theory testing and theory generation. Inherent is the belief that the event under study can be modelled or "objectified" (Schumacher and Gortner, 1992). The relevant syntax for nursing would consist of (a) generalized knowledge based on explanation of kind-phenomena; (b) human phenomena objectively identifiable and observable; and (c) predictions as well as explanation (Kim, personal communication, 1991; Schumacher and Gortner, 1992).

Because of this expectation, contemporary empiricism has the capacity for explanation that is so necessary for clinical practice. The observables (mood state, vital signs, laboratory and radiographic findings) must be linked with the unobservables, those normal and abnormal physiological and psychological processes to suggest causal factors and thus treatment. The efficacy of treatment is judged in terms of outcomes. Clinical practice has become more scientific and technologically dependent because of the need for identifying increasingly complex patient states (presumptive and competing diagnoses), which require prolonged periods of observation and assessment because of their complexity, and for which multiple therapies are needed. Acute care practitioners continually confront these complexities. Their scientific and clinical judgments are analytical, logical and empirical as often as they are intuitive and interpretive.[5] The latter forms of reasoning inform and extend the former, but generally lack specificity and logic. They answer the what of the phenomenon, not the why which is the impetus for therapeutic action. They also provide the equivalent of hypothetical counterarguments or counterfactuals, to support or weaken the clinical or scientific explanation.

Empiricism then is criticized for the very features that have made it the mainstay of scientific work. It is particularly relevant for the biological and behavioral sciences, for explicating fundamental human processes of biological and behavioral origin. It has appeal for subspecialties in acute and critical care, in which the human state is objectified and monitored painstakingly. It forces upon the investigator precision, caution and skepticism about outcomes; it seeks associations between theory and fact, acknowledging the importance of *a priori* propositions and hypothesized causal processes.

In the author's view, empiricism has been given short shrift in nursing, because of continued fallacious identification with logical positivism, because of lack of familiarity with primary sources on the perspective, and because of the critiques rendered by hermeneuticists, phenomenologists, and critical social theorists. Our historical reliance on the social sciences for our scientific base contributes to the anti-empiricist or anti-naturalist argument.[6] Also contributing to the critique of positivism is our inclination to adopt a philosopher of the month (Kuhn was our first white knight, followed by Laudan, Habermas, Toulmin and Foucault). We might take seriously Suppe's recent admonition not to take philosophy as dogma (Suppe, 1990).[7]

Hermeneutics

Hermeneutics has a century old tradition in continental philosophy (Palmer, 1969), and together with humanism is gaining appreciable interest in North American circles, especially in departments of philosophy, education, and social science (e.g., Phillips, 1987; Rosenberg, 1988). The reasons for this development are several, not the least of which is belief that the human world is one distinctly different from the natural world. Literary and artistic works are uniquely human creations, societies and cultures are human creations and so, goes the reasoning, are human responses to health and illness. Dilthey was one of the foremost proponents of a distinct human science philosophy in the last century; his "Geisteswissenschaften" was an attempt to set in place an epistemology for the human sciences that would complement that of natural science "Naturwissenshaften" (Dilthey, 1988):

The goals of the human sciences—to lay hold of the singular and the individual in historico-social reality; to recognize uniformities operative in shaping the singular; to establish goals and rules for its continued development—can be attained only by the devices of reason: analysis and abstraction (Dilthey, 1:27).

This perspective on historical consciousness and the value of humanistic and historical knowledge in understanding human existence was an important contribution to understanding and explanation. Dilthey's hermeneutics reflect an accommodation of the "scientific" and the "human"; his anti-naturalism appears less fundamental and dogmatic than that of Heidegger (1962), who took an ontological rather than an epistemological turn with his conception of "Dasein" (Palmer, 1969). It is the power of the ontological sentiment of "being as being" (Palmer, 1969) that has brought hermeneutics close to the philosophical orientations of phenomenology, existentialism, and even critical theory. Indeed, the language and semantics require disciplehood, making intersubjectivity difficult except among disciples (a phenomenon called "communicative entrophy" by Suppe, 1990). Further, some proponents of Heidegerrian philosophy have operationalized features as method, contributing to the development of new scholars as well as to programs of scholarship of their own. There are several tenets of contemporary hermeneutics that have influenced nursing theorists and scholars: the appreciation of the human state or essence as supreme; the interactive circle ("hermeneutic circle") between patient and nurse or subject and scientist; shared meaning and embedded meaning, and self-reflection and understanding ("Verstehen") as the basis of knowing.[8] There is a common requirement of social discourse, generating a text or historical record for analysis.

Nursing theories increasingly address biology, behavior, and culture, frequently in interface with one another. They depict associations among factors and may suggest explanatory variables for human health and illness. Some require partitioning, objectification, and specification of relationships, hypothetical and real. The entire area of ecological knowledge known epidemiologically as "host factors" (or "risk factors") cannot be accommodated in a hermeneutic or phenomenology perspective. Human ecology requires identification of an antecedent state in the host/human, interrupting the process of lived experience which is continuous, has no antecedent or consequent, and is the "unit of analysis". Ideologically, hermeneutics captures the ethic of caring identified with nursing; it serves history, sociology, and art well; in this respect, it can frame the artform of nursing in rich and meaningful dimensions. It can frame the nature of human suffering, human health, human recovery in terminology that can enrich human understanding and thus discourse between sufferer, loved ones and clinicians. Because it will not objectify the human state or model it, it cannot supplant empiricism in explanatory power, only in understanding. Syntax based on this view would value contextual knowledge and understanding from the agent's perspective (Collin, 1992).

Had Dilthey pre-empted Heidegger in the nursing literature, might we have seen more accommodation of the empirical/historical in our writings? Our arguments around philosophies appropriate for the natural or human sciences appear to be classically American (Gortner, 1990). Colleagues elsewhere in northern Europe employ the Diltheyan "Geisteswissenschaften" in their scholarship and are not troubled by an apparent incongruity of philosophy and method as are we. They would appear to illustrate the Suppean "radical separationist thesis".

Feminism and Critical Social Theory

Rational philosophies employing feminist perspectives and critical social theory increasingly challenge traditional epistemology in a number of fields, including the social sciences (Marshall,

1988) and nursing (Allen, 1985; Thompson, 1987; Holter, 1988; Moccia, 1988; Campbell and Bunting, 1991). While these views have quite distinct origins and hold a variety of current positions, they have in common an emphasis on the subjective, on the social construction of reality, on socio-political and economic influences on science, and on the prevalence of racism and sexism in scientific as well as social activities. In recognition of these oppressive mechanisms, both views have an emancipatory purpose with that of critical social theory emphasizing the collective, the aggregate rather than the personal and individual. Here the commonalities cease and distinctions become important.

Critical social theory arose in Germany, specifically in Frankfurt, as a philosophical reaction to early 20th century positivism and natural science and to traditional Marxism (Habermas, 1971; Marshall, 1988; Holter, 1988). Assumptions of critical social theory have been stated by Holter (1988), Stevens (1989) and Campbell and Bunting (1991) for the nursing audience. These hold that all research and theory are socio-political constructions, that human societies are inherently oppressive, and that all world interpretations (mythical, religious, scientific, practical and political) are open to criticism (Stevens, 1989). Perhaps the most powerful feature of contemporary critical theory is in the capacity and mandate for the critique; this emphasis on rationality is contrasted with the emphasis on relations, feelings and emotions among some feminist thinkers. While most contemporary scientists would acknowledge the need to consider the political and social consequences of their inquiry, there is not agreement that these features must be part of regular scientific activity (even though it is acknowledged that all theories reflect underlying ideologies and "truth" claims as an anonymous reviewer of this paper has pointed out). Opinions vary on the extent to which scientists should be obligated to consider the socio-political frameworks of their studies. In this respect critical scholars are "up

front" in stating clearly for the reader the inherent assumptions governing a given investigation. Critical theorists and critically inclined scientists take seriously the charge for action; for them inquiry is incomplete without the consequential and liberating act. In this key feature critical social theory can become the basis for political and social action; for nursing situations involving group processes and societal organization, the dialectic as rationality and method is appropriate and creative. As rationality, critical theory provides a multidimensional lens for scholarship; as method it requires that oppositional and/or underrepresented views on a given problem area are specifically represented. Syntax would acknowledge knowledge as action based.

The number of studies employing critical social theory as perspective is growing in nursing and related fields. As the findings are published and subject to scrutiny (to the process of legitimization and credentialing), the quality of the investigations will be judged. It is important that the style of presentation and argument be such as to encourage the intended discourse and debate rather than overwhelm and alienate intended audiences. In nursing's literature, critical rationality has taken a more moderate form of expression than was the case several years ago. Yet the requirement for social and liberating action remains and is one of the features this author finds troubling, especially for novice scholars. Why? Because if one knows ahead of time that one is going to undertake social action, then one does not need to carry out the justifying research. One can act as social and autonomous agent without the benefit of science.

Another feature that is troubling is the lack of modeling, and theory respecification, given the stated dissatisfaction with classical social and economic theories. Critical social theory has social, political and economic relations as the units of analysis. This feature has made its empirical application limited to date in our field. So the expectations of realism and explanatory power have yet to be demonstrated. Perhaps a new theory of rationality could be forged, incorporating some of the assumptions of postempiricist philosophy.

The feminist critique of society and science has many of the features of critical social theory, but places its emphasis on the world of women in a male dominated society (patriarchy). It shares with hermeneutics the belief in lived experience and history as the basis of knowing, generating and using language for documentation and analyses. As such it also has a requirement for social discourse and reflexivity among competent persons, presented in the context of the social situation with attendent embedded meanings. Feminist literature in nursing is seen in the writings of MacPherson (1983), Chinn and Wheeler (1985), Duffy (1985), Bunting and Campbell (1990), and Campbell and Bunting (1991). Feminist scholarship appears to be enlarging in nursing theory and research, representing liberal, cultural and radical views, which need to be differentiated for uninformed audiences. Central to the radical view is the belief that oppression (due to the patriarchy) is fundamental and pervasive; here the similarity to critical social theory is clear. Yet one perspective is based in social philosophy, and the other is moving to philosophical statements from sociopolitical arguments. Until recently, critical social theory and feminist theory were not examined for their similarities in social statements, assumptions and methodologies. Several thoughtful comparisons are now available from authors such as Marshall (1988) and Campbell and Bunting (1991). Both perspectives have too heavy a reliance on social relations and actions to serve nursing exclusively. On the other hand, feminism is attractive and meaningful for nursing as a predominantly female profession. Analyses such as that provided by McCormick (1989) and Lips (1987) can provide insights into how nursing science can contribute to improved understanding of human behavior in health and illness without forfeiting science values and strategies. Differences among men and women in moral and scientific reasoning have

been demonstrated (Gilligan, 1982) as have gender differences in recovery from illness or treatment (e.g. cardiac surgery) (Rankin, 1990). Would a theory of gender be a major contribution, as Marshall (1988) suggests? Perhaps if it includes the "rapport de force", the social context in which gender is examined (Perreault, 1990). Whether feminist and critical social theory will become part of nursing syntax will depend less on the splendor of the rhetoric and more on the quality of the research and the extent to which the studies have interdisciplinary appeal.

Recapitulation

This critique has set the dual notions of scientific realism and explanatory power as requirements for nursing's developing syntax. Admittedly, these notions reflect empiricist traditions, although they need not be so represented in the position taken by this author. No single world view should have primacy in our syntax; rather the consequences of particular world views for substantive theory development in nursing science need to be considered. The anti-naturalistic positions found within hermeneutics, critical social theory and some feminist views impose limitations on human science development even more consequential than those of empiricism and empirical inquiry.[9] Common to the hermeneutic position is the foundational place of human agency, an intensionality that has no reality outside the context of the lived experience. Central to the feminist and critical theory arguments is the foundational place of domination (in gender, social class, work place) and emancipation. These features of humanity, gender, class and society are appropriate to contemporary social science and to nursing, in so far as it is a social science. But nursing is not exclusively a social science. It has a biological science component, which it will continue to incorporate in its disciplinary structure until such time as it decides to be an exclusively social activity. Nursing will not be served well by substituting social determinism for biological determinism, any more than feminists will be so served (Marshall, 1988). We are biological as well as social beings; our cell structures and biochemistry exhibit regularities over and over; our social actions barring catastrophes tend to be more regular than otherwise. What is normative for the individual is just that, and should represent "baseline" for contrast against which to judge severity of illness or recovery.

Nursing theories must incorporate the relevant domains, including biology as well as individual and social action and specify the hypothesized links with reality that will encourage theory testing and expansion. Only one of the competing world views, hermeneutics, specifically disallows modeling of the human. In this respect, hermeneutics is as antirealist in its position as was logical positivism earlier in this century. Just as logical positivism expired by virtue of its own constraints, so too may hermeneutics if it disallows realism and explanations beyond the subjective. As Collin has argued recently (1992), an interpetive (hermeneutic) nursing science does not allow theoreticity or the building of theoretical constructs outside of the person and lived experience. A "normative" science structure would, and would use what Collin calls a "third-person" stance to explain "particular quirks in the patient's self-conceptions." Such theories would be causal theories, and we would want them to describe the mechanisms behind distorted self-conception in a way which is both conceptually simple and of general application" (Collin, 1992, p.23). In essence the case is being made for nomothetic as well as idiographic understandings and explanations. Further, nursing is defined not as idiographic activity but as "individualizing activity" (p.18), for which theorizing and specifically scientific theorizing is appropriate. "Generalized knowledge will be indispensable in the process of understanding the individual case" (p.18). For disciplinary fields must build theories about the stuff and substance that intrigues them: for nursing it is the human state during illness and in health, the ecology of human health across the life span.

We have acknowledged our need for prescriptive theories, in addition to descriptive ones (Gortner, 1984). Our developing syntax must hold that need intact.

ACKNOWLEDGEMENTS. The author is indebted to Hesook Suzie Kim, Professor of Nursing at the University of Rhode Island, Ann Whall, Professor of Nursing at the University of Michigan, Donna Wells, Assistant Professor of Nursing at the University of Toronto and an anonymous reviewer for their careful readings of earlier versions of this paper. Philosopher of science Frederick Suppe's paper immediately preceded the presentation of the original paper; his observations about 'invisible colleges', 'credentialling' of knowlwedge claims, and the 'radical separationist thesis' were important additions to the author's thinking. Colleague and professor of philosophy at the University of California, Riverside, Alex Rosenberg, reviewed the substantive critiques of the world views and reassured the author that her criticisms were valid as presented. Finally, the continued interest of colleagues Karen Schumacher, Inger Margrethe Holter and Afaf Meleis in the author's writings on philosophy of science is gratefully acknowledged. They have been compatriots in the quest for nursing's scientific philosophy and have provided immeasurable assistance.

NOTES

1. Hesook Kim comments on these requirements, noting that scientific realism and explanatory power "represent major value systems of science that have contributed to the empiricist view of scientific knowledge". She suggests that hermeneutics, feminist (relativist) and critical social theory propose a different syntax. Donna Wells agrees, noting that the expectation of scientific realism for nursing's syntax construction gives "immediate primacy to a world view of empiricism". My contention is that these requirements, or some variation thereof, should be imposed on those views proposing a different syntax, to illustrate consequences and to aid in the choice of syntax. I would agree with Wells some conjoint view would be an improvement, as against a primordial view (one asserting primacy).

2. In her review of this paper, Kim notes that credentialing knowledge claims is a function of syntax, again supporting the importance of syntactical arguments for the discipline.

3. Ann Whall's response to the "radical separationist thesis" is that such separation would make for a "very disparate and conflicting knowledge base"; perhaps

this is what nursing has at present, but "is it a valid and worthy goal?" Probably not, but it does reflect current reality. Could the theories be reframed in the light of the evidence, I ask?

4. Wells comments that more than meaning and motives would result: patterns of health and illness might be revealed through such examination, aiding explanation as well as understanding.

5. Kim comments that this argument "suggests immediate linkages between 'idiosyncratic' features of practice and nomothetic/theoretical knowledge of science". Whall argues that nursing models need to incorporate physiological patterns as well as organismic relationships; valuing of one over the other will produce variations in outcomes and explanations that are insufficient or incomplete (Fitzpatrick and Whall, 1989, p. 11).

6. Wells takes issue with this statement, noting that the social sciences have long believed that only empiricist methods will lead to progress in their disciplines. That the critical social theorist arguments were as much against scientism as against positivism is an important observation. I castigate contemporary empiricism and its proponents for the continuing equation of "good science" with "good method". This narrow view of science and scientific quality constrains novel designs and methods and accepts warrantable evidence more readily from programs of biomedical science than those of clinical or social science.

7. Was Suppe "right" or "reasonable", asks Wells. When do we turn to philosophy and under what conditions?

8. This requirement and that of the hermeneutic circle, joining investigator and subject, eliminates virtually all of basic biology as a potential scientific base for nursing; does it disenfranchise basic nurse scientists from engaging in theory development and criticism within nursing?

9. Anti-naturalist is being used here in its original philosophical sense of being distinct from natural science (thus making inappropriate the methodology of natural science for study of the person). Hermeneutics and critical theory are decidedly antinaturalistic given this definition; radical feminism is as well. Hermeneutics also is antirealist, in that the world view does not allow belief in theoretic entities (noumena) external to the lived world.

REFERENCES

Allen, D. (1985). Nursing research and social control: alternative modes of science that emphasize understanding and emancipation. *IMAGE: J. Nurs. Scholarship* **17**, 58–64.

Benner, P. (1985). Quality of life: a phenomenological perspective on explanation, prediction and understanding in nursing science. *Adv. Nurs. Sci.* **8**, 1–16.

Benner, P. and Wrubel, J. (1989). *The Primacy of Caring: Stress and Coping in Health and Illness.* Addison-Wesley, Menlo Park, CA.

Boyd, R. N. (1984). The current status of scientific realism. In *Scientific Realism* (Leplin, J., Ed.), pp. 41–82. University of California Press, Berkeley, CA.

Bunting, S. and Campbell, J. J. (1990). Feminism and nursing: historical perspectives. *Adv. Nurs. Sci.* **12**, 11–24.

Campbell, J. C. and Bunting, S. (1991). Voices and paradigms. Perspectives on critical and feminist theory in nursing. *Adv. Nurs. Sci.* **13**, 1–15.

Chinn, P. L. and Wheeler, C. E. (1985). Feminism and nursing. *Nurs. Outlook* **33**, 74–77.

Collin, F. (1992). Nursing science as an interpretive discipline: problems and challenges. *Vard I Norden* **12**, 14–23.

Dilthey, W. (1988). *Introduction to the Human Sciences. An Attempt to Lay a Foundation for the Study of Society and History* (Betanzos, R. J., Translator). Wayne State University Press, Detroit, MI.

Donaldson, S. and Crowley, D. (1978). The discipline of nursing. *Nurs. Outlook* **26**, 113–120.

Duffy, M. (1985). A critique of research: a feminist perspective. *Health Care for Women Int.* **6**, 341–352.

Eriksson, K. (1990). Systematic and contextual caring science. A study of the basic motive of caring and contest. Nursing science in a Nordic perspective. *Scand. J. Caring Sci.* **4**, 3–5.

Fitzpatrick, J. A. and Whall, A. (1989). *Conceptual Models of Nursing: Analysis and Application*, 2nd Edn. Robert J. Brady, Co. Bowie, MD.

Fraassen, B. C. van (1980). *The Scientific Image.* Clarendon Press, Oxford.

Gadow, S. (1980). Existential advocacy. Philosophical foundations of nursing. In *Nursing: Images and Ideals* (Stuart, E. and Gadow, S., Eds). Springer Publishing, New York, NY.

Gilligan, C. (1982). *In a Different Voice.* Harvard University Press, Cambridge, MA.

Glymour, C. (1980). Logical empiricist theories of confirmation. In *Theory and Evidence*, pp. 10–62. Princeton University Press, Princeton, NJ.

Gortner, S. R. (1984). Knowledge in a practice discipline: philosophy and pragmatics. In *Nursing Research and Policy Formation: The Case of Prospective Payment.* Papers of the 1983 Scientific Session of the American Academy of Nursing (pp. 5–7). American Academy of Nursing, Kansas City, MO.

Gortner, S. R. (1990). Nursing values and philosophy: toward a science philosophy. *IMAGE: J. Nurs. Scholarship* **22**, 101–105.

Gortner, S. R. and Schultz, P. R. (1988). Approaches to nursing science methods. *IMAGE: J. Nurs. Scholarship* **20**, 22–24.

Habermas, J. T. (1971). *Knowledge and Human Interests* (Shapiro, J., Translator). Beacon Press, Boston, MA.

Hacking, I. (1981). *Scientific Revolutions*. Oxford University Press, Oxford.

Hagell, E. I. (1989). Nursing knowledge: women's knowledge. A sociological perspective. *J. Adv. Nurs.* **14**, 226–233.

Heidegger, M. (1962). *Being and Time* (Macquarrie J. and Robinson, E., Translators). Harper & Row, New York, NY.

Holden, R. J. (1990). Models, muddles, and medicine. *Int. J. Nurs. Stud.* **27**, 223–234.

Holmes, C. A. (1990). Alternatives to natural science foundations for nursing. *Int. J. Nurs. Stud.* **27**, 187–198.

Holter, I. M. (1988). Critical theory: a foundation for the development of nursing theories. *Schol. Inq. Nurs. Prac.* **2**, 223–232.

Jacox, A. (1974). Theory construction in nursing: an overview. *Nurs. Res.* **23**, 4–13.

Kuhn, T. (1970). Introduction II, The route to normal science; I, The nature of normal science. In *Structure of Scientific Revolutions* (Kuhn, T., Ed.), pp. 1–34. University of Chicago Press, Chicago, IL.

Lakatos, I. (1970). Falsification and the methodology of scientific research programmes. In *Criticism and the Growth of Knowledge* (Lakatos, I. and Musgrave, A., Eds), pp. 91–196. Cambridge University Press, Cambridge.

Laudan, L. (1977). *Progress and its Problems*. University of California Press, Berkeley, CA.

Leonard, V. W. (1989). A Heideggerian phenomenologic perspective on the concept of person. *Adv. Nurs. Sci.* **11**, 40–55.

Lips, H. (1987). Toward a new science of human being and behavior. In *The Effects of Feminist Approaches on Research Methodologies* (Tomm, W., Ed.), pp. 51–69. Wilfrid Laurier Press, Waterloo, Ontario.

MacPherson, K. I. (1983). Feminist methods: A new paradigm for nursing. *Adv. Nurs. Sci.* **5**, 17–25.

Marshall, B. L. (1988). Feminist theory and critical theory. *Can. Rev. Sociol. Anthropol.* **25**, 208–230.

McCormick, T. (1989). Feminism and the new crisis in methodology. In *The Effects of Feminist Approaches on Research Methodologies* (Tomm, W., Ed.), pp. 13–31. Wilfrid Laurier Press, Waterloo, Ontario.

Meleis, A. I. (1987). Revisions in knowledge development: a passion for substance. *Schol. Inq. Nurs. Prac.* **1**, 5–19.

Meleis, A. I. (1991). *Theoretical Nursing*, 2nd Edn. Lippincott, Philadelphia.

Moccia, P. (1988). A critique of compromise: beyond the methods debate. *Adv. Nurs. Sci.* **10**, 1–9.

Nagle, L. M. and Mitchell, G. J. (1991). Theoretic diversity: evolving paradigmatic issues in research and practice. *Adv. Nurs. Sci.* **14**, 17–25.

Newman, M. A., Sime, A. M. and Corcoran-Perry, S. A. (1991). The focus of the discipline of nursing. *Adv. Nurs. Sci.* **14**, 1–6.

Norbeck, J. (1986). In defense of empiricism. *IMAGE: J. Nurs. Schol.* **19**, 28–30.

Palmer, R. E. (1969). *Hermeneutics. Interpretation Theory in Schleiermacher, Dilthey, Heidegger, and Gadamer*. Northwestern Press, Evanston, IL.

Perreault, M. (1990). Les rapports sociaux de sexe comme fondement d'analyse. Commentaire critique du texte de Gladys Simons "Les femmes-cadres dans l'univers bureaucratique". Sous presse dans le cadre du colloque international: "L'Individu dans l'organization: les dimensions oubliees". Montreal Université.

Phillips, D. (1987). The new dynamics of the sciences. In *Philosophy, Science and Social Inquiry*, pp. 20–36. Pergamon Press, New York, NY.

Rankin, S. H. (1990). Differences in recovery from cardiac surgery: a profile of male and female patients. *Heart and Lung* **19**(5), 481–485.

Roy, Sr. C. (1989). Nursing care in theory and practice: early interventions in brain injury. In *Recovery from Brain Injury* (Harris, R., Burns, R. and Rees, R., Eds). Institute for the Study of Learning Difficulties, Adelaide.

Sarnecky, M. T. (1990). Historiography: a legitimate research methodology for nursing. *Adv. Nurs. Sci.* **12**, 1–10.

Schumacher, K. L. and Gortner, S. R. (1992). (Mis)conceptions and reconceptions about traditional science. *Adv. Nurs. Sci.* **14**, 1–11.

Schwab, J. (1964). Structure of the disciplines: meanings and significance. In *The Structures of Knowledge and the Curriculum* (Ford, G. W. and Pugno, L., Eds). Rand McNally, Chicago, IL.

Stevens, P. E. (1989). A critical social reconceptualization of environment in nursing: implications for methodology. *Adv. Nurs. Sci.* **11**, 56–68.

Suppe, F. and Jacox, A. (1985). Philosophy of science and the development of nursing theory. In *Annual Review of Nursing Research* (Werley, H. and Fitzpatrick, J., Eds), Vol. 3, pp. 241–267. Springer Publishing Company, New York, NY.

Suppe, F. (1990). Knowledge development in the context of shifting world views: the philosophy–theory linkage. Paper presented at the first symposium on knowledge development in nursing. Newport, Rhode Island, September 1990.

Thompson, J. L. (1985). Practical discourse on nursing: going beyond empiricism and historicism. *Adv. Nurs. Sci.* 7, 59–71.

Thompson, J. L. (1987). Critical scholarship: the cri-tique of domination in nursing. *Adv. Nurs. Sci.* 11, 27–38.

Whall, A. (1989). The influence of logical positivism on nursing practice. *IMAGE: J. Nurs. Scholarship* 21, 243–245.

Whall, A. (1991). Personal communication, 17 April 1991.

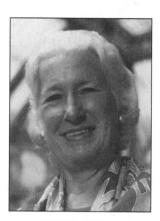

SUSAN R. GORTNER

The Pragmatics of Explanation

Bas van Fraassen

A Biased History

Current discussion of explanation draws on three decades of debate, which began with Hempel and Oppenheim's "Studies in the Logic of Explanation" (1948).[1] The literature is now voluminous, so that a retrospective must of necessity be biased. I shall bias my account in such a way that it illustrates my diagnoses of the difficulties and points suggestively to the solution I shall offer below.

HEMPEL: GROUNDS FOR BELIEF

Hempel has probably written more papers about scientific explanation than anyone; but because they are well known I shall focus on the short summary which he gave of his views in 1966.[2] There he lists two criteria for what is an explanation:

> *explanatory relevance:* the explanatory information adduced affords good grounds for believing that the phenomenon did, or does, indeed occur.

> *testability:* the statements constituting a scientific explanation must be capable of empirical test.

In each explanation, the information adduced has two components, one ("the laws"), information supplied by a theory, and the other ("the

initial or boundary conditions"), auxiliary factual information. The relationship of providing good grounds is explicated separately for statistical and nonstatistical theories. In the latter, the information *implies* the fact that is explained; in the former, it *bestows high probability* on that fact.

As Hempel himself points out, the first criterion does not provide either sufficient or necessary conditions for explanation. This was established through a series of examples given by various writers (but especially Michael Scriven and Sylvain Bromberger), which have passed into the philosophical folklore.

First, giving good grounds for belief does not always amount to explanation. This is most strikingly apparent in examples of the asymmetry of explanation. In such cases, two propositions are strictly equivalent (relative to the accepted background theory), and the one can be adduced to explain why the other is the case, but not conversely. Aristotle already gave examples of this sort (*Posterior Analytics*, Book I, Chapter 13). Hempel mentions the phenomenon of the *red shift:* Relative to accepted physics, the galaxies are receding from us if and only if the light received from them exhibits a shift toward the red end of the spectrum. While the receding of the galaxies can be cited as the reason for the red shift, it hardly makes sense to say that the red shift is the reason for their motion. A more simpleminded example is provided by the *barometer*, if we accept the simplified hypothesis that it falls exactly when a storm is coming, yet does not explain (but rather, is explained by) the fact that a storm is coming. In both examples, good grounds of belief are provided by either proposition for the other. The flagpole is perhaps the most famous asymmetry. Suppose that a flagpole, 100 feet high, casts a shadow 75 feet long. We can explain the length of the shadow by noting the angle of elevation of the sun, and appealing to the accepted theory that light travels in straight lines. For given that angle, and the height of the pole, trigonometry enables us to deduce the length of the base of the right-angled triangle formed by pole, light ray, and shadow. However, we can similarly deduce the length of the pole from the length of the shadow plus the angle of elevation. Yet if someone asks us why the pole is 100 feet high, we cannot explain that fact by saying "because it has a shadow 75 feet long." The most we could explain that way is how we *came to know*, or how he might himself verify the claim, that the pole is indeed so high.

Second, not every explanation is a case in which good grounds for belief are given. The famous example for this is *paresis:* No one contracts this dreadful illness unless he had latent, untreated syphilis. If someone asked the doctor to explain to him why he came down with this disease, the doctor would surely say, "Because you had latent syphilis which was left untreated." But only a low percentage of such cases are followed by paresis. Hence if one knew of someone that he might have syphilis, it would be reasonable to warn him that, if left untreated, he might contract paresis—but not reasonable to expect him to get it. Certainly we do not have here the high probability demanded by Hempel.

It might be replied that the doctor has only a partial explanation, that there are further factors which medical science will eventually discover. This reply is based on faith that the world is, for macroscopic phenomena at least, deterministic or nearly so. But the same point can be made with examples in which we do not believe that

there is further information to be had, even in principle. The half-life of uranium U^{238} is $(4.5) \cdot 10^9$ years. Hence the probability that a given small enough sample of uranium will emit radiation in a specified small interval of time is low. Suppose, however, that it does. We still say that atomic physics explains this, the explanation being that this material was uranium, which has a certain atomic structure, and hence is subject to spontaneous decay. Indeed, atomic physics has many more examples of events of very low probability, which are explained in terms of the structure of the atoms involved. Although there are physicists and philosophers who argue that the theory must therefore be incomplete (one of them being Einstein, who said "God does not play with dice") the prevalent view is that it is a contingent matter whether the world is ultimately deterministic or not.

In addition to the above, Wesley Salmon raised the vexing problem of *relevance*, which is mentioned in the title of the first criterion but does not enter into its explication. Two examples that meet the requirements of providing good grounds are:

> John Jones was almost certain to recover from his cold because he took vitamin C, and almost all colds clear up within a week of taking vitamin C.
> John Jones avoided becoming pregnant during the past year, for he has taken his wife's birth control pills regularly, and every man who takes birth control pills avoids pregnancy.[3]

Salmon assumed here that almost all colds spontaneously clear up within a week. There is then something seriously wrong with these "explanations," since the information adduced is wholly or partly irrelevant. So the criterion would have to be amended at least to read, "provides good and *relevant* grounds." This raises the problem of explicating relevance, also not an easy matter.

The second criterion, of testability, is met by all scientific theories, and by all the auxiliary information adduced in the above examples, so it cannot help to ameliorate these difficulties. . . .

THE DIFFICULTIES: ASYMMETRIES AND REJECTIONS

There are two main difficulties, illustrated by the old paresis and barometer examples, which none of the examined positions can handle. The first is that there are cases, clearly in a theory's domain, where the request for explanation is nevertheless rejected. We can explain why John, rather than his brothers, contracted paresis, for he had syphilis; but not why he, among all those syphilitics, got paresis. Medical science is incomplete, and hopes to find the answer some day. But the example of the uranium atom disintegrating just then rather than later is formally similar and we believe the theory to be complete. We also reject such questions as the Aristotelians asked the Galileans: Why does a body free of impressed forces retain its velocity? The importance of this sort of case, and its pervasive character, has been repeatedly discussed by Adolf Grünbaum. It was also noted, in a different context, by Thomas Kuhn.[4] Examples he gives of explanation requests that were considered legitimate in some periods and rejected in others cover a wide range of topics. They include the qualities of compounds in chemical theory (explained before Lavoisier's reform, and not considered something to be explained in the nineteenth century, but now again the subject of chemical explanation). Clerk Maxwell accepted as legitimate the request to explain electromagnetic phenomena within mechanics. As his theory became more successful and more widely accepted, scientists ceased to see the lack of this as a shortcoming. The same had happened with Newton's theory of gravitation, which did not (in the opinion of Newton or his contemporaries) contain an explanation of gravitational phenomena, but only a description. In both cases there came a stage at which such problems were classed as intrinsically illegitimate, and regarded exactly as the request for an explanation of why a body retains its velocity in the absence of impressed forces. While all of this may be interpreted in various ways (such as through Kuhn's theory of paradigms) the important fact for the theory of explanation is that not everything in a theory's domain is a legitimate topic for why-questions; and that what is, is not determinable *a priori*.

The second difficulty is the asymmetry revealed by the barometer, the red shift, and the flagpole examples: Even if the theory implies that one condition obtains when and only when another does, it may be that it explains the one in terms of the other and not vice versa. An example that combines both the first and second difficulty is this: According to atomic physics, each chemical element has a characteristic atomic structure and a characteristic spectrum (of light emitted upon excitation). Yet the spectrum is explained by the atomic structure, and the question why a substance has that structure does not arise at all (except in the trivial sense that the questioner may need to have the terms explained to him).

To be successful, a theory of explanation must accommodate, and account for, both rejections and asymmetries. I shall now examine some attempts to come to terms with these, and gather from them the clues to the correct account.

CAUSALITY: THE *CONDITIO SINE QUA NON*

Why are there no longer any Tasmanian natives? Why are the Plains Indians now living on reservations? Of course it is possible to cite relevant statistics: In many areas of the world, during many periods of history, upon the invasion by a technologically advanced people, the natives were displaced and weakened culturally, physically, and economically. But such a response will not satisfy: What we want is the story behind the event.

In Tasmania, attempts to round up and contain the natives were unsuccessful, so the white settlers simply started shooting them, man, woman, and child, until eventually there were none left. On the American Plains, the whites systematically destroyed the great buffalo herds on which the Indians relied for food and clothing, thus dooming them to starvation or surrender. There you see the story, it moves by its own internal necessity, and it explains why. . . .

CAUSALITY: SALMON'S THEORY

. . . An account of causal explanation which focuses on extended processes has recently been given by Wesley Salmon.[5]

In his earlier theory, to the effect that an explanation consists in listing statistically relevant factors, Salmon had asked "What more could one ask of an explanation?" He now answers this question:

> What does explanation offer, over and above the inferential capacity of prediction and retrodiction . . . ? It provides knowledge of the mechanisms of *production* and *propagation* of structure in the world. That goes some distance beyond mere recognition of regularities, and of the possibility of subsuming particular phenomena thereunder.[6]

The question "What is the causal relation?" is now replaced by "What is a causal process?" and "What is a causal interaction?" In his answer to these questions, Salmon relies to a large extent on Reichenbach's theory of the common cause. . . . But Salmon modifies this theory considerably.

A process is a spatio-temporally continuous series of events. The continuity is important, and Salmon blames some of Hume's difficulties on his picture of processes as chains of events with discrete links.[7] Some processes are causal, or genuine processes, and some are pseudo-processes. For example, if a car moves along a road, its shadow moves along that road too. The series of events in which the car occupies successive points on that road is a genuine causal process. But the movement of the shadow is merely a pseudo-process, because, intuitively speaking, the position of the shadow at later times is not caused by its position at earlier times. Rather, there is shadow here now because there is a car here now, and not because there was shadow *there* then.

Reichenbach tried to give a criterion for this distinction by means of probabilistic relations.[8] The series of events A_r is a causal process provided

(1) the probability of A_{r+s} given A_r is greater than or equal to the probability of A_{r+s} given A_{r-t}, which is in turn greater than the probability of A_{r+s} *simpliciter*.

This condition does not yet rule out pseudo-processes, so we add that each event in the series *screens off* the earlier ones from the later ones:

(2) the probability of A_{r+s} given both A_r and A_{r-t} is just that of A_{r+s} given A_r

and, *in addition*, there is no other series of events B_r which screens off A_{r+s} from A_r for all r. The idea in the example is that if A_{r+s} is the position of the shadow at time $r+s$, then B_r is the position of the car at time $r+s$.

This is not satisfactory for two reasons. The first is that (1) reminds one of a well-known property of stochastic processes, called the Markov property, and seems to be too strong to go into the definition of causal processes. Why should not the whole history of the process up to time r give more information about what happens later than the state at time r does by itself? The second problem is that in the addition to (2) we should surely add that B_r must itself be a genuine causal process. For otherwise the movement of the car is not a causal process either, since the movement of the shadow will screen off successive positions of the car from each other. But if we say that B_r must be a genuine process in this stipulation, we have landed in a regress.

Reichenbach suggested a second criterion, called the *mark method*, and (presumably because it stops the threatened regress) Salmon prefers that.

> If a fender is scraped as a result of a collision with a stone wall, the mark of that collision will be carried on by the car long after the interaction with the wall occurred. The shadow of a car moving along the shoulder is a pseudo-process. If it is deformed as it encounters a stone wall, it will im-

mediately resume its former shape as soon as it passes by the wall. It will not transmit a mark or modification.[9]

So if the process is genuine then interference with an earlier event will have effects on later events in that process. However, thus phrased, this statement is blatantly a causal claim. How shall we explicate "interference" and "effects"? Salmon will shortly give an account of causal interactions (see below) but begins by appealing to his "at-at" theory of motion. The movement of the car consists simply in being at all these positions at those various times. Similarly, the propagation of the mark consists simply in the mark being there, in those later events. There is not, over and above this, a special propagation relation.

However, there is more serious cause for worry. We cannot define a genuine process as one that *does* propagate a mark in this sense. There are features which the shadow carries along in that "at-at" sense, such as that its shape is related, at all times, in a certain topologically definable way to the shape of the car, and that it is black. Other special marks are not always carried—imagine part of a rocket's journey during which it encounters nothing else. So what we need to say is that the process is genuine if, *were* there to be a given sort of interaction at an early stage, there *would be* certain marks in the later stages. . . .

We can, at this point, relativize the notions used to the theory accepted. About some processes, our theory *implies* that certain interactions at an early stage will be followed by certain marks at later stages. Hence we can say that, *relative to the theory* certain processes are classifiable as genuine and others as pseudoprocesses. What this does not warrant is regarding the distinction as an objective one. However, if the distinction is introduced to play a role in the theory of explanation, and if explanation is a relation of theory to fact, this conclusion does not seem to me a variation on Salmon's theory that would defeat its purpose.[10]

Turning now to causal interactions, Salmon describes two sorts. These interactions are the "nodes" in the causal net, the "knots" that combine all those causal processes into a causal structure. Instead of "node" or "knot" Reichenbach and Salmon also use "fork" (as in "the road forks"). Reichenbach described one sort, the *conjunctive fork* which occurs when an event C, belonging to two processes, is the *common cause* of events A and B, in those separate processes, occurring after C. Here common cause is meant in Reichenbach's original sense:

$$(3) \quad P(A \,\&\, B/C) = P(A/C) \cdot P(B/C)$$
$$(4) \quad P(A \,\&\, B/\bar{C}) = P(A/\bar{C}) \cdot P(B/\bar{C})$$
$$(5) \quad P(A/C) > P(A/\bar{C})$$
$$(6) \quad P(B/C) > P(B/\bar{C})$$

which . . . entails that there is a positive correlation between A and B.

In order to accommodate the recalcitrant examples . . . Salmon introduced in addition the *interactive fork*, which is like the preceding one except that (3) is changed to

$$(3^{*}) \quad P(A \,\&\, B/C) > P(A/C) \cdot P(B/C)$$

These forks then combine the genuine causal processes, once identified, into the causal net that constitutes the natural order.

Explanation, on Salmon's new account, consists therefore in exhibiting the relevant part of the causal net that leads up to the events that are to be explained. In some cases we need only point to a single causal process that leads up to the event in question. In other cases we are asked to explain the confluence of events, or a positive correlation, and we do so by tracing them back to forks, that is, common origins of the processes that led up to them.

Various standard problems are handled. The sequence *barometer falling–storm coming* is not a causal process since the relevance of the first to the second is screened off by the common cause of atmospheric conditions. When paresis is explained by mentioning latent untreated syphilis, one is clearly pointing to the causal process, whatever it is, that leads from one to the other—or to their common cause, whatever that is. It must of course be a crucial feature of this theory that ordinary explanations are "pointers to" causal processes and interactions which would, if known or described in detail, give the full explanation.

If that is correct, then each explanation must have, as cash-value, some tracing back (which is possible in principle) of separate causal processes to the forks that connect them. There are various difficulties with this view. The first is that to be a causal process, the sequence of events must correspond to a continuous spatio-temporal trajectory. In quantum mechanics, this requirement is not met. It was exactly the crucial innovation in the transition from the Bohr atom of 1913 to the new quantum theory of 1924, that the exactly defined orbits of the electrons were discarded. Salmon mentions explicitly the limitation of this account to macroscopic phenomena (though he does discuss Compton scattering). This limitation is serious, for we have no independent reason to think that explanation in quantum mechanics is essentially different from elsewhere.

Secondly, many scientific explanations certainly do not look as if they are causal explanations in Salmon's sense. A causal law is presumably one that governs the temporal development of some process or interaction. There are also "laws of coexistence," which give limits to possible states or simultaneous configurations. A simple example is Boyle's law for gases (temperature is proportional to volume times pressure, at any given time); another, Newton's law of gravitation; another, Pauli's exclusion principle. In some of these cases we can say that they (or their improved counterparts) were later deduced from theories that replaced "action at a distance" (which is not action at all, but a constraint on simultaneous states) with "action by contact." But suppose they were not so replaceable—would that mean that they could not be used in genuine explanations?

Salmon himself gives an example of explanation "by common cause" which actually does not seem to fit his account. By observations on

Brownian motion, scientists determined Avogadro's number, that is, the number of molecules in one mole of gas. By quite different observations, on the process of electrolysis, they determined the number of electron charges equal to one Faraday, that is, to the amount of electric charge needed to deposit one mole of a monovalent metal. These two numbers are equal. On the face of it, this equality is astonishing; but physics can explain this equality by deducing it from the basic theories governing both sorts of phenomena. The common cause Salmon identifies here is the basic mechanism—atomic and molecular structure—postulated to account for these phenomena. But surely it is clear that, however much the adduced explanation may deserve the name "common cause," it does not point to a relationship between events (in Brownian motion on specific occasions and in electrolysis on specific occasions) which is traced back via causal processes to forks connecting these processes. The explanation is rather that the number found in experiment A at time t is the same as that found in totally independent experiment B at *any* other time t', because of the *similarity* in the physically independent causal processes observed on those two different occasions.

Many highly theoretical explanations at least look as if they escape Salmon's account. Examples here are explanations based on principles of least action, based on symmetry considerations, or, in relativistic theories, on information that relates to space–time as a whole, such as specification of the metric or gravitational field.

The conclusion suggested by all this is that the type of explanation characterized by Salmon, though apparently of central importance, is still at most a subspecies of explanations in general.

THE CLUES OF CAUSALITY

Let us agree that science gives us a picture of the world as a net of interconnected events, related to each other in a complex but orderly way. The difficulties we found in the preceding two sections throw some doubt on the adequacy of the terminology of cause and causality to describe that picture; but let us not press this doubt further. The account of explanation suggested by the theories examined can now be restated in general terms as follows:

1. Events are enmeshed in a net of causal relations.
2. What science describes is that causal net.
3. Explanation of why an event happens consists (typically) in an exhibition of salient factors in the part of the causal net formed by lines "leading up to" that event.
4. Those salient factors mentioned in an explanation constitute (what are ordinarily called) the *cause(s)* of that event.

There are two clear reasons why, when the topic of explanation comes up, attention is switched from the causal net as a whole (or even the part that converges on the event in question) to "salient factors." The first reason is that any account of explanation must make sense of common examples of explanation—especially cases typically cited as scientific explanations. In such actual cases, the reasons cited are particular prior events or initial conditions or combinations thereof. The second reason is that no account of explanation should imply that we can never give an explanation—and to describe the whole causal net in any connected region, however small, is in almost every case impossible. So the least concession one would have to make is to say that the explanation need say no more than that *there is* a structure of causal relations of *a certain sort*, which could *in principle* be described in detail: The salient features are what picks out the "certain sort."

Interest in causation as such focuses attention on (1) and (2), but interest in explanation requires us to concentrate on (3) and (4). Indeed, from the latter point of view, it is sufficient to guarantee the truth of (1) and (2) by *defining*

the causal net = whatever structure of relations science describes

and leaving to those interested in causation as such the problem of describing that structure in abstract but illuminating ways, if they wish.

Could it be that the explanation of a fact or event nevertheless resides solely in that causal net, and that *any* way of drawing attention to it explains? The answer is *no*; in the case of causal explanation, the *explanation* consists in drawing attention to certain ("special," "important") features of the causal net. Suppose for example that I wish to explain the extinction of the Irish elk. There is a very large class of factors that preceded this extinction and was statistically relevant to it—even very small increases in speed, contact area of the hoof, height, distribution of weight in the body, distribution of food supply, migration habits, surrounding fauna and flora—we know from selection theory that under proper conditions any variation in these can be decisive in the survival of the species. But although, if some of these had been different, the Irish elk would have survived, they are not said to provide the explanation of why it is now extinct. The explanation given is that the process of sexual selection favored males with large antlers, and that these antlers were, in the environment where they lived, encumbering and the very opposite of survival-adaptive. The other factors I mentioned are not spurious causes, or screened off by the development of these huge and cumbersome antlers, because the extinction was the total effect of many contributing factors; but those other factors are not the salient factors.

We turn then to those salient features that are cited in explanation—those referred to as "the cause(s)" or "the real cause(s)." Various philosophical writers, seeking for an objective account of explanation, have attempted to state criteria that single out those special factors. I shall not discuss their attempts. Let me just cite a small survey of their answers: Lewis White Beck says that the cause is that factor over which we have most control; Nagel argues that it is often exactly that factor which is not under our control; Braithwaite takes the salient factors to be the unknown ones; and David Bohm takes them to be the factors which are the most variable.[11]

Why should different writers have given such different answers? The reason was exhibited, I think, by Norwood Russell Hanson, in his discussion of causation:

> There are as many causes of x as there are explanations of x. Consider how the cause of death might have been set out by a physician as "multiple hemorrhage," by the barrister as "negligence on the part of the driver," by a carriage-builder as "a defect in the brakeblock construction," by a civic planner as "the presence of tall shrubbery at that turning".[12]

In other words, the salient feature picked out as "the cause" in that complex process is salient to a given person because of his orientation, his interests, and various other peculiarities in the way he approaches or comes to know the problem—contextual factors.

It is important to notice that in a certain sense these different answers cannot be combined. The civic planner "keeps fixed" the mechanical constitution of the car, and gives his answer in the conviction that regardless of the mechanical defects, which made a fast stop impossible, the accident need not have happened. The mechanic "keeps fixed" the physical environment; despite the shrubbery obscuring vision, the accident need not have happened if the brakes had been better. What the one varies, the other keeps fixed, and you cannot do both at once. In other words, the selection of the salient causal factor is not simply a matter of pointing to the most interesting one, not like the selection of a tourist attraction; it is a matter of *competing* counterfactuals.

We must accordingly agree with the Dutch philosopher P. J. Zwart who concludes, after examining the above philosophical theories,

> It is therefore not the case that the meaning of the sentence "A is the cause of B" depends on the na-

ture of the phenomena A and B, but that this meaning depends on the context in which this sentence is uttered. The nature of A and B will in most cases also play a role, indirectly, but it is in the first place the orientation or the chosen point of view of the speaker that determines what the word *cause* is used to signify.[13]

In conclusion, then, this look at accounts of causation seems to establish that explanatory factors are to be chosen from a range of factors which are (or which the scientific theory lists as) objectively relevant in certain special ways—but that the choice is then determined by other factors that vary with the context of the explanation request. To sum up: No factor is explanatorily relevant unless it is scientifically relevant; and among the scientifically relevant factors, context determines explanatorily relevant ones.

WHY-QUESTIONS

Another approach to explanation was initiated by Sylvain Bromberger in his study of why-questions.[14] After all, a why-question is a request for explanation. Consider the question:

1. Why did the conductor become warped during the short circuit?

This has the general form

2. Why (is it the case that) P?

where P is a statement. So we can think of "Why" as a function that turns statements into questions.

Question 1 *arises*, or *is in order*, only if the conductor did indeed become warped then. If that is not so, we do not try to answer the question, but say something like: "You are under a false impression, the conductor became warped much earlier," or whatever. Hence Bromberger calls the statement P the *presupposition* of the question *Why P?* One form of the rejection of explanation requests is clearly the denial of the presupposition of the corresponding why question.

I will not discuss Bromberger's theory further here, but turn instead to a criticism of it.

The following point about why-questions has been made in recent literature by Alan Garfinkel and Jon Dorling, but I think it was first made, and discussed in detail, in unpublished work by Bengt Hannson circulated in 1974.[15] Consider the question

3. Why did Adam eat the apple?

This same question can be construed in various ways, as is shown by the variants:

3a. Why was it Adam who ate the apple?
3b. Why was it the apple Adam ate?
3c. Why did Adam *eat* the apple?

In each case, the canonical form prescribed by Bromberger (as in 2 above) would be the same, namely

4. Why (is it the case that) (Adam ate the apple)?

yet there are three different explanation requests here.

The difference between these various requests is that they point to different contrasting alternatives. For example, 3b may ask why Adam ate *the apple* rather than some other fruit in the garden, while 3c asks perhaps why Adam *ate* the apple rather than give it back to Eve untouched. So to 3b, "because he was hungry" is not a good answer, whereas to 3c it is. The correct general, underlying structure of a why-question is therefore

5. Why (is it the case that) *P in contrast to* (other members of) *X*?

where *X*, the *contrast-class*, is a set of alternatives. *P* may belong to *X* or not; further examples are:

Why did the sample burn green (rather than some other color)? Why did the water and copper reach equilibrium temperature 22.5°C (rather than some other temperature)?

In these cases the contrast-classes (colors, temperatures) are "obvious." In general, the contrast-class is not explicitly described because, *in*

context, it is clear to all discussants what the intended alternatives are.

This observation explains the tension we feel in the paresis example. If a mother asks why her eldest son, a pillar of the community, mayor of his town, and best beloved of all her sons, has this dread disease, we answer: because he had latent untreated syphilis. But if that question is asked about this same person, immediately after a discussion of the fact that everyone in his country club has a history of untreated syphilis, *there is no answer*. The reason for the difference is that in the first case the contrast-class is the mother's sons, and in the second, the members of the country club, contracting paresis. Clearly, an answer to a question of form 5 must adduce information that *favors P in contrast to* other members of *X*. Sometimes the availability of such information depends strongly on the choice of *X*. . . .

THE CLUES ELABORATED

The discussions of causality and of why-questions seem to me to provide essential clues to the correct account of explanation. In the former we found that an explanation often consists in listing salient factors, which point to a complete story of how the event happened. The effect of this is to eliminate various alternative hypotheses about how this event did come about, and/or eliminate puzzlement concerning how the event could have come about. But salience is context-dependent, and the selection of the correct "important" factor depends on the range of alternatives contemplated in that context. In N. R. Hanson's example, the barrister wants this sort of weeding out of hypotheses about the death relevant to the question of legal accountability; the carriage-builder, a weeding out of hypotheses about structural defects or structural limitations under various sorts of strain. *The context*, in other words, *determines relevance* in a way that goes well beyond the statistical relevance about which our scientific theories give information. . . .

In the discussion of why-questions, we have

discovered a further contextually determined factor. The range of hypotheses about the event which the explanation must "weed out" or "cut down" is not determined solely by the interests of the discussants (legal, mechanical, medical) but also by a range of contrasting alternatives to the event. This *contrast-class* is also determined by context.

It might be thought that when we request a *scientific* explanation, the relevance of possible hypotheses, and also the contrast-class are automatically determined. But this is not so, for both the physician and the motor mechanic are asked for a scientific explanation. The physician explains the fatality *qua* death of a human organism, and the mechanic explains it *qua* automobile crash fatality. To ask that their explanations be scientific is only to demand that they rely on scientific theories and experimentation, not on old wives' tales. Since any explanation of an individual event must be an explanation of that event *qua* instance of a certain kind of event, nothing more can be asked.

The two clues must be put together. The description of some account as an explanation of a given fact or event, is incomplete. It can only be an explanation with respect to a certain *relevance relation* and a certain *contrast-class*. These are contextual factors, in that they are determined neither by the totality of accepted scientific theories, nor by the event or fact for which an explanation is requested. It is sometimes said that an Omniscient Being would have a complete explanation, whereas these contextual factors only bespeak our limitations due to which we can only grasp one part or aspect of the complete explanation at any given time. But this is a mistake. If the Omniscient Being has no specific interests (legal, medical, economic; or just an interest in optics or thermodynamics rather than chemistry) and does not abstract (so that he never thinks of Caesar's death *qua* multiple stabbing, or *qua* assassination), then no why-questions ever arise for him in any way at all— and he does not have any explanation in the sense that we have explanations. If he does have

interests, and does abstract from individual peculiarities in his thinking about the world, then his why-questions are as essentially context-dependent as ours. In either case, his advantage is that he always has all the information needed to answer any specific explanation request. But that information is, in and by itself, not an explanation; just as a person cannot be said to be older, or a neighbor, except in relation to others.

Asymmetries of Explanation: A Short Story

ASYMMETRY AND CONTEXT: THE ARISTOTELIAN SIEVE

That vexing problem about paresis, where we seem both to have and not to have an explanation, was solved by reflection on the contextually supplied contrast-class. The equally vexing, and much older, problem of the asymmetries of explanation, is illuminated by reflection on the other main contextual factor: contextual relevance.

If that is correct, if the asymmetries of explanation result from a contextually determined relation of relevance, then it must be the case that these asymmetries can at least sometimes be reversed by a change in context. In addition, it should then also be possible to account for specific asymmetries in terms of the interests of questioner and audience that determine this relevance. These considerations provide a crucial test for the account of explanation which I propose.

Fortunately, there is a precedent for this sort of account of the asymmetries, namely in Aristotle's theory of science. It is traditional to understand this part of his theory in relation to his metaphysics; but I maintain that the central aspects of his solution to the problem of asymmetry of explanations are independently usable.[16]

Aristotle gave examples of this problem in the *Posterior Analytics* I, 13, and he developed a typology of explanatory factors ("the four causes"). The solution is then simply this. Suppose there are a definite (e.g., four) number of types of explanatory factors (i.e., of relevance relations for why-questions). Suppose also that relative to our background information and accepted theories, the propositions *A* and *B* are equivalent. It may then still be that these two propositions describe factors of different types. Suppose that in a certain context, our interest is in the mode of production of an event, and "Because *B*" is an acceptable answer to "Why *A*?" Then it may well be that *A* does not describe any mode of production of anything, so that, *in this same context*, "Because *A*" would not be an acceptable answer to "Why *B*?"

Aristotle's lantern example (*Posterior Analytics* II, 11) shows that he recognized that in different contexts, verbally the same why-question may be a request for different types of explanatory factors. In modern dress the example would run as follows. Suppose a father asks his teenage son, "Why is the porch light on?" and the son replies "The porch switch is closed and the electricity is reaching the bulb through that switch." At this point you are most likely to feel that the son is being impudent. This is because you are most likely to think that the sort of answer the father needed was something like: "Because we are expecting company." But it is easy to imagine a less likely question context: The father and son are rewiring the house and the father, unexpectedly seeing the porch light on, fears that he has caused a short circuit that bypasses the porch light switch. In the second case, he is *not* interested in the human expectations or desires that led to the depressing of the switch.

Aristotle's fourfold typology of causes is probably an oversimplification of the variety of interests that can determine the selection of a range of relevant factors for a why-question. But in my opinion, appeal to some such typology will successfully illuminate the asymmetries (and also the rejections, since no factor of a *particular* type may lead to a telling answer to the why-question). If that is so then, as I said before, asymmetries must be at least sometimes reversible through a change in context. The story which follows is meant to illustrate this. As in

the lantern (or porch light) example, the relevance changes from one sort of efficient cause to another, the second being a person's desires. As in all explanations, the correct answer consists in the exhibition of a single factor in the causal net, which is made salient in that context by factors not overtly appearing in the words of the question.

"THE TOWER AND THE SHADOW"

During my travels along the Saône and Rhône last year, I spent a day and night at the ancestral home of the Chevalier de St. X . . . , an old friend of my father's. The Chevalier had in fact been the French liaison officer attached to my father's brigade in the first war, which had—if their reminiscences are to be trusted—played a not insignificant part in the battles of the Somme and Marne.

The old gentleman always had *thé à l'Anglaise* on the terrace at five o'clock in the evening, he told me. It was at this meal that a strange incident occurred; though its ramifications were of course not yet perceptible when I heard the Chevalier give his simple explanation of the length of the shadow which encroached upon us there on the terrace. I had just eaten my fifth piece of bread and butter and had begun my third cup of tea when I chanced to look up. In the dying light of that late afternoon, his profile was sharply etched against the granite background of the wall behind him, the great aquiline nose thrust forward and his eyes fixed on some point behind my left shoulder. Not understanding the situation at first, I must admit that to begin with, I was merely fascinated by the sight of that great hooked nose, recalling my father's claim that this had once served as an effective weapon in close combat with a German grenadier. But I was roused from this brown study by the Chevalier's voice.

"The shadow of the tower will soon reach us, and the terrace will turn chilly. I suggest we finish our tea and go inside."

I looked around, and the shadow of the rather curious tower I had earlier noticed in the grounds, had indeed approached to within a yard from my chair. The news rather displeased me, for it was a fine evening; I wished to remonstrate but did not well know how, without overstepping the bounds of hospitality. I exclaimed,

"Why must that tower have such a long shadow? This terrace is so pleasant!"

His eyes turned to rest on me. My question had been rhetorical, but he did not take it so.

"As you may already know, one of my ancestors mounted the scaffold with Louis XVI and Marie Antoinette. I had that tower erected in 1930 to mark the exact spot where it is said that he greeted the Queen when she first visited this house, and presented her with a peacock made of soap, then a rare substance. Since the Queen would have been one hundred and seventy-five years old in 1930, had she lived, I had the tower made exactly that many feet high."

It took me a moment to see the relevance of all this. Never quick at sums, I was at first merely puzzled as to why the measurement should have been in feet; but of course I already knew him for an Anglophile. He added drily,

"The sun not being alterable in its course, light traveling in straight lines, and the laws of trigonometry being immutable, you will perceive that the length of the shadow is determined by the height of the tower."

We rose and went inside.

I was still reading at eleven that evening when there was a knock at my door. Opening it I found the housemaid, dressed in a somewhat old-fashioned black dress and white cap, whom I had perceived hovering in the background on several occasions that day. Courtseying prettily, she asked,

"Would the gentleman like to have his bed turned down for the night?"

I stepped aside, not wishing to refuse, but remarked that it was very late—was she kept on duty to such hours? No, indeed, she answered, as she deftly turned my bed covers, but it had occurred to her that some duties might be pleasures as well. In such and similar philosophical

reflections we spent a few pleasant hours together, until eventually I mentioned casually how silly it seemed to me that the tower's shadow ruined the terrace for a prolonged, leisurely tea.

At this, her brow clouded. She sat up sharply.

"What exactly did he tell you about this?" I replied lightly, repeating the story about Marie Antoinette, which now sounded a bit farfetched even to my credulous ears.

"The *servants* have a different account," she said with a sneer that was not at all becoming, it seemed to me, on such a young and pretty face.

"The truth is quite different, and has nothing to do with ancestors. That tower marks the spot where he killed the maid with whom he had been in love to the point of madness. And the height of the tower? He vowed that shadow would cover the terrace, where he first proclaimed his love, with every setting sun—that is why the tower had to be so high."

I took this in but slowly. It is never easy to assimilate unexpected truths about people we think we know—and I have had occasion to notice this again and again.

"Why did he kill her?" I asked finally.

"Because, sir, she dallied with an English brigadier, an overnight guest in this house."

With these words she arose, collected her bodice and cap, and faded through the wall beside the doorway.

I left early the next morning, making my excuses as well as I could.

NOTES

1. C. G. Hempel and P. Oppenheim, "Studies in the Logic of Explanation." *Philosophy of Science*, 15 (1948), 135–75.
2. C. G. Hempel, *Philosophy of Natural Science* (Englewood Cliffs, N.J.: 1966), pp. 48f.: see S. Bromberger, "Why-Questions," (n. 14 below) for some of the counterexamples.
3. W. C. Salmon, *Statistical Explanation and Statistical Relevance* (Pittsburgh: University of Pittsburgh Press, 1971), pp. 33f.
4. T. Kuhn, *The Structure of Scientific Revolutions* (Chicago: University of Chicago Press, 1970), pp. 107f.

5. W. C. Salmon. "Why ask 'Why'?", presidential address to the Pacific Division of the American Philosophical Association, San Francisco, March 1978. The paper is published in *Proceedings and Addresses of the American Philosophical Association,* 51 (1978). 683–705.

6. Op. cit., p. 64.

7. Ibid., p. 57.

8. Hans Reichenbach, *The Direction of Time* (Berkeley: University of California Press, 1956), Sects. 19 and 22.

9. Salmon, op. cit., pp. 56–57.

10. But it might defeat the use of Salmon's theory in metaphysical arguments, for example, his argument for realism at the end of this paper.

11. This survey is found in Zwart, P. J., *Causaliteit* (Assen: van Gorcum, 1967), p. 135, n. 19; references are to Beck's and Nagel's papers in H. Feigi and M. Brodbeck (eds.), *Readings in the Philosophy of Science* (New York: Appleton-Century-Crofts, 1953), pp. 374 and 698; R. B. Braithwaite, *Scientific Explanation* (Cambridge: Cambridge University Press, 1953), p. 320; D. Bohm, *Causality and Chance in Modern Physics* (London: Routledge & Regan Paul, 1957), *passim.*

12. N. R. Hanson, *Patterns of Discovery* (Cambridge: Cambridge University Press, 1958), p. 54.

13. Zwart, op. cit., p. 136; mv translation.

14. S. Bromberger, 'Why-Questions', pp. 86–108, in R. G. Colodny (ed.), *Mind and Cosmos* (Pittsburgh: University of Pittsburgh Press, 1966).

15. 'Explanation-of-What?', mimeographed and circulated, Stanford University, 1974. The idea was independently developed, by Jon Dorling in a paper circulated in 1976, and reportedly by Alan Garfinkel in *Explanation and Individuals* (Yale University Press, forthcoming). I wish to express my debt to Bengt Hanson for discussion and correspondence in the autumn of 1975 which clarified these issues considerably for me.

16. For a fuller account of Aristotle's solution of the asymmetries, see my "A Reexamination of Aristotle's Philosophy of Science." *Dialogue*, 1980. The story was written in reply to searching questions and comments by Professor J.J.C. Smart, and circulated in November 1976.

The Function of General Laws in History

Carl G. Hempel

1. It is a rather widely held opinion that history, in contradistinction to the so-called physical sciences, is concerned with the description of particular events of the past rather than with the search for general laws which might govern those events. As a characterization of the type of problem in which some historians are mainly interested, this view probably can not be denied; as a statement of the theoretical function of general laws in scientific historical research, it is certainly unacceptable. The following considerations are an attempt to substantiate this point by showing in some detail that general laws have quite analogous functions in history and in the natural sciences, that they form an indispensable instrument of historical research, and that they even constitute the common basis of various procedures which are often considered as characteristic of the social in contradistinction to the natural sciences.

By a general law, we shall here understand a statement of universal conditional form which is capable of being confirmed or disconfirmed by suitable empirical findings. The term 'law' suggests the idea that the statement in question is actually well confirmed by the relevant evidence available; as this qualification is, in many cases,

irrelevant for our purpose, we shall frequently use the term 'hypothesis of universal form' or briefly 'universal hypothesis' instead of 'general law', and state the condition of satisfactory confirmation separately, if necessary. In the context of this paper, a universal hypothesis may be assumed to assert a regularity of the following type: In every case where an event of a specified kind C occurs at a certain place and time, an event of a specified kind E will occur at a place and time which is related in a specified manner to the place and time of the occurrence of the first event. (The symbols 'C' and 'E' have been chosen to suggest the terms 'cause' and 'effect', which are often, though by no means always, applied to events related by a law of the above kind.)

2.1 The main function of general laws in the natural sciences is to connect events in patterns which are usually referred to as *explanation* and *prediction*.

The explanation of the occurrence of an event of some specific kind E at a certain place and time consists, as it is usually expressed, in indicating the causes or determining factors of E. Now the assertion that a set of events—say, of the kinds $C_1, C_2, \ldots, C_n$—have caused the event to be explained, amounts to the statement that, according to certain general laws, a set of events of the kinds mentioned is regularly accompanied by an event of kind E. Thus, the scientific explanation of the event in question consists of

This article is a slightly modified version of the original text, which appeared in The Journal of Philosophy XXXIX, pp. 35–48 (1942). It is reprinted with kind permission of the Editor, The Journal of Philosophy, and Carl G. Hempel.

(1) a set of statements asserting the occurrence of certain events $C_1, \ldots C_n$ at certain times and places,
(2) a set of universal hypotheses, such that
   (*a*) the statements of both groups are reasonably well confirmed by empirical evidence,
   (*b*) from the two groups of statements the sentence asserting the occurrence of event E can be logically deduced.

In a physical explanation, group (1) would describe the initial and boundary conditions for the occurrence of the final event; generally, we shall say that group (1) states the *determining conditions* for the event to be explained, while group (2) contains the general laws on which the explanation is based; they imply the statement that whenever events of the kind described in the first group occur, an event of the kind to be explained will take place.

Illustration: Let the event to be explained consist in the cracking of an automobile radiator during a cold night. The sentences of group (1) may state the following initial and boundary conditions: The car was left in the street all night. Its radiator, which consists of iron, was completely filled with water, and the lid was screwed on tightly. The temperature during the night dropped from 39° F. in the evening to 25° F. in the morning; the air pressure was normal. The bursting pressure of the radiator material is so and so much. Group (2) would contain empirical laws such as the following: Below 32° F., under normal atmospheric pressure, water freezes. Below 39.2° F., the pressure of a mass of water increases with decreasing temperature, if the volume remains constant or decreases; when the water freezes, the pressure again increases. Finally, this group would have to include a quantitative law concerning the change of pressure of water as a function of its temperature and volume.

From statements of these two kinds, the conclusion that the radiator cracked during the night can be deduced by logical reasoning; an explanation of the considered event has been established.

2.2 It is important to bear in mind that the symbols 'E', 'C', 'C_1', 'C_2', etc., which were used above, stand for kinds or properties of events, not for what is sometimes called individual events. For the object of description and explanation in every branch of empirical science is always the occurrence of an event of a certain *kind* (such as a drop in temperature by 14° F., an eclipse of the moon, a cell-division, an earthquake, an increase in employment, a political assassination) at a given place and time, or in a given empirical object (such as the radiator of a certain car, the planetary system, a specified historical personality, etc.) at a certain time.

What is sometimes called the *complete description* of an individual event (such as the earthquake of San Francisco in 1906 or the assassination of Julius Caesar) would require a statement of all the properties exhibited by the spatial region or the individual object involved, for the period of time occupied by the event in question. Such a task can never be completely accomplished.

A fortiori, it is impossible to give a *complete explanation* of an individual event in the sense of accounting for *all* its characteristics by means of universal hypotheses, although the explanation of what happened at a specified place and time may gradually be made more and more specific and comprehensive.

But there is no difference, in this respect, between history and the natural sciences: both can give an account of their subject-matter only in terms of general concepts, and history can "grasp the unique individuality" of its objects of study no more and no less than can physics or chemistry.

3. The following points result more or less directly from the above study of scientific explanation and are of special importance for the questions here to be discussed.

3.1 A set of events can be said to have caused the event to be explained only if general laws can be indicated which connect "causes" and "effect" in the manner characterized above.

3.2 No matter whether the cause-effect terminology is used or not, a scientific explanation has been achieved only if empirical laws of the kind mentioned under (2) in 2.1 have been applied.[1]

3.3 The use of universal empirical hypotheses as explanatory principles distinguishes genuine from pseudo-explanation, such as, say, the attempt to account for certain features of organic behavior by reference to an entelechy, for whose functioning no laws are offered, or the explanation of the achievements of a given person in terms of his "mission in history", his "predestined fate," or similar notions. Accounts of this type are based on metaphors rather than laws; they convey pictorial and emotional appeals instead of insight into factual connections; they substitute vague analogies and intuitive "plausibility" for deduction from testable statements and are therefore unacceptable as scientific explanations.

Any explanation of scientific character is amenable to objective checks; these include

(a) an empirical test of the sentences which state the determining conditions;
(b) an empirical test of the universal hypotheses on which the explanation rests;
(c) an investigation of whether the explanation is logically conclusive in the sense that the sentence describing the events to be explained follows from the statements of groups (1) and (2).

4. The function of general laws in *scientific prediction* can now be stated very briefly. Quite generally, prediction in empirical science consists in deriving a statement about a certain future event (for example, the relative position of the planets to the sun, at a future date) from (1) statements describing certain known (past or present) conditions (for example, the positions and momenta of the planets at a past or present moment), and (2) suitable general laws (for example, the laws of celestial mechanics). Thus, the logical structure of a scientific prediction is

the same as that of a scientific explanation, which has been described in 2.1. In particular, prediction no less than explanation throughout empirical science involves reference to universal empirical hypotheses.

The customary distinction between explanation and prediction rests mainly on a pragmatic difference between the two: While in the case of an explanation, the final event is known to have happened, and its determining conditions have to be sought, the situation is reversed in the case of a prediction: here, the initial conditions are given, and their "effect"—which, in the typical case, has not yet taken place—is to be determined.

In view of the structural equality of explanation and prediction, it may be said that an explanation as characterized in 2.1 is not complete unless it might as well have functioned as a prediction: If the final event can be derived from the initial conditions and universal hypotheses stated in the explanation, then it might as well have been predicted, before it actually happened, on the basis of a knowledge of the initial conditions and the general laws. Thus, e.g., those initial conditions and general laws which the astronomer would adduce in explanation of a certain eclipse of the sun are such that they might also have served as a sufficient basis for a forecast of the eclipse before it took place.

However, only rarely, if ever, are explanations stated so completely as to exhibit this predictive character (which the test referred to under (c) in 3.3 would serve to reveal). Quite commonly, the explanation offered for the occurrence of an event is incomplete. Thus, we may hear the explanation that a barn burnt down "because" a burning cigarette was dropped in the hay, or that a certain political movement has spectacular success "because" it takes advantage of widespread racial prejudices. Similarly, in the case of the broken radiator, the customary way of formulating an explanation would be restricted to pointing out that the car was left in the cold, and the radiator was filled with water. In explanatory statements like these, the general laws which confer upon the stated conditions the character of "causes" or "determining factors" are completely omitted (sometimes, perhaps, as a "matter of course"), and, furthermore, the enumeration of the determining conditions of group (1) is incomplete; this is illustrated by the preceding examples, but also by the earlier analysis of the broken radiator case: as a closer examination would reveal, even that much more detailed statement of determining conditions and universal hypotheses would require amplification in order to serve as a sufficient basis for the deduction of the conclusion that the radiator broke during the night.

In some instances, the incompleteness of a given explanation may be considered as inessential. Thus, e.g., we may feel that the explanation referred to in the last example could be made complete if we so desired; for we have reasons to assume that we know the kind of determining conditions and of general laws which are relevant in this context.

Very frequently, however, we encounter "explanations" whose incompleteness can not simply be dismissed as inessential. The methodological consequences of this situation will be discussed later (especially in 5.3 and 5.4).

5.1 The preceding considerations apply to *explanation in history* as well as in any other branch of empirical science. Historical explanation, too, aims at showing that the event in question was not "a matter of chance," but was to be expected in view of certain antecedent or simultaneous conditions. The expectation referred to is not prophecy or divination, but rational scientific anticipation which rests on the assumption of general laws.

If this view is correct, it would seem strange that while most historians do suggest explanations of historical events, many of them deny the possibility of resorting to any general laws in history. It is possible, however, to account for this situation by a closer study of explanation in history, as may become clear in the course of the following analysis.

5.2 In some cases, the universal hypotheses underlying a historical explanation are rather explicitly stated, as is illustrated by the italicized passages in the following attempt to explain the tendency of government agencies to perpetuate themselves and to expand:

> As the activities of the government are enlarged, more people develop a vested interest in the continuation and expansion of governmental functions. *People who have jobs do not like to lose them; those who are habituated to certain skills do not welcome change; those who have become accustomed to the exercise of a certain kind of power do not like to relinquish their control—if anything, they want to develop greater power and correspondingly greater prestige.* . . .
>
> Thus, government offices and bureaus, once created, in turn institute drives, not only to fortify themselves against assault, but to enlarge the scope of their operations.[2]

Most explanations offered in history or sociology, however, fail to include an explicit statement of the general regularities they presuppose; and there seem to be at least two reasons which account for this:

First, the universal hypotheses in question frequently relate to individual or social psychology, which somehow is supposed to be familiar to everybody through his everyday experience; thus, they are tacitly taken for granted. This is a situation quite similar to that characterized in section 4.

Second, it would often be very difficult to formulate the underlying assumptions explicitly with sufficient precision and at the same time in such a way that they are in agreement with all the relevant empirical evidence available. It is highly instructive, in examining the adequacy of a suggested explanation, to attempt a reconstruction of the universal hypotheses on which it rests. Particularly, such terms as "hence," "therefore," "consequently," "because," "naturally," "obviously," etc., are often indicative of the tacit presupposition of some general law: they are used to tie up the initial conditions with the event to be explained; but that the latter was "naturally" to be expected as a "consequence" of the stated conditions follows only if suitable general laws are presupposed. Consider, for example, the statement that the Dust Bowl farmers migrated to California "because" continual drought and sandstorms made their existence increasingly precarious, and because California seemed to them to offer so much better living conditions. This explanation rests on some such universal hypothesis as that populations will tend to migrate to regions which offer better living conditions. But it would obviously be difficult accurately to state this hypothesis in the form of a general law which is reasonably well confirmed by all the relevant evidence available. Similarly, if a particular revolution is explained by reference to the growing discontent, on the part of a large part of the population, with certain prevailing conditions, it is clear that a general regularity is assumed in this explanation, but we are hardly in a position to state just what extent and what specific form the discontent has to assume, and what the environmental conditions have to be, to bring about a revolution. Analogous remarks apply to all historical explanations in terms of class struggle, economic or geographic conditions, vested interests of certain groups, tendency to conspicuous consumption, etc.: all of them rest on the assumption of universal hypotheses[3] which connect certain characteristics of individual or group life with others; but in many cases, the content of the hypotheses which are tacitly assumed in a given explanation can be reconstructed only quite approximately.

5.3 It might be argued that the phenomena covered by the type of explanation just mentioned are of a statistical character, and that therefore only probability hypotheses need to be assumed in their explanation, so that the question as to the "underlying general laws" would be based on a false premise. And indeed, it seems possible and justifiable to construe certain explanations offered in history as based on the assumption of probability hypotheses rather than of general "deterministic" laws, i.e., laws in the form of universal conditionals. This claim may be extended to many of the explanations offered in other fields of empirical science as well. Thus, e.g., if Tommy comes down with the measles two weeks after his brother, and if he has not been in the company of other persons having the measles, we accept the explanation that he caught the disease from his brother. Now, there is a general hypothesis underlying this explanation; but it can hardly be said to be a general law to the effect that any person who has not had the measles before will get it without fail if he stays in the company of somebody else who has the measles; that contagion will occur can be asserted only with high probability.

Many an explanation offered in history seems to admit of an analysis of this kind: if fully and explicitly formulated, it would state certain initial conditions, and certain probability hypotheses,[4] such that the occurrence of the event to be explained is made highly probable by the initial conditions in view of the probability hypotheses. But no matter whether explanations in history be construed as causal or as probabilistic, it remains true that in general the initial conditions and especially the universal hypotheses involved are not clearly indicated, and can not unambiguously be supplemented. (In the case of probability hypotheses, for example, the probability values involved will at best be known quite roughly.)

5.4 What the explanatory analyses of historical events offer is, then, in most cases not an explanation in one of the senses indicated above, but something that might be called an *explanation sketch*. Such a sketch consists of a more or less vague indication of the laws and initial conditions considered as relevant, and it needs "filling out" in order to turn into a full-fledged explanation. This filling-out requires further empirical research, for which the sketch suggests the direction. (Explanation sketches are common also outside of history; many explanations in psychoanalysis, for instance, illustrate this point.)

Obviously, an explanation sketch does not

admit of an empirical test to the same extent as does a complete explanation; and yet, there is a difference between a scientifically acceptable explanation sketch and a pseudo-explanation (or a pseudo-explanation sketch). A scientifically acceptable explanation sketch needs to be filled out by more specific statements; but it points into the direction where these statements are to be found; and concrete research may tend to confirm or to infirm those indications; i.e., it may show that the kind of initial conditions suggested are actually relevant; or it may reveal that factors of a quite different nature have to be taken into account in order to arrive at a satisfactory explanation.

The filling-out process required by an explanation sketch will in general effect a gradual increase in the precision of the formulations involved; but at any stage of this process, those formulations will have some empirical import: it will be possible to indicate, at least roughly, what kind of evidence would be relevant in testing them, and what findings would tend to confirm them. In the case of nonempirical explanations or explanation sketches, on the other hand—say, by reference to the historical destiny of a certain race, or to a principle of historical justice—the use of empirically meaningless terms makes it impossible even roughly to indicate the type of investigation that would have a bearing upon those formulations, and that might lead to evidence either confirming or infirming the suggested explanation.

5.5 In trying to appraise the soundness of a given explanation, one will first have to attempt to reconstruct as completely as possible the argument constituting the explanation or the explanation sketch. In particular, it is important to realize what the underlying explanatory hypotheses are, and to appraise their scope and empirical foundation. A resuscitation of the assumptions buried under the gravestones 'hence', 'therefore', 'because', and the like will often reveal that the explanation offered is poorly founded or downright unacceptable. In many cases, this procedure will bring to light the fallacy of claiming that a large number of details of an event have been explained when, even on a very liberal interpretation, only some broad characteristics of it have been accounted for. Thus, for example, the geographic or economic conditions under which a group lives may account for certain general features of, say, its art or its moral codes; but to grant this does not mean that the artistic achievements of the group or its system of morals has thus been explained in detail; for this would imply that from a description of the prevalent geographic or economic conditions alone, a detailed account of certain aspects of the cultural life of the group can be deduced by means of specifiable general laws.

A related error consists in singling out one of several important groups of factors which would have to be stated in the initial conditions, and then claiming that the phenomenon in question is "determined" by that one group of factors and thus can be explained in terms of it.

Occasionally, the adherents of some particular school of explanation or interpretation in history will adduce, as evidence in favor of their approach, a successful historical prediction which was made by a representative of their school. But though the predictive success of a theory is certainly relevant evidence of its soundness, it is important to make sure that the successful prediction is in fact obtainable by means of the theory in question. It happens sometimes that the prediction is actually an ingenious guess which may have been influenced by the theoretical outlook of its author, but which can not be arrived at by means of his theory alone. Thus, an adherent of a quite metaphysical "theory" of history may have a sound feeling for historical developments and may be able to make correct predictions, which he will even couch in the terminology of his theory, though they could not have been attained by means of it. To guard against such pseudo-confirming cases would be one of the functions of test (*c*) in 3.3.

6. We have tried to show that in history no less than in any other branch of empirical in-

quiry, scientific explanation can be achieved only by means of suitable general hypotheses, or by theories, which are bodies of systematically related hypotheses. This thesis is clearly in contrast with the familiar view that genuine explanation in history is obtained by a method which characteristically distinguishes the social from the natural sciences, namely, *the method of emphatic understanding:* The historian, we are told, imagines himself in the place of the persons involved in the events which he wants to explain; he tries to realize as completely as possible the circumstances under which they acted and the motives which influenced their actions; and by this imaginary self-identification with his heroes, he arrives at an understanding and thus at an adequate explanation of the events with which he is concerned.

This method of empathy is, no doubt, frequently applied by laymen and by experts in history. But it does not in itself constitute an explanation; it rather is essentially a heuristic device; its function is to suggest psychological hypotheses which might serve as explanatory principles in the case under consideration. Stated in crude terms, the idea underlying this function is the following: The historian tries to realize how he himself would act under the given conditions, and under the particular motivations of his heroes; he tentatively generalizes his findings into a general rule and uses the latter as an explanatory principle in accounting for the actions of the persons involved. Now, this procedure may sometimes prove heuristically helpful; but it does not guarantee the soundness of the historical explanation to which it leads. The latter rather depends upon the factual correctness of the generalizations which the method of understanding may have suggested.

Nor is the use of this method indispensable for historical explanation. A historian may, for example, be incapable of feeling himself into the role of a paranoiac historic personality, and yet he may well be able to explain certain of his actions by reference to the principles of abnormal psychology. Thus, whether the historian is or is not in a position to identify himself with his historical hero is irrelevant for the correctness of his explanation; what counts is the soundness of the general hypotheses involved, no matter whether they were suggested by empathy or by a strictly behavioristic procedure. Much of the appeal of the "method of understanding" seems to be due to the fact that it tends to present the phenomena in question as somehow "plausible" or "natural" to us;[5] this is often done by means of persuasive metaphors. But the kind of "understanding" thus conveyed must clearly be separated from scientific understanding. In history as anywhere else in empirical science, the explanation of a phenomenon consists in subsuming it under general empirical laws; and the criterion of its soundness is not whether it appeals to our imagination, whether it is presented in terms of suggestive analogies or is otherwise made to appear plausible—all this may occur in pseudo-explanations as well—but exclusively whether it rests on empirically well confirmed assumptions concerning initial conditions and general laws.

7.1 So far, we have discussed the importance of general laws for explanation and prediction, and for so-called understanding in history. Let us now survey more briefly some other procedures in historical research which involve the assumption of universal hypotheses.

Closely related to explanation and understanding is the so-called *interpretation of historical phenomena* in terms of some particular approach or theory. The interpretations which are actually offered in history consist either in subsuming the phenomena in question under a scientific explanation or explanation sketch; or in an attempt to subsume them under some general idea which is not amenable to any empirical test. In the former case, interpretation clearly is explanation by means of universal hypotheses; in the latter, it amounts to a pseudo-explanation which may have emotive appeal and evoke vivid pictorial associations, but which does not further our theoretical understanding of the phenomena under consideration.

7.2 Analogous remarks apply to the procedure of ascertaining the "*meaning*" of given historical events; its scientific import consists in determining what other events are relevantly connected with the event in question, be it as "causes," or as "effects"; and the statement of the relevant connections assumes, again, the form of explanations or explanation sketches which involve universal hypotheses; this will be seen more clearly in the next subsection.

7.3 In the historical explanation of some social institutions great emphasis is laid upon an analysis of the *development* of the institution up to the stage under consideration. Critics of this approach have objected that a mere description of this kind is not a genuine explanation. This argument may be given a slightly different form in terms of the preceding reflections: An account of the development of an institution is obviously not simply a description of *all* the events which temporally preceded it; only those events are meant to be included which are "*relevant*" to the formation of that institution. And whether an event is relevant to that development is not a matter of evaluative opinion, but an objective question depending upon what is sometimes called a causal analysis of the rise of that institution.[6] Now, the causal analysis of an event establishes an explanation for it, and since this requires reference to general hypotheses, so do assumptions about relevance, and, consequently, so does the adequate analysis of the historical development of an institution.

7.4 Similarly, the use of the notions of *determination* and of *dependence* in the empirical sciences, including history, involves reference to general laws.[7] Thus, e.g., we may say that the pressure of a gas depends upon its temperature and volume, or that temperature and volume determine the pressure, in virtue of Boyle's law. But unless the underlying laws are stated explicitly, the assertion of a relation of dependence or of determination between certain magnitudes or characteristics amounts at best to claiming that they are connected by some unspecified empirical law; and that is a very meager assertion indeed: If, for example, we know only that there is some empirical law connecting two metrical magnitudes (such as length and temperature of a metal bar), we can not even be sure that a change of one of the two will be accompanied by a change of the other (for the law may connect the same value of the "dependent" or "determined" magnitude with different values of the other), but only that with any specific value of one of the variables, there will always be associated one and the same value of the other; and this is obviously much less than most authors mean to assert when they speak of determination or dependence in historical analysis.

Therefore, the sweeping assertion that economic (or geographic, or any other kind of) conditions "determine" the development and change of all other aspects of human society, has explanatory value only in so far as it can be substantiated by explicit laws which state just what kind of change in human culture will regularly follow upon specific changes in the economic (geographic, etc.) conditions. Only the establishment of specific laws can fill the general thesis with scientific content, make it amenable to empirical tests, and confer upon it an explanatory function. The elaboration of such laws with as much precision as possible seems clearly to be the direction in which progress in scientific explanation and understanding has to be sought.

8. The considerations developed in this paper are entirely neutral with respect to the problem of "*specifically historical laws*": they do not presuppose a particular way of distinguishing historical from sociological and other laws, nor do they imply or deny the assumption that empirical laws can be found which are historical in some specific sense, and which are well confirmed by empirical evidence.

But it may be worth mentioning here that those universal hypotheses to which historians explicitly or tacitly refer in offering explanations, predictions, interpretations, judgments of relevance, etc., are taken from *various* fields of scientific research, in so far as they are not pre-scientific generalizations of everyday experiences. Many of the universal hypotheses underlying historical explanation, for instance, would commonly be classified as psychological, economical, sociological, and partly perhaps as historical laws; in addition, historical research has frequently to resort to general laws established in physics, chemistry, and biology. Thus, e.g., the explanation of the defeat of an army by reference to lack of food, adverse weather conditions, disease, and the like, is based on a—usually tacit—assumption of such laws. The use of tree rings in dating events in history rests on the application of certain biological regularities. Various methods of testing the authenticity of documents, paintings, coins, etc., make use of physical and chemical theories.

The last two examples illustrate another point which is relevant in this context: Even if a historian should propose to restrict his research to a "pure description" of the past, without any attempt at offering explanations or statements about relevance and determination, he would continually have to make use of general laws. For the object of his studies would be the past—forever inaccessible to his direct examination. He would have to establish his knowledge by indirect methods: by the use of universal hypotheses which connect his present data with those past events. This fact has been obscured partly because some of the regularities involved are so familiar that they are not considered worth mentioning at all; and partly because of the habit of relegating the various hypotheses and theories which are used to ascertain knowledge about past events, to the "auxiliary sciences" of history. Quite probably, some of the historians who tend to minimize, if not to deny, the importance of general laws for history, are prompted by the feeling that only "genuinely historical laws" would be of interest for history. But once it is realized that the discovery of historical laws (in some specified sense of this very vague notion) would not make history methodologically autonomous and independent

of the other branches of scientific research, it would seem that the problem of the existence of historical laws ought to lose some of its importance.

The remarks made in this section are but special illustrations of two broader principles of the theory of science: first, the separation of "pure description" and "hypothetical generalization and theory-construction" in empirical science is unwarranted; in the building of scientific knowledge the two are inseparably linked. And, second, it is similarly unwarranted and futile to attempt the demarcation of sharp boundary lines between the different fields of scientific research, and an autonomous development of each of the fields. The necessity, in historical inquiry, to make extensive use of universal hypotheses of which at least the overwhelming majority come from fields of research traditionally distinguished from history is just one of the aspects of what may be called the methodological unity of empirical science.

NOTES

1. Maurice Mandelbaum, in his generally very clarifying analysis of relevance and causation in history (*The Problem of Historical Knowledge*, New York, 1938, Chs. 7, 8) seems to hold that there is a difference between the "causal analysis" or "causal explanation" of an event and the establishment of scientific laws governing it in the sense stated above. He argues that "scientific laws can only be formulated on the basis of causal analysis," but that "they are not substitutes for full causal explanations" (*l.c.*, p. 238). For the reasons outlined above, this distinction does not appear to be justifiable: every "causal explanation" is an "explanation by scientific laws"; for in no other way than by reference to empirical laws can the assertion of a causal connection between events be scientifically substantiated.

2. Donald W. McConnell *et al.*, *Economic Behavior;* New York, 1939; pp. 894–95. (Italics supplied.)

3. What is sometimes misleadingly called an explanation by means of a certain *concept* is, in empirical science, actually an explanation in terms of *universal hypotheses* containing that concept. "Explanations" involving concepts which do not function in empirically

testable hypotheses—such as "entelechy" in biology, "historic destination of a race" or "self-unfolding of absolute reason" in history—are mere metaphors without cognitive content.

4. E. Zilsel, in a stimulating paper on "Physics and the Problem of Historico-Sociological Laws" (*Philosophy of Science*, Vol. 8, 1941, pp. 567–79), suggests that all specifically historical laws are of a statistical character similar to that of the "macro-laws" of physics. The above remarks, however, are not restricted to specifically historical laws since explanation in history rests to a large extent on nonhistorical laws (cf. section 8 of this paper).

5. For a criticism of this kind of plausibility, cf. Zilsel, *l.c.*, pp. 577–78, and sections 7 and 8 in the same author's "Problems of Empiricism," in *International Encyclopedia of United Science*, Vol. II, 8 (Chicago: University of Chicago Press, 1941).

6. See the detailed and clear exposition of this point in M. Mandelbaum's book, chapters 6–8.

7. According to Mandelbaum, history, in contradistinction to the physical sciences, consists "not in the formulation of laws of which the particular case is an instance, but in the description of the events in their actual determining relationships to each other; in seeing events as the products and producers of change" (*l.c.*, pp. 13–14). This is, in effect, a conception whose untenability has been pointed out already by Hume, namely, that a careful examination of two specific events alone, without any reference to similar cases and to general regularities, can reveal that one of the events produces or determines the other. This thesis does not only run counter to the scientific meaning of the concept of determination which clearly rests on that of general law, but it even fails to provide any objective criteria which would be indicative of the intended relationship of determination or production. Thus, to speak of empirical determination independently of any reference to general laws is to use a metaphor without cognitive content.

Explanation in Nursing Science

E. Carol Polifroni • *Sheila A. Packard*

Is it possible to explain that which we do in nursing and in most human sciences? Is explanation/prediction our goal? Instead, should the goal be understanding/interpretation? Might the goal be both understanding and explanation? Is nursing, as a human science, focused on individuality or generalizability? This paper explores the current debate in relation to explanation and understanding. The traditional view of explanation is addressed as is the dichotomous view of understanding. A third view on explanation and understanding, designed by Miller (1983), is offered as a possible middle ground between the two diverse views as an approach for nursing as a human science.

In recent years, much controversy has arisen within nursing with regard to appropriate and, therefore, fruitful methodological strategies. The frequently cited "methods debate," which purports an extant dichotomy between quantitative/empirical and qualitative/interpretive approaches, is a current example of this controversy. The most frequently posited solution to this schism is triangulated or blended methodology (Packard & Polifroni, 1991). Yet it may be contended that this response does not resolve the more fundamental problem of generalizability of findings, nor does it address basic questions regarding objectivity in scientific enterprises. Disagreement on the intentions or purposes of nursing science (in particular, whether or not to aim for explanation or understanding) is simply reflected in the use of eclectic methodological strategies, and debates about these strategies, throughout the discipline.

A large part of the controversy over methods within nursing evolves from a fundamental conflict among scholars regarding the nature of scientific explanation in a human science, and whether explanation is even possible in such a science. At the same time, frustration on the part of nurse scientists in attempting to achieve overarching predictive theory, and a pressing need for intermediate-range theory, which may serve to guide practice, lend great urgency to a discussion of explanation in nursing science.

The purpose of this paper is to briefly present the two major opposing views concerning explanation that have, in the authors' opinion, fuelled the fires of controversy regarding the methodological development in nursing. In addition, an elaborated view of the nature of explanation based on the ideas of Miller (1983) will be offered as a means of reframing the debate at this crucial juncture in the evolution of nursing as a science.

Reprinted by permission from the Canadian Journal of Nursing Research 27(2):45–58. © 1995, Canadian Journal of Nursing Research.

Perspectives on Explanation

When is a particular statement or set of propositions an adequate explanation of why a specific phenomenon occurred? Simply stated, an adequate explanation should provide true descriptions of prior conditions. However, it may be argued that this requirement is not enough. The fact that a patient had a restless night is an accurate but insufficient explanation for his falling out of bed the next afternoon. The confusion as to what additional qualifications or characteristics comprise a valid explanation constitutes a fundamental and pervasive dispute in the philosophy of science for all sciences, physical and human. The ramifications of this dispute have led to a suggestion by some scholars that nursing science should aim for understanding rather than explanation/prediction (Benner, 1985). Conversely, other nurse scholars hold that "the ultimate goal of science is to be able to explain the empirical world and, thus, to have increased control over it" (Burns & Grove, 1987, p. 11). The diverse opinions of the aim of science are perhaps best framed as follows: "The real business of inquiry was explanation, whereas interpretive practices were confined to the special domain of the human sciences, the traditional *Geisteswissenschaften*" (Bohman, Hiley, & Shusterman, 1991, pp. 2–3). For purposes of clarity, these two disparate perspectives, explanation and understanding/interpretation, will be briefly described in terms of the deductive-nomological and the hermeneutic views.

A Covering Law:
The Deductive-Nomological View

Carl Hempel (1965), in *Aspects of Scientific Explanation,* identifies four models of covering law. They are deductive nomological, causal explanation, deductive statistical, and inductive statistical. Each model is intended to represent a single law that addresses all phenomena. The deductive nomological covering-law model answers a *why* question. "The kind of explanation whose logical structure is suggested by schema will be called the deductive-nomological explanation . . . ; for it effects a deductive subsumption of the explanandum under principles that have the character of general laws" (Hempel, 1965, pp. 336–337).

Causal explanation, as a covering-law model, focuses on the underlying reason something happened as an effect. Deductive-statistical explanation and inductive-statistical explanation address explanation within the parameters of probability and the likelihood that a specific event will or will not occur. The two statistical models differ in terms of the method of probability determination: deductive or inductive.

Although Hempel addresses four models of covering law, in this century the more widely held analysis of explanation has come to be known as the deductive-nomological, or covering-law, view. For the remainder of this paper, the term *covering law* should be read as the deductive-nomological view of explanation.

Basically, this covering-law view makes explanation, whether in the human or natural sciences, a matter of subsumption under general laws. A valid explanation of an event ought to contain characteristics of the situation leading up to the event and general empirical laws indicating that when such characteristics are realized, an event of that particular kind always (or almost always) follows.

Hempel elaborates on the deductive-nomological covering law in great detail, postulating that explanation in any and all fields of science must meet the following specific conditions of adequacy: (a) the conclusion must be a logical consequence of the premises (it must be deducible from the information contained in the premises); (b) the premises must contain at least one general law, and this law must be required for derivation of the conclusion; (c) the premises must have empirical content, which is to say they must be capable (at least in principle) of test by experiment or observation; and (d) the sentences in the premises must be true.

Hempel (1965) summarizes the arguments put forth by skeptics regarding the application of this criteria to the non-physical sciences as: (a) the contention that the activities of human beings have a peculiar uniqueness and irrepeatability that make them inaccessible to causal explanation; (b) the belief that the establishment of scientific generalizations for human behaviour is not possible because reactions of an individual are at least partially dependent on the individual's previous history; and (c) the supposition that purposive behaviour calls for reference to motives and thus necessitates teleological rather than causal explanation. As a counter to these arguments emanating from social science, Hempel states that events in physical science, are no less unique than human activities. And phenomena studied in physical science also have a history, which must be taken into account in the generation of general regularities. In addition, he has submitted that motivations involved in human behaviour, while referring to the future, are actually situated prior to activity and, therefore, may be classified as among the antecedent conditions in a causal explanation.

Skeptics aside, the deductive-nomological covering law has dominated the practice of science, including that of non-physical fields (Miller, 1983). For example, major thinkers in sociology, such as Durkheim (1938) and Weber (cited in Gerth and Mills, 1946), regarded subsumption under general laws as the means for making the study of social life truly scientific. In much the way that nursing has struggled to take its place among the sciences, concern has centred to some extent on the formulation of causal explanations. Norbeck, in her 1987 article "In Defense of Empiricism," asserts that a reliance on systematically gathered objective data drawn from relatively large numbers of individuals will yield predictive models and causal explanation.

Gortner (1990) expresses the notion that meeting the requirements of the covering-law model will legitimize nursing as a science:

> Explanatory power is proposed as another premise of philosophy of science in nursing. Human science activities cannot rest only with increased understanding; nor can understanding be taken as the sole criteria for explanation. . . . Human patterns and regularities and perhaps even "laws" characterize the human state and undergird the whole enterprise of society and human life . . . explanation in the sense that is being proposed here must suggest what might occur the next time the event or phenomenon occurs. Thus temporality and predictability are assumed in scientific explanations that are within the definition of explanatory power. (p. 104)

The Hermeneutic View

Most opponents of the deductive-nomological covering-law model in nursing espouse a perspective going back at least as far as Wilhelm Dilthey (1883–1911). To Dilthey (cited in Copleston, 1965), the natural and the human sciences are both empirical, but the former deals with the outer experience of nature, while the latter are based on inner, "lived" experience, which provides a direct awareness of human life. The difference in aims of the natural versus human sciences (as opposed to the stance taken by Gortner, 1990) is characterized as that between explanation and understanding. The natural sciences seek causal explanations of nature that connect representations of outer experience through generalizations and abstract laws. The human sciences aim at an understanding of the fundamental structures of life found in the lived experience. The human sciences thus place an equal value on understanding of both individuality *and* universality. In contrast, the natural sciences are thought to place value solely on ever more comprehensive generalizations without concern for or attention to the individual.

Habermas (1989) submits that the deductive-nomological covering law does describe the goal of natural science—a pursuit of general laws with an interest in instrumental control over the environment. However, Habermas and his followers contend that this deductive-nomological approach neglects to recognize the insights offered by other sources of knowledge more important to the human sciences, such as the recognition and inclusion of understanding and interpretation.

While Bohman, Hiley, and Shusterman (1991, p. 5) do not specifically address explanation as a topic, they do state: "The issue is further compounded, because the human sciences are 'doubly hermeneutic.' They do not give interpretations, they are interpretations of interpretations." In other words, the human sciences are not necessarily concerned with general laws, but rather their focus is on interpretation of human experience to achieve understanding about the individual without concern for generalizability. Additionally, the interpretation (and subsequent understanding) is coloured and shaped by the lived experience of the interpreter (doubly hermeneutic).

The emphasis in human science is on understanding instead of on explanation, and the understanding is based on the lived experience of interpretation. Nurse disciples of Dilthey-Habermas point to the failure of the covering-law model to validate hermeneutic understanding. This understanding, felt to be the aim of a human science such as nursing, refers to the capacity to interpret the words, acts, and symbols of others in the interest of mutual understanding and self-reflection.

The opposing positions of the deductive-nomological covering law and the hermeneutic view regarding the aims of human sciences place nursing in a quandary as it moves into the 21st century. "The hermeneutic stress on the narrative features of . . . explanation aggravates rather than resolves the question of how such narrations influence behavior (on the assumption that they sometimes do)" (Roth, 1991, p. 183). This polarity of perspectives is alluded to by Moccia (1988, p. 6) in asking,

> Is science intended to legitimize nursing as a scientific discipline by expanding and refining the ability to predict and prescribe human behavior? Or is it intended to be useful in helping the non-scientific population to understand and explain their experiences in the world? Is there a science to be developed that might combine these polarities?

A Middle Ground in the Explanation Debate

In light of Moccia's query, is it possible to construct a way of looking at explanation that will allow for the future expansion of nursing science? Miller (1983) proposes such an approach in considering the position of human sciences. Fundamentally, Miller's alternative theory of adequate explanation employs causal notions, not notions of regularity or of accessibility to hermeneutic faculty. Simply put, an adequate explanation is seen as a true description of underlying causal factors sufficient to bring about the phenomenon in question. Three important distinctions from the previously discussed perspectives on explanation (model of covering law and hermeneutics) are inherent in this explication of scientific explanation: (a) an explanation must describe causal factors sufficient to bring about the phenomenon in question under the circumstances at hand, (b) causal factors must possess sufficient depth, and (c) the explanation is appropriate for only this particular event within this context (the phenomenon in question). A discussion of each of these distinctions will convey the usefulness of Miller's theory of explanation.

When might causal factors be deemed sufficient to bring about the phenomenon in question? It is suggested that particular rules of causal sufficiency are inherent in theoretical frameworks, subject to empirical debate. Value judgements may affect the assessment of explanatory adequacy, in as much as they affect the choice of research question. In other words, acceptance of sufficient explanation is inseparable from theory. Furthermore, explanation in nursing science is best viewed not from a single source, but rather from multiple sources within physical and human sciences, given that nursing science is multidimensional (Gortner, 1993).

In a pragmatic sense, an explanation must describe those factors that led to the phenomenon under study, bounded by the circumstances at hand—the context. For example, a sufficient explanation could indicate that lack of maternal experience in combination with fear of failure may lead to difficulties in establishing a breast-feeding regimen among a population of inner-city adolescents in the United States. However, to require a description of all the causally relevant factors, factors that taken together would produce the phenomenon in question no matter what the further circumstances, is to reimpose the covering-law model (Miller, 1983). In the example cited, the factors of lack of experience and fear of failure are meant to be considered causal only in the circumstances at hand. There is no statement of a general law in the explanation. Difficulties in establishing a breast-feeding regimen may arise from other factors, given other circumstances—a different group of mothers in terms of age and nationality, or a different point in time. The explanation offered may give clues pertaining to different circumstances but is not intended to serve as a universal explanation.

A causal description sufficient to bring about a phenomenon is not an explanation if the causal factors included are lacking in depth. The description may be inadequate because of two kinds of shallowness: The factors in the explanation may lack depth in that had they not been present something else would have occurred, filling in the causal role and thus producing the same effects (Miller, 1983). If it may be shown that the same sorts of difficulties in establishing a breast-feeding regimen could occur to the group of young mothers when there is a weak support system, then lack of experience and fear

do not explain the phenomenon. It must be assumed that there exists a deeper underlying cause.

The second issue related to depth of factors depends on a sort of causal priority. There are frequently relationships among the concurrent factors producing a phenomenon. It may be that a particular factor is sufficient to bring about the phenomenon of concern only because of the other factor (Miller, 1983). With regard to the case in point, it may be that fear of failure is in fact produced by maternal inexperience. Therefore, the shallower cause (fear of failure) is a means by which the deeper cause (lack of maternal experience) produces its effect.

In essence, then, any scientific explanation is intrinsically comparative. In accounting for how a phenomenon was produced, we must also deny that another, "deeper," causal process is involved. Appraisal of scientific explanation using such criteria provides an assurance that rigour prevails.

van Fraassen (cited in Rubin, 1993, p. 287) summarizes this new view of explanation by simply stating, "An explanation is not the same as a proposition, or an argument, or list of propositions; it is an *answer*." The explanation is an answer to a question, which has been framed within the context of "why." Therefore, a theory of explanation may be viewed as a theory of why-questions.

Value to Nursing

While the above example is perhaps a simplistic representation of explanatory power in nursing, it serves to illustrate the value of a different approach to the issue. Several points may be made regarding the departure from the present polarity in viewing explanation.

The proposed theory moves away from the deductive-nomological perspective, which, Hempel's (1965) arguments to the contrary, has proven to be problematic for human sciences. Phenomena of concern to nursing often comprise numerous factors. In addition, it is hard to imagine situations that are not too idiosyncratic to be governed by universal laws. In reality, this is frequently the case in physical science as well. Explaining why there are topographical formations on earth in no way implies an identical process on Mars. The covering-law model has placed nursing science in a seemingly impossible situation. Gortner (1990) acknowledges the frustration involved in trying to accommodate the science of nursing to standards derived for physical science. She states that "perhaps concern with the mechanistic philosophy of science has prompted the reaction against explication of patterns" in nursing science (p. 104).

Furthermore, the proposed theory of explanation provides an avenue for scientific aims beyond that of hermeneutic interpretation. It is submitted that this alternative stance does not nullify or oppose the potential contribution of hermeneutic understanding, but rather allows for the value placed on the identification of universal experience. Explanation appraised through empirical debate as opposed to rules of logic (as in the deductive-nomological view) anticipates diversity in theoretical grounding. Opportunity is provided for a variety of conceptual approaches in the recognition that all are not equally valid. The governing principle is simply that a theoretical approach is invalid if the science guided by it is an inferior source of further discoveries. It is assumed that over time the more relevant frameworks will be the more productive. When one is searching for an answer, the context of the phenomenon becomes the guiding principle and the answer is the explanation.

Perhaps the greatest benefit of a different notion of scientific explanation has to do with shifting the attention of the discipline away from debates on methodology. Focus may then be placed on the aims and the products of science in nursing.

REFERENCES

Benner, P. (1985). Quality of life: A phenomenological perspective on explanation, prediction and understanding in nursing science. *Advances in Nursing Science, 8(1)*, 1–16.

Bohman, J., Hiley, D., & Shusterman, R. (1991). Introduction: The interpretive turn. In D. Hiley, J. Bohman, & R. Shusterman (Eds.), *The interpretive turn: Philosophy, science and culture* (pp. 1–14). New York: Cornell University Press.

Burns, N., & Grove, S. (1987). *The practice of nursing research: Conduct, critique and utilization.* Philadelphia: Saunders.

Copleston, F. (1965). *A history of philosophy.* New York: Image.

Durkheim, E. (1938). *The rules of sociological method.* New York: Macmillan.

Gerth, H. H., & Mills, C. W. (Eds.). (1946). *From Max Weber: Essays in sociology.* New York: Oxford University Press.

Gortner, S. (1990). Nursing values and science: Toward a science of philosophy. *Image: Journal of Nursing Scholarship, 22,* 101–105.

Gortner, S. (1992). Nursing's syntax revisited: A critique of philosophies said to influence nursing theories. *International Journal of Nursing Studies, 30, 6,* 477–488.

Habermas, J. (1989). *On the logic of the social sciences.* Cambridge, MA: MIT Press.

Hempel, C. (1965). *Aspects of scientific explanation.* New York: Macmillan.

Hiley, D., Bohman, J., & Shusterman, R. (Eds.). (1991). *The interpretive turn: Philosophy, science and culture.* New York: Cornell University Press.

Miller, R. (1983). Fact and method in the social sciences. In R. Boyd, P. Gasper, & J. D. Trout (Eds.), *The philosophy of science* (pp. 743–762). Cambridge, MA: MIT Press.

Moccia, P. (1988). A critique of compromise: Beyond the methods debate. *Advances in Nursing Science, 10,* 1–9.

Norbeck, J. S. (1987). In defense of empiricism. *Image: Journal of Nursing Scholarship, 19,* 28–30.

Packard, S., & Polifroni, E. C. (1991). Dilemmas in nursing science. *Nursing Science Quarterly, 5,* 7–13.

Polifroni, E. C., & Packard, S. (1994). Explanation in nursing science. In *The contribution of nursing research: Past-present-future proceedings* (pp. 805–812). Oslo, Norway: Workgroup of European Nurse Researchers.

Roth, P. (1991). Interpretation as explanation. In D. Hiley, J. Bohman, & R. Shusterman (Eds.), *The interpretive turn: Philosophy, science and culture* (pp. 179–196). New York: Cornell University Press.

Rubin, David-Hillel. (1993). *Explanation.* New York: Oxford University Press.

In Memoriam

Sheila Packard died peacefully, April 23, 1995, after a courageous battle with metastatic cancer. Sheila will be remembered for her keen intellect, her wit, her love of life and her pursuit of truth.

She was a dedicated and committed nurse and educator who envisioned the nurse/professor as a healer engaged in a dialectic with those whom s/he served. Sheila will be deeply missed, but her legacy will last forever.

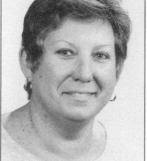

E. CAROL POLIFRONI

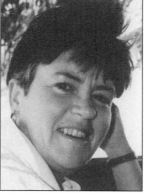

SHEILA A. PACKARD

Free Will or Determinism

E. Carol Polifroni

In Western culture, and most particularly the United States, the notion of freedom reigns supreme. The political perspective of freedom includes a system or worldview wherein an individual is not constrained from doing those things or engaging in activities in which s/he believes. The pure form of freedom often causes controversy in that one has a freedom to do something even if that something is against the beliefs of someone else; for example, the burning of the flag. As of this writing, one is free to burn the flag if one so desires even though others believe the act to be wrong. Within this perspective, freedom is seen as choice: the opportunity to make a decision and to act on that decision.

FREE WILL

Within the philosophical world, the notion of freedom is viewed from a different perspective. The reader needs to visualize a straight line and mark one end with determinism and the other with chaoticism. Along this line lies the entire philosophical debate of determinism, free will and chaos. There are those who subscribe to the belief that freedom does not really exist because the world and the events within the world structure are determined. By virtue of what has happened before, the future is essentially constrained by the past. William James (1842–1910) was an American philosopher and psychologist whose most famous works address issues of truth, pragmatism and psychology. Throughout his life and career, James was pulled in different directions. In one area, his work on *The Principles of Psychology* (1890) drew him to the direction of a functional theory of consciousness. In another area, he was drawn to the religious world. In trying to juxtapose the two directions, James began to address the idea of freedom and truth. James (1979) stated that

> those parts of the universe already laid down absolutely appoint and decree what the other past shall be. The future has no ambiguous possibilities hidden in its womb; the part we call the present is compatible with only one totality (p. 117).

In this view, the future is anything but shapeless and ambiguous; it has been determined by the past. In other words, there is a linear operation of cause and effect. When making decisions, the decision is bound by the history of previous events and the decision is not free but rather determined.

The opposite of determinism is the view of chaos, wherein events occur completely independent of sufficient causal conditions. In this condition, neither the past nor the present participate, bind or influence the future. The chaoticist view is that the events occur as a result of absolute freedom and the inherent absence of causality and connectedness.

INDETERMINISM

The middle ground between these polar opposites is known as the indeterminist perspective. For James (1979), the indeterminist view is that

> the parts of the universe have a certain amount of loose play on one another, so that laying down of one of them does not necessarily determine what the others shall be. It admits the possibilities may be in excess of actualities and that things not yet revealed to our knowledge may really in themselves be ambiguous (p. 118).

In the indeterminist perspective, antecedent conditions and actions are acknowledged. However, the indeterminist does not then believe that the antecedent conditions dictate the present and the future. Rather, through acknowledgment, the antecedent conditions are simply known. The influence of the antecedent conditions is neither necessary nor accepted as a given.

ANTECEDENT CONDITIONS

Repeatedly, the construct of causal conditions has been addressed. What are causal antecedent conditions? For this definition, two elements must be in place. First, the states or events have occurred in the past prior to the event at hand. In other words, an event from the past is known and accepted as being known and true. Secondly, the events or states to be explained or understood (the issue at hand, the present) are shaped by the past. The shaping of the present must be both sufficient and efficient. That is, to have acknowledged a past event but neither identify nor be able to define the role it fulfills in shaping the present is not a causal antecedent condition. The past must determine the event at hand (the future) and the test is both sufficient and efficient. Thus, the reader understands that efficient causal conditions imply the potential influence of the past on the future.

Knowing the past is not a sufficient causal condition to explain the present in all instances. For example, knowing that it rained yesterday is insufficient to explain why it is sunny today; thus, yesterday's rain is not a sufficient antecedent causal condition of sun. On the other hand, knowing it rained two inches yesterday explains the dampness one feels in the basement; yesterday's quantity of rain is a sufficient causal antecedent condition of dampness.

To summarize the discussion in regard to determinism and chaoticism, the determinist accepts the causal nature of human order as an absolute (the existence and adherence to antecedent causal conditions), the indeterminist does not view antecedent causal conditions as absolutes (but does not deny their existence either) and the chaoticist rejects all notions of antecedent causal conditions. For the determinist, the order of all present and future events is absolutely and irrevocably dictated by the past events.

The indeterminist believes that the past must be acknowledged but the future and present are not inextricably woven or wedded to the events of the past and thus, are not necessarily determined by it. The chaoticist view, as the polar opposite of determinism rejects both determinism and indeterminism by simply stating that all events occur at random and are independent of each other as well as independent and free of past events and occurrences.

FREEDOM

This introduction began with a brief discussion on freedom. The reader needs to turn his/her attention to the notion of free will as a form of human freedom. There is great debate about free will. Is freedom an absolute or is freedom mitigated by the past? Are there other conditions which must be present in order to be truly free?

James (1979) categorizes the determinists as either hard or soft. The hard determinist (the pure determinist) rejects the notion of free will and believes free will and determinism are irreconcilable. For the soft determinist, on the other hand, free will and determinism are not polar opposites, but rather can exist in harmony. The notion of antecedent conditions holds constant for the soft determinist (Mill, 1975). However, even though the antecedent conditions are known, the compatabilist (soft determinist) posits that freedom is both possible and probable. The soft determinist also does not reject the causal notion of the past but rather makes decisions based on the causality of the past. The past is a part of the decision-making process and thus the decision making is influenced by the past. For the soft determinist, the absoluteness of the causality of nature exists but humans make decisions within that causality. This view is difficult to understand. How can one be bound to the absolute of the past and be simultaneously wedded to the notion of free will and human choice? The soft determinist posits that the two are not irreconcilable but rather interconnected. There is human choice but it is conditioned by the past and the antecedent conditions are sufficient and causal to determine the future. However, within that determinism, there is choice on what to do. The soft determinist believes that a person can make a different decision when the antecedent conditions are different, but the same decision, even with free will, will be made every time the antecedent conditions are identical.

The libertarian view, on the other hand, embraces the dichotomy between free will and determinism and rejects the notion that the two can exist together. From the libertarian view, one can only be truly free if the opportunity and possibility to choose a different course truly existed regardless of the same sufficient and efficient antecedent causal conditions. Thus, the libertarian view subscribes to the tenets of indeterminism as discussed previously.

The issues of both power and persuasion/preference (Viney and Crosby, 1994) are raised within the condition of free will. Viney and Crosby (as indeterminists) argue that free will can not occur unless an individual has both the power and the persuasion to act on a specific belief. In other words, to simply say you have free will is not truly free will. The condition does not become real unless one has the associated power to enact the free will option and the preference to do so. The power to act means possession of the means and wherewithal to perform. One has the choice to purchase a multimillion dollar home but it is not an act of free will unless one has the power, the means (a million-dollar income), to actually buy the property. Free will is not to be considered within a vacuum but rather grounded in the construct of power or ability.

Concurrently, the notion of persuasion or preference must also be present for the act of free-will decisions to be possible. Building on the million-dollar home above, one is not fulfilling free will if the home is not something the person is interested in. If the preference does not exist, then neither does free will. Even if the ability is present, the construct of free will is only fully operationalized when both the power and the persuasion to act are present.

Another view of free will is the concept of situated freedom as introduced by Dilthey (1988) and enlarged and expanded by Parse (1987). Wilhelm Dilthey (1833–1911), a German neo-Kantian philosopher, separated the physical sciences from those that deal with the human spirit. For him, the spirit within and that of science guides one to a contextual perspective. Additionally, the essence of the science of spirit (human science) must be attended through *verstehen,* a method of understanding.

Situated freedom is the notion and belief that one's base of freedom is grounded in the experience of the moment. The focal point of situated freedom is the phenomenon of presence bounded by the past and the horizons of the future. Situated freedom relies on an understanding and an acceptance of the past but it is not dictated by the past unless the individual chooses to be so dictated and controlled. In other words, the notion of situated freedom is a contextual process wherein the knower, the person, determines the boundaries of his or her own freedom and acts accordingly. Antecedent conditions exist and are acknowledged, perhaps, but they do not determine the actions of the person. Freedom is an attitude as much as it is a state within situated freedom. The person, the human being, is situated (grounded) in a phenomenon and chooses to act in a specific way colored by the events s/he chooses to include in the decision-making process. Situated freedom is clearly neither deterministic nor chaotic but rather indeterminate, like the libertarian view. The individual, not antecedent conditions, determines his or her own future.

CONCLUSIONS AND READINGS

In conclusion, free will and determinism are mutually exclusive concepts for most individuals. Determinism is a reliance on and is tied to the events of the past in the shaping of the future; the antecedent conditions essentially dictate the present and ultimately the future. For the individual believing in free will, the past is acknowledged but choices are possible and probable. The past is recognized as a component of both the here and now and the yet to be. However, the past is not directly and inextricably causal. The past is simply acknowledged and addressed as one factor in the present choice.

The readings direct or guide the reader to review these ideas and beliefs in greater detail. Mitchell and Cody introduce the notion of situated freedom through the eyes and words of Dilthey (1988). Polifroni and Packard explore the notion of free will and its relationship to borrowed theories within nursing care. Viney and Crosby compare and contrast different types of free will and determinism. In each instance, the readings provide greater depth as well as provide the reader with sources of and guides for discussion.

DISCUSSION GUIDE

1. What makes the world go round? Is it free will or predetermined?
2. In order for one to have free will, what other elements must be present?
3. Compare and contrast chaos and determinism. Fatalism and determinism. Free will and determinism. Indeterminism and determinism.
4. What is compatabilism? Soft determinism?
5. What is the relationship of free will or determinism to compliance with a health regimen?
6. Compare and contrast one's views on free will or determinism and relate them to the decision to undergo an organ transplant.

REFERENCES

Dilthey, W. (1988). *Introduction to human sciences* (R. J. Betanzos, Trans.). Detroit: Wayne State University.

James, W. (1979). *The will to believe and other essays in popular philosophy* (F. H. Burkhardt, F. Bowers, & I. K. Skrupskelis, Eds.). Cambridge: Harvard University Press.

Mill, J. S. (1975). *On liberty.* (D. Spitz, Ed.). New York: Norton.

Parse, R. R. (1987). *Nursing science: Major paradigms, theories and critiques.* Philadelphia: Saunders.

Viney, D., & Crosby, D. (1994). Free will in process perspective. *New Ideas in Psychology, 12*(2), 129–141.

BIBLIOGRAPHY

Bergson, H. (1960). *Time and free will.* New York: Harper Torchbooks.

James, W. (1884). The dilemma of determinism. *Unitarian Review, 22,* 193–224.

Kenny, A. (1988). *Free will and responsibility.* London: Routledge.

Mitchell, G., & Cody, W. (1992). Nursing knowledge and human science: Ontological and epistemological considerations. *Nursing Science Quarterly, 5*(2), 54–61.

Polifroni, E. C., & Packard, S. (1993). Psychological determinism and the evolving nursing paradigm. *Nursing Science Quarterly, 6*(2), 63–68.

Rychlak, J. (1994). Four kinds of 'determinism' and free will: A response to Viney and Crosby. *New Ideas in Psychology, 12*(2), 143–146.

Rychlak, J. F., & Rychlak, R. J. (1990). The insanity defense and the question of human agency. *New Ideas in Psychology, 8,* 3–24.

Sappington, A. (1990). Recent psychological approaches to the free will versus determinism issue. *Psychological Bulletin, 108,* 19–29.

Viney, D. (1986). William James on free will and determinism. *The Journal of Mind and Behavior, 7*(4), 555–566.

Viney, D. W. (Ed.). (1989). *Questions of value.* Needham Heights, MA: Ginn Press.

Weatherford, R. (1991). *The implications of determinism.* London: Routledge.

Williams, C. (1988). *Free will and determinism.* Indianapolis: Hackett.

Nursing Knowledge and Human Science: Ontological and Epistemological Considerations

Gail J. Mitchell ● *William K. Cody*

This article examines the meaning of human science in relation to extant nursing knowledge. The origins of the human science tradition are traced to the philosopher Wilhelm Dilthey, who challenged the dominance of the positivist perspective for generating knowledge of the human lifeworld. Specific ontological and epistemological criteria for human science are proposed. Four nursing frameworks, Paterson and Zderad's humanistic nursing, Newman's model of health as expanding consciousness, Watson's human science and human care, and Parse's theory of human becoming, are found to have consistencies and inconsistencies with the human science tradition. It is proposed that the human science perspective is present in and will continue to be reflected in the evolution of nursing science.

Increasingly, nursing is being referred to as a human science (Connors, 1988; Gortner & Schultz, 1988; Meleis, 1990; Munhall, 1989; Parse, 1981, 1987; Watson, 1985). The meaning of this term as it is used in the literature, however, is not clear. Munhall (1989), Parse (1981) and Watson (1985) refer to human science as distinct from natural science and as bearing specific views, concepts, and methods. Contrary to this position, Connors (1988) and Gortner and Schultz (1988) refer to human science as the fields of biology, psychology, anthropology, and sociology. Is human science inclusive of any inquiry about human beings, or is it a distinctive philosophical foundation for science? Is nursing currently a human science or is this an ideal to be esteemed and aspired to? The purpose of this article is to examine the meaning of human science as originated by Dilthey (1961, 1976, 1977a, 1977b, 1988) and explicated by Giorgi (1970, 1971, 1985) and to compare selected works from nursing's extant theoretical base to the explicit attributes that constitute "human" science.

Defining Human Science

The origins of the term human science can be traced to the philosopher Wilhelm Dilthey (1833–1911). The German term for human science, *Geisteswissenschaften*, has also been translated as "human studies." Translators frequently note the linguistic challenge involved in capturing the meaning of freshly coined and esoteric German expressions in English. Also noted in Dilthey's works is his tendency to refer to "psychic" life in a nineteenth-century fashion while

Reprinted by permission from Nursing Science Quarterly 5(2):54–61. © 1992, Chestnut House Publications.

writing of the coherent whole of lived experience. Dilthey did, however, describe life as unity, a living nexus. And he consistently referred to individuals as wholes and to human life as interconnected with others and history. The intent of the authors here is to offer an admittedly hermeneutical interpretation of Dilthey's view, in what is believed to be the unitary perspective of human beings that he intended.

Dilthey in the late 1800s was very concerned about what he called a "crisis in science," a crisis of modern consciousness, thought, and values (Ermarth, 1978). The industrial society had already concretized the successes of the natural sciences, and the developing science of *Anthropologie,* with no other model, was rapidly abandoning any interest in human consciousness in favor of a crude "mindless" naturalism (Ermarth, 1978). Dilthey (1977a) described what he saw as a sterile empiricism that disconnected life from knowledge. His fears were stoked by the growing trend to regard human behavior and culture as susceptible to the methods of natural science, which, he thought, stripped life of human meaning and purpose (Dilthey, 1977a). He proposed that "the deepest problem of modern thought and culture is to understand life as it is lived by man" (Ermarth, 1978, p. 17).

Dilthey (1977a, 1977b, 1988) believed that the development of a human science held the only hope for understanding life as it is humanly lived. He proposed that the human sciences required concepts, methods, and theories which were fundamentally different from those of the natural sciences (Dilthey, 1977a, 1988). Dilthey viewed human beings as the preeminent source of knowledge. His philosophy took as its basis the whole of lived experience, the coherent nexus of life as it is humanly lived (Dilthey, 1977a). He wrote about "living" knowledge and "reflective" life. History and culture were, for Dilthey, manifestations of patterns of human life, pervaded with meaning. The natural sciences, concerned with the elaboration of physical laws from observation and experimentation,

were, for Dilthey, very different from the concerns a true human science would focus on: meaning, values, and relationships within the coherent texture of humanly lived experience. The subject matter of the human sciences is "the interrelation of life, expression, and understanding" (Dilthey, 1976, p. 175).

Dilthey proposed that the lived experience should be "the basic empirical datum of the human sciences" (Ermarth, 1978, p. 97). Further, the researcher, a living being too, is inexorably and unequivocally "in" and "of" what is investigated. There could be no meaningful objective/subjective dichotomy and no analytic reduction beyond experience as humanly lived. Human experience is a coherent whole to which subjectivity is fundamental; objectivity is a human creation. Dilthey maintained that life is a process, a continuous becoming which manifests itself in the dynamic unity of experience (Dilthey, 1976). Human beings were described as individual wholes with intrinsic value (Dilthey, 1977b). Dilthey (1977b) referred to the self as a "life-unity" that is free yet also determined by history. The concept of free will is a fundamental assumption of human science. On free will, Dilthey (1988) wrote, "This is an immediately given actuality. *It cannot be denied* . . . [O]ne *cannot explain* the fact of free will, for it is precisely its hallmark that we cannot break it down in a conceptual system" (p. 270).

More recently, the psychologist Giorgi (1970, 1971, 1985) has reasserted the need for an approach to the human sciences fundamentally different from conventional empirical methods. He proposed to study human beings as persons, as experiencing participants. He challenged the prevailing positivistic methods of psychology, contending that human experience must be understood in the way that it reveals itself, and he maintained that the study of lived experience could be done scientifically (Giorgi, 1985).

According to Giorgi, understanding life experiences requires a focus on meaning within the context of the person's experience of the phenomenon. Human beings cannot be known as objects, nor as separate from their lives. Echoing Dilthey, Giorgi maintained that a person is not "a passive receiver of physical energies, but rather his or her behavior reflects intentionality" (Giorgi, 1971, p. 23). Giorgi also addressed the influence of the researcher in conceptualizing research and the impact of the researcher on study findings. For Giorgi, the most important variable in the human sciences is the meaning of the lived experience for the subject. An exposition of the major thinkers and scholars, such as Gadamer (1976), Geertz (1973), Heidegger (1962), Ricoeur (1974), Schutz (1967), and Winch (1958), who have built on the tradition of which Dilthey is the foremost progenitor, is beyond the scope of this article.

The domination of twentieth-century social science by positivistic approaches in stark contrast to human science philosophy has been well documented (Polkinghorne, 1983) and contributes to the contextual situation in which this article emerges. The philosophical stance of human science outlined here has underpinned or strongly influenced the works of the six seminal scholars mentioned above and many others in the tradition of human science. These scholars have recognized the manifest necessity for the human sciences to explore and understand lived experience, the full complexity of human meanings and values, with no more fundamental reference than the human lives which are the phenomena of concern; indeed this formidable undertaking is the very mission of human science.

Based on the above explications of human science by Dilthey and Giorgi, specific ontological and epistemological attributes emerge as crucial to this approach for nursing science. Human science, in view of its origins and its philosophical foundations, cannot be viewed as a generic term for any and all disciplines studying human beings. It is proposed here that for a scientific discipline to be considered a "human science" logically it must incorporate the ontology and epistemology of its philosophical underpinnings, as described in Table 16-1.

A distinction must be made between a "humanistic" philosophy of science and "human science." According to Webster (1985), "humanism" entails a rejection of supernaturalism and asserts "the essential dignity and worth of man and his capacity to achieve self-realization through the use of reason and scientific

TABLE 16-1. Ontology and Epistemology of the Human Science Paradigm

Ontology	Epistemology
Human beings are unitary wholes in continuous inter-relationship with their dynamic, temporal, historical, cultural worlds.	Research and practice focus on the coherent experience of the person's meanings, relations, values, patterns, and themes.
Human experience is preeminent and fundamental and reality is the whole complex of what is experienced and elaborated in thinking, feeling, and willing.	Lived experience is the basic empirical datum, as gleaned from the participant's description free of comparison to objective realities or predefined norms.
Human beings are intentional, free-willed beings who actively participate in life continuously.	The person's coparticipation in generating knowledge of lived experience is respected, and no more fundamental reference than what is disclosed by the person is sought.
The researcher is inextricably involved with any phenomenon investigated.	The researcher seeks knowledge and understanding of lived experience and is cognizant of the other's lived reality as a unitary whole.

Synthesized and condensed from Dilthey, 1961, 1976, 1977a, 1977b, 1988; and Giorgi, 1970, 1971, 1985.

method." Humanism thus is seen to acknowledge human values and potentialities without requiring a critique of "scientific method." Human science, in contrast, unequivocally rejects the methods of natural science (Dilthey, 1976, 1977a, 1988; Giorgi, 1985) and asserts from the outset that lived experience, the world as experienced, meaning, and understanding are all aspects of a unitary process of human life and cannot be adequately described, explained, or analyzed through objectification, measurement, or reduction.

Significance of Human Science for Nursing

If nurses embrace the human science paradigm, activities in theory development, research, and practice will change to reflect the new philosophical perspective. An examination of nursing's philosophical and theoretical body of literature reveals that, in the past decade, such a change has already begun. In order to explore to what extent nurses are incorporating beliefs of the human science paradigm in theory, research and practice, four nursing frameworks were selected for analysis. These frameworks are: Paterson and Zderad's (1988) humanistic nursing, Newman's (1986a, 1990) model of health as expanding consciousness, Watson's (1985) human science and human care, and Parse's (1981, 1987, 1990a) theory of human becoming (formerly man-living-health, 1981). These frameworks were selected because all their authors claim a unitary conceptualization of human beings, thereby evincing some degree of interfacing with the human science perspective. Further, these authors have publicly renounced the natural science approach and have called for new and different methods more congruent with nursing's philosophical foundations.

Critical to the development of nursing theories underpinned by the human sciences would be the acknowledgment of human beings as individual wholes who are situated in-the-world and who are respected as intentional, free-willed persons. Any theoretical principles and concepts used to structure a theory would need to incorporate these beliefs. Also essential would be approaches which view the individual's lived experience as the focus in both practice and research and which honor the person's lived experience as reality. Researchers and practitioners would be regarded as coparticipants with persons in inquiry and practice in a human science paradigm.

Analysis of the Nursing Frameworks

Inquiry into the four frameworks above revealed a definite commitment to the human science paradigm. Parse's theory of human becoming was found not only to be consistent with the human science beliefs but to clarify, expand, and develop this approach. Consequently, an indepth analysis of Parse's theory will be offered at a later point. Analysis of the works of Newman, Paterson and Zderad, and Watson illuminated consistencies and inconsistencies in relation to the beliefs of human science. Consistencies and commonalities included affirmation, to varying degrees, of the wholeness of the human being, the significance of subjective experience, and mutual participation in the creation of reality.

The inconsistencies took two main forms. In some instances, the author(s) acknowledged an inability to reconcile traditional objectivist beliefs with beliefs congruent with human science, and consequently they incorporated conflicting beliefs in theoretical conceptualizations. Alternately, the author(s) extended and elaborated on beliefs essential to the human science tradition, leading to significant dissidence with the core philosophy. These two inconsistencies are discussed with specific examples to illustrate logical incongruencies with the human science tradition. The intent here is not to rebuke the nursing theorists for their philosophical obscurities, for obscurity engenders clarification. Rather, the intent is to illuminate the inconsistencies in order to foster clarity and further the development of nursing science.

Incorporating Diverging Beliefs

As previously noted, the nursing frameworks revealed both consistencies and inconsistencies with the foundational beliefs of the human science paradigm. Perhaps reflecting the evolutionary nature of knowledge and theory development, several of the authors incorporated diverging beliefs in their work, leaving the reader unclear as to their philosophical underpinnings. The inconsistencies arise in three main areas: the human being's wholeness, the intentionality and free will of the person, and the nature of reality. Each of these will be explored in relation to the works of Paterson and Zderad (1988), Newman (1986a, 1990), and Watson (1985).

WHOLENESS OF HUMAN BEINGS

Paterson and Zderad (1988) in their humanistic nursing practice propose that "the nurse sees the patient as a whole, a gestalt" (p. 25). Human beings are described as "in the-world" and nurses are guided to recognize the complexity and uniqueness of each person's relating and experiencing. Paterson and Zderad note, however, that this view of the person as a whole conflicts with the evaluative stance of the conventional nursing process. They address this conflict by positing that "both subject-subject and subject-object relationships are essential for clinical nursing" (Paterson & Zderad, 1988, p. 27) in which focusing on discrete parts rather than the whole person is sometimes necessary. This attempt to incorporate human science beliefs with biomedical traditions leads to conceptual inconsistencies. It is suggested here that nurses cannot switch their very beliefs according to the nature of the practice situation. What seems to be overlooked by Paterson and Zderad is that nurses can live according to human science beliefs and still perform tasks related to the execution of medical orders. There need not be the subject-subject, subject-object dilemma as espoused by these authors. Though Paterson and Zderad reflect on the inadequacy of the labelling process for capturing lived experiences,

they accept the linear, causal nursing process and the diagnosing of human responses as necessary evils, required for economic reasons. Paterson and Zderad maintain that the natural science tradition is inappropriate for nursing, yet they do not reconcile the inconsistencies between reductionistic and unitary approaches with human beings.

Newman explicitly expresses a belief in the unitary nature of human beings, yet she also discusses the human being as a "system" made up of physiological structures and functions, such as the immune system and the genetic code, reflecting a natural science orientation. The unity of the human "system," for Newman, is predicated on the idea that "mind and matter are made of the same basic stuff" (1986a, p. 37). It is apparently quite appropriate within Newman's model to discuss the physiological, psychological, and emotional processes of the "human system" in conventional terms, so long as one remembers that everything, from the atom to the human being and beyond, is a manifestation of the implicate order, or "absolute consciousness" (pp. 33–37). Similarly, Watson (1985) maintains that the person is conceptualized as an irreducible whole, yet she repeatedly refers to body, mind, spirit and soul, and physical, emotional, and spiritual spheres. Her definitions of health and illness are dependent on the harmony or disharmony within these aspects. Watson also refers to several selves; the "real self," the "inner self," and the "ideal self" are presented as distinct entities. She refers to the "I" and the "Me" of the person and the potential disharmony of these aspects. It is not consistent to maintain that a person is a unitary whole and then to define the person according to these separate parts or spheres. Dilthey (1977a) maintained that "we continually experience a sense of connectedness and totality in ourselves" (p. 53). The authors' struggles to incorporate the concept of the unitary human being into nursing theory and practice parallel a long and complex tradition of discourse in the human sciences.

Intentional Free-Willed Beings

Human science conceptualizes human beings as intentional and inherently free-willed; therefore the nurse would seek no more fundamental reference than the lived experience of the person. Paterson and Zderad (1988) address the *nurse's* intention and free will to commit authentically to another. The authors also regard the human being as free-willed, yet they suggest, "The nurse is alert to opportunities for the patient to exercise his freedom of choice within the limits of safe and sound practice" (p. 17). The nurse is guided to monitor the patient's choices and to determine if they are responsible ones. To carry out this monitoring, the nurse would have to rely on some schema of normative standards or beliefs in order to judge what is "responsible," which is an inconsistent practice if the nurse wishes to respect the human science belief that the individual is an intentional being possessing free will.

Newman's (1986a) conceptualization of freedom describes an arc-like progression as consciousness expands. Human beings first *lose* freedom as they "come into being," are "bound in time" and "find . . . identity in space," until they reach a stage in which choice is engendered through movement (p. 46). "Restriction of movement forces one into a realm beyond space and time" (p. 62). Thereafter one throws off self-concerns, recognizes one's own "boundarylessness" and "timelessness" and *gains* the freedom of returning to "absolute consciousness" (p. 46). It is essentially the movement toward spirituality that imbues the human being with freedom, which is relative to the extent that consciousness is expanded.

The notion that human freedom underpins human science is quite different, in that freedom is never "lost," and there is no requisite for expanding consciousness to "gain" it. Human beings are believed to be free to choose meaning and direction because they make such choices continuously in living everyday life (Dilthey, 1988). "It is true," writes Dilthey (1988), "that the will depends on intellect, but the will can choose or not choose what the intellect understands . . . in fact the will is free precisely inasmuch as in it the search for a reason ends" (p. 270). Newman's (1986b) proposal for "the diagnosis of pattern" would appear to be hinged on her notion of freedom as relative to expanded consciousness. She states, "The role of the nurse within a paradigm of pattern is to help clients recognize their own patterns," a process in which a "burst of insight" occurs that "opens up" a "pathway of action" (pp. 55–56). From a human science perspective, by contrast, the pathway of action is always open.

Watson (1985) says that human beings are free to self-determine and free to choose. Nurses are guided to hold nonpaternalistic values which respect human autonomy and freedom. Yet this belief is violated in two ways. First, there are references to the nurse's helping, integrating, and "correcting" the patient's condition to increase harmony and to try to find meaning in the situation. Second, Watson maintains that "*ideally* [italics added], a person should have the opportunity for self-determination of the meaning of a health-illness experience *before professionals make decisions* [italics added] about treatments and interventions" (1985, p. 66). Human science philosophy abdicates the position of science as the arbiter of truth; the human scientist is a seeker of truth, a seeker rather than a dispenser of wisdom. Dilthey maintained that "understanding constitutes the goal of the human studies in the way that explanation defines the natural sciences" (cited in Makkreel, 1977, p. 7). Knowledge is not used or applied to the person, but rather knowledge enhances understanding for participating with the person in the process of becoming. Dilthey (1976) proposed, "In everything there is the same limitation of possibilities and yet freedom to choose between them, and the beautiful feeling of being able to move forward and to realize new potentialities in one's own existence" (p. 245).

The Nature of Reality

In a human science ontology, human beings and their worlds as experienced cannot be separated. Human science does not distinguish between subjective and objective realities because the focus of scientific activities is the humanly lived experience of the world, in which subjectivity is primal. Paterson and Zderad suggest that "nurses are drawn toward two realities—the reality of the objective scientific world and the reality of the subjective-objective world" (p. 36). The authors' endorsement of the traditional nursing process automatically places the person in the position of object and the nurse in the role of arbiter of truth. Again this reflects the conflicting views proposed with respect to the nurse-patient relationship.

Newman's (1986a) view of the nature of reality draws on Bohm's (1980) theory of the implicate order. All humanly experienced phenomena comprising the explicate order are posited as manifestations of an unseen, unknowable implicate order which comprises the unity of all that is. According to this view, patterns of human experience are reflective of this underlying primary reality. Newman writes, "We need to remind ourselves that our manifest reality is a small portion of the total enfoldment of the pattern in time-space" (1986a, p. 15). Her model theoretically eliminates the subject-object duality, according to its ontology. However, Newman's (1986a, 1986b) view is that neither objectivity nor subjectivity has any validity, since the perspective adapted from Bohm says there are no boundaries to (physical) reality. From a human science perspective, this is still essentially an objectivist reality, founded on the basis of the speculations of physical scientists that the nature of reality is a complex, multidimensional whole. The human being in such a model is defined by what physical science says about matter and energy. By contrast, human science directly asserts that human reality as lived is itself a complex multidimensional whole (Dilthey, 1977a).

The preeminence of the human experience is ostensibly highly valued in Watson's theory. She speaks of developing knowledge about the lived world of human experience and contends that the phenomenological research method is most congruent with her theoretical perspective.

However, Watson distinguishes the person's experience of the world (phenomenal field) from the world as it actually is. For example, she proposes that nurses "help integrate the person's subjective experience and emotions with the objective external view of the situation" (Watson, 1985, p. 65). Watson also suggests that there can be incongruencies between the person and nature (world). For example, she states, "If a person does not feel congruent with mind, body, and soul . . . or rejects the self . . . or is obsessed with an ideal self, the person will be dissatisfied and maladjusted" (p. 57). These distinctions reveal a belief in an objective reality separate from the person's experience of it. This essentially dichotomous view is inconsistent with human science philosophy, in which being human means participating in the creation of reality. Human consciousness already is the unity of the person's subjective-objective relationship with the world; it is not something to be aspired to (Dilthey, 1977a). The use of the conventional subjective-objective constructs speaks to the exigencies of traditional science but is inconsistent with the understanding of humanly lived reality that underpins human science.

Extending Essential Beliefs

In several instances within the frameworks examined, departures from the human science tradition were noted in areas where some congruence might be expected based on the overall presentation and central concepts. Paterson and Zderad (1988) move from focusing on the human being's lived experience to focusing on nurses' lived experiences and their descriptions of human beings. Both Newman (1986a) and Watson (1985) go well beyond the lived experience as the primal foundation of human knowledge by assigning higher order importance to metaphysical concepts.

It is clear that the basic empirical datum in Paterson and Zderad's humanistic nursing is the nurse's experience, "the between" of existentially experienced nursing situations. The authors address the importance of meanings, patterns, values, and themes, but it is not clear whose experiences are paramount, the nurse's or the patient's. Paterson and Zderad contend that nursing must be described phenomenologically, that nurses' descriptions of nursing situations with patients will build the knowledge and "make explicit a science of nursing" (1988, p. 3). This is a description of the practice of nursing, however, not of a nursing science based on the health experience of human beings. Giorgi (1985) proposed that a discipline is not ready-made in the world and simply viewed and studied. Rather, it is created by a unique knowledge base that is housed within its theories. Thus, to study the nursing act phenomenologically as Paterson and Zderad suggest is to study the particular nurse's view of nursing. It is suggested in this article that nursing science focuses on the concepts of human-environment and health, not the nurse's views of the between. To be consistent with the human science approach nurses must rely on the person's description as it is given, and not on what that experience is assumed to be. Paterson and Zderad's focus on the practitioner's experience reflects a serious departure from beliefs related to the practice of a human science, which investigates lived experiences and life expressions of human beings.

Human consciousness is an important concept in human science; it is the origin of all knowledge about lived experience (Dilthey, 1988). The ontology of Newman's theory is largely metaphysical, in that the key concept of "absolute consciousness" is beyond the realm of lived experience. Newman (1986a) ascribes consciousness to atoms, rocks, plants, animals, and unspecified "astral" and "spiritual" entities (pp. 33–37). In human science philosophy there is no way of knowing a more fundamental ground behind or beyond the lived experience of the person. One wonders why Newman (1986a), whose central thesis is "health as expanding consciousness," has completely ignored continental European philosophy and theory on consciousness throughout her work. Instead, Newman

cites works of speculative physics as underpinning her theory, even when addressing human experience. Dilthey (1977a) maintained that "consciousness cannot go behind itself" (p. 75). It is the structure of consciousness that sheds light on the coherent unity of human life.

In human science, humanly lived experiences elaborated in thinking, feeling, and willing are the complex whole of reality. Watson emphasizes the significance of human experience as it is lived. However, her emphasis on the metaphysical, spiritual realm clouds the issue of the primacy of lived experience. Watson (1985) states that "the human soul is more than physical, mental, emotional existence . . . the soul exists for something larger than physical life" (p. 45). She maintains, "The soul, inner self, spiritual self is tied to a higher degree of consciousness . . . that transcends time and space" (p. 46). This soul, which "may be underdeveloped and in need of reawakening" (p. 45), reflects a reality beyond that which is directly experienced by human beings and is in conflict with the purported human science origins of Watson's theory.

Watson explicitly presents her framework as emerging from the human science paradigm. Paterson and Zderad refer to their work as humanistic, a related term but not synonymous with human science. Although the concepts Newman uses are abundantly addressed in human science, the ontology underpinning her theory is derived instead from speculative physics. The selective extraction of inconsistencies with the human science paradigm in these authors' works is not intended to suggest a failing on their part but is intended to foster greater conceptual clarity and is offered in the spirit of scholarly questioning and debate. The purpose of this analysis was to determine to what extent the values and beliefs of the human science paradigm were currently evident in nursing's extant knowledge base. The authors conclude that the human science tradition is present to varying degrees in nursing science.

Of the four theories explored here, Parse's

(1981, 1987, 1990a) theory of human becoming remained consistent with the fundamental ontology and epistemology of the human science tradition. The theory can be seen to have expanded and clarified major ideas of the human science tradition. Parse's (1981) work was the first publication in nursing to specify nursing as a human science in Dilthey's traditional sense. Parse's theory is analyzed here with regard to both its adherence to and expansion of the human science tradition.

Parse's Theory of Human Becoming

Parse's first chapter begins, "To posit the idea of nursing rooted in the human sciences is to make explicit an alternative to the traditional practice of nursing as a medical model grounded in the natural sciences" (1981, p. 3). Parse describes nursing as a human science focusing on the unitary human being's experience of living and creating health, and she cites Dilthey in her explication of the concepts of her theory. She states that the methodologies of human sciences focus on "uncovering the meaning of phenomena as humanly experienced" and "on understanding the connectedness of life itself" (1981, p. 11). Dilthey (1977b) suggested that explicating human interrelatedness connects that which is universally human with that which is individual.

Parse (1981) synthesized concepts from Rogers' (1970) science of unitary human beings and tenets of contemporary existential phenomenology in such a way that the fundamental notion of human science proposed by Dilthey was brought to fruition for nursing science in the theory of human becoming. The tenets of human subjectivity and intentionality, and the concepts of human coexistence, coconstitution, and situated freedom, drawn from existential phenomenology, reflect the development of ideas germinated by Dilthey and others in the philosophy of human science. The synthesis of concepts from Rogers' work with concepts from existential phenomenology to form a unique, coherent theory of nursing underscores the compelling fit between human science philosophy and nursing as a unique and autonomous discipline. Parse (1987) avoided conceptual inconsistencies by inventing nursing practice and research methodologies which flow directly from the ontological and epistemological foundations of her theory. In this way there is no need to reconcile human science beliefs with biomedical traditions. Parse's theory and her practice and research methodologies express and structure the beliefs which underpin human science in a new way specifically for nursing science.

Parse's (1981, 1987, 1990a) theory of human becoming has three central themes: meaning, rhythmicity, and cotranscendence. Her explication of these themes moves her theory beyond human science as described by Dilthey (1961). Parse describes the human being as an open unity who freely chooses meaning in situations, bears responsibility for choices, and coconstitutes with the environment rhythmical patterns of relating in the process of cotranscending with emerging possibilities. Health is described as a "process of becoming, a cocreated process of living value priorities" (1981, p. 31). Health is the day-to-day living of rhythmical patterns reflecting the person's unfolding and cotranscending with the possibles (the moving onward in life in a chosen way) (Parse, 1981).

The goal of practice in Parse's theory is the quality of life from the person's perspective (1987). Nurses in true presence with people live the practice method, which revolves around the all-at-once of illuminating meaning through "explicating," synchronizing rhythms through "dwelling with," and mobilizing transcendence through "moving beyond" (1987, p. 167). Parse's research method is rooted in phenomenology and is structured to be congruent with the assumptions and principles of the human becoming theory. It focuses on uncovering the structures of universal lived experiences in the human-universe-health interrelationship. The goal of the method is to enhance understanding of lived experiences of health.

Critique of the Theory of Human Becoming

Parse presents her theory as emerging from the human science paradigm and she remains congruent with those philosophical underpinnings throughout her work. The human being is viewed as unitary, mutually interrelating with environment, and there is no reference to human beings other than as living unities. The person's lived experience is clearly regarded as the preeminent ground of human health. The researcher explores universal lived experiences of health, with the goal of enhancing understanding. This is consistent with Dilthey's concern "to understand life as it is lived by man" (Ermarth, 1978, p. 17). Both the research and practice methods focus on the lived experience of human beings. There is no subject-object dichotomy; reality is viewed as cocreated with the universe and others while experienced uniquely by the person. Nursing is seen as a scientific discipline in which the concepts of unitary human beings, mutual unfolding, human coexistence, intentionality, free will, and intersubjective sharing of meaning may at last be fully elaborated and incorporated in praxis. Dilthey consistently maintained that all theory was theory for praxis (Ermarth, 1978).

Parse suggests that persons "unfold with contemporaries the ideas of predecessors . . . in a continuity that connects past with future" (1981, p. 26). The "way the person lives in interrelationship with others reflects chosen meanings and reveals cherished values" (1981, p. 48). Individuals freely choose the meaning of situations and freely live personal values by choosing ways of being/becoming from among possibilities. Again, this is consistent with Dilthey's (1961) view of human interconnectedness, yet it goes beyond his view.

Guided by Parse's theory, the nurse in true presence with the person focuses on the individual's own meaning without judging, labelling, or trying to change the person. The nurse goes with the person as he or she explores options, images consequences of choices, and plans to live hopes and dreams. In the true presence of the nurse the individual clarifies the meaning of the situation and new meanings are uncovered; new insights generate new possibles, the understanding of opportunities and limitations in light of what is truly valued. The nurse coparticipates with the person in the process of moving beyond the now moment, guided by the theory to understand that the person chooses his or her own way (Parse, 1987). Parse maintains that individuals know their own way, reflectively and prereflectively. The nurse in true presence bears witness to the person's unfolding and becoming (Parse, 1990b). In creating the theory of human becoming, Parse has uncovered the intrinsic relevance of the human science perspective, which is centrally concerned with what it means to be human for the discipline of nursing.

In Parse's (1987) research methodology, the researcher "lives" dialogical engagements with participants. This is described as "an intersubjective being with, in which the researcher and participant live the I-Thou process as they move through an unstructured discussion about the lived experience" (1987, p. 176). The researcher views the participant as the expert on the lived experience being explored and remains focused on the phenomenon as it is revealed by the person. The researcher participates in generating enhanced understanding of the phenomenon by creatively abstracting the structure of the lived experience in the language of science.

In summary, Parse's theory, intentionally structured as a human science theory of nursing, accurately reflects the ontology and epistemology of human science philosophy. Parse's theory lays a foundation for a nursing science that is grounded in the meaning of lived experiences in the human-universe process. The theory focuses on the lived experience of unitary human beings in continuous interrelationship with their worlds. Reality as perceived by the person is not compared to an "objective" reality but is respected, as is the free will of the person, in choosing ways of becoming. Parse's theory is thus congruent with yet goes beyond the ontology and epistemology of human science as posited in this article and is an emergent, a newly created theory for praxis that uncompromisingly incorporates the beliefs of human science into nursing research and practice.

Conclusion

Nursing science is currently undergoing change as new views emerge which challenge the traditional methods of natural science-based, biomedical nursing. The human science paradigm is one such view. This perspective is surfacing in nursing at a time when nurse scholars are questioning the precepts of the natural science paradigm and, in doing so, are expressing many of the concerns which led Dilthey to propose a different approach to human science over a hundred years ago. It has been suggested in this article that the human science tradition is not merely any study of human beings, but a particular way of studying human life which values the lived experience of unitary persons and seeks to understand life in all its interwoven patterns of meanings and values.

Nurse scientists are defining boundaries and seeking knowledge which is unique to nursing. This knowledge is currently organized in conceptual and theoretical frameworks, some of which reflect the values and beliefs of the human science paradigm. Of the four frameworks explored here, one, Parse's theory of human becoming, was found not only to be congruent with but to go beyond the human science perspective. The other three frameworks, Paterson and Zderad's humanistic nursing, Newman's model of expanding consciousness, and Watson's human science and human care, demonstrated both consistencies and inconsistencies with the philosophy of human science. Continued explication of the assumptions, values, and beliefs which underpin different theoretical approaches is needed, so that nurses can understand with depth and clarity the foundations of the unique knowledge base of nursing. Only

through contemplative consideration of the philosophical basis of the extant body of theory and through open critique and discourse can nurses choose which paths to follow in the quest for knowledge.

REFERENCES

Bohm, D. (1980). *Wholeness and the implicate order.* London: Routledge.

Connors, D. (1988). A continuum of researcher-participant relationships: An analysis and critique. *Advances in Nursing Science, 10*(4), 32–42.

Dilthey, W. (1961). *Pattern and meaning in history: Thoughts on history and society* (H.P. Rickman, Ed. and Trans.). New York: Harper & Row.

Dilthey, W. (1976). *Selected writings* (H.P. Rickman, Trans.). Cambridge: Cambridge University Press.

Dilthey, W. (1977a). Ideas concerning a descriptive and analytic psychology. (Original work published 1894). In R.M. Zaner & K.L. Heiges (Trans.), *Descriptive psychology and historical understanding* (pp. 23–120). The Hague, Netherlands: Nijhoff.

Dilthey, W. (1977b). The understanding of other persons and their expressions of life. (Original work published 1927). In R.M. Zaner & K.L. Heiges (Trans.), *Descriptive psychology and historical understanding* (pp. 123–144). The Hague, Netherlands: Nijhoff.

Dilthey, W. (1988). *Introduction to the human sciences* (R.J. Betanzos, Trans.). Detroit: Wayne State University Press. (Original work published 1883)

Ermarth, M. (1978). *Wilhelm Dilthey: The critique of historical reason.* Chicago: University of Chicago Press.

Gadamer, H.G. (1976). *Philosophical hermeneutics* (D.E. Linge, Trans.). Berkeley: University of California Press.

Geertz, C. (1973). *The interpretation of cultures.* New York: Basic Books.

Giorgi, A. (1970). *Psychology as a human science.* New York: Harper & Row.

Giorgi, A. (1971). Phenomenology and experimental psychology: II. In A. Giorgi, W. Fischer & R. von Eckartsberg (Eds.), *Duquesne studies in phenomenological psychology*, (Vol. 1, pp. 3–29). Pittsburgh, PA: Duquesne University Press.

Giorgi, A. (1985). Sketch of a psychological phenomenological method. In A. Giorgi (Ed.), *Phenomenology and psychological research* (pp. 8–22). Pittsburgh: Duquesne University Press.

Gortner, S.R., & Schultz, P.R. (1988). Approaches to nursing science methods. *Image: Journal of Nursing Scholarship, 20*, 22–24.

Heidegger, M. (1962). *Being and time* (J. Macquarrie & E. Robinson, Trans.). New York: Harper & Row.

Makkreel, R.A. (1977). Introduction. In R.M. Zaner & K.L. Heiges (Trans.), *Descriptive psychology and historical understanding* (pp. 1–20). The Hague, Netherlands: Nijhoff.

Meleis, A. (1990, September). *Directions for nursing theory development.* Paper presented at the National Nursing Theory Conference, Los Angeles, CA.

Munhall, P. (1989). Philosophical ponderings on qualitative research methods in nursing. *Nursing Science Quarterly, 2,* 20–28.

Newman, M. (1986a). *Health as expanding consciousness.* St. Louis: Mosby.

Newman, M. (1986b). Nursing's emerging paradigm: The diagnosis of pattern. In A.M. McLane (Ed.), *Classification of nursing diagnoses: Proceedings of the seventh conference.* St. Louis: Mosby.

Newman, M. (1990). Newman's theory of health as praxis. *Nursing Science Quarterly, 3,* 37–41.

Parse, R.R. (1981). *Man-living-health: A theory of nursing.* New York: Wiley.

Parse, R.R. (1987). *Nursing science: Major paradigms, theories and critiques.* Philadelphia: Saunders.

Parse, R.R. (1990a, September). [Speaker on] *Panel of nursing theorists.* National Nursing Theory Conference, Los Angeles, CA.

Parse, R.R. (1990b). Health: A personal commitment. *Nursing Science Quarterly, 3,* 136–140.

Paterson, J.G., & Zderad, L.T. (1988). *Humanistic nursing.* New York: National League for Nursing.

Polkinghorne, D. (1983). *Methodology for the human sciences: Systems of inquiry.* Albany: State University of New York Press.

Ricoeur, P. (1974). *The conflict of interpretations: Essays in hermeneutics* (W. Domingo et al., Trans.). Evanston, IL: Northwestern University Press.

Rogers, M.E. (1970). *An introduction to the theoretical basis of nursing.* Philadelphia: Davis.

Schutz, A. (1967). *The phenomenology of the social world* (G. Walsh & F. Lehnert, Trans.). Evanston, IL: Northwestern University Press.

Watson, J. (1985). *Nursing: Human science and human care.* Norwalk, CT: Appleton-Century-Crofts.

Webster's ninth new collegiate dictionary. (1985). Springfield, MA: Merriam-Webster.

Winch, P. (1958). *The idea of a social science and its relation to philosophy.* London: Routledge & Kegan Paul.

Psychological Determinism and the Evolving Nursing Paradigm

E. Carol Polifroni • Sheila Packard

The purpose of this article is to explore three behaviorist theories and their roles within the evolving paradigm of nursing. The authors suggest that the behaviorist theories of locus of control, self-efficacy, and the health belief model are derived from deterministic philosophical premises. These premises are in direct conflict with the premise of free will. As interpreted by the authors and many others, the emerging paradigm of nursing relies on the free will of the individual, the ability of the individual to choose for himself/herself what course of action to take, to avoid, or to pursue. The authors address the psychological deterministic philosophical premises within the three theories and utilize nursing theories to compare and contrast the views of free will and determinism. Finally, they suggest that the use of borrowed and applied theories should decline when nurse scientists are true to the philosophical assumptions of theories within nursing science.

Nursing has rather commonly been called an applied science. One usage of the term *applied* refers to the fact that a reciprocity exists between praxis and scholarship within the discipline. For example, the *process* of caring is influenced by research and theoretical developments which in turn are mediated and inspired by the *phenomenon* of caring. A second meaning exists, however, with regard to the term *applied*. This is the idea that nursing epistemology borrows theoretical constructs from other fields and adapts these constructs to the nursing situation. These adaptations may then be utilized to frame both practice and research endeavors (Packard & Polifroni, 1991).

It is the purpose of this article to demonstrate that the assumption of borrowed theories may

conflict with the philosophical foundations of the evolving paradigm in nursing. Of particular import with this regard are notions pertaining to determinism and free will. Three theories chosen to illustrate this point are: locus-of-control orientation, the health belief model, and self-efficacy theory.

Borrowed Theories

Locus-of-control orientation is a construct developed in psychology to address beliefs about individual control (Rotter, 1966) and expanded to include expectancies concerning health outcomes (Wallston, Wallston, & DeVillis, 1978; Wallston, Wallston, Kaplan, & Maides, 1976). It is hypothesized that persons with an external locus-of-control orientation are apt to feel that health and health-related outcomes are determined by chance, fate or powerful others. This orientation can lead to the behavioral outcomes

Reprinted by permission from Nursing Science Quarterly 6(2):63–68. © 1993, Chestnut House Publications.

of surrendering or passively relying on others with regard to health matters. On the other hand, persons with an internal locus-of-control orientation are expected to feel more personally in control of health and associated outcomes. It has been asserted that individual control beliefs affect perception of stressful events and therefore influence choices of coping strategies (Johnson, Christman, & Stitt, 1985). Specifically, research has sought to demonstrate that an internal locus-of-control orientation is associated with more positive outcomes (Strickland, 1978) than an external locus-of-control orientation (Belgrave, 1991; Johnson et al., 1985; Levenson, 1973; Rock, Myerowitz, Maisto, & Wallston, 1987; Saudia, Kinney, Brown, & Young-Ward, 1991; Wallston & Wallston, 1982). Once a person's locus-of-control orientation is ascertained, it can then be used to predict behavioral outcomes.

The health belief model was developed to explain health-related behavior at the individual level from a psychological perspective (Maiman & Becker, 1974; Rosenstock, 1966). It has been used to explain and predict compliance with prescribed regimens. The model purports that attitudinal variables precede a health-related action and influence the course of that action (Becker & Maiman, 1975; Rosenstock, 1966). Fundamental to this construct is the assumption that human behavior is determined by an objective, logical thought process (Salazar, 1991). Originally, the health belief model espoused four specific attitudinal variables: perceived susceptibility, perceived seriousness, perceived benefits, and perceived barriers. It is believed that a health behavior is more likely to result when an individual believes herself/himself susceptible to a given condition, perceives the condition to be of at least moderate severity, believes that a particular action would be of benefit in reducing susceptibility, and feels that the action would not involve overcoming important barriers such as high cost, pain or embarrassment (Champion, 1988; Salazar, 1991). In the early 1970s, the additional variables of general health motivation

(as measured by preventive health practices) and perceived control (an aspect of self-efficacy) were included in the health belief model. Nurse investigators have framed their studies on this model in an effort to identify factors that explain and predict a particular behavioral outcome salient to clinical practice (Champion, 1985; Hallal, 1982; Huebsch, 1991; Murdaugh & Verran, 1987; Rutledge, 1987).

Self-efficacy refers to the personal convictions people have regarding their ability to successfully execute particular behaviors in order to produce certain outcomes. The theory was developed by Bandura and colleagues in the 1970s to predict and explain individual health behaviors (Bandura, 1977). According to Bandura (1977), a person's expectation of success and personal mastery determines whether or not she or he will engage in a particular behavior. Thus, self-judgments of efficacy partly determine which activities an individual will attempt and which activities an individual will avoid. Two types of expectations are hypothesized to exert powerful influences on behavior: *outcome expectancy*, which is the conviction that certain behaviors will lead to specific outcomes, and *self-efficacy expectancy*, which is the conviction that one can successfully execute the behavior required to produce the outcomes. It is asserted that expectations are based on four major sources of information: performance accomplishments, vicarious experiences, verbal persuasion, and emotional/psychological arousal. In a review of self-efficacy studies Lawrance and McLeroy (1986) concluded that ratings of self-efficacy can help identify individuals at risk for certain unhealthful behaviors. In a separate re-

> ❝Do not go gentle into
> that good night
> Rage, rage against the
> dying of the light.❞
>
> *(Dylan Thomas)*

view, Strecher, De Vellis, Becker, and Rosenstock (1986) contend that for all health-related areas, self-efficacy appears to be a consistent predictor of short- and long-term success and that in experimental studies, manipulations of self-efficacy have proven consistently powerful in initiating and maintaining change. Salazar (1991) has called for the use of self-efficacy theory in occupational health nursing practice.

An important assumption common to locus-of-control orientation, the health belief model, and self-efficacy theory is that human behavior is linear. Each of the aforementioned constructs seeks to predict behavioral outcomes through the identification of individual psychological attributes. In a very simple form, this is to say that A does indeed (at least partly) cause B. If an individual's locus-of-control orientation, or health beliefs, or self-efficacy scores are known, then the nurse in a given situation would to some degree be assured of a particular patient outcome. (Additionally, if the most favorable orientation, beliefs, and perceptions could be infused, then behavior could be manipulated so as to comply with the views of the health care provider.) It is assumed that human behavior is the result of objective and logical thought which is not unique to the individual but rather can be generalized to include all persons. This assumption originates in the philosophical stance of determinism and in particular may be posited in the class designated as psychological determinism (Kenny, 1978).

Positions on Freedom

Determinism may be defined as the view that every event has a cause (Kenny, 1978; Weatherford, 1991; Williams, 1988). Generally determinists hold that the future of the world is fixed in one unavoidable pattern. Various forms of determinism evoke different explanations of why and how it is fixed (Weatherford, 1991, p. 3). With regard to human beings, the term *event* refers to bodily movements and thoughts that pass through human minds. The term *cause*

connotes sufficient antecedent conditions (a state or occurrence preceding in time the event to be explained, such that it is a sufficient condition for the happening of such an event). Psychological determinism is a particular brand of determinism in which action is considered to be determined by the wants and beliefs of agents; behavior is the outward result of internal motivating forces operating in the mind. The characteristic laws of psychological determinism contain mentalistic terms, terms for mental events and states of mind (Kenny, 1978).

The converse of determinism is the belief that human behavior arises out of free will. Some analyses of the freedom concept place most emphasis on the notion of choice or desire; others place most emphasis on the notion of ability or power. On the one hand, a person does something freely if she or he does it because she or he wants to; on the other hand, one does something freely if she or he does it even though it is within his or her power not to do it. Freedom conceived in terms of choice or wanting is liberty of spontaneity; freedom conceived in terms of power to do otherwise is liberty of indifference (Kenny, 1978; Williams, 1988). The more fundamental of these two notions of freedom is the latter. In this case, in order to do something freely, an individual must have both the power and the ability to do otherwise even if everything (the facts, own values, and other aspects) were exactly the same in all respects.

Compatabilism is a philosophical stance which argues that human actions can be both free and determined. This particular point of view is also known as *soft determinism* (James, 1923). Compatabilists hold that there is a difference between causally determined behavior and constrained behavior. Since it is constraint that is the opposite of freedom, it is possible for action to be both free and causally determined (Weatherford, 1991). The soft determinists' position asserts that human actions are determined in the metaphysical sense but are seemingly free (undetermined) from the perspective of the individual (Hume, 1739/1967; Mill, 1859/

1975). Hume (1739/1967) held that humans possess the freedom of spontaneity, that a person is usually free from constraint or outside coercion but ultimately everything is determined by an absolute fate. The kind of freedom that Mill (1859/1975) embraced includes the assertion that an individual can never do other than what she or he in fact does. However, Mill mentioned that humans possess a sense of having chosen one course of action over another.

The argument concerning the type or amount of freedom involved in human behavior remains moot. That is to say, the debate continues in philosophy and is considered to be irresolvable in the same way that an absolute definition of truth may be irresolvable (Packard & Polifroni, 1992). Kenny (1978) states:

> Most people who have a firm belief in determinism or indeterminism seem to me to base their conviction on an act of faith, or at best on an extrapolation from the history of science, or the particular period of history of science may incline one to determinism or to indeterminism in accordance with the particular science, or the particular period of history from which one decides to extrapolate. (p. 33)

It is beyond the scope of this article to put the debate over freedom to rest. However, it is contended that at least one particular sort of determinism, psychological determinism, is both logically flawed and unsuited to the human science of nursing.

Inherent Problems of Psychological Determinism

According to the psychological determinists, wants and beliefs are mental states or processes which stand in causal connection with bodily movements. For this to be the case, the mental events must be capable of separate identification from the physical units. Moreover, these two kinds of events must be related by a causal law. It may be argued that neither of these two conditions hold (Kenny, 1978). Every voluntary action is in some sense wanted by the actor (if it were in no way wanted it would not be voluntary). But an action may be voluntary without there being any mental event, separate from the action which precedes or coincides with it.

Several different types of actions may be considered to be voluntary, based upon the idea that they are wanted. Thus the meaning of the term *want* may be classified in one of the following ways.

1. There are sensual wants such as the desire for food, drink, sex and sleep which are indeed mental processes in that they originate in sensations that have intensity, duration, and universal characteristics.
2. There are wants for long and short-term goals. Such wants need not be present in a person's mind whenever they are operative (an intention to become a nurse might influence one's actions without being an item of consciousness).
3. There are wants to adopt means to specific ends. These also may influence conduct without conscious thought. But unlike the wants for goals, they may entail things not wanted for their own sake (taking a test so as to pass a course).
4. There is the kind of want which is necessary if an action is to be voluntary. This type of want is known as consent. The person chooses it neither as a means nor an end, but it would not take place were it not for the pursuit of a purpose (a nurse may break a patient's rib in the process of cardiopulmonary resuscitation).

In each of these cases except the first, the wants can occur without any mental event separate from the action which manifests the want. The mental and physical events, therefore, are not capable of separate identification as they must be if the relation between them is causal in nature (Kenny, 1978).

Wants explain actions; they are the person's reasons for acting. According to the psychological determinist, it is the reasons for action which provide the causes for actions. However, there is a difference between the operation of causes and the explanations of reason. If there is an adequate cause for an effect, then the effect must follow. A cause is a sufficient antecedent condition for the effect. If the cause is present without the effect, then the cause is not sufficient. Yet, there may be a good reason for performing a certain action, but the action does not follow without casting doubt on the adequacy of the reason. Rules pertaining to practical reasoning differ from those applied to causal laws (Kenny, 1978; Williams, 1988).

In essence, psychological forms of determinism are incoherent because they misconstrue the nature of the mental phenomenon upon which they explicitly or implicitly base their formulation. It may be noted that even devout determinists express doubt regarding the claims made in this arena.

> I believe that psychology—if it is a science at all—will turn out to be reducible to chemistry, physics, and information theory. It may, of course, turn out that there are no such things as psychological laws at all, in which case physical determinism might be true and psychological determinism false. . . . If physical determinism is true and if we are physical systems, then our psyches must also be determined (although our future states might be predictable only by physical not psychological laws). (Weatherford, 1991, p. 187)

The will is the capacity to behave in pursuit of long-term goals and in light of the comparative attractiveness of alternative courses of action. How and why choices are made regarding health, the recognition of patterns in human experience, and the depiction of inner reality are of great importance to nursing. Newman, Sime, and Corcoran-Perry (1991) have described the stance espoused in psychological determinism as follows:

> From the particular deterministic perspective phenomena can be viewed as isolatable, reducible entities having defendable properties that can be measured. These entities have orderly and predictable connectedness to each other. Change is assumed to be a consequence of antecedent conditions—conditions that if sufficiently identified and understood, could be used to predict and control change in the phenomena. Relationships within and among entities are viewed as linear and causal. Kinds of knowledge sought include facts and universal laws. (p. 4)

It is contended that this view aside from its inherent flaws is ultimately unsuited to the evolving paradigm in nursing.

Free Will and the Evolving Nursing Paradigm

Theories borrowed from other disciplines such as locus-of-control orientation, the health belief model, and self-efficacy theory share the intrinsic problems of psychological determinism as delineated above. In addition, they do not offer a perspective which is consistent with the evolving paradigm in nursing.

Newman et al. (1991) have proposed that nursing is the study of caring in the human health experience. In discussing the different approaches which might be utilized in the tasks of nursing inquiry they submit that a unitary-transformative perspective is essential for the full explication of knowledge. This perspective, a specification of the simultaneity paradigm (Parse, Coyne, & Smith, 1985) which views change as unpredictable and unidirectional, is the evolving paradigm of nursing. Newman et al. (1991) note that knowledge is personal, involves pattern recognition, and is a function of both the viewer and the phenomenon viewed. It is not the particular-deterministic perspective that offers promise to the study of caring in the human health experience. Phillips (1990) asserts "emerging research methods are breaking the restraints imposed by research methods inconsistent with nursing's basic philosophy and theoretical perspectives of humans. . . . The old methods simply do not fit the new paradigm" (p. 1). A major source of conflict between psychological determinism and the evolving epistemology in nursing centers on philosophical notions pertaining to the situated freedom of human beings. In order to depict this conflict, it is useful to briefly discuss the ideas of several major contributors to the more recent theoretical development of nursing.

In 1976, Paterson and Zderad proposed that nurses consciously and deliberately approach nursing as an existential experience. They suggested that the science of nursing would be built over time by compilation and complementary synthesis of phenomenological descriptions of experiences in the nursing situation. They spoke of humanistic nursing which recognizes the uniqueness of each human being. Fundamental to this uniqueness is an appreciation of freedom. They state:

> With such uniqueness of each human being as a given, an assumed fact, only each person can describe or choose the evolvement of the project which is himself-in-his-situation. This awesome and lonely capacity for choice and novel evolvement presents both hope and fear as regards the unfolding of human "moreness." (Paterson & Zderad, 1976, p. 4)

Over the past decade other thinkers have explicitly addressed this idea of personal freedom as it pertains to nursing.

Parse's (1981) man-living-health theory, now the theory of human becoming (Parse, 1992), asserts that humans have situated freedom. Situated freedom means that an individual participates in choosing her/his situations as well as her/his attitudes toward situations. Through this choosing a person expresses value priorities. In and through her/his choices, an individual gives meaning to her/his world. In actuality, humans are always choosing. The choices "are made without full acknowledgement of the outcomes, yet with full responsibility for the consequences" (Parse, 1981, p. 21). The options from which a person chooses are always contextual in nature. They arise from experiences which are multidimensional (Parse, 1988).

In a similar vein, Newman (cited in Clements & Roberts, 1983) alludes to freedom in her theory of health as expanding consciousness. Health is viewed as the pattern of the whole person as he/she progresses toward higher levels of consciousness. Newman submits that health is the "developing awareness of self and environment together with increasing ability to perceive alternatives and respond in a variety of ways" (p. 164).

Benner and Wrubel (1989) take on the issue of freedom in some depth. They believe that a person is neither radically free nor radically unfree. By this they mean that individuals do not choose all of their meanings all of the time. Rather, they contend that the individual has situated freedom. "Situated freedom is the view that persons come to situations with their own meanings, habits, and perspectives and that this history actually sets up the possibilities in the situation" (p. 54). Benner and Wrubel point out that simple homeostatic theories fail to capture the situated possibility because these theories ignore individual meaning and history.

Utilizing cognitivism as an example, Benner and Wrubel (1989) elaborate on the inadequacies of mechanistic models for explaining human activity. They caution that the use of such models can lead to a non-caring stance in health care givers. Specifically, Benner and Wrubel describe and critique four assumptions that underlie the mechanistic model: (a) the primacy of efficient causality in scientific inquiry; (b) the person as a reactive organism; (c) the necessity for reductionism; and (d) knowing as representing. A brief description of each of these assumptions is worthy of note.

The primacy of efficient causality in scientific inquiry refers to the idea that human sciences have strived to appear as "scientific" as the physical sciences through a focus on antecedent conditions which move an object (person). This view has negated the physiological causality, formal causality (pertaining to forms or patterns), and final causality (purposes) of human behavior. Personhood is understood only in terms of achieving particular circumscribed ends. The result is an extremely reductive approach to human science. The assumption that *a person is a reactive organism* signifies the thought that an individual is a passive receptor of stimuli from the external environment. The mind is seen as being incapable of creating or originating. All knowing comes from the outside. The person is assumed to passively receive and accordingly respond.

Of the assumption pertaining to *reductionism*, Benner and Wrubel (1989) state:

> If social scientists must look to efficient causality in their explanations (that is, the external force, antecedent condition, or independent variable) and if all complex ideas can be seen as combinations of simple ideas originating in the external world, then, to understand people, researchers need to discover the basic atomic terms (the simple ideas) that precede behavior. (p. 32)

This reduction in scientific inquiry fails to capture human actions, human concerns, and complex physiology. Qualitative differences are then lost in the emphasizing of simple terms.

Knowing as representing refers to the assumption that meaning is idiosyncratic (Benner & Wrubel, 1989). The human mind is assumed to be both personal and inaccessible. Because meaning is *idiosyncratic*, it is not considered to be a relevant subject for investigation. Idiosyncratic meaning reveals only aspects of a single person but nothing about people in general. Subjective data are therefore rejected in favor of objective (behavior) data. Persons are viewed as objects for study, and methods used in investigation must meet criteria of objectivity. This assumption results in a science which denies that individuals are creative and generating and live their lives embedded in a context of meaning. It negates a perspective that views human actions and understandings within a comprehensive whole.

Each of the four assumptions basic to mechanistic models conflict with the emerging image of person in the human science of nursing. Yet, each of these assumptions is consistent with the philosophical stance of psychological determinism as previously discussed. The nursing theories mentioned above (Newman, 1986; Parse, 1981, 1992; Paterson & Zderad, 1976) convey a notion of personhood which is different from and more than a sum of parts. The personhood is characterized by freedom wherein the individual, given her or his unique history, actively participates in the choices without full knowledge of the outcome. Human actions cannot be understood through the identification of overly simplified antecedent conditions. The laws of explanation which govern the physical sciences do not apply if human beings are seen as possessing essential freedom of any sort in the situation.

Psychological determinism is based on the premise that the cause of human action may be identified. If this cause (antecedent condition) exists, the result is inevitable and therefore predictable. The antecedent mental state (locus-of-control orientation, health belief, self-judgement of efficacy) will cause an individual to act a certain way regardless of her or his history. Psychological determinism is directed at reducing personhood to a set of simplified rules. These rules necessitate the denial of free will.

Conclusion

It is not alleged that all borrowed theories must be avoided in the evolution of nursing epistemology. Thorne (1991), in discussing methodological orthodoxy, speaks to the contributions of ethnography, phenomenology, and grounded theory to nursing science. Each of these perspectives comes from a different discipline (anthropology, philosophy, and sociology, respectively). However, Thorne (1991) emphasizes the need to adapt aspects of each of these theoretical traditions to the study of phenomena uniquely of interest to nursing. She states that nursing is "a scientific enterprise with an identity distinct from philosophy, sociology, and anthropology in its (a) central values, (b) capacity for ambiguity,

(c) complexity, and (d) insistence on practical application" (Thorne, 1991, p. 191). In essence, theories from other sciences which are consistent with what Parse et al. (1985) have called the simultaneity paradigm or what Newman et al. (1991) term the unitary-transformative perspective may indeed be useful to nursing science.

It is the purpose of this article to call attention to the philosophical underpinnings of certain borrowed theories. Locus-of-control orientation, the health belief model, and self-efficacy theory were chosen as examples of theoretical constructs whose fundamental premises are in conflict with the evolving nursing paradigm. It is suggested that theories taken from other disciplines be examined in light of philosophical assumptions. It is perhaps important to be reminded that use of a particular theory implies ontological commitment to the concepts in that theory. Nurse scientists should exercise caution in making such commitments. The evolving paradigm in nursing which includes the acknowledgement of situated freedom should guide research endeavors.

REFERENCES

Bandura, A.B. (1977). *Social learning theory.* Englewood Cliffs, NJ: Prentice Hall.

Becker, M.H., & Maiman, L.A. (1975). Sociobehavioral determinants of compliance with health and medical care recommendations. *Medical Care, 13,* 10–24.

Belgrave, F.Z. (1991). Psychological predictors of adjustment to disability in African Americans. *Journal of Rehabilitation, 57,* 37–40.

Benner, P., & Wrubel, J. (1989). *The primacy of caring: Stress and coping in health and illness.* Menlo Park, CA: Addison-Wesley.

Champion, V.L. (1985). Use of the health belief model in determining the frequency of self breast exam. *Research in Nursing & Health, 8,* 373–379.

Champion, V.L. (1988). Attitudinal variables related to intention, frequency, and proficiency of breast self-examination in women 35 and over. *Research in Nursing & Health, 11,* 283–291.

Clements, I.W., & Roberts, F.B. (1983). *Family health: A theoretical approach to nursing care.* New York: Wiley.

Hallal, J. (1982). The relationship of health beliefs, health locus of control and self concept to the practice of breast self-examination in adult women. *Nursing Research, 31,* 137–142.

Huebsch, J.A. (1991). Educational and behavioral strategies for successful cholesterol management. *Journal of Cardiovascular Nursing, 5* (2), 44–54.

Hume, D. (1967). *A treatise of human nature.* L.A. Selby-Brigge (Ed.). Oxford: Clarendon. (Original work published 1739)

James, W. (1923). The dilemma of determinism. *The will to believe and other essays in popular philosophy.* New York: Longmans & Green.

Johnson, J.E., Christman, N.J., & Stitt, C. (1985). Personal control interventions: Short and long term effects on surgical patients. *Research in Nursing and Health, 8*(1), 131–145.

Kenny, A. (1978). *Free will and responsibility.* London: Routledge & Kegan Paul.

Lawrance, L., & McLeroy, K.R. (1986). Self efficacy and health education. *Journal of School Health, 56* (8), 317–321.

Levenson, H. (1973). Multidimensional locus of control in psychiatric patients. *Journal of Consulting and Clinical Psychology, 41,* 397–404.

Maiman, L.A., & Becker, M.H. (1974). The health belief model: Origins and correlates in psychological theory. *Health Education Monographs, 2,* 336–353.

Mill, J.S. (1975). *On liberty.* D. Spitz (Ed.). New York: W.W. Norton. (Original work published 1859)

Murdaugh, C.L., & Verran, J.A. (1987). Theoretical modeling to predict physiological incidents of cardiac preventive behaviors. *Nursing Research, 36,* 384–391.

Newman, M.A., Sime, A.M., & Corcoran-Perry, S.A. (1991). The focus of the discipline of nursing. *Advances in Nursing Science, 14*(1), 1–6.

Packard, S., & Polifroni, E.C. (1991). The dilemma of nursing science: Current quandaries and lack of direction. *Nursing Science Quarterly, 4,* 7–13.

Packard, S., & Polifroni, E.C. (1992). The nature of scientific truth. *Nursing Science Quarterly, 5,* 158–163.

Parse, R.R. (1981). *Man-living-health: A theory of nursing.* New York: Wiley.

Parse, R.R. (1988). Caring from a human science perspective. In M.M. Leininger (Ed.), *Caring: An essential human need.* Proceedings of the three national caring conferences. Detroit: Wayne State University Press.

Parse, R.R. (1992). Human becoming: Parse's theory of nursing. *Nursing Science Quarterly, 5,* 35–42.

Parse, R.R., Coyne, A.B., & Smith, M.J. (1985). *Nursing research: Qualitative methods.* Bowie, MD: Brady.

Paterson, J.G., & Zderad, L.T. (1976). *Humanistic nursing*. New York: National League for Nursing.

Phillips, J.R. (1990). New methods of research: Beyond the shadows of nursing science. *Nursing Science Quarterly, 3*, 1–2.

Rock, D.L., Myerowitz, B.E., Maisto, S.A., & Wallston, K.A. (1987). The derivation and validation of six multidimensional health locus of control clusters. *Research in Nursing and Health, 10*, 185–195.

Rosenstock, L.M. (1966). Why people use health services. *Millbank Memorial Fund Quarterly, 44*, 94–121.

Rotter, J.B. (1966). Generalized expectancies for internal versus external control of reinforcement. *Psychology Monographs, 80* (1), 1–28.

Rutledge, D. (1987). Factors related to women's practices of breast self examination. *Nursing Research, 36*, 117–121.

Salazar, M.K. (1991). Comparisons of four behavioral theories: A literature review. *American Association of Occupational Health Nursing Journal, 39* (3), 128–135.

Saudia, T.L., Kinney, M.R., Brown, K.C., & Young-Ward, L. (1991). Health locus of control and helpfulness of prayer. *Heart and Lung, 20* (1), 60–65.

Strecher, V.I., De Vellis, B.M., Becker, M.H., & Rosenstock, I.M. (1986). The role of self-efficacy in achieving health behavior changes. *Health Education Quarterly, 13* (1), 73–91.

Strickland, B.R. (1978). Internal-external expectancies and health related behaviors. *Journal of Consulting and Clinical Psychology, 46*, 1192–1211.

Thomas, D. (1957). *The collected poems of Dylan Thomas* (p. 128). New York: New Directions.

Thorne, S.E. (1991). Methodological orthodoxy in qualitative nursing research: Analysis of the issues. *Qualitative Health Research, 1* (2), 178–197.

Wallston, B.S., Wallston, K.A., Kaplan, G.D., & Maides, S.A. (1976). Development and validation of the health locus of control (HLC) scales. *Journal of Consulting and Clinical Psychology, 44*, 580–585.

Wallston, K.A., & Wallston, B.S. (1982). Who is responsible for health? The construct of health locus of control. In G. Sanders & J. Suls (Eds.), *Social psychology of health and illness* (pp. 65–95). Hillsdale, NJ: Lawrence Erlbaum.

Wallston, K.A., Wallston, B.S., & DeVillis, R. (1978). Development of the multidimensional health locus of control (MHLC) scales. *Health Education Monographs, 6*, 161–170.

Weatherford, R. (1991). *The implications of determinism*. London: Routledge.

Williams, C. (1988). *Free will and determinism*. Indianapolis, IN: Hackett.

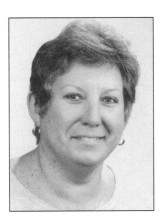

E. CAROL POLIFRONI

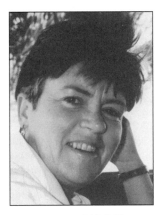

SHEILA A. PACKARD

Free Will in Process Perspective

Donald Wayne Viney ● *Donald A. Crosby*

Positions in the ongoing debate about free will are characterized and compared, that is, determinism, indeterminism, chaoticism, stronger and weaker versions of indeterminism and chaoticism, hard and soft determinism, and libertarianism. Libertarianism is claimed to be the most adequate of these alternatives and defended from the process perspectives of Alfred North Whitehead, Charles Hartshorne, and the psychologist–philosopher, William James. The defense is developed by responding to three objections to libertarianism: (1) that scientific explanations in psychology and other disciplines require belief in causal determinism; (2) that indeterminism, assumed by libertarianism, makes impossible moral or other kinds of responsibility for human acts; and (3) that libertarianism must assume an untenable mind–body dualism. The article concludes that libertarianism is a more subtle and cogent position than most of its opponents have recognized, that determinism has glaring deficiencies of its own, and that libertarianism is an appropriate position for psychology—even for a scientific psychology.

I. Introduction

Crossing disciplinary boundaries, like crossing international ones, can raise problems of communication. Differences of assumption, method, conceptualization, and language often pose formidable barriers to understanding. Fortunately, philosophers and psychologists can find common ground in the thought of William James, who was conversant with both disciplines. His writings, and especially his seminal article "The dilemma of determinism" (James, 1884), have helped to map various positions in the vigorous debate about free will that has continued in both psychology and philosophy since his time.

In the first section of this article we briefly

Reprinted from New Ideas in Psychology 12(2): 129–141, 1994, with permission from Elsevier Science.

characterize several of these positions, comparing and contrasting them with one another. In that context, we define our own position of libertarianism, paving the way for our responses, in subsequent sections, to three objections to the libertarian view (as so characterized) that we judge to be especially germane to the field of psychology. We develop our responses largely under the inspiration of a tradition of thought within our own discipline, that of process philosophy—a tradition to which James made substantial contributions.

II. Definitions and Clarifications

James realized that progress in addressing the issue of free will is unlikely unless the distinction between determinism and indeterminism is clearly understood. He identified determinism, or necessitarianism, as the view that those parts of the universe already laid down absolutely appoint and decree what the other parts shall be. The future has no ambiguous possibilities hidden in its womb: the part we call the present is compatible with only one totality. (James, 1979, p. 117)

More prosaically, determinism is the thesis that every feature of every event in the universe is the necessary outcome of a set of antecedent efficient causal conditions.[1] Thus, for any event E (including whatever qualities it possesses) there is a set of antecedent efficient causal conditions C such that, if C obtains, nothing but E could have occurred.

The logical contradictory of determinism is indeterminism. James describes indeterminism in these terms.

Indeterminism . . . says that the parts [of the universe] have a certain amount of loose play on one another, so that the laying down of one of them does not necessarily determine what the others shall be. It admits that possibilities may be in excess of actualities, and that things not yet revealed to our knowledge may really in themselves be ambiguous. (James, 1979, p. 118)

If indeterminism is true, then it is not the case that every feature of every event is the necessary outcome of a set of antecedent efficient causal conditions. For at least some events, the antecedent conditions C are compatible with the occurrence of E or with not-E (where not-E is understood to be any deviation from E and its qualities).

Indeterminism must not be confused, however, with the view that at least some, if not all, events (or features of events) occur in *complete independence* of efficient causal conditions. Let us call this view *chaoticism*, in order to keep it distinct from indeterminism. Chaoticism posits a universe in which at least some events have no causal relations with each other, meaning that, in at least some instances, literally anything can happen and that some, if not all, regularities in nature may be completely fortuitous.

It is crucial that we understand the difference between indeterminism and chaoticism, because the two concepts are often confused. Indeterminism does not deny efficient causal conditions or contexts for any events (or choices, or actions); it simply denies the deterministic claim that those conditions or contexts are adequate in all cases to exhaustively explain or account for events. To put the point somewhat differently, indeterminism is the position that, while efficient causal conditions are always necessary for explaining the occurrence of an event, they are at least sometimes not sufficient for explaining its occurrence. Other factors, such as chance or free choice, may also have to be taken into account. By contrast, chaoticism denies that efficient causal conditions are always necessary conditions for the occurrence of events. At least some events, it holds, occur in complete independence of such conditions, that is, such conditions are *neither necessary nor sufficient* for explaining the occurrence of those events.

Given these definitions, it follows that indeterminism is similar to determinism in holding that efficient causal conditions are necessary for the occurrence of events, although it differs from determinism in denying that those conditions are always sufficient to account for the occurrence of events. It also follows that indeterminism is similar to chaoticism in holding that efficient causal conditions are not sufficient to explain the occurrence of at least some events, while it differs from chaoticism in its insistence that such conditions are always necessary for the occurrence of events.

We can also note the possibility of stronger versions of both indeterminism and chaoticism. The stronger version of indeterminism is the view that efficient causal conditions are *never* sufficient for explaining the occurrence of any event; in other words, that such factors as chance, freedom, or novelty are always operative in events. Charles Hartshorne (1962, 1970) and Alfred North Whitehead (1978) are process philosophers who have taken this position. The stronger version of chaoticism is that *all* events occur in complete independence of efficient causal conditions, implying a helter-skelter universe in which no events have any causal connections with any other events.

Strong chaoticism lies at the opposite end of the scale from determinism, showing these two views to be the extremes, while indeterminism, whether in its stronger or weaker forms, lies between the two extremes. We can sum up the differences among determinism, indeterminism (whether in its weaker or stronger forms), and strong chaoticism in this way: determinism says that the efficient causal order of the universe is absolute; indeterminism says that the efficient causal order of the universe is not absolute; and strong chaoticism says that there is absolutely no efficient causal order in the universe.[2]

The fact that indeterminism (in either of its forms) is a moderate position between the extremes of determinism and strong chaoticism is rarely noticed. While strong chaoticism implausibly assumes a universe of nothing but chance, randomness, or spontaneity—a universe totally devoid of efficient causal connections—determinism requires acceptance of the staggering idea that everything that happens in the universe stretches by an unbroken chain into the infinite past, or up to the very beginning of the universe, if there was such. A heavy burden of proof must rest on those who would seek to defend either of these two extremes.

Determinism's theoretical extravagance is not its only liability. In addition, prima facie it is incompatible with belief in free will. James notes that determinists fall into two camps on the question of human freedom. Some determinists deny the freedom of the will, and others do not. Hard determinists reject free will out of hand, while soft determinists believe that human freedom is compatible with determinism. James chose the words "hard" and "soft" partly for their polemical value. "Hard" suggests rigidity of thought, and "soft" implies muddled thinking. For this reason, these two kinds of determinist are not always happy with James's labels. In any case, it is essential to recognize that soft determinists are no less convinced of the truth

of determinism than hard determinists; they are not "soft on" determinism. The difference between them has to do with whether human freedom is believed to be compatible with complete determinism.[3]

Soft determinists (e.g., Mill, 1884) opt for a definition of freedom that does not conflict with determinism. Persons are free, they say, when persons are capable of doing what they want to do, of carrying out their desires, wishes, aims, or motivations. And this is true even though all their wants are themselves wholly determined by efficient causal conditions. Just as an engine runs freely when nothing inhibits the proper functioning of its parts, so persons act freely when nothing inhibits them from doing what they want to do. Having acted, could a person have done differently? Yes, say soft determinists, but only if the efficient causal conditions had been different, allowing for the person's pattern of motivations to have been different.

The remaining position in the free will debate to be identified here is customarily called libertarianism. Like hard determinists, libertarians maintain that free will and determinism are irreconcilable. Hence, because they support free will, they reject determinism and endorse indeterminism in either the strong or weak senses of that term, as characterized above. Determinism and freedom are irreconcilable, according to libertarians, because one can be said to be truly free only if it was possible to have chosen differently from the way one did, *given relevantly identical efficient causal circumstances* (any circumstance not relevant to the choice need not be identical).

James illustrates this concept of freedom with his Oxford Street/Divinity Avenue thought experiment. He must decide which road to take on his way home. He makes a decision and acts accordingly. Could he, under the same efficient causal circumstances, have chosen differently? All parties agree that under different causal circumstances he could have. But libertarians maintain that he must have been able to choose differently under the relevantly same causal circumstances if we are to call him free in the most meaningful and robust sense of that term. This is not to suggest that the efficient causal circumstances have nothing to do with his action in either case, but it is to insist that they are not sufficient to explain it. A factor of free choice among the relevant alternatives, in one and the same context of relevant efficient causes, must also be taken into account if his action is to be termed a free action.

Libertarianism, with its assumption of indeterminism, is the position we take in the free will debate.[4] In the sections to follow, we consider three basic objections to the libertarian view and defend it against these objections. In so doing, we not only want to contribute toward an exhibition of the soundness of libertarianism as a psychological and philosophical position, but also to further explore its implications and meaning.

III. Libertarianism and Scientific Explanations

The first objection to libertarianism runs as follows. If scientific explanations of human behavior are possible, then determinism has to be true. Scientific explanations of human behavior are clearly possible, given the substantial strides of psychology to date in providing such explanations. Therefore, determinism must be true. And since libertarians acknowledge determinism to be irreconcilable with their view, it follows that libertarianism is false.

We respond to this argument by questioning the truth of its first premise, which is of the form, if p, then q. Any statement of this form, by the rules of symbolic logic, means that the truth of q is necessary to the truth of p. But is the truth of determinism really a necessary condition for the possibility of scientific explanations? There are several reasons for thinking that it is not.

First, libertarians are quite willing to concede that much in human behavior tends to be regular and predictable, especially when we study

general patterns of behavior among large numbers of people. Thus, in many instances, given a certain set of circumstances a particular outcome is highly likely. This does not mean that none of the human beings in question could have done otherwise, the causal circumstances remaining the same, only that they did not do otherwise and are unlikely to do so in the future. The pervasive role in human life of factors such as habit, acculturation, and social expectation is especially relevant here, as is the fact that humans have a common biological makeup. A scientific psychology is quite capable of analyzing, predicting, and explaining human behavior, then, to the significant extent that such behavior tends to be regular and predictable. This capability provides ample scope for its inquiries without implying any resolution of the issue between determinists and libertarians.

Second, if it turns out that a small number of a set of persons under study at a particular time act differently than a scientific hypothesis predicts they will, this fact is often seen as a tolerable "margin of error" or slight aberration in the empirical data, with no disconfirming statistical significance. Therefore, the attempt at scientific explanation for the type of behavior in question can still be deemed to have been successful. But such "aberrations" could also be viewed as evidence of free choice, of a capacity in persons to follow the lines of most resistance in a given situation, however unlikely it may be that the bulk of people will choose to do so.

Third, while psychology may have been successful in providing scientific explanations of some aspects of human behavior, it is a long way from having thus explained everything about human beings. It is also far from having explained enough about them to date to warrant the generalization that everything about them is, in principle, capable of being accounted for by science. Some psychologists may assume that, eventually, their discipline will be able to produce scientific accounts for every type of human activity, in the sense of identifying sets of efficient causes that are both necessary and sufficient to explain the activity and allow for its complete predictability.

At best this assumption is a promissory note, an expression of these psychologists' faith in determinism. The stupendous leap from presently available evidence such faith requires is brought home to us in a perceptive comment by William James: "However closely psychical changes may conform to law, it is safe to say that individual histories and biographies will never be written in advance no matter how 'evolved' psychology may become" (James, 1981, vol. II, p. 1179). At worst, the assumption represents an impossible, because incoherent, ideal. No theory could predict human creative achievements in detail without co-opting those achievements for itself. For instance, if we could now predict the precise cure for AIDS to be discovered in the future we would, by virtue of the prediction, already have the cure—in which case it could no longer be an achievement of the future! Hence, the partial successes of a scientific psychology do not give persuasive evidence for the truth of determinism or show the necessity of determinism for the enterprise of science.

Fourth, even if libertarians are right and efficient causal conditions are necessary but not sufficient conditions for human activity, psychology could still be a highly respectable science in its search for the necessary causal conditions for certain forms of human activity, that is, for the causal contexts within which certain kinds of choices are, or can be, exercised. There is no compelling reason to assume that scientific explanations must, by definition, always be complete or all-encompassing. We could view them as significant contributions to more inclusive ways of seeking to understand why particular persons or groups of persons tend to act as they do. There more inclusive ways might take into account, for example, their conscious assessment of alternatives posed by causal contexts and exercise of a power of choice among those alternatives, together with their expressed intentional reasons (not mere causal motives) for the choices made. Causal explanations would thus

be supplemented by intentional explanations in the search for more complete understandings.

A scientific psychology operating within the context of libertarianism could go further than this. It could develop hypotheses about when the necessary causal conditions are also likely to be sufficient for purposes of explanation, and its predictions in those cases might turn out to be ones of high probability, though not of the kind of certitude that would be possible if the causal conditions for human actions were always both necessary and sufficient. This high probability might pertain especially to predictions about specific acts of large aggregates of persons in certain clearly defined situations.

Fifth, we argue that working toward scientific explanations and testing explanatory hypotheses with carefully controlled experiments, as scientific psychologists are rightly committed to doing, is itself a type of purposeful, reasoned activity that is possible only if we assume the truth of libertarianism. Thus, instead of accepting the key premise of this first objection, namely, that the truth of determinism is a necessary condition for the enterprise of science, we conclude that it would be *fatal* to that enterprise.

Our argument turns on the crucial distinction between reasons and causes, a distinction that cannot consistently be made by determinism. Rational adjudication among contending claims to truth, whether in the domain of science or not, requires that we be free to weigh the strength of reasons for or against those claims, and that we be able to do so independently of what may motivate or causally incline us to accept or reject the claims. But if our causal motivations are in all cases sufficient to account for the ways in which we select among contending claims, as determinists allege, then it would make no sense to urge that we evaluate the reasons for the claims independently of what may causally incline us to accept or reject them. In other words, for determinism there can be no such thing as rationally justifying or criticizing a belief; all we can do is to give causal explanations for it. We may think that we can freely choose among alternative claims, hypotheses, or theories by reasoning about them in light of the available evidence, but we are really capable of making but one choice, the one determined by our underlying pattern of motives.

Thus, if determinism is true, there can be no way of demonstrating the truth or falsity of scientific claims. Whether we accept or reject them has nothing to do with the strength of the evidence. We cannot help deciding about them as we do, so long as our motives remain the same. And should we change our "judgment" about them at some future date, that is only because the motives themselves have been caused to change. We might happen in some cases to accept claims that are true or to reject ones that are false, but we would have no way of knowing this to be the case. It would just be a matter of luck.

The life of reason presupposes a capacity to transcend one's strong inclinations to believe something in light of reasons for not believing it, or to transcend one's strong inclinations not to believe something in light of reasons for believing it. But determinism makes such rational transcendence of inclinations impossible and thereby renders null and void the whole enterprise of assessing scientific hypotheses strictly on their logical and empirical merits. Instead, it makes all of us captive to likes and dislikes stemming from our fixed hereditary makeups and the causal influences of our environments. Persons so described are not capable of scientific reasoning in the commonly accepted sense of that term.[5]

IV. Libertarianism and Responsibility

We lead into the second objection to libertarianism by first noting that one of libertarianism's assumed selling points is that it alone among the positions in the free will debate can make sense out of holding humans responsible for their choices. In a deterministic world, according to this reasoning, the concept of *agency*, of being the source of one's choices, can have no mean-

ing. It is not that persons in a deterministic world cannot make choices, but that their choices are links—albeit conscious links—in an unbroken causal chain. Frederick Ferré (1973) puts the point this way:

> In the narrow perspective it is possible for a determinist to isolate a human person as contributory cause of some event; in the wider perspective, however, the "fixity of past inputs" that *ex hypothesi* has determined every attribute, motive, and reaction of the individual makes such an isolation from the entire relevant region of the universe arbitrary. (p. 166)

Ferré is merely describing the "block universe" of determinism in which no single cause is more or less essential than any other to what occurs. To hold people responsible for their decisions, however, requires belief that "the buck stops" with the free agent.

Determinists often seek to turn the tables on libertarians by arguing for the opposing view that if indeterminism is true there can be no such thing as moral or other types of responsibility. This second basic objection to libertarianism contends that the libertarian concept of free will is indistinguishable from randomness or utter inexplicability, and that choices that happen randomly or inexplicably are not choices for which any one can be held accountable. Libertarian replies to this objection vary depending on how it is formulated.

In one of its forms, the objection turns on a confusion between indeterminism and chaoticism. For example, in the course of arguing for a compatabilist understanding of freedom, Schlick (1939) claims that "[t]he opposite of the universal validity of a formula, of the existence of a law, is the nonexistence of a law, indeterminism, acausality" (p. 149). When he speaks of acausality, Schlick clearly has in mind some form of chaoticism, not indeterminism. Free choices that were completely separated from causal conditions would indeed be arbitrary or random. But libertarians do not assert that free choices are made independently of efficient causal conditions, only that those conditions do not absolutely determine choices. Were it not for causal regularities in our brains and many other parts of our bodies, for example, we would have no capacity for choice. Without dependable regularities in our environments and awareness of those regularities, we would be incapable of executing our choices, of consistently carrying them out in actions. So we could hardly be termed free. For libertarians, free will is not, and cannot be, exercised in a causal vacuum.

A second way in which this objection to libertarianism has been framed is the complaint that libertarianism bars the way to conclusive explanations for free decisions and thereby deprives persons of accountability for their decisions. Thus, in James's day Georg Von Gizycki asked,

> *Why* did [someone] act as he did, and not *otherwise?* How is it that he, under these external conditions, did his duty while others in his position would have ignored it? He did so, we are told, because he wished to, because it was his free will to do so! Yes, but *why* did he wish to, *why* did his free will determine him to do right? What caused him to come to the conclusion he reached and no other? (Von Gizycki, 1888, p. 758)

But Von Gizycki begs the question by calling for the sort of explanation that could only be an efficient causal explanation for free choices. His "why's" are all implicit demands for such an explanation.

Jules Lequier, a philosopher from whom James learned much about how to think of free will, argued that one should guard against the temptation to look to the causal antecedents of a free choice for a complete understanding of why it occurred. When libertarians state that a choice was made because a person deliberated about the available alternatives and decided to act upon one of them, determinists may object, "But that is no answer!" Lequier's riposte to their question-begging query about sufficient causal conditions that could fully account for the choice is, "But that is no question!"

(Lequier, 1952, p. 47). According to libertarianism, a free choice by its very nature cannot be completely explained by antecedent causal conditions.

Ironically, a libertarian named Robert Kane has given the second objection to libertarianism its most precise and intriguing formulation:

> If we say . . . that the agent did A rather than B here and now because the agent had such and such reasons or motives and engaged in such and such a deliberation before choosing to act, how would we have explained the doing of B rather than A given exactly the same reasons or motives and the same prior deliberation? If the deliberation rationalized the doing of A rather than B (or vice versa), would not the doing of B rather than A (or vice versa) as an outcome of the same deliberation be arbitrary or capricious relative to the agent's past—a kind of fluke or accident? (Kane, 1989, p. 229)

Libertarians claim that one is free only if one could have chosen differently under the relevantly identical causal circumstances. This entails that different choices can be made on the basis of a single process of deliberation. Kane sees this entailment as posing what he calls the problem of dual rationality.

Kane's version of the objection does not fall prey to the misunderstandings we have noted in other writers. However, what he refers to as a problem is, in truth, a defining feature of libertarian free will. In James's Oxford Street/Divinity Avenue thought experiment, either choice between the routes homeward would be rational and consistent with the desires, motives, and other psychological states of the agent prior to the decision. James's example was designed, in part, to illustrate this idea. Instead of speaking of the *problem* of dual rationality, then, we should speak of the *characteristic* of dual rationality.

Regarding dual rationality as a problem may result from the mistaken assumption that, given the agent's beliefs, motives, deliberations, and so forth, there must always be only one reasonable choice to be made. For example, in the game of chess the goal is to put the opponent's King in checkmate. If a player has a choice between checkmating the opponent's King or taking another piece, it would be unreasonable, given the player's knowledge of the rules and desire to win the game, not to checkmate the King. However, if, as sometimes happens, there is more than one way to put the King in checkmate, then there is no single rational answer to the question of which move should be made.

This chess example is not unlike other times in our lives where decisions are called for. The arena of moral decision making is replete with examples of alternatives that are equally reasonable in light of the evidence and commonly accepted moral principles. It is not always a question of choosing between absolute good and absolute evil. There are often greater and lesser goods and even goods of comparable value. Try as they may, moral philosophers have failed to discover a set of algorithms for resolving all ethical conflicts or telling us how to decide in all situations of moral choice.

Another, deeper, misunderstanding may underlie the claim that dual rationality is a problem. This is the confusion of deliberation with mere calculation. For instance, Richard Double asks, "why bother to deliberate if you are just as likely to opt for either of two contradictory alternatives?" (Double, 1991, p. 195). To illustrate his point, however, he uses an example of simple problem solving (in elementary logic) rather than an example of complex deliberation. To solve such a simple problem is to have a predetermined goal to which one aspires. We have already seen that, even at this level, there is often room for more than one rational response. But the question also arises, in some circumstances, of which goals one chooses to make one's own. For example, we deliberate about goals when we balance prudential considerations against moral ideals, or when enlightened self-interest comes into conflict with habits or immediate desires. James notes that in these critical moments, "[t]he problem with the man is less what act he shall now choose to do, than what being he shall now resolve to become"

(James, 1981, vol. I, p. 227). A carefully deliberated choice among alternative goals is arbitrary only in the harmless sense of its not being predetermined by efficient causal conditions. But it is not arbitrary in the sense of being irrational or somehow incompatible with the agent's psychological makeup.[6]

The upshot of our responses to the three forms of the second objection considered here is that free choices, in the libertarian sense of "free," are ones for which persons can clearly be held responsible. There is no convincing reason to regard such choices as capricious, out of control, or unintelligible, despite their not being wholly amenable to efficient causal explanations.

V. Libertarianism and Dualism

The third fundamental objection to libertarianism we shall consider argues that freedom in the libertarian sense can be made intelligible only if a sharp dualism of mind and body is assumed, and that the position of mind–body dualism must be rejected. The basic argument runs this way: libertarian freedom entails that some bodily movements (and probably some neural events) are produced by mental events which traditionally are described as acts of the will. However, this implied dualism between body and mind is radically flawed for a number of reasons, including the notorious problem of how two completely different orders of reality can interact. A purely mental cause having a physical effect is tantamount to telekenesis.[7] Since there are good reasons for thinking that mind–body dualism is false, and since libertarian freedom presupposes such a dualism, it follows that there are good reasons for thinking that libertarian freedom is not possible.

We are not proponents of mind–body dualism, so we have no intention of defending it here. What we will do is to reject the major premise of the argument by showing that mind–body dualism is not a necessary condition for the existence of libertarian freedom. The objection we are considering presupposes that a self capable of choosing or acting in even relative independence of antecedent causal conditions, as libertarians claim, would have to be somehow outside the network of causal relations that constitutes the realm of matter and, hence, be nonmaterial or of an entirely different order of being from anything in the natural world.

The first thing to notice about this objection to libertarian freedom is that it assumes the natural world to be a closed system of efficient causes, a view that libertarians reject. Hence, it begs a fundamental question. As we saw earlier, indeterminists such as James believe that there is "a certain amount of loose play" of the parts of the universe upon one another, meaning that events in the world are not completely controlled or constrained by efficient causes. For the human self to have the capability of choosing in more than one way, the relevant causal conditions remaining the same, is, therefore, not wholly different from its being possible for events outside the human sphere to exhibit a relative independence of antecedent causal conditions (or, as James puts it, a factor of chance). In this indeterministic vision, the prospect of novel or unpredictable occurrences is not confined to human choices or actions; it is prevalent in the universe (and, if the strong version of indeterminism is true, present in everything that occurs).

This is not to say that there is no difference between an event that occurs by chance, or at least some element of chance, and a purposefully directed free choice or action. However, were the universe not marked by some such looseness or contingency, some genuine openness of the future, human choices could not be efficacious in the way libertarians believe them to be. The truth of indeterminism is not a sufficient condition for libertarian freedom, but it is a necessary condition. Hence, there is a continuum, rather than a sharp break, between novelties or uncertainties that humans introduce into the universe by their free choices, on the one hand, and the contingencies of a universe not wholly bound together by efficient causes, on the other. No hard-and-fast dualism is required here.

Libertarianism conceived along nondualistic lines posits no trans-empirical or nonmaterial self as the source of free decisions. Human beings are products of an evolutionary development, and whatever special abilities they possess are augmented features of natural processes. Free will, in the sense of informed, purposeful choice among alternative courses of action, is an emergent phenomenon, different from but continuous with similar abilities found in related species in the animal kingdom. The libertarian who conceives freedom in this nondualistic fashion can look to comparative and developmental psychologies to explore the empirical dimensions of freedom and creativity, for example, their origins, limits, and degrees.

Although libertarianism is not necessarily tied to mind–body dualism, it is definitely committed to a nonreductionistic account of human behavior. Talk of neural events or bodily movements as though they were the sum and substance of human choices and actions inevitably distorts or destroys any meaningful concept of human freedom. Agents, the ones who make choices, can readily be conceived by libertarians—especially those standing within the tradition of process philosophy—as physical beings subject to a variety of conditions and stimuli. But they are seen as all this and more; the "more" is the measure of their freedom.

It is beyond the scope of this essay to do more than suggest, in outline, how a nondualistic and nonreductionistic libertarianism would look. Suffice it to say that thinkers such as James, Whitehead, and Hartshorne, to say nothing of Aristotle, have developed sophisticated metaphysical outlooks or systems in which these two conditions are kept in view. It is fitting that we end by appealing to their example as a final defense against the objection that libertarianism and mind–body dualism necessarily go together.

VI. Conclusion

The three objections to libertarianism that we have presented and responded to here are not, of course, the only ones that might be made. But they are objections of substantial importance and ones that frequently recur. By exposing their weaknesses, we have not only shown libertarianism to be a more subtle, tenable position than its opponents have generally assumed it to be, but have also shown determinism to have glaring deficiencies of its own. Most importantly, we have given reasons for our strong conviction that libertarianism merits careful consideration as a theory of human choice and behavior, a theory entirely appropriate for the fields of philosophy and psychology—even for a scientific psychology.

NOTES

1. There is a version of determinism holding that final causes are real but that these, no less than efficient causes, completely determine their effects. Blanshard (1961) takes this position, for example, and it seems to be implicit in Rychlak and Rychlak (1990). In our view, however, reference to final causes introduces a note of *indeterminacy* into an efficient causal situation, implying a factor of self-determination or self-resolution by entities standing within that situation. In the case of human individuals, which are our principal concern in this essay, to choose in light of final causes is to envision alternative paths of choice allowed by a given context of efficient causes. This means that there is such a thing as a relatively open future whose indeterminacy can be resolved by the free choices of those individuals.

2. The weaker version of chaoticism joins with indeterminism in denying that the efficient causal order of the universe is absolute, while still allowing for a significant amount of such order. It differs from indeterminism, however, in stipulating that some events can occur in complete independence of efficient causal conditions, that is, be completely spontaneous or random.

3. Because soft determinists hold that determinism and the freedom necessary to moral responsibility are compatible, they are sometimes called compatibilists. However, soft determinism and compatibilism are not identical. Compatibilism is the view that determinism and freedom *can* both be true. Soft determinism adds that determinism and freedom *are* true. Some soft determinists make the stronger claim that the truth of determinism is a necessary condition of freedom.

4. We shall here assume the weaker version of indeterminism, although we happen to agree with the stronger version. The latter requires more defense, or at least a more complex defense, and we need not take on that task for the purpose of this essay. Decision on whether an element of chance, freedom, or novelty enters into *every* event in the universe is not required for defense of the libertarian claim that, while efficient causal conditions are necessary for genuinely free human actions, they are not sufficient to account for them. This claim entails rejection of the deterministic thesis that every event, choice, or act can be exhaustively explained in terms of efficient causes.

5. Our fifth response to the first objection to libertarianism owes much to Jordan (1969). Jordan argues convincingly that, if determinism is true, there could be no way to show that it is true. He points out that his "argument does not assume or imply that determinism is false." It simply raises and answers negatively the question of whether, if every thought is conditioned by necessary and sufficient causes, "we could have recognizably good reasons to entertain anything, including the methodological principle or empirical generalization that every thought is so conditioned" (pp. 63–64).

6. Joseph and Ronald Rychlak identify free will with the capacity to "*choose* the grounds *for the sake of which* [persons] will be determined (final-cause determinism)," what the two call a *telesponse* (Rychlak & Rychlak, 1990, p. 15; Sappington 1990, p. 21). Although, talk of "final-cause determinism" obscures the fact that libertarianism is antithetical to any form of determinism, the writers are correct that telesponsive ability, in the sense of being capable of choosing grounds for the sake of which one acts, is a necessary characteristic of free will.

7. The dualist's inability to account for alleged interactions of two wholly different substances or kinds of being is implicit in the most famous treatise on mind–body dualism, the *Meditations on First Philosophy* by René Descartes. Descartes's failure to answer this objection is embarrassingly evident in his exchange of letters with Elisabeth of Bohemia, who first formulated this objection to his dualism (see Viney's translation of the letters of May 16, May 21, June 20, and June 28, 1643, in Viney, 1989, pp. 103–111).

REFERENCES

Blanshard, B. (1961). The case for determinism. In S. Hook (Ed.), *Determinism and freedom* (pp. 19–30). New York: Collier-Macmillan.

Double, R. (1991). *The non-reality of free will.* New York: Oxford University Press.

Ferré, F. (1973). Self-determinism. *American Philosophical Quarterly*, **10**, 165–176.

Hartshorne, C. (1962). *The logic of perfection.* LaSalle, IL: Open Court.

Hartshorne, C. (1970). *Creative synthesis and philosophic method*. LaSalle, IL: Open Court.

James, W. (1884). The dilemma of determinism. *Unitarian Review*, **22**, 193–224.

James, W. (1979). *The will to believe and other essays in popular philosophy* (F. H. Burkhardt, F. Bowers, & I. K. Skrupskelis, Eds.). Cambridge, MA: Harvard University Press.

James, W. (1981). *The principles of psychology* (3 vols., F. Burkhardt & F. Bowers, Eds.). Cambridge, MA: Harvard University Press.

Jordan, J. N. (1969). Determinism's dilemma. *Review of Metaphysics, 23*, 48–66.

Kane, R. (1989). Two kinds of incompatibilism. *Philosophy and Phenomenological Research*, **50**, 219–254.

Lequier, J. (1952). *Oeuvres Completes* (Jean Grenier, Ed.). Neuchâtel, Switzerland: Editions de la Baconniere.

Mill, J. S. (1884). *An examination of Sir William Hamilton's philosophy, and of the principal philosophical questions discussed in his writings* (2 vols. in 1 ed.). New York: Henry Holt and Company.

Rychlak, J. F., & Rychlak, R. J. (1990). The insanity defense and the question of human agency. *New Ideas in Psychology*, **8**, 3–24.

Sappington, A. A. (1990). Recent psychological approaches to the free will versus determinism issue. *Psychological Bulletin*, **108**, 19–29.

Schlick, M. (1939). *Problems of ethics*. New York: Prentice-Hall.

Viney, D. W. (Ed.). (1989). *Questions of value*. Needham Heights, MA: Ginn Press.

Von Gizycki, G. (1888). Determinism versus indeterminism: an answer to William James. *The Open Court*, **I**, 729–734, 758–762.

Whitehead, A. N. (1978). *Process and reality: an essay in cosmology* (corr. ed., D. R. Griffin, & D. Sherburne, Eds.). New York: The Free Press.

Phenomenology and Hermeneutics

Marylouise Welch

The history of philosophical thought had a significant impact on the development of phenomenology and hermeneutics. This book is not the place for a review of the history of philosophy but a few grounding comments are essential to understand the context that gave rise to phenomenology. Although the major developments occurred in the twentieth century they were directly connected to the problems set out by eighteenth- and nineteenth-century thinkers. In the eighteenth century Kant tried to weave a middle ground synthesizing the rationalism of Descartes and the empiricism of the British thinkers. He described an impersonal philosophy seeking universals and claiming that knowing must be explicated before we can understand the nature of being. Kant used the term phenomena for objects and events as they appear in our experience or our consciousness. Another eighteenth-century philosopher to use the term phenomena was Hegel, the German idealist. He viewed phenomenology as the science in which we come to know the mind as it is in itself through the study of the ways in which it appears to us. He contended that this should be the only concern of philosophy.

Nineteenth-century influences include the contemporaries Wilhelm Dilthey (1833–1911) and Franz Brentano (1838–1917), a teacher of Husserl who developed the intentional theory of the mind which characterizes mental acts such as judgments, beliefs, meanings and values. For Brentano the concept of intentionality made the distinction between the mental and the physical; intentionality belongs to mental acts. Dilthey, also a nineteenth-century philosopher and additionally an historian, attempted to establish the conditions of historical knowledge. He tried to set forth the humanities as interpretive disciplines and was the first person to espouse the notion of human science, *geisteswissenschaften*, concerned with understanding the structures of life as given in lived experience (Dilthey, 1975).

Dilthey believed explanation to be the method of the natural sciences and understanding to be the method of the human sciences. Human sciences shared the techniques of observation and description with the natural sciences but added to these *verstehen*, the understanding of mental acts like thoughts and emotions. Dilthey suggested that the researcher be interested in the expression of what is inside the person and what that person finds meaningful to living life. From this starting point he moved to reintroduce hermeneutics, the art of interpretation, into philosophy.

Hermeneutics, a concept derived from the Greek word, *hermeneia*, to express, interpret and translate (Klemm, 1983), had existed since the time of Luther when it referred to the process of interpreting the Bible in lay terms. It was originally a systematic, historical and critical scientific method specific to the interpretation of theological and philosophical exegesis. As it was reintroduced by Dilthey, it broadened its focus to history and in the twentieth century has come to include art, symbols and importantly for nursing, human action. Hermeneutics has moved from a technique used for understanding texts to a general philosophy of how humans understand experience. This chapter uses the writings of Husserl, Heidegger, Merleau-Ponty and Gadamer to trace the development and the various tangents that this view of philosophy has traveled in the twentieth century.

PHENOMENOLOGY, EXISTENTIALISM AND THE HERMENEUTIC TURN

Phenomenology, a twentieth-century philosophical movement begun by Edmund Husserl (1859–1938), has as its primary objective the direct investigation and description of phenomena as consciously experienced free from unexamined preconceptions and free of causal theories. Husserl's goal was to develop a method for the analysis of consciousness through which philosophy would gain the character of a strict rigorous science. One of his main tenets was a return to the things themselves *zu den Sachen selbst*, by which he meant the actual phenomena and problems as they appear and exist. One clears out the metaphysical assumptions by returning to the things themselves and this allows the person to describe what is directly given to consciousness. This perspective is in contrast to the natural science stance which begins with created theories removed from the everyday reality of life.

In order to understand the philosophical underpinnings of phenomenology and hermeneutics there are some basic themes that must be understood. For Husserl, philosophy was transcendental phenomenology. He first worked with this concept in the lectures that he developed for his students in Gottingen. It is his notes for these lectures which is the reading included in this anthology, in which he conceives of a universal phenomenology as the ultimate foundation for and critique of all knowledge. According to Spiegelberg (1982), he never fully explained the notion of transcendental but it seems to mean a reaching back to the ultimate source of all knowledge, which is consciousness. The science of the essential structures of pure consciousness became transcendental phenomenology.

In Frieberg, Martin Heidegger worked as an assistant to Husserl but very quickly began to steer a different course. Heidegger built on the ideas of both Dilthey and Husserl. From Dilthey he expanded the epistemological thinking about how we know, to include understanding. Husserl's phenomenology, with its focus on the things themselves and its attempt to describe phenomena of consciousness accurately, suggested to Heidegger to relook at the Aristotelean problem of being. Heidegger labored over the meaning of the things themselves from a Greek perspective, without the epistemological baggage of centuries of European thought (Krell, 1977). The result was a radical move by Heidegger to change the central focus of philosophy from epistemology to ontology. It is no longer how we know as humans, but rather, what does it mean to be that is the central question. Heidegger conceived of knowing not as understanding but as of being (Ricoeur, 1981).

Existentialism is a philosophical movement that focuses on the uniqueness of each individual and that abandons the search for universal human qualities. Heidegger is classified as an existentialist in part because he discarded Husserl's search for universal structures of consciousness as he looked to the particulars and the uniqueness of the person living in the world, and also because of his early concerns with care, anxiety and our thrownness into an existing world. For most existentialists, one comes to understand humans through the analysis of critically difficult situations like death and anxiety. Heidegger saw the world as given *a priori* and the existential view that a person arrives into a preconceived existence was consonant with that belief.

From these two perspective arrived Maurice Merleau-Ponty (1908–1961). He retained many of Heidegger's existential analyses while discarding the metaphysical ones (Merleau-Ponty, 1962). He combined Husserl's transcendental approach to epistemological questions with an existential orientation derived from Heidegger, among others. He not only discussed the existential nature of the human subject but also its bodily nature. He wanted to move beyond sense data and return to the world as we actually experience it. That is why he liked Husserl's call to return to the things themselves (Spiegelberg, 1982). His main argument was that the lived body was not an object in the world but it was the person's own point of view of the world; the body was itself the knowing subject.

Merleau-Ponty began with a more phenomenological than ontological perspective. As he wrote *The Phenomenology of Perception* he was mostly influenced by Husserl and the lived experience and was much less concerned with the ontological question of being as posed by Heidegger. He built on Husserl's idealism but focused on the perceptual experience. He believed experience remains murky and confusing and bracketing would not help to bring it into the light. We need to understand experience in its confusion and flux.

Finally, with Hans-Georg Gadamer (1900–1996) phenomenology makes its complete hermeneutic turn. He extended hermeneutics to practical philosophy (Bernstein, 1983). He believed that consciousness was not universal and transcendental but rather cultural and historical. This view is closer to Heidegger, his professor, than to Husserl. Gadamerian hermeneutics has as its main tasks the study of documents and artifacts that give evidence to what being human has meant and the analysis of how different interpretations and understandings are variable depending upon their forestructure, cultural world and context. In his work he was concerned with the notion of effective historical consciousness, in which he saw the person connected to the text or the tradition that s/he seeks to understand. The interpreter actually belongs to the culture or the context. Therefore, the interpreter, through language or dialogue, seeks to mediate this relationship to gain a richer understanding.

In contemporary philosophy, phenomenology is not a school of thought but rather a movement with various meanings for different people. Most would agree that phenomenology is a search for knowledge leading to description, not explanation, and that in the search for understanding, subjectivity is given a privileged position. Some phenomenologists such as Husserl focused on epistemology and others following Heidegger have concentrated on ontology.

IMPORTANT PHENOMENOLOGIC AND HERMENEUTIC THEMES

Lived Experience, *Lebenswelt*

In 1932 Husserl published *The Crisis of European Sciences and Transcendental Phenomenology* (1962), in which he pulled together his transcendental reduction into one systematic philosophical framework. It was in this later book that he moved from a focus on science to a focus on the lifeworld (*lebenswelt*). He was very self-critical in his later work as he tried to address the situatedness of perceptual experience by broadening his inquiry to the study of the lifeworld. The concept of the lifeworld is a return to early Husserl, when he told philosophers to return to the things themselves; in other words, to return to the everyday practical world of living in order to best understand the human condition without the blinders of theories. This is the world of lived experience and science is derivative of this world. The lifeworld, unexamined and undisclosed, is taken for granted in our everyday world. The positivistic scientific approach, according to Husserl, presupposed a lifeworld, *lebenswelt*, and one that remained unexamined. He tries to give a description of the lifeworld.

His existential followers, Heidegger and Merleau-Ponty, were less concerned with the cognition and consciousness of the *lebenswelt* and more interested in its action. But the seminal notion of *lebenswelt*, begun by Husserl, is apparent in their works and has remained an important feature in the evolution of philosophy.

Intentionality, Consciousness and Perception

Most phenomenologists ascribe to some view of intentionality. Husserl probably devoted the most attention to the concept, building on the concept of intentionality that had been described by his mentor, Brentano. It refers to the directedness of consciousness toward its objects. Expanding on Descartes he says, "I think and what I am thinking of are the objects of my thoughts." Thinking to Husserl (1960; 1962) means to be conscious, which is, as he describes it, a meeting of subject and object and all consciousness is consciousness of something.

Intentionality includes the meaning that we have for and intend toward something we perceive. It refers to the directedness of consciousness toward its objects. Husserl used the example of the cube where we only view three sides and then we assume the other three sides. We have been intentionally active in presuming the sides that we cannot see. We apprehend the object as a cube because of all of our presuppositions (other experiences of what constitutes a cube). We construct the intentional object. For Husserl this intended object gets meaning from the observer's (the subject's) perceptions.

To summarize, the notion of intentionality suggests perception as an active process in two ways. First, consciousness knows its objects by filling out hidden sides, projecting assumptions about what is not given. Second, we construct by creating a pattern from pieces which are not necessarily present, or in view, but are necessary to understand that which is being presented, for example, the cube.

Related to the notion of intentionality is the idea of essential structures. In our everyday life or "lived experience" there are always variations of size, shape and culture but the essence, what makes a cube a cube, remains unchangeable. When we view a cube drawn on paper we also simultaneously perceive the geometric principles of a cube. For Husserl (1960; 1962), this is an immediate, nonreflective perception because of our consciousness of the essential principles of the cube. The goal of phenomenology then is to unearth the essential structure of the conscious act and the objective entity that corresponds to it and then to describe it as faithfully as possible.

Imbedded in Husserl's description of intentionality is his notion that all that is important occurs through the structures of consciousness. It is these universal structures (essences) that the phenomenological reduction will help to disclose. For Merleau-Ponty, intentionality has as its goal the revelation of the world as ready-made and already existing. But Merleau-Ponty does not focus on this concept. Building not on Husserl's early work on structures, consciousness and intentionally, but on the lifeworld, he views all meaning as occurring through perception. It is perception that constitutes the ground level of knowledge and it occurs before there is scientific knowledge. For Husserl the reduction to the essential structures of consciousness is foundational to science; for Merleau-Ponty the phenomenology of perception is foundational (Merleau-Ponty, 1962). Intentionality can only reveal the world as it exists, ready-made, and this is done through reflection rather than the unveiling of universal structures.

An arch opponent of Cartesian rationalism, Merleau-Ponty was the first philosopher to make the body the central feature of a philosophy. For him, consciousness was always embodied and incarnate. In *The Phenomenology of Perception* Merleau-Ponty (1962) located consciousness in the body and described all consciousness as perceptual, even the consciousness of ourselves. This was a significant step beyond Husserl. He wanted to avoid splitting the mind and the body so he defined perception as engaged and embodied knowledge of the world. This opening up of experiences through our bodies has held an appeal for nurse theorists, as can be seen in the works of Benner (1984; 1985) and Benner and Wrukel (1989).

For Heidegger and Gadamer, intentionality was of almost no import as such. It was the human reality itself that was intentional. Gadamer, who drew from Heidegger, did not really discuss intentionality or structures but rather his main focus was on dialogue and language. With a new emphasis on the changing picture of phenomenology and hermeneutics, Gadamer returned to the concept of consciousness from Husserl. In *Truth and Method*, Gadamer (1975) discussed at length his concern with historical consciousness. In this discussion he has returned to some of the points of Dilthey's philosophy while retaining the ontology of Heidegger.

Being Qua Being

What it means to be is the fundamental question for Heidegger. Gelven (1970) used the example of a jail to illustrate this point. He discussed the difference in description of a jail from a physical perspective—the coldness, the bars, the concrete—to the understanding derived from the question, What does it mean to be in jail? The response contains a description of loneliness, fear and loss of freedom. Drawing on Gelven's example for nursing, the question might revolve around illness. I may ask, What is an illness? And the reply may include a physical description of disruption, anatomical damage and physiological malfunction. If I change the question to, What does it mean to be ill?, the answer is different and may include feelings of pain, difficulty, limitation or loss, hope or spirituality, as well as the effects on significant others. What it means to be ill is more primordial than what an illness is.

Therefore, for Heidegger, the question of what it means to be is the essential question to be posed and he is convinced that man lives completely oblivious to this question of being (Spiegelberg, 1982). There are several important concepts involved in understanding being in Heidegger's work. The first is *dasein*, from the German, meaning experience, or being which emphasizes the situatedness of human reality. *Dasein* is collective beings in a historical temporal world, constituted by the past and the future and it makes possible a clearing in which the history of the entities can appear (Cohen & Omery, 1994). Heidegger describes *dasein* in the everyday world, that is, atheoretical and unanalyzed. It is a happening during the life course.

Dasein is distinguished by the fact that it provides the foundation for an interpretation of being in general (Spiegelberg, 1982). *Dasein* is the human being but it is also more than that. It is an openness in which entities are revealed in the light of being. It is both a human structure (human reality) and a structure of the world. The world is always revelatory of *dasein*. The world and the person co-constitute one another. In summary, a basic characteristic of *dasein* is that things show up as significant and the significance is the background for more reflective understanding. It is through understanding the person in a context that what a person values and finds significant shows up (Dreyfus, 1991).

Time is another central concept. For Heidegger time is constitutive of being. Temporality is the term Heidegger used to describe a notion of time that was prior to or more original than our common sense of time as a linear succession of nows.

Heidegger uses the term thrownness to express the idea of the person as always already situated as being-in-the-world. Our destiny involves us making choices and creating possibilities from within the world into which we have been thrown by virtue of our being. World is defined as the relationships, practices, and language that we have from the moment we are born. It is a priori.

The person, for Heidegger, is self-interpreting in an atheoretical way. Contrary to Husserl's claims that these interpretations are a product of individual consciousness of subjects, Heidegger claims that these interpretations are not generated in individual consciousness as subjects related to objects but rather are given in our linguistic and cultural traditions and make sense only against a background of significance. Nothing can be known independent of our background.

METHOD

Husserl believed that the base of scientific knowledge was consciousness and science had ignored this in its attempt to discover facts (Spiegelberg, 1982). Heidegger's monumental *Being and Time* (1962) can be seen as an extension of Husserl's project from its narrow focus on epistemology (How do I know?) to that of ontology (What does it mean to be?), as described earlier, but it can also be seen as an abandonment of Husserl's method.

The criticism of Husserl is that he described an elaborate method but never tried to use it in research with humans. He attempted to create a rigorous science in which one investigates in a systematic manner all the ideas (presuppositions and intentions) that we have taken for granted in everyday life (natural attitude). He believed that we can transcend our natural attitudes when we bracket our presuppositions of the everyday world in order to get at the essences. In bracketing one holds in abeyance one's presuppositions so that what remains is the process of human consciousness and its intended objects.

It was through his systematic method that Husserl hoped to establish phenomenology as a rigorous science interested in the conscious experience by returning to things themselves *zu den Sachen selbst*. He saw his goal as epistemologic and hoped to reveal the universal structures of consciousness that would guarantee the certainty required for good scientific research. He thought one could do this through the process of reduction or bracketing (Husserl, 1960; 1962). Subsequent phenomenologists have discarded some of Husserl's steps and many have added others. The main notion is to bracket the everyday world and our presuppositions to get to a privileged position of intuition. For Husserl the goal was to describe the essence of phenomena as faithfully as possible. The following is a brief description of the method as articulated by him.

Phenomenological Reduction

There are three steps involved in the phenomenological investigative process. The first step is the reduction, the epoche, in which the mental acts are described as free as possible of theories and presuppositions. One suspends the natural attitude and one brackets both subject and object and describes what is left. The second step is the eidetic reduction through which, reflecting on a particular act, the essence of it may be intuited. It is an analysis to reveal the defining form. This is done through comparison, observation and imagination by examining the variations of what is presented to uncover what is left unchanged, the invariant essence. The invariants this process discloses would be the forms, the eidetic structures, of consciousness, meaning and experience. The last step is the phenomenological reduction, which is to get at the essence of the object of the conscious process.

Merleau-Ponty builds on Husserl's phenomenological reduction with his own reinterpretation (Spiegelberg, 1982). He views the Husserlian concept of transcendental phenomenology as rigorous reflection, where bracketing helps us to set aside our history and culture so that we can uncover our lived experiences as we perceive them (Merleau-Ponty, 1962). He expands the goal of the reduction to include an understanding of the relationship between consciousness and nature. However, he is not advocating a return to consciousness, as described by Husserl, but through perception a description of the here and now. This method then permits the discovery of the lifeworld. The term essence is conspicuous by its absence.

Hermeneutical Interpretation

Hermeneutic phenomenology illuminates what is and brings out that which is taken for granted. It uncovers the hidden meanings. Knowledge is the result of reflective hermeneutic thinking but reflection can not specify a clear method with procedural steps. In *Being and Time* (1962) Heidegger leaves open many possibilities. Most authors refer to a hermeneutical circle of understanding which is a metaphor for a dialectic of moving between parts and whole (Leonard, 1989). It is a way of articulating what occurs in understanding.

The concept of the hermeneutic circle of understanding began with Dilthey as a useful mode to comprehend historical experiences. There exists an exchange between an individual lived experience and the text. Heidegger took this notion of the circle and transformed it to represent a circle in which we understand and interpret something because we have a shared knowledge of our cultural and historical experiences. As we understand something we are involved and as we are involved we understand. He is making an ontological turn as the hermeneutic circle becomes interpretive of human beings. He uses hermeneutics to interpret *dasein*.

The hermeneutic circle is a shifting from the parts to the whole to the parts in order to accurately understand the experience being investigated. It is a dialectical process in which the meaning of the parts is determined by the foreknowledge of the whole. One then deepens the understanding of the whole through increased knowledge of the parts.

Gadamer takes up the hermeneutic circle in a description of a circular relationship between explanation and understanding that involves seeing something familiar in a new light. Like Heidegger, he is emphasizing the importance of the ontological existential side of the dialogue as the source of truth. He is not seeking absolute truth but rather an understanding of understanding. Understanding is a forestructure of assumptions and beliefs that guides interpretation, is never without presuppositions and is prescientific. Understanding is always ahead of itself because it projects expectations that interpretation then makes explicit. This conception of understanding is similar to Husserl's definition of intentionality.

For Gadamer the interpretation occurs through the fusion of horizons of the observed and of the interpreter. The horizon is "the range of vision that includes everything that can be seen from a particular vantage point" (Gadamer, 1975, p. 111). The task then becomes to understand how the horizon of the interpreter and the horizon of the interpreted become fused and create meaning in that context. Through dialogue each person loses a little of the self to the other and the new horizon that they co-create becomes part of the investigative process. According to Hekman (1986) there are three methodological implications for a Gadamerian approach. First, the interpreter must define the cultural and historical horizon. Second, the researcher must articulate the different horizon that is in play during the research. Third, the researcher requires a self-awareness of his/her own. However, hermeneutics remains more as a process of understanding than a specific method. For Heidegger hermeneutic phenomenology and science are incompatible.

CONCLUSION

Phenomenology is less a monolithic school than a family of ideas. Its diversity makes it difficult to understand but also explains its endurance and appeal over the past hundred years. In general terms it is a philosophy of experience. It attempts to understand how meaning is made in human experience, and it sees our lived experience of the world as the foundation of meaning. It began with Husserl, who believed that science had failed to be exact because it had not clearly described the essence of things before they were put into theoretical statements (Spiegelberg, 1982). For Husserl philosophy is foundational to science and they have a reciprocal relationship. His goal was a reform of science and he continued to view science and philosophy as sharing a mutual reciprocal relationship.

Contemporary phenomenologists discarded many of Husserl's assumptions though they have done so by exploring them and altering them. They respected the pioneering effort to understand and describe the human consciousness and as a result many of his basic ideas remain, though changed. In the twentieth century phenomenology is a philosophical movement whose primary objective is the direct investigation and description of phenomena as consciously experienced. It remains different from and in opposition to positivism because it is atheoretical, noncausal and attempts to be free of presupposition. For most phenomenologists experience explains the world rather than the world helping to shape and explain experience. Hermeneutic phenomenology as a method illuminates the normally hidden, taken for granted purposes and meanings of humans.

For Husserl phenomenology contains two important features: a descriptive method and an a priori science derived from the method. The basic method is the reduction which puts one in a privileged position to be able to intuit—in the eidetic reduction the essences can be grasped. These are the universal structures that remain unchanged but are hidden and taken for granted in the everyday world. Husserl's method was used differently by Merleau-Ponty, with his emphasis on perceptions and not on consciousness and universals. He is looking at particulars from an existential perspective. The lifeworld is mediated through perception.

It is difficult to place Heidegger because he is difficult to classify. He is a phenomenologist though the word no longer appeared in his later works. He is also an existentialist but not in the way of the existentialists like Merleau-Ponty. Heidegger is suggesting a hermeneutical interpretation but not with the purity of Gadamer. He is probably the most eclectic thinker in these two sections. All three, Merleau-Ponty, Heidegger and Gadamer, studied experience to know the world as it is lived by revealing the hidden, unexamined meanings that dwell in our everyday world of experience and practice. Beginning with Merleau-Ponty's description of perception they have left the realm of thought (consciousness) and moved to world as lived. For Gadamer the lifeworld is mediated by language (Gadamer, 1976).

Patricia Benner has been a leader in the movement to draw nursing's attention to what hermeneutics has to offer. In her seminal article (1985) she differentiates the questions and answers that arise from a natural science approach from those that come from a hermeneutical stance. Leonard (1989) joined Benner (1985) in stressing the importance of identifying the appropriate philosophical/ontological perspective before choosing a methodology when one is designing a research project. Both authors give examples of why a Heideggerian hermeneutical position offers a philosophy with specific methods suitable to certain types of nursing questions.

Benner (1985) described the types of questions that emerge when one is looking at how a person lives and experiences health and illness. These questions are very different from ones that emanate from wanting to know the effects of "maternal hyperglycemia on idiopathic neonatal hypoglycemia" (Leonard, 1989, p. 42). "The goal is to understand everyday practices and the experiences of health and illness" (p. 5). Finally,

Leonard describes the hermeneutic circle and how it will lead to new insights and "practical knowledge that eludes traditional empirical research" (p. 52).

As nurses have felt a connection to Heidegger, perhaps because his descriptions of the meaning of being human are close to the central issues in nursing, Drew (1998) is concerned that nurses have overlooked some important contributions of Husserl. From Husserl we can gain direction about how to answer certain epistemological questions by reexamining his discussions of phenomenological method and the concern for the researcher's stance in the examination and description of findings. Through researcher self-reflection the importance of the researcher's experiences as being included in the data will strengthen future phenomenological research.

DISCUSSION GUIDE

1. Identify an area of interest to nursing science and develop a research question reflecting the four perspectives described in this chapter. What are the similarities and differences in the questions?
2. Define phenomenology and hermeneutics as philosophies and as methods.
3. Discuss whether or not it is possible for the investigator to eliminate completely what s/he brings to the object in order to reveal and describe accurately its true essence.
4. Discuss whether or not nursing should follow Husserl and use transcendental phenomenology to describe universals.
5. If one uses Gadamerian hermeneutics, what is truth? Can it be verified?
6. Hermeneutics views the social world as separate and distinct from the natural world. To use this approach for knowledge development to one have to agree with this position?
7. If one uses Gadamerian hermeneutics, how will it be known which prejudice is illuminating and which one blinding?
8. Is it possible for the investigator to eliminate completely what s/he brings to the object in order to reveal and describe accurately its true essence?

REFERENCES

Benner, P. (1984). *From novice to expert: Excellence and power in clinical nursing practice.* Reading, MA: Addison-Wesley.

Benner, P. (1985). Quality of life: Phenomenological perspective on explanation, prediction, and understanding in nursing science. *Advances in Nursing Science, 8*(1), 7–14.

Benner, P., & Wrubel, J. (1989). *The primacy of caring.* Reading, MA: Addison-Wesley.

Bernstein, R. (1983). *Beyond objectivism and relativism: Science, hermeneutics and praxis.* Philadelphia: University of Pennsylvania Press.

Cohen, M., & Omery, A. (1994). Schools of phenomenology: Implications for research. In J. Morse (Ed.), *Critical issues in qualitative research* (pp. 136–156). Thousand Oaks, CA: Sage.

Dilthey, W. (1975). *Philosophy of the human sciences* (R. Makreel, Trans.). Princeton, NJ: Princeton University Press.

Drew, N. (1998). A return to Husserl and researcher self-awareness. In E. C. Polifroni, & M.

Welch (Eds.), *Perspectives on philosophy of science in nursing: An historical and contemporary anthology* (pp. 263–272). Philadelphia: Lippincott.

Dreyfus, H. L. (1991). *Being-in-the-world: A commentary on division I of* Being and time. Cambridge, MA: MIT Press.

Gadamer, H-G. (1975). *Truth and method* (B. Garrett, & J. Cunning, Trans.). New York: Seabury.

———. (1976). *Philosophical hermeneutics.* Berkeley: University of California Press.

Gelven, M. (1970). *A commentary on Heidegger's* Being and time. New York: Harper & Row.

Heidegger, M. (1962). *Being and time* (J. Macquarrie, & E. Robinson, Trans.). New York: Harper & Row. (Originally published in 1927).

Hekman, S. (1986). *Hermeneutics and the sociology of knowledge.* Notre Dame: University of Notre Dame Press.

Husserl, E. (1960). *Cartesian meditations* (D. Cairns, Trans.). The Hague: Martinus Nijhoff.

———. (1962). *Ideas: General introduction to pure phenomenology* (R. B. Gibson, Trans.). New York: Collier.

Klemm, D. (1983). *The hermeneutical theory of Paul Ricoeur.* East Brunswick, NJ: Associated University Press, Inc.

Krell, D. F. (1977). General introduction: "The question of being." In J. Glenn Gray (Ed.), *Martin Heidegger: Basic writings.* New York: Harper & Row.

Leonard, V. (1989). A Heideggerian phenomenological perspective on the concept of person. *Advances in Nursing Science, 11*(4), 40–55.

Merleau-Ponty, M. (1962). *The phenomenology of perception.* London: Routledge & Kegan Paul.

Ricoeur, P. (1981). *Hermeneutics and the human sciences* (J. B. Thompson, Trans.). Cambridge: Cambridge University Press.

Spiegelberg, H. (1982). *The phenomenological movement.* (3rd ed.). The Hague: Martinus Nijhoff.

BIBLIOGRAPHY

Allen, D. G. (1995). Hermeneutics: Philosophical traditions and nursing practice research. *Nursing Science Quarterly, 8*(4), 174–183.

Bleicher, J. (1980). *Contemporary hermeneutics: Hermeneutics as a method, philosophy and critique.* London: Routledge & Kegan Paul.

Colaizzi, P. (1978). Psychological research as the phenomenologist views it. In R. Valle, & M. King, (Eds.), *Existential-phenomenological alternatives for psychology* (pp. 48–71). London: Oxford University Press.

Gadamer, H-G. (1981). *Reason in the age of science* (F. G. Lawrence, Trans.). Cambridge, MA: MIT Press. (Original work published 1976.)

Giorgi, A. (1985). *Phenomenology and psychological research.* Pittsburgh: Duquesne University Press.

Grondin, J. (1994). *Introduction to philosophical hermeneutics* (J. Weinsheimer, Trans.). New Haven: Yale University Press.

Guignon, C. (1983). *Heidegger and the problem of knowledge.* Indianapolis: Hackett.

Heidegger, M. (1971). *Poetry, language, thought* (A. Hofstadter, Trans.). New York: Harper & Row.

———. (1975). *The basic problems of phenomenology* (A. Hofstadter, Trans.). Bloomington: Indiana University Press.

———. (1977). *The question concerning technology and other essays* (W. Lovitt, Trans.). New York: Harper & Row.

Hiley, D. R., Bohman, J. F., & Shusterman, R. (Eds.). (1991). *The interpretive turn: Philosophy, science and culture*. Ithaca, NY: Cornell University Press.

Husserl, E. (1970). *The crisis of European sciences and transcendental phenomenology* (D. Carr, Trans.). Evanston, IL: Northwestern University Press.

———. (1982). *General introduction to a pure phenomenology* (F. Kersten, Trans.). The Hague: Martinus Nijhoff.

———. (1990). *The idea of phenomenology*. (W. Alston, & G. Naknihian, Trans.). Boston: Kluwer Academic Publishers.

Jasper, M. A. (1994). Issues in phenomenology for researchers of nursing. *Journal of Advanced Nursing 19*, 309–314.

Koch, T. (1995). Interpretive approaches in nursing research; The influence of Husserl and Heidegger. *Journal of Advanced Nursing, 21*, 827–836.

Kockelmans, J. J. (1994). *Edmund Husserl's phenomenology*. West Lafayette, IN: Purdue University Press.

Madison, G. B. (1988). *The hermeneutics of postmodernity*. Indianapolis: Indiana University Press.

Merleau-Ponty, M. (1973). *Consciousness and the acquisition of language* (H. Silverman, trans.). Evanston, IL: Northwestern University Press.

Mitchell, G. J. (1994). Discipline-specific inquiry: The hermeneutics of theory-guided nursing research. *Nursing Outlook 42*, 224–228.

Morse, J. (Ed.). *Critical issues in qualitative research methods*. New York: Sage.

Nelms, T. P. (1996). Living a caring presence in nursing: A Heideggerian hermeneutical analysis. *Journal of Advanced Nursing, 24*, 368–374.

Oiler, C. (1982). The phenomenological approach in research. *Nursing Research 31*, 178–181.

Omery, A., Kasper, G., & Page, G. (Eds.). (1995). *In search of nursing science*. Thousand Oaks, CA: Sage.

Packer, M., & Addison, R. B. (Eds.). (1989). *Entering the circle: Hermeneutic investigation in psychology*. Albany: State University of New York Press.

Paley, J. (1997). Husserl, phenomenology and nursing. *Journal of Advanced Nursing, 26*, 187–193.

Polkinghorne, D. (1983). *Methodology for the human sciences*. Albany: State University of New York Press.

Rabinow, P., & Sullivan, W. M. (Eds.). (1987). *Interpretative social sciences: A second look*. Berkeley: University of California Press.

Reeder, R. (1988). Hermeneutics. In B. Sarter (Ed.), *Paths to knowledge: Innovative research methods in nursing* (pp. 193–238). New York: National League for Nursing.

Ricoeur, P. (1965). *History and truth* (C. A. Kelbely, trans.). Evanston, IL: Northwestern University Press.

Schutz, A. (1967). *The phenomenology of the social world*. (G. Walsh, & E. Lehnert, trans.). Chicago: Northwestern University Press. (Original work published 1932.)

Strasser, S. (1985). *Understanding and explanation: Basic ideas concerning the humanity of the human sciences*. Pittsburgh: Duquesne University Press.

Taylor, C. (1985). *Human agency and language*. Philosophical papers (Vol. 1). Cambridge: Cambridge University Press.

———. (1985). *Philosophy and the human sciences:* Philosophical papers (Vol. 2). Cambridge: Cambridge University Press.

Thompson, J. L. (1990). Hermeneutic inquiry. In L. E. Moody (Ed.), *Advancing nursing science through research* (Vol. 2, pp. 223–280). Newbury Park, CA: Sage.

Van Manen, M. (1990). *Researching lived experience: Human science for action sensitive pedagogy*. New York: State University of New York Press.

Reading 19

The Train of Thoughts in the Lectures

Edmund Husserl

<41> **Lecture III**

[The carrying out of the epistemological reduction: Bracketing everything transcendent. Theme of the investigation: The pure phenomenon. The question of the "objective validity" of the absolute phenomenon. The impossibility of limiting ourselves to singular data; phenomenological cognition as a cognition of essences. Two senses of the concept of the *a priori*.]

<43> By these considerations what the critique of cognition may and may not use has been precisely and adequately determined. What is especially puzzling for such a critique is the possibility of transcendence, but it may never under any conditions exploit for its purposes the actuality of transcendent things. Obviously the sphere of usable objects or of cognitions is limited to those which present themselves as valid, and which can remain free of the marks of epistemological vacuity; but this sphere is not empty. We have indubitably secured the whole realm of *cogitationes*. The existence of the *cogitatio*, more precisely the phenomenon of cognition itself, is beyond question; and it is free from the riddle of transcendence. These existing things are already presupposed in the statement of the problem of cognition. The question as to how transcendent things come into cognition would lose its sense

Reprinted with permission of Kluwer Academic Publishers and Professor Rudolf Bernet, Director, Husserl-Archives Leuven. This work originally appeared in *The Idea of Phenomenology*, pp. 3–12, 1964.

if cognition itself, as well as the transcendent object, were put in question. It is also clear that the *cogitationes* present a sphere of *absolutely immanent data; it is in this sense that we understand "immanence."* In the "seeing" pure phenomena the object is not outside cognition or outside "consciousness," while being given in the sense of the absolute self-givenness of something which is simply "seen."

But here we need assurance through *epistemological reduction*, the methodological essence of which we now want to examine *in concreto* for the first time. We need the reduction at this point in order to prevent the evidence of the existence of the *cogitatio* from being confused with the evidence that *my cogitatio* exists, with the evidence of the *sum cogitans*, and the like. One must guard himself from the fundamental confusion between the *pure phenomenon*, in the sense of phenomenology, and the *psychological phenomenon*, the object of empirical psychology. If I, as a human being employing my natural modes of thought, look at the perception which I am undergoing at the moment, then I immediately and almost inevitably apperceive it (that <44> is a fact) in relation to my ego. It stands there as a mental process of this mentally living person, as his state, his act; the sensory content stands there as what is given or sensed, as that of which I am conscious; and it integrates itself with the perception of objective time. Perception, and any other *cogitatio*, so apperceived, is a *psychological fact*. Thus it is apperceived as a datum in objective time, belonging to the mentally living ego, the ego which is in the world and lasts through its duration (a duration which is measured by means of empirically calibrated timepieces). This, then, is the phenomenon which is investigated by that natural science we call "psychology."

The phenomenon in this sense falls under the principle to which we must subject ourselves in the critique of cognition, the principle of the ἐποχή, which holds for everything transcendent. The ego as a person, as a thing in the world, and the mental life as the mental life of this person, are arranged—no matter even if quite indefinitely—on objective time; they are all transcendent and epistemologically null. Only through a reduction, the same one we have already called *phenomenological reduction*, do I attain an absolute datum which no longer presents anything transcendent. Even if I should put in question the ego and the world and the ego's mental life as such, still my simply "seeing" reflection on what is given in the apperception of the relevant mental process and on my ego, yields the *phenomenon* of this apperception; the phenomenon, so to say, of "perception construed as my perception." Of course, I can also make use of the natural mode of reflection here, and relate this phenomenon to my ego, postulating this ego as an empirical reality through saying again: I have this phenomenon, it is mine. Then, in order to get back to the pure phenomenon, I would have to put the ego, as well as time and the world once more into question, and thereby display a pure phenomenon, the pure *cogitatio*. But while I am perceiving I can also look, by way of purely "seeing," at the perception, at it itself as it is there, and ignore its relation to the ego, or at least abstract from it. Then the perception which is thereby grasped and delimited in "seeing," is an absolutely given, pure phenomenon in the phenomenological sense, renouncing anything transcendent.

<45> *Thus to each psychic lived process there corresponds through the device of phenomenological reduction a pure phenomenon, which exhibits its intrinsic (immanent) essence (taken individually) as an absolute datum.* Every postulation of a "non-immanent actuality," of anything which is not contained in the phenomenon, even if intended by the phenomenon, and which is therefore not given in the second sense, is bracketed, i.e., suspended.

If it is possible to take such phenomena for objects of investigation, then it is obvious that we are now no longer within psychology, within a natural, transcendently "objectivizing" science. Then we do not investigate and speak of psychological phenomena, of certain happenings in so-called real actuality (the existence of which remains throughout in question), but of that which exists and is valid whether there is such a thing as objective actuality or not, whether the postulation of such transcendent entities is justifiable or not. Thus at this point we speak of such absolute data; even if these data are related to objective actuality via their intentions, their intrinsic character is *within* them; nothing is assumed concerning *the existence or non-existence of actuality*. And so we have dropped anchor on the shore of phenomenology, the existence of the objects of which is assured, as the objects of a scientific investigation should be; not, however, in the manner of components of the ego or of the temporal world, but rather as absolute data grasped in purely immanent "seeing." And this pure immanence is first of all to be characterized, in our approach, through *phenomenological reduction*: I mean, not with respect to what it refers to beyond itself, but with respect to what it is in itself and to what it is given as. All this discussion is, of course, only a roundabout way of helping one to see what is to be seen in this regard, viz., the distinction between the quasi-givenness of transcendent objects and the absolute givenness of the phenomenon itself.

But we must take new steps, enter onto new considerations, so that we may gain a firm foothold in the new land and not finally run aground on its shore. For this shore has its <46> rocks, and over it lie clouds of obscurity which threaten us with stormy gales of scepticism. What we have said up to this point holds for all phenomena, although for purposes of the critique of reason, we are, naturally, interested only in cognitive phenomena. Thus the results set forth below can just as well be applied to all phenomena, as they hold *mutatis mutandis* for all of them.

In our quest for a critique of cognition, we have been led to a beginning, to a stronghold of data which is at our disposal, and it appears that this is what we need above all. If I am to fathom the essence of cognition, then I must, of course, possess cognition in all its questionable forms, *as a datum*, and possess it in such a way that this datum has in itself nothing of the problematic character which other cognitions bring with them, however much they seem to offer us data.

Having assured ourselves of the field of pure cognition, we can now investigate it and start a science of pure phenomena, a *phenomenology*. Is it not obvious that this must be the basis for the solution to the problems which have been agitating us? Thus it is clear that I can only attain insight into the essence of cognition if I look at it myself, and if it itself is given to me to "see," as it really is. I must study it immanently and by pure inspection within the pure phenomenon, within "pure consciousness." To be sure, its transcendence is doubtful; the existence of objects to which it is related insofar as it is transcendent, is not given to me; and questions are raised precisely as to how, in spite of this, they can be postulated, and as to what significance it has and must have if such postulation is to be possible. On the other hand, even if I raise questions about the existence and reaching the object of this relation to transcendent things, still it has something which can be grasped in the pure phenomenon. The relating-itself-to-transcendent-things, whether it is meant in this or that way, is still an inner feature of the phenomenon. It almost seems as if it would depend only on a science of absolute *cogitationes*. Since I have to cancel out any previous acceptance of the intended transcendent objects, where else could I investigate both the *meaning* of this intending-something-beyond, and also, along with this meaning, its possible *validity*, or the meaning of such validity? Where else but the place at which this meaning is unqualifiedly given and at which in the pure phenomenon of <47> relation, corroboration, justification the meaning of validity, for its part, comes to absolute givenness.

To be sure, we are overtaken here once more by the doubt whether there is not still a surplus which must pass over into action, whether the datum of validity does not carry with it the givenness of the object, which, on the other hand, could not be the givenness of the *cogitatio*, at least insofar as there is really such a thing as valid transcendence. Nevertheless a science of absolute phenomena, understood as *cogitationes*, is the first thing we need, and this has to produce at least a major part of the solution.

Thus, it must be our aim to set up a phenomenology, more specifically a phenomenology of cognitions, construed as a theory of the essence of pure cognitive phenomena. The outlook is favorable. But how is phenomenology to proceed? How is it possible? I am supposed to make assertions, indeed objectively valid assertions; I am supposed to cognize pure phenomena scientifically. *But does all science not lead to the establishing of objects existing in themselves, i.e., to transcendent objects?* What is scientifically established is something which is what it is in itself; it is to be accepted just as existing whether I, in my cognition, postulate it as existing or not. Does not science by its very essence have as its correlate the objectivity of that which is known only in science, and which is scientifically established? And that which is scientifically established is universally valid, is it not? But what is the situation here? We move in the field of pure phenomena. But why do I say *field*? It is more nearly a *Heraclitean flux* of phenomena. What assertions can I make about it? Now, while "seeing," I can say: this here: No doubt it is. Perhaps I can further say that this phenomenon includes that one as a part, or is connected to that one; this one spreads over that one, etc.

But obviously there is no "objective validity" to these assertions; they have *no "objective meaning"*; they have a merely *"subjective"* truth. Now we do not wish to become involved here in an attempt to determine whether there is not a sense in which these assertions have a certain objectivity, even while they can be pronounced "subjectively" true. But it is already clear to a fleeting glance that higher dignity of objectivity, <48> which the prescientific natural judgment dramatizes, so to speak, and which the considered judgments of the exact sciences bring to an incomparably higher fulfillment, is altogether lacking here. We shall not attribute any special value to such assertions—that this is here, etc.—which we make on the basis of pure "seeing."

Moreover we are reminded here of the famous Kantian distinction between *judgments of perceptions* and *judgments of experience*. The relationship is obvious. However, as Kant lacked the concepts of phenomenology and phenomenological reduction, and as he had not been able to completely escape psychologism and anthropologism, he did not arrive at the ultimate significance of the distinction which is necessary here. Naturally with us it is not a question of merely subjectively valid judgments which are limited in their validity to the empirical subject, or even of objective validity in the sense of validity for every subject without restriction. Indeed we have bracketed the empirical subject; and the transcendental apperception, consciousness as such, will soon acquire for us a completely different meaning, one which is not at all mysterious.

Let us now return to the main theme of our discussion. Phenomenological judgments, if restricted to singular judgments, do not have very much to teach us. But how are judgments, particularly scientifically valid judgments, to be established? And the word *scientific* immediately puts us into an embarassing position. Does objectivity not carry *transcendence* with it, and along with this also the doubt as to what it is

supposed to signify, as to *whether* and how it is possible? Through *epistemological reduction* we exclude transcendent presuppositions, because transcendence is in question with respect to its possible validity and its meaning. But then are the scientific or transcendent conclusions of the theory of knowledge themselves still possible? Is it not obvious that before the possibility of transcendence is established no transcendent result of the theory of knowledge can itself be secure? But if, as it might seem, the epistemological ἐποχή demands that we accept nothing transcendent until we have established its possibility, and if the establishing of the possibility of transcendence itself, as an objective result, requires transcendent postulations, then it seems that we <49> are faced with the prospect of a circle, which makes phenomenology and the theory of knowledge impossible; and the labor of love in which we have been engaged up to this point will have been in vain.

We cannot, without more ado, despair of the possibility of a phenomenology and of what is obviously bound up with that in this discussion—a critique of cognition. What we need at this point is a further step which will unroll this spurious circle for us. We have already accomplished this in principle, for we distinguished two senses of transcendence and of immanence. After Descartes had established the evidence of the *cogitatio* (or rather of the *cogito ergo sum*, a conception which we have not adopted), he asked, as you will recall: *What is it which assures me of these fundamental data?* The answer is: the *clara et distincta perceptio*.[1] We can carry this further. I need not claim that we already have a purer and deeper grasp of the matter than Descartes, and that thereby we grasp and understand [the concept of] evidence, the *clara et distincta perceptio*, in a more exact sense. With Descartes we can now take the further step (*mutatis mutandis*): to whatever is given through a *clara et distincta perceptio*, as each *cogitatio* is, we may accord an equal validity. To be sure, if we recall the third and fourth Meditations, the proofs of the existence of God, the appeal to the *veracitas dei*,[2] etc., we can expect difficulties. Therefore, be very sceptical, or rather critical.

We have the givenness of the pure *cogitatio* as an absolute possession, but not the givenness of outer things in external perception, although such perception makes a claim to be giving the existence of these things. The transcendence of things requires that we put them in question. We do not understand how perception can reach transcendent objects, but we understand how perception can reach the immanent, provided it is reflective and purely immanent perception which has undergone reduction. But what enables us to understand this? Well, we directly "see," we directly grasp what we intend in the act of "seeing" and grasping. To have a phenomenon before one's eyes, which points to something which is not itself given in the phenomenon, and then to doubt whether such an object exists, and if so how it is to be understood that it exists—this is meaningful. But to "see" and to intend absolutely nothing more than what is grasped in "seeing," and then still <50> to question and doubt, that is nonsense. Basically what I am saying amounts to this. The "seeing" or grasping of what is given, insofar as it is actual "seeing," actual self-givenness in the strictest sense and not another sort of givenness which points to something which is not given— that is an ultimate. That is *absolute self-evidence;* if you are looking for what is not self-evident, what is problematic, or perhaps entirely mysterious, consider the reference to something transcendent, i.e., intention, belief, even a detailed proof of something not given. And it does not help us that even here an absolute datum can be found—the givenness of intention and belief themselves. To be sure, if we only reflect we will find this before us; but what is given here is not what was intended.

But can it be that absolute self-evidence, self-givenness in "seeing," is realized only in particular mental processes and their particular abstract aspects and parts, i.e., only in the "seeing" grasp of the *here and now?* Would there not have to be a "seeing" grasp of other data as absolute data, e.g., universals, in such a way that were a universal to attain self-evident givenness within "seeing," any doubt about it would then be absurd?

How remarkable it would be to limit the *cogitatio* to phenomenologically singular data can be seen from this fact, that the whole doctrine of evidence, which we, following Descartes, have set forth, and which certainly is illuminated with absolute clarity and self-evidence, would lose its value. That is, concerning the case of a *cogitatio* which lies before us as something particular, perhaps a feeling which we are now undergoing, one might say: this is given. But we would by no means dare to put forward the most universal proposition: *the givenness of any reduced phenomenon is an absolute and indubitable givenness.*

But this is only to help you along. In any event, it is illuminating that the possibility of a critique of cognition depends on the demonstration of absolute data which are different from even the reduced *cogitationes.* To view the matter more precisely, in the subject-predicate judgments which we make concerning them, we have already gone beyond them. If we say: this phenomenon of judgment underlies this or that phenomenon of imagination, this perceptual <51> phenomenon contains this or that aspect, color content, etc., and even if, just for the sake of argument, we make these assertions in the most exact conformity with the givenness of the *cogitatio,* then the logical forms which we employ, and which are reflected in the linguistic expressions themselves, already go beyond the mere *cogitationes.* A "something more" is involved which does not at all consist of a mere agglomeration of new *cogitationes.* And even if predicational thinking gives rise to new *cogitationes,* which are joined to those concerning which we made the assertions, nevertheless they are not what constitute the predicational facts which are the objective correlates of the assertions.

That cognition, which can bring to *absolute self-givenness* not only particulars, but also *universals, universal objects, and universal states of affairs*, is more easily conceivable, at least for anyone who can assume the position of pure "seeing" and can hold all natural prejudices at arm's length. This cognition is of decisive significance for the possibility of phenomenology. For its special character consists in the fact that it is the analysis of essence and the investigation into essence in the area of pure "seeing" thought and absolute self-givenness. That is necessarily its character; it sets out to be a science and a method which will explain possibilities—possibilities of cognition and possibilities of valuation—and will explain them in terms of their fundamental essence. They are generally questionable possibilities, and investigations of them must take on the character of general investigations of essence. Analysis of essence is *eo ipso* general analysis; cognition of essence in terms of essence, in terms of essential nature, in terms of cognition which is directed to universal objects. It is here that talk of the *a priori* has its legitimate place. For what does *a priori* cognition mean except a cognition which is directed to general essences, and which entirely bases its absolute validity on essence, at least insofar as we exclude the discredited empiricist concept of the *a priori*.

In any event, although this may be the only justifiable concept of the *a priori*, another one can be found if we range under the heading of the *a priori* all concepts which as categories have a principal meaning in a certain sense, and then in addition the essential principles which are based on these concepts.

<52>   If we concentrate here on the first concept of the *a priori*, then phenomenology will have to do with the *a priori* in the sphere of origins and of absolute data, with species grasped in general "seeing," and with the *a priori* truths which these species render immediately "seeable." When we engage in the critique of reason, not only the theoretical, but also the practical and any other kind, the chief goal is certainly the *a priori* in the second sense; it is to establish the principal self-given forms and facts and, by means of this self-givenness, to develop, inter-

pret, and evaluate the concepts which come forward with a claim to crucial significance, as well as the principles of logic, ethics, and theory of value.

Lecture IV   <53>

[Extension of the sphere of investigation through a consideration of intentionality. The self-givenness of the universal; the philosophical method of the analysis of essence. Critique of the interpretation of evidence as feelings; evidence as self-givenness. No limitation on the sphere of genuine (*Reell*) immanence; the theme of all self-givenness.]

If we restrict ourselves to the pure phenome-   <55> nology of cognition, then we will be concerned with the *essence of cognition* as revealed in direct "seeing," i.e., with a demonstration of it which is carried out by way of "seeing" in the sphere of phenomenological reduction and self-givenness, and with an analytical distinction between the various sorts of phenomena which are embraced by the very broad term "cognition." Then the question is as to what is essentially contained and grounded in them, from what factors they are built up, what possibilities of combination can be found while remaining purely within their essential natures, and what general interrelations flow from their essences.

And it is not merely concerned with the genuinely (*reell*) immanent, but also with what is *immanent in the intentional sense*. Cognitive mental processes (and this belongs to their essence) have an *intentio*, they refer to something, they are related in this or that way to an object. This activity of relating itself to an object belongs to them even if the object itself does not. And what is objective can appear, can have a certain kind of givenness in appearance, even though it is at the same time neither genuinely (*reell*) within the cognitive phenomenon, nor does it exist in any other way as a *cogitatio*. To explain the essence of cognition and the essential connections which belong to it and to bring this to self-givenness, this involves examining both these sides of the matter; it involves investigating this relatedness which belongs to the essence of cognition. And just here lie the puzzles, the mysteries, the problems concerning the ultimate meaning of the objectivity of cognition, including its reaching or failing to reach the object, if it is judgmental cognition and its adequacy, if it is evident cognition, etc.

In any case, the whole investigation into essence is, in fact, obviously a general investigation. The particular cognitive phenomenon, coming and going in the stream of consciousness, is not the sort of thing about which phenomenology establishes its conclusions. Phe-<56> nomenology is directed to the "sources of cognition," to general origins which can be "seen," to general absolute data which present the universal basic criteria in terms of which all meaning, and also the correctness, of confused thinking is to be evaluated, and by which all the riddles which have to do with the objectivity of cognition are to be solved.

Still, are real *universality*, universal essences, and the universal states of affairs attaching to them capable of self-givenness in the same sense as a *cogitatio? Does not the universal as such transcend knowledge?* Knowledge of universals is certainly given as an absolute phenomenon; but in this we shall seek in vain for the universal which is to be identical, in the strictest sense, in the equally immanent contents of innumerable possible cases of cognition.

Of course, we answer, as we have already answered: to be sure, the universal has this kind of transcendence. Every genuine (*reell*) constituent of the cognitive phenomenon, this phenomenological particular, is also a particular; and so the universal, which certainly is no particular, cannot be really contained in the consciousness of the universal. But the objection to *this* kind of transcendence is nothing more than a prejudice, which stems from an inappropriate interpretation of cognition, one which is not based on the source of cognition. Thus one has to get especially clear about the fact that we accord the status of absolute self-givenness to the absolute

phenomenon, the *cogitatio* which has undergone reduction, not because it is a particular, but because it displays itself in pure "seeing" after phenomenological reduction, *precisely as absolute self-givenness.* But in pure "seeing" we find that universality no less displays *just* such an absolute givenness.

Is this actually the case? Let us now consider some cases in which a universal is given, i.e., cases where a purely immanent consciousness of the universal is built up on the basis of some "seen" and self-given particular. I have a particular intuition of redness, or rather several such intuitions. I stick strictly to the pure immanence; I am careful to perform the phenomenological reduction. I snip off any further significance of redness, any way in which it may be viewed as something transcendent, e.g., as the redness of a piece of blotting paper on my table, <57> etc. And now I fully grasp in pure "seeing" the *meaning* of the concept of redness in general, redness *in specie*, the *universal* "seen" as *identical* in this and that. No longer is it the particular as such which is referred to, not this or that red thing, but redness in general. If we really did this in pure "seeing," could we then still intelligibly doubt what redness is in general, what is meant by this expression, what it may be in its very essence? We truly "see" it; there it is, the very object of our intent, this species of redness. Could a deity, an infinite intellect, do more to lay hold of the essence of redness than to "see" it as a universal?

And if now perhaps two species of redness are given to us, two shades of red, can we not judge that this and that are similar to each other, not this particular, individual phenomenon of redness, but the type, the shade as such? Is not the relation of similarity here a general absolute datum?

Again, this givenness is also something purely immanent, not immanent in the spurious sense, i.e., existing in the sphere of an individual consciousness. We are not speaking at all of the act of abstraction in the psychological subject, and of the psychological conditions under which this takes place. We are speaking of the general essence of meaning of redness and its givenness in general "seeing."

Thus it is now senseless still to raise questions and doubts as to what the essence of redness is, or what the meaning of redness is, provided that while one "sees" redness and grasps it in its specific character, one means by the word "red" just exactly that which is being grasped and "seen" there. And in the same way it is senseless, with respect to the essence of cognition and the fundamental structure of cognition, to wonder what its meaning is, provided one is immediately given the paradigmatic phenomena and the type in question in a purely "seeing" and eidetic (*ideierender*) reflection within the sphere of phenomenological reduction. However, cognition is certainly not so simple a thing as redness; a great many forms and types of it are to be distinguished. And not only that; their essential relations to one another need to be investigated. For to understand cognition we must generally clarify the *teleological interconnections* within <58> cognition, which amount to certain essential relations of different essential types of intellectual forms. And here belongs also the ultimate explanation of the principles which, as ideal conditions of the possibility of scientific objectivity, function as norms governing the whole enterprise of empirical science. This whole attempt at the explanation of principles moves throughout in the sphere of essence, which is repeatedly built up (*konstituiert*) on the basis of particular phenomena through phenomenological reduction.

At every point this analysis is an analysis of essences and an investigation of the general states of affairs which are to be built up in immediate intuition. Thus the whole investigation is an *a priori* one, though, of course, it is not *a priori* in the sense of mathematical deductions. What distinguishes it from the "objectivizing" *a priori* sciences is its methods and its goal. *Phenomenology proceeds by "seeing," clarifying, and determining meaning, and by distinguishing meanings.* It compares, it distinguishes, it forms

connections, it puts into relation, divides into parts, or distinguishes abstract aspects. But all within pure "seeing." It does not theorize or carry out mathematical operations; that is to say, it carries through no explanations in the sense of deductive theory. As it explains the basic concepts and propositions which function as principles governing the possibility of "objectivizing" science (but finally it also takes its own basic concepts and principles as objects of reflective explanation), it ends where "objectivizing" science begins. Hence it is a science in a completely different sense, and with completely different problems and methods. *The procedure of "seeing" and eidetic abstraction within the strictest phenomenological reduction is exclusively its own: it is the specifically philosophical method, insofar as this method belongs essentially to the meaning of the critique of cognition and so generally to every sort of critique of reason* (hence also evaluative and practical reason). But whatever is called philosophy in addition to the critique of reason in the strict sense, is intimately related to this: metaphysics of nature and metaphysics of all <59> forms of mental life, and thus metaphysics in general in the widest sense.

In such cases one speaks of seeing something *evident*, and in fact those who recognize the pregnant concept of evidence and take a firm grip on the essence of such evidence have these kinds of occurrences exclusively in mind. The basic point is that one must not overlook the fact that evidence is this consciousness which is truly [a] "seeing" [consciousness] and which has a direct and adequate grasp of itself and that signifies nothing other than adequate self-givenness. The empiricist epistemologists, who speak so much about the virtues of investigating origins, and with all this remain as far from true origins as the most extreme rationalist, would have us believe that the whole distinction between judgments that are evident and those that are not consists of a certain feeling through which the former are marked out. But what can a feeling do to give us an understanding of this matter? What is it supposed to accomplish? Is it, so to speak, supposed to call out to us: "Stop! Here is the truth?" But why then do we have to trust this call? Must this trust also carry its credentials in feeling? And why does a judgment with the meaning 2 times 2 equals 5 never have this mark in feeling? and why is it impossible for it to have such a mark? Exactly how does one come to the theory that the mark of truth resides in feeling? Well, one says to oneself: "The same judgment, in the logical sense, e.g., the judgment that 2 times 2 equals 4, can at one time be evident to me and at another time not; the same concept of 4 can at one time be given to me in luminous intuition (*intuitiv in Evidenz*) and at another time in a merely symbolic representation. Thus with respect to content, on both occasions we have the same phenomenon, but on the one occasion there is a feeling which marks it out and thereby lends it a superior status, a character of validity." Have I in fact the same object on both occasions, except that on one occasion a feeling is given along with it, on the other not? But if one directs his attention to the phenomenon, he will notice at once that in actuality it is not the same phenomenon which lies before him on these two occasions, but two essentially different phenomena, which have only one feature in common. If I see that 2 times 2 equals 4, and then assert it in a vague symbolic assertion, in the latter case I am referring to an equality; but to refer to equality, that is not to have that phenomenon. The content of the two is different. One time I "see," and in "seeing" the interrelation itself is given; the other time I perform a symbolic reference. One time I have intuition; the other time I have an empty intention.

<60> Thus does the distinction amount to this, that in both cases something common is present, the same "meaning," once with a feeling-label and once without? Let one attend to the phenomenon itself, instead of going beyond to talk about it and interpret it. Let us take a simpler example: if I at a certain time have redness in a living intuition and at another time think about redness in terms merely of symbols with

empty intention, is it then the case that both times the same phenomenon of redness is really present, only once with a feeling and once without?

Thus one needs only to look at the phenomena in order to recognize that they are completely different, united only through what identifies them as two cases of the same thing, which we call "meaning." But if the difference is to be found in the phenomena themselves, then what need have we of feeling as a principle of distinction? And does the distinction not lie precisely in this, that in one case the self-givenness of redness lies before us, the self-givenness of number and of the general equality of number— or, subjectively expressed, the adequate "seeing" grasp and possession of the entities themselves—while in the other case we have a mere reference to these things? And so we have no sympathy with this notion of feeling as evidence. It could be justified only if it were to display itself in pure "seeing," and if pure "seeing" were to signify just that which *we* attribute to it and which contradicts it.

Thus with respect to the application of the concept of evidence, we can now say: in the existence of the *cogitatio* we find evidence, and for that reason the *cogitatio* engenders no puzzles, not even the puzzle of transcendence. We accord it the status of something unquestionable, on the basis of which we may proceed further. No less do we find evidence in the universal; we recognize that *universal objects* and *states of affairs* attain self-givenness. And they are unquestionably given in the same sense; hence they are adequately self-given in the strictest sense of the term.

Hence phenomenological reduction does not entail a limitation of the investigation to the sphere of genuine (*reell*) immanence, to the sphere of that which is genuinely contained within the absolute this of the *cogitatio*. It entails no limitation to the sphere of the *cogitatio*. Rather it entails a limitation to the sphere of things that are *purely self-given*, to the sphere of those things which are not merely spoken about,

<61> meant, or perceived, but instead to the sphere of those things that are given in just exactly the sense in which they are thought of, and moreover are self-given in the strictest sense—in such a way that nothing which is meant fails to be given. In a word, we are restricted to the sphere of pure evidence, but understanding this term in a certain strict sense, which definitely excludes any "mediate evidence," and especially excludes all evidence in a loose sense.

Absolute givenness is an ultimate. Of course one can easily say and insist that something is absolutely given to him when it is not really the case. Again, absolute givenness can either be vaguely spoken of, or can itself be given in absolute givenness. Just as I can "see" a phenomenon of redness, and also can merely talk about it without "seeing," so I can also either talk about the "seeing" of redness or direct my "seeing" to the "seeing" of redness, and so grasp the "seeing" of redness itself in "seeing." On the other hand, to deny self-givenness in general is to deny every ultimate norm, every basic criterion which gives significance to cognition. But in that case one would have to construe everything as illusion, and, in a nonsensical way, also take illusion as such to be an illusion; and so one would altogether relapse into the absurdities of scepticism. However, it is obvious that the only one who can argue in this way against the sceptic is the man who "*sees*" the ultimate basis of knowledge, who is willing to assign a significance to "seeing," inspecting evidence. Whoever does not see or will not see, who talks and argues, but always remains at the place where he accepts all conflicting points of view and at the same time denies them all, there is nothing we can do with him. We cannot answer: "obviously" it is the case. For he denies that there is any such thing as "obviously." It is as if a blind man wished to deny that there is such a thing as seeing, or still better, as if one who has sight wished to deny that he himself sees and that there is any such thing as seeing. How could we convince him, assuming that he has no other mode of perception?

Thus if we hold fast to the absolute self-givenness of which we already know that it does not signify the self-givenness of genuine (*reell*) particulars, not even the absolute particulars of the *cogitatio*, then the question arises as to how far it extends and as to the extent to which, and the sense in which, it ties itself down to the sphere of *cogitationes* and the universals which <62> are abstracted from them. If one has cast off the first and most immediate prejudice, which sees the only absolute datum in the particular *cogitatio* and in the sphere of genuinely (*reell*) immanent things, one must now also do away with the further and no less immediate prejudice, according to which newly self-given objects spring up *only* in general intuitions derived from the sphere of *cogitationes*.

"In reflective perception, the *cogitationes* are absolutely given to us in that we consciously undergo them," so one would like to begin. And then we can inspect universals which are singled out within them and within their genuinely (*reell*) abstract aspects; we can, in a "seeing" abstraction, grasp universals and the essential connections which are solely grounded in them as self-given states of affairs, constituted in "seeing"-interrelating thought. That is the end of the matter.

Meanwhile no inclination is more dangerous to the "seeing" cognition of origins and absolute data than to think too much, and from these reflections in thought to create supposed self-evident principles. Principles which for the most part are not at all explicitly formulated and hence are not subject to any critique based on "seeing" but rather implicitly determine and unjustifiably limit the direction of investigation. *"Seeing" cognition is that form of reason which sets itself the task of converting the understanding into reason.* The understanding is not to be allowed to interrupt and to insert its unredeemed bank notes among the certified ones; and its method of convertion and exchange, based on mere treasury bonds, is not questioned here.

Thus as little interpretation as possible, but as pure an intuition as possible (*intuitio sine com-*

prehensione). In fact, we will hark back to the speech of the mystics when they describe the intellectual seeing which is supposed not to be a discursive knowledge. And the whole trick consists in this—to give free rein to the seeing eye and to bracket the references which go beyond the "seeing" and are entangled with the seeing, along with the entities which are supposedly given and thought along with the "seeing," and, finally, to bracket what is read into them through the accompanying reflections. The crucial question is: Is the supposed object given in <63> the proper sense? Is it, in the strictest sense, "seen" and grasped, or does the intention go beyond that?

Supposing this to be the case, we soon recognize that it would be a *fiction* to believe that investigation by way of "seeing" moves in the sphere of a so-called *inner perception* and in the sphere of the purely immanent abstractions based on the phenomena and phenomenal aspects of inner perception. There are many sorts of objectivity and, correlatively, many sorts of so-called givenness. Perhaps the givenness of existents in the sense of the so-called "inner perception," and again the givenness of the existents in the natural, "objectivizing" sciences, is only one sort of givenness; while the others, although labeled as nonexistent, are still types of givenness. And it is only because they are, that they can be set over against the other sorts and distinguished from them in evidence.

<65> **Lecture V**

[The constitution (*Konstitution*) of time-consciousness. Apprehension of essences as an evident givenness of essence; the constitution of the individual essence and of the consciousness of universality. Categoreal data. The symbolically thought as such. The field of research in its widest extent: the constitution of different modes of objectivity in cognition. The problem of the correlation of cognition and the object of cognition.]

<67>   If we have firmly established the evidence of the *cogitatio*, and then have conceded the fur-

ther step of recognizing the evident givenness of the universal, this step will at once lead us further.

By perceiving color and exercising reduction on this perception I arrive at the pure phenomenon of color. And if I now achieve a pure abstraction, I will get to the essence of phenomenological color as such. But am I not equally in full possession of this essence if I have a clear image?

As far as *memory* is concerned it is not anything simple, and from the start it presents different forms of objects and, interconnected with these, different forms of givenness. Thus one could refer to the so-called *primary memory*, the *retention* which is necessarily bound up with every perception. The mental process which we are now undergoing becomes objective to us in immediate reflection, and thenceforth it displays in reflection the same objectivity: the self-same tone which has just existed as an actual "now" remains henceforth the same tone, but moving back into the past and there continually constituting the same objective point in time. And if the tone does not cease but continues, and during its continuation presents itself as the same in content or else as changing content, can we not grasp this fact—that it remains the same or changes—evidently (within certain limits)? And again, does this not mean that "seeing" *extends* beyond the strictly present moment and hence is capable of grasping intentionally, in continually new moments, what is no longer existing, and that it is capable of becoming certain of a stretch of past time in the manner of evident givenness? And again we must distinguish, on the one hand, the pertinent object which is and was, which endures and changes and, on the other hand, the pertinent phenomenon of presentness and pastness, of duration and change, which is from time to time a "now." It is in the latter, and in the gradations it contains and the continual changes it undergoes, that *temporal existence* <68> is brought into appearance and presented. The object is not a genuinely concrete part of the phenomenon; in its temporality it has something which cannot at all be found in the phenomenon or reduced to the phenomenon. And yet it is constituted within the phenomenon. It is presented therein and is evidently given as "existing" there.

Further, as to the givenness of essences, it is constituted not only on the basis of perception and the retention which is bound up with it, in such a way that we, so to speak, pluck a universal from the phenomenon itself; it is also constituted by *universalizing* the object of appearance, positing a universal while gazing on it, e.g., temporal content in general, duration in general, change in general. Moreover, imagination and memory can also serve as its foundation; they themselves present pure possibilities to be grasped. In a similar way we can take from these acts universals which, for their part, are not genuinely contained in these acts.

It is obvious that a fully evident grasp of essence *refers back* to some particular intuition on the basis of which it must be built up, but therefore *not necessarily to a particular perception*, which has given us the paradigm of an individual thing as something present in a genuine "now." The essence of phenomenological tone-quality, tone-intensity, of color quality, of brightness, etc., is itself given whether the eidetic abstraction carries out its operation on the basis of a *perception* or on that of a *realization in imagination;* and it is *irrelevant* to either of these whether we suppose the objects to *exist* in actuality or in some other way. The same holds for an apprehension of essences which has to do with various sorts of psychic data in the proper sense, e.g., judgment, assertion, denial, perception, inference, etc. And of course it holds also for the general states of affairs which appertain to such universals. The realization that of two tones one is lower, the other higher, and that this relation is asymmetrical, is developed within "seeing." The instances must stand before our eyes, but not necessarily in the manner of facts of perception. For a consideration of essence, perception and imagination are to be treated exactly alike; the same essence can equally well be

"seen" in either, or abstracted from either, and <69> any interpolated suppositions about existence are irrelevant. That the perceived tone together with its intensity, pitch, etc., *exists* in a certain sense, that the imagined tone, to put it bluntly, the fictitious tone, *does not exist,* that the former is obviously present in a genuine sense, the latter not, that in the case of memory the tone is posited as having existed rather than as existing now and is only presented at this moment—all this belongs to another investigation. In a consideration of essence none of this is to the point, unless that investigation turns its attention to the presentation of just these distinctions, which also are capable of being given, and to establishing general principles concerning them.

Moreover it is quite clear that even if the underlying instances are given in perception, the actual existence which sets perceptual givenness off from other kinds has no bearing on the matter. It is not just that imagination is as suitable as perception for the consideration of essence; it is also the case that imagination appears to contain *individual data* within itself, and even actually evident data.

Let us consider *mere imagination*, even without this being fixed in memory. An imagined color is not a datum in the way a sensed color is. We distinguish the imagined color from the mental process of imagining the color. The hovering of the color before me (to put it roughly) is a "now," a presently existing *cogitatio*, but the color itself is not a presently existing color; it is not perceived. On the other hand, it is given in a certain way, it stands before my gaze. Just like the perceived color it can be reduced through the exclusion of all transcendent significance, so that it no longer signifies for me the color of the paper, the house, etc. It is possible here too to refrain from positing the existence of anything empirical; in that case I consider it just exactly as I "see" it, or, as it were, "live" it. But in spite of that it is not a genuine part of the mental process of imagining; it is not a present, but a presented color. It stands, *as it were*, before our eyes, but not as a genuine presence. But with all this, it is "seen" and as "seen" it is, in a certain sense, given. Thus I do not take it to be a physical or psychical *existent*. Nor do I take it to be existent in the sense of a proper *cogitatio*, which is a genuine "now," a datum which is, as a matter of evidence, characterized as given now. Still, <70> the fact that the imagined color is not given in this or that sense does not mean that it is given in no sense. It appears and in appearing presents itself in such a way that "seeing" it itself in its presentation I can make judgments concerning the abstract aspects which constitute it and the ways in which these aspects cohere. Naturally these are also given in the same sense, and likewise they do not "actually" exist anywhere in the mental process of imagining. They are not genuinely present; they are only "represented." The pure judgment of imagination, the mere expression of the *content*, the specific essence of that which appears, can assert: this is found in this way, contains these aspects, is changed in such and such a way—without saying anything at all about existence as really involved in objective time, about the actual present, past, and future. We could therefore say that it is concerning the *individual essence* that we make judgments and not concerning existence. Just on that account is the general judgment of essence, which we usually just call the judgment of essence, independent of the distinction between perception and imagination. Perception posits *existence*, but it also has an *essence* which as *content* posited as existing can also be the same in representation.

But the contrast of *existence* and *essence* signifies nothing else than that here two modes of being manifest themselves in two modes of self-givenness and are to be distinguished. In merely imagining a color, the existence which attaches to that color as an actuality in time is not in question; no judgment is made concerning it, and nothing concerning it is given in the *content* of the imagination. But this color appears; it stands there; it is a "this", it can become the subject of a judgment, and an evident judgment. Thus a mode of givenness is displayed in the in-

tuitions in imagination and the evident judgments which are grounded on them. To be sure, if we restrict ourselves to the sphere of particular individuals, then we can hardly get started with this kind of judgment. Only if we construct general judgments of essence, can we attain the secure objectivity which science demands. But that does not matter here. Hence we seem to get into a pretty kettle of fish.

The earliest stage was the *evidence of the cogitatio*. There it seemed first of all as if we were on solid ground—*being pure and simple*. Here one <71> would only have to grasp and "see" it. That one could, in reflecting on these data, compare and distinguish, that one could separate out the specific universals and so put forward judgments of essence, all this could be easily managed. But now it becomes clear that the pure being of the *cogitatio* reveals itself, on closer inspection, to be something which is not as simple as all that. It becomes clear that in the Cartesian sphere itself *different types* of objectivity are "constituted." And to say that they are constituted implies that immanent data are not, as it first seemed, simply in consciousness in the sense in which things are in a box, but that all the time they are displayed in something like "appearances." These appearances neither are nor genuinely contain the objects themselves. Rather in their shifting and remarkable structure they create objects in a certain way for the ego, insofar as appearances of just such a sort and just such a construction belong to that in which what we call "givenness" has been lying all along.

The *primary temporal object* is constituted in perception, along with the retention of consciousness of what is perceived; only in that sort of consciousness can time be given. Thus the universal is constituted in the *consciousness of universality* which is built up from perception and imagination. The content of intuition, in the sense of a particular *essence*, is constituted in either imagination or perception indifferently, while abstracting from existential claims. And, to remind you of this right away, from this proceed the categoreal acts, which are always presupposed in any evident assertions. The categoreal forms which we encounter here, which find expression in words like "is" and "not," "same" and "other," "one" and "many," "and" and "or," and in the forms of predication and attribution, etc., point to the forms of thinking by means of which thought-forms, when they have been appropriately constructed, come to consciousness on the basis of synthetic data which tie together the simplest acts: states of affairs of this and that ontological form. It is also at this point that the "self-constitution" of the actual objects takes place in the cognitive acts which have been so formed. The consciousness in which the given object as well as the pure "seeing" of things is brought to fulfillment is, how-

<72> ever, not like an empty box in which these data are simply lying; it is the *"seeing" consciousness*, which, apart from attention, consists of mental acts which are *formed in such and such ways;* and the things which are not mental acts are nevertheless constituted in these acts, and come to be given in such acts. It is only as so constituted that they display themselves as what they are.

But is this not an absolute marvel? And where does this constituting of objects begin and where does it end? Are there any actual limits to it? Isn't it true that in every representation or judgment we get at a datum in a certain sense? Isn't each object a datum, and an evident datum, just insofar as it is intuited, represented, or thought in such and such a way? In the perception of an external thing, just that thing, let us say a house standing before our eyes, is said to be perceived. The house is a transcendent thing, and forfeits its existence after the phenomenological reduction. The house-appearance, this *cognitatio*, emerging and disappearing in the stream of consciousness, is given as actually evident. In this house-phenomenon we find a phenomenon of redness, of extension, etc. These are evident data. But is it not also evident that a house appears in the house-phenomenon, and that it is just on that account that we call it a perception of a house? And what appears is not only a house in general, but just exactly this

house, determined in such and such a way and appearing in that determination. Can I not make an evidently true judgment as follows: on the basis of the appearance or in the content of this perception, the house is thus and so, a brick building, with a slate roof, etc.?

And if I give free rein to fantasy, so that, e.g., perhaps I see a knight like St. George killing a dragon, is it not evident that the fantasy-phenomenon represents precisely St. George, and even St. George as described in such and such a way, and that thus it here represents something transcendent? Can I not make evident judgments here, not about the genuine content of the appearance in fantasy, but about the object which appears? To be sure, only one aspect of the object comes within the purview of this realization in imagination, although more and more aspects can be brought therein; but nevertheless it is still evident that this object, this knight St. George, lies within the meaning of the phenomenon, and is manifested there "as a datum" of a sort proper to appearance.

And finally we come to so-called *symbolic* <73> *thinking*. Let us say that without any intuition I think that 2 times 2 equals 4. Can I doubt that I have directed my thought to this arithmetical proposition and that what is thought does not concern, e.g., today's weather? If this is evidently so, is there not also something functioning as a datum here? And if we go this far, nothing can prevent us from recognizing that the paradoxical, the completely absurd, is also "given" in a certain way. A round square does not appear in imagination as a dragon killer appears to me, nor does it appear in perception as an arbitrary external thing; but an intentional object is still obviously there. I can describe the phenomenon, "thinking of a round square," in terms of its genuine content. The round square itself cannot be found there, and still it is evident that it is thought in this mental act and that in the object so thought roundness and squareness as such are thought. In other words, the object of this thought is both round and square.

Above all, it must not be said that the data to

which we have finally been led in these considerations are actual data in the true sense; in that case everything perceived, imagined, pretended, or symbolically thought, every fiction and absurdity, would be "evidently given." But all that would be indicated by all this would be that *great difficulties are involved here.* It cannot hinder us in our quest for enlightenment to hold fast to the principle: *givenness extends just as far as actual evidence.* But of course the basic question will be this. In the achievement of pure evidence what is actually given in it and what is not? What is it that is produced therein only be an alien mode of thought? What interpretations are introduced without any basis in the data themselves?

And in general it is not primarily a matter of clinging to certain selected appearances as data, but rather of getting insight into the nature of givenness and of the self-constitution of different modes of objectivity. Certainly each mental phenomenon has its relation to objects; and (this is the most fundamental fact about it) each has its genuine (*reellen*) content, which is a *belief*[3] in those aspects which compose it in the genuine sense. But on the other hand there is its intentional object, an object which it intends to constitute in such and such a way according to its essential kind.

<74>   In order to bring this matter to actual evidence, we must get everything we need from the evidence itself. Within it we must become clear as to what this "intentional inexistence" really signifies and how it is related to the genuine content of the mental phenomenon. We must see in what connections it appears as actual and proper evidence, and what in these connections actual and proper givenness is. We will then be in a position to *set forth the different modes of givenness in the proper sense, and likewise the constitution of different modes of objectivity and their relations to one another:* the givenness of the *cogitatio,* the givenness of the *cogitatio preserved in a fresh recollection,* the givenness of the *unity of appearance* enduring in the phenomenal flux, the givenness of *change* itself, the

givenness of *things* to the "outer" sense, the givenness of the different forms of imagination and memory, as well as the givenness of *perceptions* and other sorts of *representations* which unify themselves synthetically in many ways in fitting associations. Of course there is also *logical givenness,* the givenness of *universals,* of *predicates,* of *states of affairs,* etc.; also the givenness of *something absurd,* of *something contradictory,* of *something which does not exist.* In general, whether a datum manifests what is merely represented or what truly exists, what is real or what is ideal, what is possible or what is impossible, it is *a datum in the cognitive phenomenon,* in the phenomenon of a thought, in the widest sense of the term. And, *generally speaking, it is in the consideration of essences that this correlation, which seems so wonderful at first sight, is to be investigated.*

It is only in cognition that the essence of objectivity can be studied at all, with respect to all its basic forms; only in cognition is it truly given, is it evidently "seen." This *evident "seeing"* itself is truly *cognition in the fullest sense.* And the object is not a thing which is put into cognition as into a sack, as if cognition were a completely empty form, one and the same empty sack in which now this, now that is   <75> placed. But in givenness we see *that the object is constituted in cognition,* that a number of different basic forms of objectivity are to be distinguished, as well as an equal number of different forms of the given cognitive acts and of clusters and interconnections of cognitive acts. And cognitive acts, more generally any mental acts, are not isolated particulars, coming and going in the stream of consciousness without any interconnections. As they are essentially related to one another, they display a teleological *coherence* and corresponding connections of realization, corroboration, verification, and their opposites. And on these connections, which present an intelligible unity, a great deal depends. They themselves are involved in the constitution of objects. They logically bring together acts which are and acts which are not given in the proper sense, acts of mere representation (or rather of mere belief) and acts of insight. And they bring together the multiplicity of acts which are relative to this same objectivity, whether they take place in intuitive or in nonintuitive thought.

And it is in these interconnections that the objectivity involved in the objective sciences is first constituted, not in one stroke but in a gradually ascending process—and especially the objectivity of real spatio-temporal actuality.

All this is to be investigated, and investigated in the sphere of pure evidence, in order to throw light on the great problems of the nature of cognition and the meaning of the *correlation of cognition and the object of cognition*. Originally the problem concerned *the relation between subjective psychological experience and the actuality grasped therein, as it is in itself*—first of all actual reality, and then also the mathematical and other sorts of ideal realities. But first we need the insight that the *crucial problem* must rather have to do with the *relation between cognition and its object*, but in the *reduced* sense, according to which we are dealing not with human cognition, but with cognition in general, apart from any existential assumptions either of the empirical ego or of a real world. We need the insight that the truly significant problem is that of the *ultimate bearing of cognition*, including the problem of objectivity in general, which only is what it is in correlation with possible cognition. Further, we need the insight that this problem can only be solved within the sphere of pure evidence, the sphere of data which are ultimate norms because they are absolutely given. And finally we need the realization that we must then investigate one by one, by the strict process of "seeing," all the fundamental forms of cognition and of the objects which fully or partially attain givenness within cognition, in order to determine the meaning of all the correlations which have to be explicated. <76>

NOTES

1. Tr. note: Clear and distinct perception.
2. Tr. note: The veracity of God.
3. English in the original.

A Return to Husserl and Researcher Self-Awareness

Nancy Drew

Over the last two decades, nurse researchers have found Heidegger's (1962) phenomenology strikingly relevant and have quite naturally gravitated to it as an arena for research because its ontological content identifies and expresses what nursing is most concerned about, the nature of Being: what it means to be human, to be a patient or to be a caregiver. In this respect Heideggerian phenemonology is a rich source of insight and subject matter for human sciences research. Heidegger (1962) set phenomenology on an ontological path because he believed that before we can effectively attend to epistemological concerns, that is, understanding how it is possible to know something, we must first understand ourselves and what it means to be human. His ontology is not entirely without epistemology, however. He also saw that understanding what it means to be human involves recognizing that our daily, uncritical immersion in the world is the foundation of any subsequent intellectual maneuvers that we may undertake as researchers, or scientists. Heidegger's hermeneutic "circle" insists that understanding is always already structured before we embark on scientific method. Prior to any theories that are created to explain it, we already have an implicit understanding of the phenomenon as the thing we see it to be. Whatever is being explored sci-entifically is viewed first from within the common-sense, everyday world that we live non-critically, and pre-reflectively.

Aside from the notion of the hermeneutic circle, however, researchers will find in Heidegger's study of being little direction for addressing epistemological concerns in phenomenological research. Husserl, who was Heidegger's teacher, focused on the epistemological aspects of phenomenology, and, although his work did not culminate in a protocol for phenomenological research, he returned repeatedly to philosophy of method and to the primary methodological goal of understanding how consciousness constitutes experience. Although Heidegger's ontological concerns of existence, care, death and time have been important themes for our studies, nursing research needs now to return to Husserl's ideas about phenomenological method.

The protocols which have been developed by the human sciences for phenomenological research over the past two decades—Spiegleberg (1984), Colaizzi (1978), Polkinghorne (1989), Giorgi (1985), Lynch-Sauer (1985), Munhall & Oiler-Boyd (1993), among others—have provided nursing researchers with guidance for conducting phenomenological studies. Much of what is reported as phenomenological research, however, lacks a component crucial to the phenomenological method as Husserl conceived it. Phenomenological studies as reported in nursing journals consist of compilations of themes that describe, often quite elegantly, the phenomena of a caring profession. Although these descriptions have contributed to understanding the world of patients and their caregivers, they are too often offered without adequate consideration for the researchers' own involvement with the data, and with resultant description. A reintroduction of Husserl's ideas about the reflectivity that is a necessary component of phenomenological method could open up a fruitful discourse about the primacy of phenomenological research and contribute to the missing element in the scholarship of nursing's phenomenological studies.

Over a lifetime Husserl developed his phenomenological philosophy and is considered its founder. His understanding of human conscious processes led him to take a critical stance regarding science. He cautioned the mid-twentieth century western cultures that the prevailing positivistic paradigm of science would lead to increasing dehumanization of society. He insisted that any projects designed to explain and control the natural world properly begin with awareness of the scientist's own experience of the phenomenon under study (Husserl, 1970b).

Following are five texts [not included here] that are important reading for anyone who is interested in understanding Husserl's phenomenology. *Logical Investigations*, translated in 1970, was his first major work, and is a study of the meaning-giving aspect of consciousness and the relationship between consciousness and its objects. The *Idea of Phenomenology* (1990), first translated in 1964, is a brief introduction to phenomenology. The progression of Husserl's conception of phenomenology as a transcendental activity, to that in which he recognized the primacy of the lifeworld from which such studies arise, can be seen in three of his best-known works: *Ideas I* (1962), originally published in

English in 1931, *Cartesian Meditations* (1977) and *The Crisis of European Sciences* (1970b), his final work, reveal his prescient awareness of the need for a foundational philosophy for the sciences. He saw phenomenology as such a philosophy.

Husserl's works give us the epistemological elements of phenomenology: the notions of intentional consciousness, transcendency and intersubjectivity. However, these ideas are addressed philosophically, leaving to the ingenuity of the researcher the manner in which one addresses the human capacity for reflecting on our pre-theoretical and uncritical involvement with the subject matter of a study. If researchers want to conduct truly phenomenological research, we need to begin developing concrete ways to examine the researcher's influence, as a resident of the lifeworld, upon research results. Although the following discussion about Husserl's ideas is organized by sections, the concepts of lifeworld, intersubjectivity and intentionality are part of a larger gestalt, interconnected and in relation to each other within the phenomenological paradigm. I hope to convey the interrelatedness of these concepts despite having to present them in a discrete fashion.

Lifeworld

In *Ideas I* (1962) Husserl implies that the lifeworld is the arena of phenomenological investigations, but the focus of his thinking in this, and subsequent works, was primarily on explicating the relationship between consciousness and its objects, as well as the phenomenologist's methodological attitude. Husserl's (1962) early discussions of consciousness as the noematic process seem to dismiss the everyday world of conscious experience, or to relegate it to the background. In his later work, the *lebenswelt* is clearly acknowledged as having priority over any seemingly isolated processes of consciousness (1970b). It is as if he had sensed by then that his highly abstract depiction of phenomenology as transcendental consciousness needed grounding in order to be recognized and acknowledged as the crucial philosophy that it is. Husserl saw phenomenology as the first philosophy, that is, the guiding stance or attitude for all scientific thinking because phenomenology takes into account the scientist's relationship with research projects, thereby assuring the objectivity upon which science is founded. He also understood that phenomenology provides the way for the human sciences to explore the "spiritual," the non-empirical domain of the lifeworld, a task which the natural sciences are ill-equipped to do (Husserl, 1970b).

Ultimately Husserl moved beyond a seemingly mechanistic and abstract rendering of conscious processes to attest to experiencing as the primordial nature of consciousness, that is, a straightforward, non-critical involvement with the things that we study. In his return to everyday reality and the lifeworld, he saw that it is not enough to explicate consciousness as simply a process or relationship between perception and its objects, but that the environment of perception, the everyday world in which consciousness lives and functions, is the concern and realm of phenomenology. It would be a mistake, however, for us to dismiss Husserl's initial preoccupation with conscious processes and miss the significance that consciousness has for phenomenology. The goal of understanding lived experience depends on thoughtful consideration of the reciprocity between perception and the lifeworld, how perception contributes to lived experience.

Experience equates with the lifeworld; experience can only be considered within the lifeworld, for that is where we live and conduct our ordinary, day to day tasks and projects, the walking, eating, musing, that make up the lifeworld. It is only in the lifeworld that we find the truth about being, our ontology, for the lifeworld is the home of both our subjective experiencing and our scientific role as logically objective observers. Phenomenology always takes us from the objectivism that science breeds and returns us to the lifeworld and to ourselves (Merleau-

Ponty, 1964). Merleau-Ponty (1962) describes the lifeworld as

. . . the world which precedes knowledge, of which knowledge always speaks, and in relation to which every scientific schematization is an abstract and derivative sign-language, as is geography in relation to the countryside in which we have learned beforehand what a forest, a prairie or a river is. (p. ix)

The lifeworld is constituted by the never-ending experiencing of the daily lives of its members, thus, the subject matter of phenomenological research is limitless. For meaning that can be understood from the lifeworld is never finally complete, but always potentially expandable (Merleau-Ponty, 1973). The lifeworld concept reminds us of what we know instinctively, that the immediate, the concrete—that particular experience of a flower, or that particular moment of understanding between nurse and dying patient—has a primacy and significance that outweighs any theorizing.

Intersubjectivity

Phenomenology's realm is the lifeworld, the moment to moment experiencing that goes on in our daily lives. Phenomenology is concerned with subjective experience of the lifeworld; and because we can think about, reflect on, our experiencing, phenomenology is further understood as concerned with transcendental subjectivity. Husserl spent a great deal of time explicating the notion of the transcendental, that uniquely human capacity to look at oneself, to think about thinking, i.e., the capacity for awareness of the meaning of one's experience. But more important to our purposes here is Husserl's recognition that transcendental, reflexive activity itself can and should be a focus for study. Phenomenological investigative processes can be explored phenomenologically (Husserl, 1962, section 65). This means that for phenomenologists, self-awareness is an integral aspect of exploring phenomena.

The idea of transcendency ultimately leads to the notion of intersubjectivity. Understanding that I can look at and reflect on myself leads to the inescapable realization that you, too, can look at and reflect on yourself, i.e., that all human beings have the same capacity for self-awareness, that they can think about their thinking as I do, and furthermore, that they are aware of my capacity to do so (and therein reappears the notion of the lifeworld). Our shared world is co-constituted by all of us as reflective subjects, beings whose awareness allows us to continually expand understanding of the world and our relation with it and with each other. As phenomenological researchers, when we study the events and things of the world we are inevitably returned to ourselves because the phenomena of the lifeworld are an amalgam of the concrete world and of our perceiving, experiencing of it. Furthermore, being returned to ourselves means that we cannot escape awareness of our fellow lifeworld members; "self-consciousness and consciousness of others are inseparable" (Husserl, 1970b, p. 253). The significance of this recognition of others and the community of the lifeworld is that it brings Husserl's phenomenology into conjunction with Heidegger's ontology, although taking up the task of describing our ontology was left to Heidegger. With the discovery that reflexivity and self-awareness invoke the presence of others, we can complete the circle, closing the gap between ontology and epistemology. They are no longer disparate concepts, placed in sequence with each other, or prioritized one over the other. Instead we see the relationship between knowing and being, between concern for reliable and valid knowledge and the fact that our knowing is always tied up with understanding who we are, which is, in part, that we are always in relation with others.

Husserl's phenomenological philosophy emphasizes transcendental subjectivity, the ability to self-reflect, and intersubjectivity, the inevitable awareness that others have this same self-reflective capacity. His phenomenology acknowledges the lifeworld community that intersubjectivity creates. At the same time, it holds that the ground of all community, the foundation of the lifeworld, is the singular person, the individual and his or her experience. Recognition of the centrality of intersubjectivity keeps us, as scientists, grounded in the lifeworld and in relationships among persons; it makes us keep our research historically aware, contextually sensitive. Additionally, because phenomenological research seeks out and uncovers the principles of experience, the essential structures of it, it makes others' experience understandable, thus strengthening community (Kohák, 1978).

Intentionality

Husserl saw that Descartes' radical doubt, and Kant's categories of the mind, particularly synthetic a priori judgments, had opened the door to phenomenology, but neither of these early philosophers had reached it. Kant had introduced the idea that we are not just passive recipients of impressions sent to us by objects, but that we understand the world around us because of mental structures that are the organizing framework for our perceptions and experience. Husserl took up this idea of implicit involvement with that which we experience and set about to explicate consciousness as a constitutive process. He did this by pursuing a concept which his mentor, Franz Brentano, had introduced: intentionality.

The notion of intentionality, or intentional consciousness is crucial to understanding Husserl's phenomenological philosophy and method; In *Ideas I* (1962) he states clearly that intentionality is the main theme of phenomenology. Intentionality refers to the relationship between persons and the object or events of their experience, or more simply, one's directed awareness of an object or event (Husserl, 1962). There is always an intentional relationship with the things that make up our everyday lives, that is, we understand the meaning of the things that we use and that we see around us as the things and places that belong to and signify our world. A phenomenologist is interested in the way that consciousness grasps an object or event as something, as meant (Natanson, 1973). To say that something is understood as meant, indicates an historical relationship with the thing; because I have had previous experience with a phenomenon, it has meaning for me and I bring this meaning to subsequent perceptions and interactions with it.

Within the realm of the lifeworld phenomenology looks not simply at objects and events as such, but at the way that they are experienced. Phenomenology seeks essences, or the universal patterns of experiencing, which are then described as faithfully as possible. The discovery of patterns of experiencing sets us on a path different from that of traditional positivistic science's processes which conveys the notion that we are separate from, unconnected to, the things that we observe, explore and manipulate. Phenomenology makes clear that consciousness is a creative participant in the relationship between ourselves and the world that we call experience. Our residency in the lifeworld places us in the position of creative contributors to that world so that the things that we study as researchers might be seen, in part, as products of our perceptions. Phenomenological research, if it is true to phenomenological philosophy, gives us clear information about how we are connected to the world that we study.

To say that a phenomenon is experienced implies an active relationship between consciousness and its objects. An active relationship between consciousness and its objects suggests a duality in which experiencing depends on the objects, events of the lifeworld; indeed one cannot have experience apart from the lifeworld and its things and situations. Consciousness is dependent on the world for content. But in a way, the content of consciousness, the things and situations which consciousness ponders, sees, understands, is constituted by it. It is a creative relationship. This is not to say that consciousness creates the things it sees, but only that it understands and it is this understanding that is unique to each consciousness, each perceiver. Bringing my past experience and understanding of an event or object to the present

moment, the phenomenon before me is the product of co-creation by me, and by it, as experience. In the moment of perceiving we experience the lifeworld in an all-at-once way, intuitively understanding what it means. We see the particular characteristics of the object or event, whatever it may be, but more important, in the phenomenological frame of mind, we can also see the universal aspects of the phenomenon that let us grasp the essence of the experience of surviving cancer, or raising a diabetic child, for example. This active relationship in which we experience the things and events of our world as endowed with meaning, as meant, is the intentionality of which Husserl spoke. The significance of this for researchers is that unless we acknowledge our already meaning-endowed relationship with the topics of our research, we are deluded about grasping the essence of any phenomenon.

INTENTIONALITY AND SELF-AWARENESS

Written description is the relatively easy part of phenomenology. Description is created from the rich data that interviewees provide from their lived experience. Phenomenological researchers take great care to faithfully describe the experiences that research participants have shared with them. The difficult part of phenomenology is scrutiny of the researcher's interaction with the data—influencing, and being influenced by, the data. Husserl understood that the phenomenological method could and should be used to understand the phenomenologist's own part in the descriptions that are created (Husserl, 1962, section 65). Phenomenological descriptions are created amidst the researcher's past and present experiencing. The researcher's intentional consciousness is integrally involved in the account of any phenomenon. If such intentionality is neglected in phenomenological research, then the labors of what we call phenomenological research are nothing more than the sorting, classifying and describing that scientists have done since Aristotle. Zaner (1970), speaking of the phenomenologist, says that ". . . since his aim is to develop his discipline as rigorously as possible, and since that signifies that he must obtain the best possible evidence for the things to be studied, then clearly, the phenomenologist must turn to his own mental life" (p. 122). Husserl repeatedly presents us with the understanding that phenomenologists look at their own conscious processes as well as the phenomena they describe (1962, 1970b). He saw science as naïve about methods, unaware of the destructiveness of its objectivism, which is that detachment from, and dismissal of, the subjectivity, the self-interest, that launches all scientific projects (Husserl, 1970b). He believed that in phenomenology he had developed a first philosophy of science, and conveyed a caveat to all scientists and researchers for the necessity of self-awareness.

Bracketing

Any discussion about intentionality invokes the term bracketing. Bracketing is about objectivity. Objectivity (as opposed to objectivism, which means being caught in the belief that subjective experience can produce no true knowledge) in phenomenology means maintaining touch with one's intentionality, one's unique perspective of the phenomenon being studied. Bracketing is a frequently used term in reports of phenomenological studies and in the literature about phenomenological research methods. Husserl introduced the term, which recalls his mathematical background, as an analogy for the mental activity in which one puts out of play one's assumptions about the phenomenon under investigation. Bracketing is also a term associated with descriptive phenomenology as opposed to hermeneutic phenomenology and is a source of disagreement between the two perspectives (Giorgi, 1992). Descriptive phenomenologists, often regarded as Husserlian, aim for pure description in which past knowledge about a phenomenon is bracketed, allowing the phenomenon to been seen "precisely as it presents itself" (Giorgi, 1992, p. 121). Hermeneutic phenomenologists, frequently referred to as Heideggerian, see bracketing as a misnomer for the reflex-

ive processes occurring in interpretive research, and reject the idea that one can bracket one's unique viewpoint in order to see a phenomenon apart from the encumbrances of one's experience of it. Phenomenologists who see themselves as hermeneutical researchers believe that total objectivity, or neutrality, is not possible because of the impossibility of freeing oneself completely of involvement as a member of the lifeworld, the bedrock from which all research arises. Explication of these philosophical viewpoints is beyond our purpose here, however. The important point is not whether bracketing is possible, but the activity itself, i.e., the ongoing attempt to identify and explicate one's unique and particular experience of a phenomenon in order to see how such experience influences the results of one's research. Merleau-Ponty (1968) is clear that absolute objectivity, however desirable it may be, is an unreachable goal, that is, bracketing, with the aim of a total phenomenological reduction, is impossible. The reflexive activity that the term bracketing signifies, however, is essential to all phenomenological research. Reflexive consideration of one's experience with the subject matter of any scientific research project is essential for the validity of that research.

A Concrete Approach to Intentionality and Bracketing

Objectivity in positivistically oriented research is sought by attempting to purge a study of the researcher's personal connections to it and by reliance on statistical theory to account for significance. Objectivity in phenomenological research is approached directly by identifying and examining the researcher's subjective involvement with, experiencing of, the phenomenon being investigated. Gadamer (1994) and Heidegger (1962) refer to subjective involvement with the terms historicity, pre-understanding, assumptions. Such involvement can be a deterrent to grasping the principle or the essence of the phenomenon. As a researcher, I may have my own particular experience of a phenomenon and the impact of my experience may obscure the essence of the phenomenon, that is, those patterns of experiencing that can be recognized by others as their experience as well (Kohák, 1978). Because personal involvement with a phenomenon has its own uniqueness, phenomenology calls for a temporary setting aside, as nearly as possible, one's individual experience of the thing being explored. This reflexive activity is what Husserl called bracketing. But just how does one bracket, that is, reflect on one's assumptions? What does the term suggest, concretely? Burns & Grove (1993, 1997), who have been more inclusive of qualitative research methods than other authors of nursing research texts, have emphasized the need for researcher reflexivity. However, their recognition of the importance of researcher self-awareness stops short of concrete guidelines. In the 1993 edition of their nursing research text, they formulated guidelines for conducting credible phenomenological studies. They identified the pitfalls to be avoided during the analysis and writing phase of a study. They observed that the researcher's reasoning process which leads to decisions about categories and themes is usually neglected in research reports, and urged researchers to make "intense efforts" to account for the decision-making process during analysis of data (1993, p. 661). An exhortation to intensify efforts suggests that the will to perform the necessary step can substitute for lack of clear ways to proceed in uncovering the conscious processes involved in phenomenological interpretation and description. Clearly, there is a need for guidelines that show us how to proceed in this crucial aspect of phenomenological research.

Bracketing means setting aside one's assumptions and preunderstanding. How do we go about doing this? How are personal assumptions recognized? First, bracketing is not a research step that, once done, can be dispensed with. Bracketing goes on throughout a study, from the first moment that the topic or theme of a study is chosen, to the final discussion of the study's findings. Second, in order to set something aside, we have to be able to recognize and identify it. In phenomenological research we start by choosing a phenomenon that we want to understand more fully, and then begin the process of gathering information, usually through interviewing, or descriptive writing. Although examining one's assumptions should be on-going throughout a study, the bracketing that we will focus on here is that which occurs during the analysis phase of phenomenological research when themes are identified. Understanding how themes get recognized and selected for conceptual transformation can reveal aspects of the researcher's decision process that may not have been immediately apparent.

Typically, when we conduct phenomenological research we transcribe interview dialogue, and then undertake repeated reviews of the transcripts. We transform our interviewees' accounts of their experience into conceptual form and select language with which to describe the phenomenon under investigation, for example, the experience of chronic illness. In the process of examining a transcript and recalling the interview, some passages of the dialogue will stand out to us as important; the phenomenon shows itself to us. It is this "standing out" that phenomenological researchers then must consider, for it signifies the intentionality that Husserl repeatedly emphasized as central to phenomenology. Natanson (1973), discussing Husserl's insight, makes the point that when we look at an object or event in phenomenological research, we must do more than simply consider what is going on and then describe it, the researcher must also look at his or her own process of seeing, perceiving the phenomenon. "Intentionality carries with it a reflexive dimension which distinguishes it from what otherwise might be thought of as simple, straightforward inspection of data—the kind of close, painstakingly accurate description of animals done by some naturalists" (p. 13). The phenomenon of standing out is the initial part of the decision-making process through which themes emerge, and ultimately, phenomenological description is created. The researcher's account of this decision-making process is a crucial component for the validity and credibility of a phenomenological study. Recognizing and understanding what stands out to us in interview transcripts, in written or verbal data, is, in large part, what makes a study phenomenological because what stands out to us, if we look closely, indicates our own experiencing of the phenomenon under investigation. The next step in phenomenological research is setting aside, or bracketing the portions of data that stand out in order to grasp the principle or essence of the experience. We bracket our personal, particular history in order to see the experience "as such" (Kohák, 1978). The act of grasping the essence of a phenomenon goes beyond counting, or naming; it involves seeing as Husserl meant it—intuition—grasping the larger point, the meaning of the experience as such. This is what Husserl means by eidetic seeing.

Intentionality and Meaningfulness

When a passage in an interview transcript stands out, it does so because it signifies inherent meaningfulness for the reader. Such meaningfulness invites explication; it holds the key to the researcher's experience of the study and the way that the researcher's experience has contributed to the study's outcome. "Phenomena, unlike gods, are not self-generating; they point back to where they have come from and to how they have traversed their constitutive path" (Natanson, 1973, p. 98). When we understand our personal connection to a theme then we have begun to look at our own consciousness of the phenomenon under investigation, and we have begun the interpretive process. If we simply describe a phenomenon, however succinct and exquisite the description, we have not given a phenomenological account of it. It is not enough to write about our participants' experiencing; our own experiencing of the study belongs to the data as well.

What stands out to us does so because we have already been involved with it; it already holds meaning for us (Heidegger, 1962, 1967;

Gendlin, 1967). But the meaning needs explication so that it can emerge from an implicit to an explicit state and reveal how it influences our ability to be objective. The themes that suggest themselves to us as we read a transcript do so because our implicit understanding of the phenomenon we are studying is what allowed us to see it as a research topic in the first place. What appears as meaningful to me? This is the first question asked during inspection of an interview transcript. (If someone other than the interviewer transcribed the tape-recording, the transcript should be reviewed as the tape is replayed.) Identifying something as meaningful inevitably leads to the second, and more difficult question, "why?" Understanding why something is meaningful requires thoughtful reflecting on one's experience with the phenomenon under investigation. Such reflecting will inevitably call forth our values and beliefs, requiring that we examine them in light of the project at hand. As researchers we need to know why we have chosen to study particular problems or topics, why they are meaningful to us, because the answer provides additional information that is crucial to researcher objectivity.

All true phenomenological research invokes self-awareness in the researcher, if he or she is ready for such awareness. Self-awareness in phenomenological research is more than setting aside preconceptions. In a larger sense, it is self-discovery. Natanson (1973) states, "Husserlian reason is committed to the responsibility of man for sustaining and honoring philosophical reflection: the integral person seeking to know himself" (p. 18). Researcher self-awareness means literally discovering, in the act of perceiving the phenomenon under investigation, the deep, foundational basis of personal meaningfulness that is always implicitly present in one's research interests.

Reflection on meaningfulness returns the researcher to the lifeworld and particular experiences found meaningful. Meaningfulness always involves intersubjectivity, relating to others. Meaningfulness equates with intentionality. Meaningfulness guides our relating to the world and to others. The meaning that we bring to our interacting with the world and others is intentionality as Husserl saw it. If we understand what we find meaningful we understand how we are connected to the things that we study and how this connection must be taken into account if we are to produce research that enhances understanding of others and our mutual lifeworld.

We can now begin to formulate guidelines for undertaking the interpretive process in phenomenological research. The concrete activity of bracketing in the analysis phase of a phenemonological study begins with the search for one's relationship with the phenomenon by returning to the transcription passages that have stood out to us as significant. Some of these passages will be immediately identifiable as pointing to particular experiences that we have had relevant to the phenomenon. Connections to personal experience for other passages will be more difficult to name. At this point, it is not necessary to understand why a passage seems important, only that it is meaningful. As these passages are identified, it is important to be aware of one's emotional reactions and to record any thoughts to that effect. With the assistance of a colleague who is an expert listener, one who can listen unconditionally and take notes of the process at hand, one can identify the personal connections that particular passages hold. Gendlin's (1978) work with pre-verbal understanding, one's "felt sense," offers good preparation for this phase of phenomenological research, for what is meaningful to us makes its appearance first in the bodily understanding mode before it is articulated with language. In the process of searching for and identifying personally meaningful transcript passages, nothing is considered irrelevant, or trivial. One's bodily responses to, and seemingly random thoughts about, the ideas, memories, beliefs, hopes, convictions, values, etc. that are associated with the phenomenon guide the process, much in the same way that free association is done. The guiding question as one proceeds through the selected passages is: What is the significance that this line or passage holds for me? As researchers,

we need to keep in mind that we always have a personal history with that which we choose to study, otherwise, we would never have considered it worth pursuing (Heidegger, 1967, Gendlin, 1967). Arising from one's personal history with the phenomenon will be some assumptions that have been made about it, taken for granted as the way that this particular phenomenon is. These are the assumptions, the pre-understanding that will be placed in brackets, scrutinized for influence on the decisions made regarding the themes and conclusions drawn in the study.

Summary

We have noted Heidegger's contributions to phenomenology, particularly his ontology, and his restatement of Husserl's insistence that we are implicitly involved with whatever we seek to know. We have highlighted a missing element in much of phenomenological research today—the researcher's experience—and noted that neglect of the phenomenologist's conscious process points to a return to Husserl's philosophy. The task that lies before phenomenological researchers now is to expand existing protocols to include Husserl's insight that the researcher's experience, when considered as data, is crucial to any study purporting to be phenomenological.

Our research as phenomenologists begins in the lifeworld, of which we are members, and situates us in the realm of the intersubjective where we discover our fellow lifeworld members' experiencing to be akin to our own. In the course of our discoveries, if we are truly phenomenologically oriented, we gain appreciation for our own creative relationship with the phenomena that we study.

REFERENCES

Burns, N., & Grove, S. (1993). *The practice of nursing research: Conduct, critique & utilization* (2nd ed.). Philadelphia: Saunders.

Burns, N., & Grove, S. (1997). *The practice of nursing research: Conduct, critique & utilization* (3rd ed.). Philadelphia: Saunders.

Colaizzi, P. (1978). Psychological research as the phenomenologist views it. In R. Valle & M. King (Eds.), *Existential-phenomenological alternatives for psychology* (pp. 48–71). New York: Oxford University Press.

Gadamer, H-G. (1994). *Truth and method* (2nd ed.). (J. Weinsheimer & D. Marshall, trans.). New York: Continuum.

Gendlin, E. (1967). *An analysis of Martin Heidegger's* What is a thing? (monograph). Chicago: Regnery.

Gendlin, E. (1978). *Focusing*. New York: Everest House.

Giorgi, A (Ed.). (1985). *Phenomenology and psychological research*. Pittsburgh: Duquesne University Press.

Giorgi, A. (1992). Description versus interpretation: Competing alternative strategies for qualitative research. *Journal of Phenomenological Psychology 23*(2), 119–135.

Heidegger, M. (1962). *Being and time*. (J. Macquarrie & E. Robinson, trans.). New York: Harper & Row.

Heidegger, M. (1967). What is a thing? (W. B. Barton, Jr. & V. Deutsch, trans.). South Bend, IN: Regnery/Gateway.

Husserl, E. (1962). *Ideas: General introduction to pure phenomenology*. (W. R. B. Gibson, trans.). New York: Collier Macmillan. (Originally published 1931.)

Husserl, E. (1970a). *Logical investigations* (2 vols.). (J. Findlay, trans.). New York: Humanities Press.

Husserl, E. (1970b). *The crisis of European sciences and transcendental phenomenology*. (D. Carr, trans.). Evanston, IL: Northwestern University Press.

Husserl, E. (1977). *Cartesian meditations*. (D. Cairns, trans.). The Hague: Martinus Nijhoff.

Husserl, E. (1990). *The idea of phenomenology*. (W. Alston & G. Nakhnikian, trans.). Boston: Kluwer Academic Publishers.

Kohák, E. (1978). *Idea & experience: Edmund Husserl's project of phenomenology in* Ideas I. Chicago: University of Chicago Press.

Lynch-Sauer, J. (1985). Using a phenomenological research method to study nursing phenomena. In M. Leininger (Ed.), *Qualitative research methods in nursing* (pp. 93–107). New York: Grune & Stratton.

Merleau-Ponty, M. (1962). *Phenomenology of perception*. (C. Smith, trans.). London: Routledge & Kegan Paul.

Merleau-Ponty, M. (1964). *Signs*. (R. McCleary, trans.). Evanston, IL: Northwestern University Press.

Merleau-Ponty, M. (1968). *The visible and the invisible*. (A. Lingis, trans.). Evanston, IL: Northwestern University Press.

Merleau-Ponty, M. (1973). *Consciousness and the acquisition of language*. (H. Silverman, Trans.). Evanston, IL: Northwestern University Press.

Munhall, P., & Oiler-Boyd, C. (1993). *Nursing research: A qualitative perspective*. New York: National League for Nursing.

Natanson, M. (1973). *Edmund Husserl: Philosopher of infinite tasks*. Evanston, IL: Northwestern University Press.

Polkinghorne, D. (1989). Phenomenological research methods. In R. Valle & S. Halling (Eds.), *Existential-phenomenological perspectives in psychology* (pp. 41–59). New York: Plenum.

Spiegelberg, H. (1984). *The phenomenological movement* (3rd ed.). Boston: Martinus Nijhoff.

Zaner, R. (1970). *The way of phenomenology*. Indianapolis: Bobbs-Merrill.

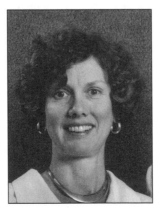

NANCY DREW

Exposition of the Question of the Meaning of Being

Martin Heidegger

The Necessity, Structure, and Priority of the Question of Being

1. The Necessity for Explicitly Restating the Question of Being

This question has today been forgotten. Even though in our time we deem it progressive to give our approval to 'metaphysics' again, it is held that we have been exempted from the exertions of a newly rekindled γιγαντομαχία περὶ τῆς οὐσίας. Yet the question we are touching upon is not just any question. It is one which provided a stimulus for the researchers of Plato and Aristotle, only to subside from then on *as a theme for actual investigation.*[1] What these two men achieved was to persist through many alterations and 'retouchings' down to the 'logic' of Hegel. And what they wrested with the utmost intellectual effort from the phenomena, fragmentary and incipient though it was, has long since become trivialized.

Not only that. On the basis of the Greeks' initial contributions towards an Interpretation of Being, a dogma has been developed which not only declares the question about the meaning of Being to be superfluous, but sanctions its

complete neglect. It is said that 'Being' is the most universal and the emptiest of concepts. As such it resists every attempt at definition. Nor does this most universal and hence indefinable concept require any definition, for everyone uses it constantly and already understands what he means by it. In this way, that which the ancient philosophers found continually disturbing as something obscure and hidden has taken on a clarity and self-evidence such that if anyone continues to ask about it he is charged with an error of method.

At the beginning of our investigation it is not possible to give a detailed account of the presuppositions and prejudices which are constantly reimplanting and fostering the belief that an inquiry into Being is unnecessary. They are rooted in ancient ontology itself, and it will not be possible to interpret that ontology adequately until the question of Being has been clarified and answered and taken as a clue—at least, if we are to have regard for the soil from which the basic ontological concepts developed, and if we are to see whether the categories have been demonstrated in a way that is appropriate and complete. We shall therefore carry the discussion of these presuppositions only to the point at which the necessity for restating the question about the meaning of Being becomes plain. There are three such presuppositions.

1. First, it has been maintained that 'Being' is the 'most universal' concept: τὸ ὄν ἐστι

καθόλου μάλιστα πάντων. Illud quod primo cadit sub apprehensione est ens, cuius intellectus includitur in omnibus, quaecumque quis apprehendit. 'An understanding of Being is already included in conceiving anything which one apprehends in entities.'[2] But the 'universality' of 'Being' is not that of a *class* or *genus*. The term 'Being' does not define that realm of entities which is uppermost when these are Articulated conceptually according to genus and species: *οὔτε τὸ ὂν γένος.* The 'universality' of Being 'transcends' any universality of genus. In medieval ontology 'Being' is designated as a '*transcendens*'. Aristotle himself knew the unity of this transcendental 'universal' as a *unity of analogy* in contrast to the multiplicity of the highest generic concepts applicable to things. With this discovery, in spite of his dependence on the way in which the ontological question had been formulated by Plato, he put the problem of Being on what was, in principle, a new basis. To be sure, even Aristotle failed to clear away the darkness of these categorial interconnections. In medieval ontology this problem was widely discussed, especially in the Thomist and Scotist schools, without reaching clarity as to principles. And when Hegel at last defines 'Being' as the 'indeterminate immediate' and makes this definition basic for all the further categorial explications of his 'logic', he keeps looking in the same direction as ancient ontology, except that he no longer pays heed to Aristotle's problem of the unity of Being as over against the multiplicity of 'categories' applicable to things. So if it is said that 'Being' is the most universal concept, this cannot mean that it is the one which is clearest or that it needs no further discussion. It is rather the darkest of all.

4   2. It has been maintained secondly that the concept of 'Being' is indefinable. This is deduced from its supreme universality, and rightly so, if *definitio fit per genus proximum et differentiam specificam.* 'Being' cannot indeed be conceived as an entity; *enti non additur aliqua natura*: nor can it acquire such a character as to have the term "entity" applied to it. "Being" cannot be derived from higher concepts by definition, nor can it be presented through lower ones. But does this imply that 'Being' no longer offers a problem? Not at all. We can infer only that 'Being' cannot have the character of an entity. Thus we cannot apply to Being the concept of 'definition' as presented in traditional logic, which itself has its foundations in ancient ontology and which, within certain limits, provides a justifiable way of characterizing "entities". The indefinability of Being does not eliminate the question of its meaning; it demands that we look that question in the face.

3. Thirdly, it is held that 'Being' is of all concepts the one that is self-evident. Whenever one cognizes anything or makes an assertion, whenever one comports oneself towards entities, even towards oneself,[3] some use is made of 'Being'; and this expression is held to be intelligible 'without further ado', just as everyone understands 'The sky *is* blue', 'I *am* merry', and the like. But here we have an average kind of intelligibility, which merely demonstrates that this is unintelligible. It makes manifest that in any way of comporting oneself towards entities as entities—even in any Being towards entities as entities—there lies *a priori* an enigma.[4] The very fact that we already live in an understanding of Being and that the meaning of Being is still veiled in darkness proves that it is necessary in principle to raise this question again.

Within the range of basic philosophical concepts—especially when we come to the concept of 'Being'—it is a dubious procedure to invoke self-evidence, if indeed the 'self-evident' (Kant's 'covert judgments of the common reason')[5] is to become the sole explicit and abiding theme for one's analytic—'the business of philosophers'.

By considering these prejudices, however, we have made plain not only that the question of Being lacks an *answer*, but that the question itself is obscure and without direction. So if it is to be revived, this means that we must first work out an adequate way of *formulating* it.

5   ## 2. THE FORMAL STRUCTURE OF THE QUESTION OF BEING

The question of the meaning of Being must be *formulated*. If it is a fundamental question, or indeed *the* fundamental question, it must be made transparent, and in an appropriate way.[6] We must therefore explain briefly what belongs to any question whatsoever, so that from this standpoint the question of Being can be made visible as a *very special* one with its own distinctive character.

Every inquiry is a seeking [Suchen]. Every seeking gets guided beforehand by what is sought. Inquiry is a cognizant seeking for an entity both with regard to the fact that it is and with regard to its Being as it is.[7] This cognizant seeking can take the form of 'investigating' ["Untersuchen"], in which one lays bare that which the question is about and ascertains its character. Any inquiry, as an inquiry about something, has *that which is asked about* [sein Gefragtes]. But all inquiry about something is somehow a questioning of something [Anfragen bei . . .]. So in addition to what is asked about, an inquiry has *that which is interrogated* [ein Befragtes]. In investigative questions—that is, in questions which are specifically theoretical—what is asked about is determined and conceptualized. Furthermore, in what is asked about there lies also *that which is to be found out by the asking* [das Erfragte]; this is what is really intended:[8] with this the inquiry reaches its goal. Inquiry itself is the behaviour of a questioner, and therefore of an entity, and as such has its own character of Being. When one makes an in-

quiry one may do so 'just casually' or one may formulate the question explicitly. The latter case is peculiar in that the inquiry does not become transparent to itself until all these constitutive factors of the question have themselves become transparent.

The question about the meaning of Being is to be *formulated*. We must therefore discuss it with an eye to these structural items.

Inquiry, as a kind of seeking, must be guided beforehand by what is sought. So the meaning of Being must already be available to us in some way. As we have intimated, we always conduct our activities in an understanding of Being. Out of this understanding arise both the explicit question of the meaning of Being and the tendency that leads us towards its conception. We do not *know* what 'Being' means. But even if we ask, 'What *is* "Being"?', we keep within an understanding of the 'is', though we are unable to fix conceptually what that 'is' signifies. We do not even know the horizon in terms of which that meaning is to be grasped and fixed. *But this vague average understanding of Being is still a Fact.*

However much this understanding of Being (an understanding which is already available to us) may fluctuate and grow dim, and border on mere acquaintance with a word, its very indefiniteness is itself a positive phenomenon which needs to be clarified. An investigation of the   6 meaning of Being cannot be expected to give this clarification at the outset. If we are to obtain the clue we need for Interpreting this average understanding of Being, we must first develop the concept of Being. In the light of this concept and the ways in which it may be explicitly understood, we can make out what this obscured or still unillumined understanding of Being means, and what kinds of obscuration—or hindrance to an explicit illumination—of the meaning of Being are possible and even inevitable.

Further, this vague average understanding of Being may be so infiltrated with traditional theories and opinions about Being that these remain hidden as sources of the way in which it is prevalently understood. What we seek when we inquire into Being is not something entirely unfamiliar, even if at first[9] we cannot grasp it at all.

In the question which we are to work out, *what is asked about* is Being—that which determines entities as entities, that on the basis of which [woraufhin] entities are already understood, however we may discuss them in detail. The Being of entities 'is' not itself an entity. If we are to understand the problem of Being, our first philosophical step consists in not μῦθόν τινα διηγεῖσθαι, in not 'telling a story'—that is to say, in not defining entities as entities by tracing them back in their origin to some other entities, as if Being had the character of some possible entity. Hence Being, as that which is asked about, must be exhibited in a way of its own, essentially different from the way in which entities are discovered. Accordingly, *what is to be found out by the asking*—the meaning of Being—also demands that it be conceived in a way of its own, essentially contrasting with the concepts in which entities acquire their determinate signification.

In so far as Being constitutes what is asked about, and "Being" means the Being of entities, then entities themselves turn out to be *what is interrogated*. These are, so to speak, questioned as regards their Being. But if the characteristics of their Being can be yielded without falsification, then these entities must, on their part, have become accessible as they are in themselves. When we come to what is to be interrogated, the question of Being requires that the right way of access to entities shall have been obtained and secured in advance. But there are many things which we designate as 'being' ["seiend"], and we do so in various senses. Everything we talk about, everything we have in view, everything towards which we comport ourselves in any way, is being; what we are is being, and so is how we are. Being lies in the fact that something is, and in its Being as it is; in Reality; in presence-at-hand; in subsistence; in validity; in Dasein; in the 'there is'.[10] In *which* en-

tities is the meaning of Being to be discerned? From which entities is the disclosure of Being to take its departure? Is the starting-point optional, or does some particular entity have priority when we come to work out the question of Being? Which entity shall we take for our example, and in what sense does it have priority?

If the question about Being is to be explicitly formulated and carried through in such a manner as to be completely transparent to itself, then any treatment of it in line with the elucidations we have given requires us to explain how Being is to be looked at, how its meaning is to be understood and conceptually grasped; it requires us to prepare the way for choosing the right entity for our example, and to work out the genuine way of access to it. Looking at something, understanding and conceiving it, choosing, access to it—all these ways of behaving are constitutive for our inquiry, and therefore are modes of Being for those particular entities which we, the inquirers, are ourselves. Thus to work out the question of Being adequately, we must make an entity—the inquirer—transparent in his own Being. The very asking of this question is an entity's mode of *Being*; and as such it gets its essential character from what is inquired about—namely, Being. This entity which each of us is himself and which includes inquiring as one of the possibilities of its Being, we shall denote by the term "*Dasein*".[11] If we are to formulate our question explicitly and transparently, we must first give a proper explication of an entity (Dasein), with regard to its Being.

Is there not, however, a manifest circularity in such an undertaking? If we must first define an entity *in its Being*, and if we want to formulate the question of Being only on this basis, what is this but going in a circle? In working out our question, have we not 'presupposed' something which only the answer can bring? Formal objections such as the argument about 'circular reasoning', which can easily be cited at any time in the study of first principles, are always sterile when one is considering concrete ways of investigating. When it comes to understanding the matter at hand, they carry no weight and keep us from penetrating into the field of study.

But factically[12] there is no circle at all in formulating our question as we have described. One can determine the nature of entities in their Being without necessarily having the explicit concept of the meaning of Being at one's disposal. Otherwise there could have been no ontological knowledge heretofore. One would hardly deny that factically there has been such knowledge.[13] Of course 'Being' has been presupposed in all ontology up till now, but not as a *concept* at one's disposal—not as the sort of thing we are seeking. This 'presupposing' of Being has rather the character of taking a look at it beforehand, so that in the light of it the entities presented to us get provisionally Articulated in their Being. This guiding activity of taking a look at Being arises from the average understanding of Being in which we always operate and *which in the end belongs to the essential constitution*[14] *of Dasein itself.* Such 'presupposing' has nothing to do with laying down an axiom from which a sequence of propositions is deductively derived. It is quite impossible for there to be any 'circular argument' in formulating the question about the meaning of Being; for in answering this question, the issue is not one of grounding something by such a derivation; it is rather one of laving bare the grounds for it and exhibiting them.[15]

In the question of the meaning of Being there is no 'circular reasoning' but rather a remarkable 'relatedness backward or forward' which what we are asking about (Being) bears to the inquiry itself as a mode of Being of an entity. Here what is asked about has an essential pertinence to the inquiry itself, and this belongs to the ownmost meaning [eigensten Sinn] of the question of Being. This only means, however, that there is a way—perhaps even a very special one—in which entities with the character of Dasein are related to the question of Being. But have we not thus demonstrated that a certain kind of entity has a priority with regard to its

Being? And have we not thus presented that entity which shall serve as the primary example to be *interrogated* in the question of Being? So far our discussion has not demonstrated Dasein's priority, nor has it shown decisively whether Dasein may possibly or even necessarily serve as the primary entity to be interrogated. But indeed something like a priority of Dasein has announced itself.

3. THE ONTOLOGICAL PRIORITY OF THE QUESTION OF BEING

When we pointed out the characteristics of the question of Being, taking as our clue the formal structure of the question as such, we made it clear that this question is a peculiar one, in that a series of fundamental considerations is required for working it out, not to mention for solving it. But its distinctive features will come fully to light only when we have delimited it adequately with regard to its function, its aim, and its motives.

Hitherto our arguments for showing that the question must be restated have been motivated in part by its venerable origin but chiefly by the lack of a definite answer and even by the absence of any satisfactory formulation of the question itself. One may, however, ask what purpose this question is supposed to serve. Does it simply remain—or *is* it at all—a mere matter for soaring speculation about the most general of generalities, *or is it rather, of all questions, both the most basic and the most concrete?*

Being is always the Being of an entity. The totality of entities can, in accordance with its various domains, become a field for laying bare and delimiting certain definite areas of subject-matter. These areas, on their part (for instance, history, Nature, space, life, Dasein, language, and the like), can serve as objects which corresponding scientific investigations may take as their respective themes. Scientific research accomplishes, roughly and naively, the demarcation and initial fixing of the areas of subject-matter. The basic structures of any such area have already been worked out after a fashion in our pre-scientific ways of experiencing and interpreting that domain of Being in which the area of subject-matter is itself confined. The 'basic concepts' which thus arise remain our proximal clues for disclosing this area concretely for the first time. And although research may always lean towards this positive approach, its real progress comes not so much from collecting results and storing them away in 'manuals' as from inquiring into the ways in which each particular area is basically constituted [Grundverfassungen]—an inquiry to which we have been driven mostly by reacting against just such an increase in information.

The real 'movement' of the sciences takes place when their basic concepts undergo a more or less radical revision which is transparent to itself. The level which a science has reached is determined by how far it is *capable* of a crisis in its basic concepts. In such immanent crises the very relationship between positively investigative inquiry and those things themselves that are under interrogation comes to a point where it begins to totter. Among the various disciplines everywhere today there are freshly awakened tendencies to put research on new foundations.

Mathematics, which is seemingly the most rigorous and most firmly constructed of the sciences, has reached a crisis in its 'foundations'. In the controversy between the formalists and the intuitionists, the issue is one of obtaining and securing the primary way of access to what are supposedly the objects of this science. The relativity theory of *physics* arises from the tendency to exhibit the interconnectedness of Nature as it is 'in itself'. As a theory of the conditions under which we have access to Nature itself, it seeks to 10 preserve the changelessness of the laws of motion by ascertaining all relativities, and thus comes up against the question of the structure of its own given area of study—the problem of matter. In *biology* there is an awakening tendency to inquire beyond the definitions which mechanism and vitalism have given for "life" and "organism", and to define anew the kind of Being which belongs to the living as such. In those *humane sciences which are historiological in character*,[16] the urge towards historical actuality itself has been strengthened in the course of time by tradition and by the way tradition has been presented and handed down: the history of literature is to become the history of problems. *Theology* is seeking a more primordial interpretation of man's Being towards God, prescribed by the meaning of faith itself and remaining within it. It is slowly beginning to understand once more Luther's insight that the 'foundation' on which its system of dogma rests has not arisen from an inquiry in which faith is primary, and that conceptually this 'foundation' not only is inadequate for the problematic of theology, but conceals and distorts it.

Basic concepts determine the way in which we get an understanding beforehand of the area of subject-matter underlying all the objects a science takes as its theme, and all positive investigation is guided by this understanding. Only after the area itself has been explored beforehand in a corresponding manner do these concepts become genuinely demonstrated and 'grounded'. But since every such area is itself obtained from the domain of entities themselves, this preliminary research, from which the basic concepts are drawn, signifies nothing else than an interpretation of those entities with regard to their basic state of Being. Such research must run ahead of the positive sciences, and it *can*. Here the work of Plato and Aristotle is evidence enough. Laying the foundations for the sciences in this way is different in principle from the kind of 'logic' which limps along after, investigating the status of some science as it chances to find it, in order to discover its 'method'. Laying the foundations, as we have described it, is rather a productive logic—in the sense that it leaps ahead, as it were, into some area of Being, discloses it for the first time in the constitution of its Being, and, after thus arriving at the structures within it, makes these available to the positive sciences as transparent assignments for their inquiry.[17] To give an example, what is philosophically primary is neither a theory of the concept-formation of historiology nor the theory of historiological knowledge, nor yet the theory of history as the Object of historiology; what is primary is rather the Interpretation of authentically historical entities as regards their historicality.[18] Similarly the positive outcome of Kant's *Critique of Pure Reason* lies in what it has contributed towards the working out 11 of what belongs to any Nature whatsoever, not in a 'theory' of knowledge. His transcendental logic is an *a priori* logic for the subject-matter of that area of Being called "Nature".

But such an inquiry itself—ontology taken in the widest sense without favouring any particular ontological directions or tendencies—requires a further clue. Ontological inquiry is indeed more primordial, as over against the ontical[19] inquiry of the positive sciences. But it remains itself naive and opaque if in its researches into the Being of entities it fails to discuss the meaning of Being in general. And the ontological task of a genealogy of the different possible ways of Being (which is not to be constructed deductively) is precisely of such a sort as to require that we first come to an understanding of 'what we really mean by this expression "Being"'.

The question of Being aims therefore at ascertaining the *a priori* conditions not only for the possibility of the sciences which examine entities as entities of such and such a type, and, in so doing, already operate with an understanding of Being, but also for the possibility of those ontologies themselves which are prior to the ontical sciences and which provide their foundations. *Basically, all ontology, no matter how rich and firmly compacted a system of categories it has at its disposal, remains blind and perverted from its ownmost aim, if it has not first adequately clarified the meaning of Being, and conceived this clarification as its fundamental task.*

Ontological research itself, when properly understood, gives to the question of Being an ontological priority which goes beyond mere resumption of a venerable tradition and advancement with a problem that has hitherto been opaque. But this objectively scientific priority is not the only one.

4. THE ONTICAL PRIORITY OF THE QUESTION OF BEING

Science in general may be defined as the totality established through an interconnection of true propositions.[20] This definition is not complete, nor does it reach the meaning of science. As ways in which man behaves, sciences have the manner of Being which this entity—man himself—possesses. This entity we denote by the term "*Dasein*". Scientific research is not the only manner of Being which this entity can have, nor is it the one which lies closest. Moreover, Dasein itself has a special distinctiveness as compared with other entities, and it is worth 12 our while to bring this to view in a provisional way. Here our discussion must anticipate later analyses, in which our results will be authentically exhibited for the first time.

Dasein is an entity which does not just occur among other entities. Rather it is ontically distinguished by the fact that, in its very Being, that Being is an *issue* for it. But in that case, this is a constitutive state of Dasein's Being, and this implies that Dasein, in its Being, has a relationship towards that Being—a relationship which itself is one of Being.[21] And this means further that there is some way in which Dasein understands itself in its Being, and that to some degree it does so explicitly. It is peculiar to this entity that with and through its Being, this Being is disclosed to it. *Understanding of Being is itself a definite characteristic of Dasein's Being.* Dasein is ontically distinctive in that it *is* ontological.[22]

Here "Being-ontological" is not yet tantamount to "developing an ontology". So if we should reserve the term "ontology" for that theoretical inquiry which is explicitly devoted to the meaning of entities, then what we have had in mind in speaking of Dasein's "Being-ontological" is to be designated as something "preontological". It does not signify simply "being-ontical", however, but rather "being in such a way that one has an understanding of Being".

That kind of Being towards which Dasein can comport itself in one way or another, and always does comport itself somehow, we call "*existence*" [*Existenz*]. And because we cannot define Dasein's essence by citing a "what" of the kind that pertains to a subject-matter [eines sachhaltigen Was], and because its essence lies rather in the fact that in each case it has its Being to be, and has it as its own,[23] we have chosen to designate this entity as "Dasein", a term which is purely an expression of its Being [als reiner Seinsausdruck].

Dasein always understands itself in terms of its existence—in terms of a possibility of itself: to be itself or not itself. Dasein has either chosen these possibilities itself, or got itself into them, or grown up in them already. Only the particular Dasein decides its existence, whether it does so by taking hold or by neglecting. The question of existence never gets straightened out except through existing itself. The understanding of oneself which leads *along this way* we call "*existentiell*".[24] The question of existence is one of Dasein's ontical 'affairs'. This does not require that the ontological structure of existence should be theoretically transparent. The question about that structure aims at the analysis [Auseinanderlegung] of what constitutes existence. The context [Zusammenhang] of such structures we call "*existentiality*". Its analytic has the character of an understanding which is not existentiell, but rather *existential*. The task
13 of an existential analytic of Dasein has been delineated in advance, as regards both its possibility and its necessity, in Dasein's ontical constitution.

So far as existence is the determining character of Dasein, the ontological analytic of this entity always requires that existentiality be considered beforehand. By "existentiality" we understand the state of Being that is constitutive for those entities that exist. But in the idea of such a constitutive state of Being, the idea of Being is already included. And thus even the possibility of carrying through the analytic of Dasein depends on working out beforehand the question about the meaning of Being in general.

Sciences are ways of Being in which Dasein comports itself towards entities which it need not be itself. But to Dasein, Being in a world is something that belongs essentially. Thus Dasein's understanding of Being pertains with equal primordiality both to an understanding of something like a 'world', and to the understanding of the Being of those entities which become accessible within the world.[25] So whenever an ontology takes for its theme entities whose character of Being is other than that of Dasein, it has its own foundation and motivation in Dasein's own ontical structure, in which a pre-ontological understanding of Being is comprised as a definite characteristic.

Therefore *fundamental ontology*, from which alone all other ontologies can take their rise, must be sought in the *existential analytic of Dasein*.

Dasein accordingly takes priority over all other entities in several ways. The first priority is an *ontical* one: Dasein is an entity whose Being has the determinate character of existence. The second priority is an *ontological* one: Dasein is in itself 'ontological', because existence is thus determinative for it. But with equal primordiality Dasein also possesses—as constitutive for its understanding of existence—an understanding of the Being of all entities of a character other than its own. Dasein has therefore a third priority as providing the ontico-ontological condition for the possibility of any ontologies. Thus Dasein has turned out to be, more than any other entity, the one which must first be interrogated ontologically.

But the roots of the existential analytic, on its part, are ultimately *existentiell*, that is, *ontical*. Only if the inquiry of philosophical research is itself seized upon in an existentiell manner as a possibility of the Being of each existing Dasein, does it become at all possible to disclose the existentiality of existence and to undertake an adequately founded ontological problematic. But 14 with this, the ontical priority of the question of being has also become plain.

Dasein's ontico-ontological priority was seen quite early, though Dasein itself was not grasped in its genuine ontological structure, and did not even become a problem in which this structure was sought. Aristotle says: ἡ ψυχὴ τὰ ὄντα πώς ἐστιν. "Man's soul is, in a certain way, entities." The 'soul' which makes up the Being of man has αἴσθησις and νόησις among its ways of Being, and in these it discovers all entities, both in the fact that they are, and in their Being as they are—that is, always in their Being. Aristotle's principle, which points back to the ontological thesis of Parmenides, is one which Thomas Aquinas has taken up in a characteristic discussion. Thomas is engaged in the task of deriving the '*transcendentia*'—those characters of Being which lie beyond every possible way in which an entity may be classified as coming under some generic kind of subject-matter (every *modus specialis entis*), and which belong necessarily to anything, whatever it may be. Thomas has to demonstrate that the *verum* is such a *transcendens*. He does this by invoking an entity which, in accordance with its very manner of Being, is properly suited to 'come together with' entities of any sort whatever. This distinctive entity, the *ens quod natum est convenire cum omni ente*, is the soul (*anima*). Here the priority of 'Dasein' over all other entities emerges, although it has not been ontologically clarified. This priority has obviously nothing in common with a vicious subjectivizing of the totality of entities.

By indicating Dasein's ontico-ontological priority in this provisional manner, we have grounded our demonstration that the question of Being is ontico-ontologically distinctive. But when we analysed the structure of this question as such (Section 2), we came up against a distinctive way in which this entity functions in the very formulation of that question. Dasein then revealed itself as that entity which must first be worked out in an ontologically adequate manner, if the inquiry is to become a transparent one. But now it has been shown that the ontological analytic of Dasein in general is what makes up fundamental ontology, so that Dasein functions as that entity which in principle is to be *interrogated* beforehand as to its Being.

If to Interpret the meaning of Being becomes our task, Dasein is not only the primary entity to be interrogated; it is also that entity which already comports itself, in its Being, towards what we are asking about when we ask this question. But in that case the question of Being is nothing other than the radicalization of an essential tendency-of-Being which belongs to Dasein itself—the pre-ontological understanding of Being.

The Twofold Task in Working Out the Question of Being. Method and Design of Our Investigation

5. THE ONTOLOGICAL ANALYTIC OF DASEIN AS LAYING BARE THE HORIZON FOR AN INTERPRETATION OF THE MEANING OF BEING IN GENERAL

In designating the tasks of 'formulating' the question of Being, we have shown not only that we must establish which entity is to serve as our primary object of interrogation, but also that the right way of access to this entity is one which we must explicitly make our own and hold secure. We have already discussed which entity takes over the principal role within the question of Being. But how are we, as it were, to set our sights towards this entity, Dasein, both as something accessible to us and as something to be understood and interpreted?

In demonstrating that Dasein is ontico-ontologically prior, we may have misled the reader into supposing that this entity must also be what is given as ontico-ontologically primary not only in the sense that it can itself be grasped 'immediately', but also in that the kind of Being which it possesses is presented just as 'immediately'. Ontically, of course, Dasein is not only close to us—even that which is closest: we *are* it, each of us, we ourselves. In spite of this, or rather for just this reason, it is ontologically that which is farthest. To be sure, its ownmost Being is such that it has an understanding of that Being, and already maintains itself in each case as if its Being has been interpreted in some manner. But we are certainly not saying that when Dasein's own Being is thus interpreted pre-ontologically in the way which lies closest, this interpretation can be taken over as an appropriate clue, as if this way of understanding Being is what must emerge when one's ownmost state of Being is considered[26] as an ontological theme. The kind of Being which belongs to Dasein is rather such that, in understanding its own Being, it has a tendency to do so in terms of that entity towards which it comports itself proximally and in a way which is essentially constant—in terms of the 'world'. In Dasein itself, and therefore in its own understanding of Being, the way the world is understood is, as we shall show, reflected back ontologically upon the way in which Dasein itself gets interpreted.

Thus because Dasein is ontico-ontologically prior, its own specific state of Being (if we understand this in the sense of Dasein's 'categorial structure') remains concealed from it. Dasein is ontically 'closest' to itself and ontologically farthest; but pre-ontologically it is surely not a stranger.

Here we have merely indicated provisionally that an Interpretation of this entity is confronted with peculiar difficulties grounded in the kind of Being which belongs to the object taken as our theme and to the very behaviour of so taking it. These difficulties are not grounded in any shortcomings of the cognitive powers with which we are endowed, or in the lack of a suitable way of conceiving—a lack which seemingly would not be hard to remedy.

Not only, however, does an understanding of Being belong to Dasein, but this understanding develops or decays along with whatever kind of Being Dasein may possess at the time; accordingly there are many ways in which it has been interpreted, and these are all at Dasein's disposal. Dasein's ways of behaviour, its capacities, powers, possibilities, and vicissitudes, have been studied with varying extent in philosophical psychology, in anthropology, ethics, and 'political science', in poetry, biography, and the writing of history, each in a different fashion. But the question remains whether these interpretations of Dasein have been carried through with a primordial existentiality comparable to whatever

existentiell primordiality they may have possessed. Neither of these excludes the other but they do not necessarily go together. Existentiell interpretation can demand an existential analytic, if indeed we conceive of philosophical cognition as something possible and necessary. Only when the basic structures of Dasein have been adequately worked out with explicit orientation towards the problem of Being itself, will what we have hitherto gained in interpreting Dasein get its existential justification.

Thus an analytic of Dasein must remain our first requirement in the question of Being. But in that case the problem of obtaining and securing the kind of access which will lead to Dasein, becomes even more a burning one. To put it negatively, we have no right to resort to dogmatic constructions and to apply just any idea of Being and actuality to this entity, no matter how 'self-evident' that idea may be; nor may any of the 'categories' which such an idea prescribes be forced upon Dasein without proper ontological consideration. We must rather choose such a way of access and such a kind of interpretation that this entity can show itself in itself and from itself [an ihm selbst von ihm selbst her]. And this means that it is to be shown as it is *proximally and for the most part*—in its average *everydayness*.[27] In this everydayness there are certain structures which we shall exhibit—not just any accidental structures, but essential ones which, in every kind of Being that factical Dasein may possess, persist as determinative for the character of its Being. Thus by having regard for the basic state of Dasein's everydayness, we shall bring out the Being of this entity in a preparatory fashion.

When taken in this way, the analytic of Dasein remains wholly oriented towards the guiding task of working out the question of Being. Its limits are thus determined. It cannot attempt to provide a complete ontology of Dasein, which assuredly must be constructed if anything like a 'philosophical' anthropology is to have a philosophically adequate basis.[28]

If our purpose is to make such an anthropol-

ogy possible, or to lay its ontological foundations, our Interpretation will provide only some
of the 'pieces', even though they are by no
means inessential ones. Our analysis of Dasein,
however, is not only incomplete; it is also, in the
first instance, *provisional*. It merely brings out
the Being of this entity, without Interpreting its
meaning. It is rather a preparatory procedure by
which the horizon for the most primordial way
of interpreting Being may be laid bare. Once we
have arrived at that horizon, this preparatory analytic of Dasein will have to be repeated on a
higher and authentically ontological basis.

We shall point to *temporality*[29] as the meaning
of the Being of that entity which we call "Dasein". If this is to be demonstrated, those structures of Dasein which we shall provisionally exhibit must be Interpreted over again as modes of
temporality. In thus interpreting Dasein as temporality, however, we shall not give the answer
to our leading question as to the meaning of Being in general. But the ground will have been
prepared for obtaining such an answer.

We have already intimated that Dasein has a
pre-ontological Being as its ontically constitutive state. Dasein *is* in such a way as to be something which understands something like Being.[30]
Keeping this interconnection firmly in mind, we
shall show that whenever Dasein tacitly understands and interprets something like Being, it
does so with *time* as its standpoint. Time must
be brought to light—and genuinely conceived—as the horizon for all understanding of
Being and for any way of interpreting it. In order for us to discern this, *time* needs to be *explicated primordially as the horizon for the understanding of Being, and in terms of temporality
as the Being of Dasein, which understands Being*.
This task as a whole requires that the conception
of time thus obtained shall be distinguished
from the way in which it is ordinarily under-
18 stood. This ordinary way of understanding it has
become explicit in an interpretation precipitated
in the traditional concept of time, which has
persisted from Aristotle to Bergson and even
later. Here we must make clear that this conception of time and, in general, the ordinary way of
understanding it, have sprung from temporality,
and we must show how this has come about. We
shall thereby restore to the ordinary conception
the autonomy which is its rightful due, as
against Bergson's thesis that the time one has in
mind in this conception is space.

'Time' has long functioned as an ontological—or rather an ontical—criterion for naively
discriminating various realms of entities. A distinction has been made between 'temporal' entities (natural processes and historical happenings) and 'non-temporal' entities (spatial and
numerical relationships). We are accustomed to
contrasting the 'timeless' meaning of propositions with the 'temporal' course of propositional
assertions. It is also held that there is a 'cleavage'
between 'temporal' entities and the 'supra-temporal' eternal, and efforts are made to bridge
this over. Here 'temporal' always means simply
being [seiend] 'in time'—a designation which,
admittedly, is still pretty obscure. The Fact remains that time, in the sense of 'being [sein] in
time', functions as a criterion for distinguishing
realms of Being. Hitherto no one has asked or
troubled to investigate how time has come to
have this distinctive ontological function, or
with what right anything like time functions as
such a criterion; nor has anyone asked whether
the authentic ontological relevance which is
possible for it, gets expressed when "time" is
used in so naively ontological a manner. 'Time'
has acquired this 'self-evident' ontological function 'of its own accord', so to speak; indeed it
has done so within the horizon of the way it is
ordinarily understood. And it has maintained itself in this function to this day.

In contrast to all this, our treatment of the
question of the meaning of Being must enable
us to show that *the central problematic of all ontology is rooted in the phenomenon of time, if
rightly seen and rigthly explained*, and we must
show *how* this is the case.

If Being is to be conceived in terms of time,
and if, indeed, its various modes and derivatives
are to become intelligible in their respective

modifications and derivations by taking time into consideration, then Being itself (and not merely entities, let us say, as entities 'in time') is thus made visible in its 'temporal' character. But in that case, 'temporal' can no longer mean simply 'being in time'. Even the 'non-temporal' and the 'supra-temporal' are 'temporal' with regard to their Being, and not just privatively by contrast with something 'temporal' as an entity 'in time', but in a *positive* sense, though it is one which we must first explain. In both pre-philosophical and philosophical usage the expression 'temporal' has been pre-empted by the signification we have cited; in the following investigations, however, we shall employ it for another signification. Thus the way in which Being and its modes and characteristics have their meaning determined primordially in terms of time, is what we shall call its "*Temporal*" determinateness.[31] Thus the fundamental ontological task of Interpreting Being as such includes working out the *Temporality of Being*. In the exposition of the problematic of Temporality the question of the meaning of Being will first be concretely answered.

Because Being cannot be grasped except by taking time into consideration, the answer to the question of Being cannot lie in any proposition that is blind and isolated. The answer is not properly conceived if what it asserts propositionally is just passed along, especially if it gets circulated as a free-floating result, so that we merely get informed about a 'standpoint' which may perhaps differ from the way this has hitherto been treated. Whether the answer is a 'new' one remains quite superficial and is of no importance. Its positive character must lie in its being *ancient* enough for us to learn to conceive the possibilities which the 'Ancients' have made ready for us. In its ownmost meaning this answer tells us that concrete ontological research must begin with an investigative inquiry which keeps within the horizon we have laid bare; and this is all that it tells us.

If, then, the answer to the question of Being is to provide the clues for our research, it cannot

be adequate until it brings us the insight that the specific kind of Being of ontology hitherto, and the vicissitudes of its inquiries, its findings, and its failures, have been necessitated in the very character of Dasein.

6. The Task of Destroying the History of Ontology

All research—and not least that which operates within the range of the central question of Being—is an ontical possibility of Dasein. Dasein's Being finds its meaning in temporality. But temporality is also the condition which makes historicality possible as a temporal kind of Being which Dasein itself possesses, regardless of whether or how Dasein is an entity 'in time'. Historicality, as a determinate character, is prior to what is called "history" (world-historical historizing).[32]

"Historicality" stands for the state of Being that is constitutive for Dasein's 'historizing' as such; only on the basis of such 'historizing' is anything like 'world-history' possible or can anything belong historically to world-history. In its factical Being, any Dasein is as it already was, and it is 'what' it already was. It *is* its past, whether explicitly or not. And this is so not only in that its past is, as it were, pushing itself along 'behind' it, and that Dasein possesses what is past as a property which is still present-at-hand and which sometimes has after-effects upon it: Dasein 'is' its past in the way of *its* own Being, which, to put it roughly, 'historizes' out of its future on each occasion.[33] Whatever the way of being it may have at the time, and thus with whatever understanding of Being it may possess, Dasein has grown up both into and in a traditional way of interpreting itself: in terms of this it understands itself proximally and, within a certain range, constantly. By this understanding, the possibilities of its Being are disclosed and regulated. Its own past—and this always means the past of its 'generation'—is not something which *follows along after* Dasein, but something which already goes ahead of it.

This elemental historicality of Dasein may remain hidden from Dasein itself. But there is a way by which it can be discovered and given proper attention. Dasein can discover tradition, preserve it, and study it explicitly. The discovery of tradition and the disclosure of what it 'transmits' and how this is transmitted, can be taken hold of as a task in its own right. In this way Dasein brings itself into the kind of Being which consists in historiological inquiry and research. But historiology—or more precisely historicity[34]—is possible as a kind of Being which the inquiring Dasein may possess, only because historicality is a determining characteristic for Dasein in the very basis of its Being. If this historicality remains hidden from Dasein, and as long as it so remains, Dasein is also denied the possibility of historiological inquiry or the discovery of history. If historiology is wanting, this is not evidence *against* Dasein's historicality; on the contrary, as a deficient mode[35] of this state of Being, it is evidence for it. Only because it is 'historical' can an era be unhistoriological.

On the other hand, if Dasein has seized upon its latent possibility not only of making its own existence transparent to itself but also of inquiring into the meaning of existentiality itself (that is to say, of previously inquiring into the meaning of Being in general), and if by such inquiry its eyes have been opened to its own essential historicality, then one cannot fail to see that the inquiry into Being (the ontico-ontological necessity of which we have already indicated) is itself characterized by historicality. The ownmost meaning of Being which belongs to the inquiry into Being as an historical inquiry, gives us the

21   assignment [Anweisung] of inquiring into the history of that inquiry itself, that is, of becoming historiological. In working out the question of Being, we must heed this assignment, so that by positively making the past our own, we may bring ourselves into full possession of the ownmost possibilities of such inquiry. The question of the meaning of Being must be carried through by explicating Dasein beforehand in its temporality and historicality; the question thus

brings itself to the point where it understands itself as historiological.

Our preparatory Interpretation of the fundamental structures of Dasein with regard to the average kind of Being which is closest to it (a kind of Being in which it is therefore proximally historical as well), will make manifest, however, not only that Dasein is inclined to fall back upon its world (the world in which it is) and to interpret itself in terms of that world by its reflected light, but also that Dasein simultaneously falls prey to the tradition of which it has more or less explicitly taken hold.[36] This tradition keeps it from providing its own guidance, whether in inquiring or in choosing. This holds true—and by no means least—for that understanding which is rooted in Dasein's ownmost Being, and for the possibility of developing it—namely, for ontological understanding.

When tradition thus becomes master, it does so in such a way that what it 'transmits' is made so inaccessible, proximally and for the most part, that it rather becomes concealed. Tradition takes what has come down to us and delivers it over to self-evidence; it blocks our access to those primordial 'sources' from which the categories and concepts handed down to us have been in part quite genuinely drawn.[37] Indeed it makes us forget that they have had such an origin, and makes us suppose that the necessity of going back to these sources is something which we need not even understand. Dasein has had its historicality so thoroughly uprooted by tradition that it confines its interest to the multiformity of possible types, directions, and standpoints of philosophical activity in the most exotic and alien of cultures; and by this very interest it seeks to veil the fact that it has no ground of its own to stand on. Consequently, despite all its historiological interests and all its zeal for an Interpretation which is philologically 'objective' ["sachliche"], Dasein no longer understands the most elementary conditions which would alone enable it to go back to the past in a positive manner and make it productively its own.

We have shown at the outset (Section I) not only that the question of the meaning of Being is one that has not been attended to and one that has been inadequately formulated, but that it has become quite forgotten in spite of all our interest in 'metaphysics'. Greek ontology and its history—which, in their numerous filiations and distortions, determine the conceptual character of philosophy even today—prove that when Dasein understands either itself or Being in general, it does so in terms of the 'world', and that the ontology which has thus arisen has deteriorated [verfällt] to a tradition in which it gets reduced to something self-evident—merely material for reworking, as it was for Hegel. In the Middle Ages this uprooted Greek ontology became a fixed body of doctrine. Its systematics, however, is by no means a mere joining together of traditional pieces into a single edifice. Though its basic conceptions of Being have been taken over dogmatically from the Greeks, a great deal of unpretentious work has been carried on further within these limits. With the peculiar character which the Scholastics gave it, Greek ontology has, in its essentials, travelled the path that leads through the *Disputationes metaphysicae* of Suarez to the 'metaphysics' and transcendental philosophy of modern times, determining even the foundations and the aims of Hegel's 'logic'. In the course of this history certain distinctive domains of Being have come into view and have served as the primary guides for subsequent problematics: the *ego cogito* of Descartes, the subject, the "I", reason, spirit, person. But these all remain uninterrogated as to their Being and its structure, in accordance with the thoroughgoing way in which the question of Being has been neglected. It is rather the case that the categorial content of the traditional ontology has been carried over to these entities with corresponding formalizations and purely negative restrictions, or else dialectic has been called in for the purpose of Interpreting the substantiality of the subject ontologically.

If the question of Being is to have its own history made transparent, then this hardened tradition must be loosened up, and the concealments which it has brought about[38] must be dissolved. We understand this task as one in which by taking *the question of Being as our clue*, we are to *destroy* the traditional content of ancient ontology until we arrive at those primordial experiences in which we achieved our first ways of determining the nature of Being—the ways which have guided us ever since.

In thus demonstrating the origin of our basic ontological concepts by an investigation in which their 'birth certificate' is displayed, we have nothing to do with a vicious relativizing of ontological standpoints. But this destruction is just as far from having the *negative* sense of shaking off the ontological tradition. We must, on the contrary, stake out the positive possibilities of that tradition, and this always means keeping it within its *limits*; these in turn are given factically in the way the question is formulated at the time, and in the way the possible field for investigation is thus bounded off. On its negative side, this destruction does not relate itself towards the past; its criticism is aimed at 'today' and at the prevalent way of treating the history of ontology, whether it is headed towards doxography, towards intellectual history, or towards a history of problems. But to bury the past in nullity [Nichtigkeit] is not the purpose of this destruction; its aim is *positive*; its negative function remains unexpressed and indirect.

The destruction of the history of ontology is essentially bound up with the way the question of Being is formulated, and it is possible only within such a formulation. In the framework of our treatise, which aims at working out that question in principle, we can carry out this destruction only with regard to stages of that history which are in principle decisive.

In line with the positive tendencies of this destruction, we must in the first instance raise the question whether and to what extent the Interpretation of Being and the phenomenon of time have been brought together thematically in the course of the history of ontology, and whether the problematic of Temporality required for this has ever been worked out in principle or ever could have been. The first and only person who has gone any stretch of the way towards investigating the dimension of Temporality or has even let himself be drawn hither by the coercion of the phenomena themselves is Kant. Only when we have established the problematic of Temporality, can we succeed in casting light on the obscurity of his doctrine of the schematism. But this will also show us *why* this area is one which had to remain closed off to him in its real dimensions and its central ontological function. Kant himself was aware that he was venturing into an area of obscurity: 'This schematism of our understanding as regards appearances and their mere form is an art hidden in the depths of the human soul, the true devices of which are hardly ever to be divined from Nature and laid uncovered before our eyes.' Here Kant shrinks back, as it were, in the face of something which must be brought to light as a theme and a principle if the expression "Being" is to have any demonstrable meaning. In the end, those very phenomena which will be exhibited under the heading of 'Temporality' in our analysis, are precisely those *most covert* judgments of the 'common reason' for which Kant says it is the 'business of philosophers' to provide an analytic.

24 In pursuing this task of destruction with the problematic of Temporality as our clue, we shall try to Interpret the chapter on the schematism and the Kantian doctrine of time, taking that chapter as our point of departure. At the same time we shall show why Kant could never achieve an insight into the problematic of Temporality. There were two things that stood in his way: in the first place, he altogether neglected the problem of Being; and, in connection with this, he failed to provide an ontology with Dasein as its theme or (to put this in Kantian language) to give a preliminary ontological analytic of the subjectivity of the subject. Instead of this, Kant took over Descartes' position quite dogmatically, notwithstanding all the essential respects in which he had gone beyond him. Furthermore, in spite of the fact that he was bringing the phenomenon of time back into the subject again, his analysis of it remained oriented towards the traditional way in which time had been ordinarily understood; in the long run this kept him from working out the phenomenon of a 'transcendental determination of time' in its own structure and function. Because of this double effect of tradition the decisive *connection* between *time* and the '*I think*' was shrouded in utter darkness; it did not even become a problem.

In taking over Descartes' ontological position Kant made an essential omission: he failed to provide an ontology of Dasein. This omission was a decisive one in the spirit [im Sinne] of Descartes' ownmost tendencies. With the '*cogito sum*' Descartes had claimed that he was putting philosophy on a new and firm footing. But what he left undetermined when he began in this 'radical' way, was the kind of Being which belongs to the *res cogitans*, or—more precisely—the *meaning of the Being of the 'sum'*.[39] By working out the unexpressed ontological foundations of the '*cogito sum*', we shall complete our sojourn at the second station along the path of our destructive retrospect of the history of ontology. Our Interpretation will not only prove that Descartes had to neglect the question of Being altogether; it will also show why he came to suppose that the absolute 'Being-certain' ["Gewissein"] of the *cogito* exempted him from raising the question of the meaning of the Being which this entity possesses.

Yet Descartes not only continued to neglect this and thus to accept a completely indefinite ontological status for the *res cogitans sive mens sive animus* ['the thing which cognizes, whether it be a mind or spirit']: he regarded this entity as a *fundamentum inconcussum*, and applied the medieval ontology to it in carrying through the fundamental considerations of his *Meditationes*. He defined the *res cogitans* ontologically as an *ens*; and in the medieval ontology the meaning of Being for such an *ens* had been fixed by understanding it as an *ens creatum*. God, as *ens in-*

finitum, was the *ens increatum*. But createdness [Geschaffenheit] in the widest sense of something's having been produced [Hergestelltheit], was an essential item in the structure of the ancient conception of Being. The seemingly new beginning which Descartes proposed for philosophizing has revealed itself as the implantation of a baleful prejudice, which has kept later generations from making any thematic ontological analytic of the 'mind' ["Gemütes"] such as would take the question of Being as a clue and would at the same time come to grips critically with the traditional ancient ontology.

Everyone who is acquainted with the middle ages sees that Descartes is 'dependent' upon medieval scholasticism and employs its terminology. But with this 'discovery' nothing is achieved philosophically as long as it remains obscure to what a profound extent the medieval ontology has influenced the way in which posterity has determined or failed to determine the ontological character of the *res cogitans*. The full extent of this cannot be estimated until both the meaning and the limitations of the ancient ontology have been exhibited in terms of an orientation directed towards the question of Being. In other words, in our process of destruction we find ourselves faced with the task of Interpreting the basis of the ancient ontology in the light of the problematic of Temporality. When this is done, it will be manifest that the ancient way of interpreting the Being of entities is oriented towards the 'world' or 'Nature' in the widest sense, and that it is indeed in terms of 'time' that its understanding of Being is obtained. The outward evidence for this (though of course it is *merely* outward evidence) is the treatment of the meaning of Being as παρουσία or οὐσία, which signifies, in ontologico-Temporal terms, 'presence' ["Anwesenheit"].[40] Entities are grasped in their Being as 'presence'; this means that they are understood with regard to a definite mode of time—the '*Present*'.[41]

The problematic of Greek ontology, like that of any other, must take its clues from Dasein itself. In both ordinary and philosophical usage, Dasein, man's Being, is 'defined' as the ζῷον λόγον ἔχον—as that living thing whose Being is essentially determined by the potentiality for discourse.[42] λέγειν is the clue for arriving at those structures of Being which belong to the entities we encounter in addressing ourselves to anything or speaking about it [im Ansprechen und Besprechen]. (Cf. Section 7 B.) This is why the ancient ontology as developed by Plato turns into 'dialectic'. As the ontological clue gets progressively worked out—namely, in the 'hermeneutic' of the λόγος—it becomes increasingly possible to grasp the problem of Being in a more radical fashion. The 'dialectic', which has been a genuine philosophical embarrassment, becomes superfluous. That is *why* Aristotle 'no longer has any understanding' of it, for he has put it on a more radical footing and raised it to a new level [aufhob]. λέγειν itself—or rather νοεῖν, that simple awareness of something present-at-hand in its sheer presence-at-hand,[43] which Parmenides had already taken to guide him in his own interpretation of Being—has the Temporal structure of a pure 'making-present' of something.[44] Those entities which show themselves in this and for it, and which are understood as entities in the most authentic sense, thus get interpreted with regard to the Present; that is, they are conceived as presence (οὐσία).[45]

Yet the Greeks have managed to interpret Being in this way without any explicit knowledge of the clues which function here, without any acquaintance with the fundamental ontological function of time or even any understanding of it, and without any insight into the reason why this function is possible. On the contrary, they take time itself as one entity among other entities, and try to grasp it in the structure of its Being, though that way of understanding Being which they have taken as their horizon is one which is itself naively and inexplicitly oriented towards time.

Within the framework in which we are about to work out the principles of the question of Being, we cannot present a detailed Temporal Interpretation of the foundations of ancient ontology, particularly not of its loftiest and purest scientific stage, which is reached in Aristotle. Instead we shall give an interpretation of Aristotle's essay on time, which may be chosen as providing a way of *discriminating* the basis and the limitations of the ancient science of Being.

Aristotle's essay on time is the first detailed Interpretation of this phenomenon which has come down to us. Every subsequent account of time, including Bergson's, has been essentially determined by it. When we analyse the Aristotelian conception, it will likewise become clear, as we go back, that the Kantian account of time operates within the structures which Aristotle has set forth; this means that Kant's basic ontological orientation remains that of the Greeks, in spite of all the distinctions which arise in a new inquiry.

The question of Being does not achieve its true concreteness until we have carried through the process of destroying the ontological tradition. In this way we can fully prove that the question of the meaning of Being is one that we cannot avoid, and we can demonstrate what it means to talk about 'restating' this question.

In any investigation in this field, where 'the thing itself is deeply veiled' one must take pains not to overestimate the results. For in such an inquiry one is constantly compelled to face the possibility of disclosing an even more primordial and more universal horizon from which we may 27 draw the answer to the question, "What is '*Being*'?" We can discuss such possibilities seriously and with positive results only if the question of Being has been reawakened and we have arrived at a field where we can come to terms with it in a way that can be controlled.

7. THE PHENOMENOLOGICAL METHOD OF INVESTIGATION

In provisionally characterizing the object which serves as the theme of our investigation (the Being of entities, or the meaning of Being in general), it seems that we have also delineated the method to be employed. The task of ontology is to explain Being itself and to make the Being of entities stand out in full relief. And the method of ontology remains questionable in the highest degree as long as we merely consult those ontologies which have come down to us historically, or other essays of that character. Since the term "ontology" is used in this investigation in a sense which is formally broad, any attempt to clarify the method of ontology by tracing its history is automatically ruled out.

When, moreover, we use the term "ontology", we are not talking about some definite philosophical discipline standing in interconnection with the others. Here one does not have to measure up to the tasks of some discipline that has been presented beforehand; on the contrary, only in terms of the objective necessities of definite questions and the kind of treatment which the 'things themselves' require, can one develop such a discipline.

With the question of the meaning of Being, our investigation comes up against the fundamental question of philosophy. This is one that must be treated *phenomenologically*. Thus our treatise does not subscribe to a 'standpoint' or represent any special 'direction'; for phenomenology is nothing of either sort, nor can it become so as long as it understands itself. The expression 'phenomenology' signifies primarily a *methodological conception*. This expression does not characterize the what of the objects of philosophical research as subject-matter, but rather the *how* of that research. The more genuinely a methodological concept is worked out and the more comprehensively it determines the principles on which a science is to be conducted, all the more primordially is it rooted in the way we come to terms with the things themselves,[46] and the farther is it removed from what we call "technical devices", though there are many such devices even in the theoretical disciplines.

Thus the term 'phenomenology' expresses a maxim which can be formulated as 'To the 28 things themselves!' It is opposed to all free-floating constructions and accidental findings; it is opposed to taking over any conceptions which only seem to have been demonstrated; it is opposed to those pseudo-questions which parade themselves as 'problems', often for generations at a time. Yet this maxim, one may rejoin, is abundantly self-evident, and it expresses, moreover, the underlying principle of any scientific knowledge whatsoever. Why should anything so self-evident be taken up explicitly in giving a title to a branch of research? In point of fact, the issue here is a kind of 'self-evidence' which we should like to bring closer to us, so far as it is important to do so in casting light upon the procedure of our treatise. We shall expound only the preliminary conception [Vorbegriff] of phenomenology.

This expression has two components: "phenomenon" and "logos". Both of these go back to terms from the Greek: φαινόμενον and λόγος. Taken superficially, the term "phenomenology" is formed like "theology", "biology", "sociology"—names which may be translated as "science of God", "science of life", "science of society". This would make phenomenology the *science of phenomena*. We shall set forth the preliminary conception of phenomenology by characterizing what one has in mind in the term's two components, 'phenomenon' and 'logos', and by establishing the meaning of the name in which these are *put together*. The history of the word itself, which presumably arose in the Wolffian school, is here of no significance.

A. The Concept of Phenomenon

The Greek expression φαινόμενον, to which the term 'phenomenon' goes back, is derived from the verb φαίνεσθαι, which signifies "to show itself". Thus φαινόμενον means that which shows itself, the manifest [das, was sich zeigt, das Sichzeigende, das Offenbare]. φαίνεσθαι itself is a *middle-voiced* form which comes from φαίνω—to bring to the light of day, to put in the light. Φαίνω comes from the stem φα—, like φῶς, the light, that which is bright—in other words, that wherein something can become manifest, visible in itself. Thus we must *keep in mind* that the expression '*phenomenon*' signifies *that which shows itself in itself*, the manifest. Ac-

cordingly the φαινόμενα or 'phenomena' are the totality of what lies in the light of day or can be brought to the light—what the Greeks sometimes identified simply with τα ὄντα (entities). Now an entity can show itself from itself [von ihm selbst her] in many ways, depending in each case on the kind of access we have to it. Indeed it is even possible for an entity to show itself as something which in itself it is *not*. When it shows itself in this way, it 'looks like something or other' ["sieht" . . . "so aus wie . . ."]. This kind of showing-itself is what we call "*seeming*" [*Scheinen*]. Thus in Greek too the expression φαινόμενον ("phenomenon") signifies that which looks like something, that which is 'semblant', 'semblance' [das "Scheinbare", der "Schein"]. Φαινόμενον ἀγαθόν means something good which looks like, but 'in actuality' is not, what it gives itself out to be. If we are to have any further understanding of the concept of phenomenon, everything depends on our seeing how what is designated in the first signification of φαινόμενον ('phenomenon' as that which shows itself) and what is designated in the second ('phenomenon' as semblance) are structurally interconnected. Only when the meaning of something is such that it makes a pretension of showing itself—that is, of being a phenomenon—*can* it show itself *as* something which it is *not*; only then *can* it 'merely look like so-and-so'. When φαινόμενον signifies 'semblance', the primordial signification (the phenomenon as the manifest) is already included as that upon which the second signification is founded. We shall allot the term 'phenomenon' to this positive and primordial signification of φαινόμενον, and distinguish "phenomenon" from "semblance", which is the privative modification of "phenomenon" as thus defined. But what *both* these terms express has proximally nothing at all to do with what is called an 'appearance', or still less a 'mere appearance'.[47]

This is what one is talking about when one speaks of the 'symptoms of a disease' ["Krankheitserscheinungen"]. Here one has in mind certain occurrences in the body which show themselves and which, in showing themselves as thus showing themselves, 'indicate' ["indizieren"] something which does *not* show itself. The emergence [Auftreten] of such occurrences, their showing-themselves, goes together with the Being-present-at-hand of disturbances which do not show themselves. Thus appearance, as the appearance 'of something', does *not* mean showing-itself; it means rather the announcing-itself by [von] something which does not show itself, but which announces itself through something which does show itself. Appearing is a *not-showing-itself*. But the 'not' we find here is by no means to be confused with the privative "not" which we used in defining the structure of semblance.[48] What appears does *not* show itself; and anything which thus fails to show itself, is also something which can never seem.[49] All indications, presentations, symptoms, and symbols have this basic formal structure of appearing, even though they differ among themselves.

In spite of the fact that 'appearing' is never a showing-itself in the sense of "phenomenon," appearing is possible only *by reason of a showing-itself* of something. But this showing-itself, which helps to make possible the appearing, is not the appearing itself. Appearing is an *announcing*-itself [das Sich-*melden*] through something that shows itself. If one then says that with the word 'appearance' we allude to something wherein something appears without being itself an appearance, one has not thereby defined the concept of phenomenon: one has rather *presupposed* it. This presupposition, however, remains concealed; for when one says this sort of thing about 'appearance,' the expression 'appear' gets used in two ways. "That wherein something 'appears'" means that wherein something announces itself, and therefore does not show itself; and in the words [Rede] 'without being itself an "appearance"', "appearance" signifies the *showing-itself*. But this showing-itself belongs essentially to the 'wherein' in which something announces itself. According to this, phenomena are *never* appearances,

though on the other hand every appearance is dependent on phenomena. If one defines "phenomenon" with the aid of a conception of 'appearance' which is still unclear, then everything is stood on its head, and a 'critique' of phenomenology on this basis is surely a remarkable undertaking.

So again the expression 'appearance' itself can have a double signification: first, *appearing*, in the sense of announcing-itself, as not-showing-itself; and next, that which does the announcing [das Meldende selbst]—that which in its showing-itself indicates something which does not show itself. And finally one can use "appearing" as a term for the genuine sense of "phenomenon" as showing-itself. If one designates these three different things as 'appearance,' bewilderment is unavoidable.

But this bewilderment is essentially increased by the fact that 'appearance' can take on still another signification. That which does the announcing—that which, in its showing-itself, indicates something non-manifest—may be taken as that which emerges in what is itself non-manifest, and which emanates [ausstrahlt] from it in such a way indeed that the non-manifest gets thought of as something that is essentially *never* manifest. When that which does the announcing is taken this way, "appearance" is tantamount to a "bringing forth" or "something brought forth," but something which does not make up the real Being of what brings it forth: here we have an appearance in the sense of 'mere appearance.' That which does the announcing and is brought forth does, of course, show itself, and in such a way that, as an emanation of what it announces, it keeps this very thing constantly veiled in itself. On the other hand, this not-showing which veils is not a semblance. Kant uses the term "appearance" in this twofold way. According to him "appearances" are, in the first place, the 'objects of empirical intuition': they are what shows itself in such intuition. But what thus shows itself (the "phenomenon" in the genuine primordial sense) is at the same time an 'appearance' as an emanation of something which *hides* itself in that appearance—an emanation which announces.

In so far as a phenomenon is constitutive for 'appearance' in the signification of announcing itself through something which shows itself, though such a phenomenon can privatively take the variant form of semblance, appearance too can become mere semblance. In a certain kind of lighting someone can look as if his cheeks were flushed with red; and the redness which shows itself can be taken as an announcement of the Being-present-at-hand of a fever, which in turn indicates some disturbance in the organism.

31

"*Phenomenon*", the showing-itself-in-itself, signifies a distinctive way in which something can be encountered.[50] "*Appearance*", on the other hand, means a reference-relationship which is in an entity itself,[51] and which is such that what *does the referring* (or the announcing) can fulfil its possible function only if it shows itself in itself and is thus a 'phenomenon'. Both appearance and semblance are founded upon the phenomenon, though in different ways. The bewildering multiplicity of 'phenomena' designated by the words "phenomenon", "semblance", "appearance", "mere appearance", cannot be disentangled unless the concept of the phenomenon is understood from the beginning as that which shows itself in itself.

If in taking the concept of "phenomenon" this way, we leave indefinite which entities we consider as "phenomena", and leave it open whether what shows itself is an entity or rather some characteristic which an entity may have in its Being, then we have merely arrived at the *formal* conception of "phenomenon". If by "that which shows itself" we understand those entities which are accessible through the empirical "intuition" in, let us say, Kant's sense, then the formal conception of "phenomenon" will indeed be legitimately employed. In this usage "phenomenon" has the signification of the *ordinary* conception of phenomenon. But this ordinary conception is not the phenomenological conception. If we keep within the horizon of the Kantian problematic, we can give an illustration of what is conceived phenomenologically as a "phenomenon", with reservations as to other differences; for we may then say that that which already shows itself in the appearance as prior to the "phenomenon" as ordinarily understood and as accompanying it in every case, can, even though it thus shows itself unthematically, be brought thematically to show itself; and what thus shows itself in itself (the 'forms of the intuition') will be the "phenomena" of phenomenology. For manifestly space and time must be able to show themselves in this way—they must be able to become phenomena—if Kant is claiming to make a transcendental assertion grounded in the facts when he says that space is the *a priori* "inside-which" of an ordering.[52]

If, however, the phenomenological conception of phenomenon is to be understood at all, regardless of how much closer we may come to determining the nature of that which shows itself, this presupposes inevitably that we must have an insight into the meaning of the formal conception of phenomenon and its legitimate employment in an ordinary signification.—But before setting up our preliminary conception of phenomenology, we must also define the signification of λόγος so as to make clear in what sense phenomenology can be a 'science of' phenomena at all.

B. The Concept of the Logos

32

In Plato and Aristotle the concept of the λόγος has many competing significations, with no basic signification positively taking the lead. In fact, however, this is only a semblance, which will maintain itself as long as our Interpretation is unable to grasp the basic signification properly in its primary content. If we say that the basic signification of λόγος is "discourse",[53] then this word-for-word translation will not be validated until we have determined what is meant by "discourse" itself. The real signification of "discourse", which is obvious enough, gets constantly covered up by the later history of the word λόγος, and especially by the numerous and arbitrary Interpretations which subsequent philosophy has provided. *Λόγος* gets 'translated' (and this means that it is always getting interpreted) as "reason", "judgment", "concept", "definition", "ground", or "relationship".⁵⁴ But how can 'discourse' be so susceptible of modification that *λόγος* can signify all the things we have listed, and in good scholarly usage? Even if *λόγος* is understood in the sense of "assertion", but of "assertion" as 'judgment', this seemingly legitimate translation may still miss the fundamental signification, especially if "judgment" is conceived in a sense taken over from some contemporary 'theory of judgment'. *Λόγος* does not mean "judgment", and it certainly does not mean this primarily—if one understands by "judgment" a way of 'binding' something with something else, or the 'taking of a stand' (whether by acceptance or by rejection). *Λόγος* as "discourse" means rather the same as *δηλοῦν*: to make manifest what one is 'talking about' in one's discourse.⁵⁵ Aristotle has explicated this function of discourse more precisely as *ἀποφαίνεσθαι*. The *λόγος* lets something be seen (*φαίνεσθαι*), namely, what the discourse is about; and it does so either *for* the one who is doing the talking (the *medium*) or for persons who are talking with one another, as the case may be. Discourse 'lets something be seen' *ἀπό* . . .: that is, it lets us see something from the very thing which the discourse is about.⁵⁶ In discourse (*ἀπόφανσις*), so far as it is genuine, *what is said [was geredet ist]* is drawn *from* what the talk is about, so that discursive communication, in what it says [in ihrem Gesagten], makes manifest what it is talking about, and thus makes this accessible to the other party. This is the structure of the *λόγος* as *ἀπόφανσις*. This mode of making manifest in the sense of letting something be seen by pointing it out, does not go with all kinds of 'discourse'. Requesting (*εὐχή*), for instance, also makes manifest, but in a different way.

When fully concrete, discoursing (letting something be seen) has the character of speaking [Sprechens]—vocal proclamation in words.

The *λόγος* is *φωνή*, and indeed, *φωνή μετὰ* **33** *φαντασίας*—an utterance in which something is sighted in each case.

And only *because* the function of the *λόγος* as *ἀπόφανσις* lies in letting something be seen by pointing it out, can the *λόγος* have the structural form of *σύνθεσις*. Here "synthesis" does not mean a binding and linking together of representations, a manipulation of psychical occurrences where the 'problem' arises of how these bindings, as something inside, agree with something physical outside. Here the *συν* has a purely apophantical signification and means letting something be seen in its *togetherness* [Beisammen] with something—letting it be seen *as* something.

Furthermore, because the *λόγος* is a letting-something-be-seen, it can *therefore* be true or false. But here everything depends on our steering clear of any conception of truth which is construed in the sense of 'agreement'. This idea is by no means the primary one in the concept of *ἀλήθεια*. The 'Being-true' of the *λόγος* as *ἀληθεύειν* means that in *λέγειν* as *ἀποφαίνεσθαι* the entities *of which* one is talking must be taken out of their hiddenness; one must let them be seen as something unhidden (*ἀληθές*); that is, they must be *discovered*.⁵⁷ Similarly, 'Being false' (*ψεύδεσθαι*) amounts to deceiving in the sense of *covering up* [verdecken]: putting something in front of something (in such a way as to let it be seen) and thereby passing it off *as* something which it is *not*.

But because 'truth' has this meaning, and because the *λόγος* is a definite mode of letting something be seen, the *λόγος* is just *not* the kind of thing that can be considered as the primary 'locus' of truth. If, as has become quite customary nowadays, one defines "truth" as something that 'really' pertains to judgment,⁵⁸ and if one then invokes the support of Aristotle with this thesis, not only is this unjustified, but, above all, the Greek conception of truth has been misunderstood. *Αἴσθησις*, the sheer sensory perception of something, is 'true' in the Greek sense, and indeed more primordially than the *λόγος* which we have been discussing. Just as seeing aims at colours, any αἴσθησις aims at its ἴδια (those entities which are genuinely accessible only *through* it and *for* it); and to that extent this perception is always true. This means that seeing always discovers colours, and hearing always discovers sounds. Pure νοεῖν is the perception of the simplest determinate ways of Being which entities as such may possess, and it perceives them just by looking at them.[59] This νοεῖν is what is 'true' in the purest and most primordial sense; that is to say, it merely discovers, and it does so in such a way that it can never cover up. This νοεῖν can never cover up; it can never be false; it can at worst remain a *non-perceiving*, ἀγνοεῖν, not sufficing for straightforward and appropriate access.

34   When something no longer takes the form of just letting something be seen, but is always harking back to something else to which it points, so that it lets something be seen *as* something, it thus acquires a synthesis-structure, and with this it takes over the possibility of covering up.[60] The 'truth of judgments', however, is merely the opposite of this covering-up, a secondary phenomenon of truth, *with more than one kind of foundation*.[61] Both realism and idealism have—with equal thoroughness—missed the meaning of the Greek conception of truth, in terms of which only the possibility of something like a 'doctrine of ideas' can be understood as philosophical *knowledge*.

And because the function of the λόγος lies in merely letting something be seen, in *letting* entities be *perceived* [im *Vernehmenlassen des Seienden*], λόγος can signify the *reason* [*Vernunft*]. And because, moreover, λόγος is used not only with the signification of λέγειν but also with that of λεγόμενον (that which is exhibited, as such), and because the latter is nothing else than the ὑποκείμενον which, as present-at-hand, already lies at the *bottom* [zum *Grunde*] of any procedure of addressing oneself to it or discussing it, λόγος qua λεγόμενον means the ground, the *ratio*. And finally, because λόγος as λεγόμενον can also signify that which, as some-

thing to which one addresses oneself, becomes visible in its relation to something in its 'relatedness', λόγος acquires the signification of *relation* and *relationship*.[62]

This Interpretation of 'apophantical discourse' may suffice to clarify the primary function of the λόγος.

C. The Preliminary Conception of Phenomenology

When we envisage concretely what we have set forth in our Interpretation of 'phenomenon' and 'logos', we are struck by an inner relationship between the things meant by these terms. The expression "phenomenology" may be formulated in Greek as λέγειν τὰ φαινόμενα, where λέγειν means ἀποφαίνεσθαι. Thus "phenomenology" means ἀποφαίνεσθαι τὰ φαινόμενα—to let that which shows itself be seen from itself in the very way in which it shows itself from itself. This is the formal meaning of that branch of research which calls itself "phenomenology". But here we are expressing nothing else than the maxim formulated above: 'To the things themselves!'

Thus the term "phenomenology" is quite different in its meaning from expressions such as "theology" and the like. Those terms designate the objects of their respective sciences according to the subject-matter which they comprise at the time [in ihrer jeweiligen Sachhaltigkeit]. 'Phenomenology' neither designates the object of its researches, nor characterizes the subject-matter thus comprised. The word merely informs us of the "*how*" with which *what* is to be treated in 35 this science gets exhibited and handled. To have a science 'of' phenomena means to grasp its objects *in such a way* that everything about them which is up for discussion must be treated by exhibiting it directly and demonstrating it directly.[63] The expression 'descriptive phenomenology', which is at bottom tautological, has the same meaning. Here "description" does not signify such a procedure as we find, let us say, in botanical morphology; the term has rather the sense of a prohibition—the avoidance of characterizing anything without such demonstration.

The character of this description itself, the specific meaning of the λόγος, can be established first of all in terms of the 'thinghood' ["Sachheit"] of what is to be 'described'—that is to say, of what is to be given scientific definiteness as we encounter it phenomenally. The signification of "phenomenon", as conceived both formally and in the ordinary manner, is such that any exhibiting of an entity as it shows itself in itself, may be called "phenomenology" with formal justification.

Now what must be taken into account if the formal conception of phenomenon is to be deformalized into the phenomenological one, and how is this latter to be distinguished from the ordinary conception? What is it that phenomenology is to 'let us see'? What is it that must be called a 'phenomenon' in a distinctive sense? What is it that by its very essence is *necessarily* the theme whenever we exhibit something *explicitly*? Manifestly, it is something that proximally and for the most part does *not* show itself at all: it is something that lies *hidden*, in contrast to that which proximally and for the most part does show itself; but at the same time it is something that belongs to what thus shows itself, and it belongs to it so essentially as to constitute its meaning and its ground.

Yet that which remains *hidden* in an egregious sense, or which relapses and gets *covered up* again, or which shows itself only 'in disguise', is not just this entity or that, but rather the *Being* of entities, as our previous observations have shown. This Being can be covered up so extensively that it becomes forgotten and no question arises about it or about its meaning. Thus that which demands that it become a phenomenon, and which demands this in a distinctive sense and in terms of its ownmost content as a thing, is what phenomenology has taken into its grasp thematically as its object.

Phenomenology is our way of access to what is to be the theme of ontology, and it is our way of giving it demonstrative precision. *Only as phenomenology, is ontology possible.* In the phenomenological conception of "phenomenon" what

one has in mind as that which shows itself is the Being of entities, its meaning, its modifications and derivatives.[64] And this showing-itself is not just any showing-itself, nor is it some such thing as appearing. Least of all can the Being of entities ever be anything such that 'behind it' stands something else 'which does not appear'.

'Behind' the phenomena of phenomenology there is essentially nothing else; on the other hand, what is to become a phenomenon can be hidden. And just because the phenomena are proximally and for the most part *not* given, there is need for phenomenology. Covered-upness is the counter concept to 'phenomenon'.

There are various ways in which phenomena can be covered up. In the first place, a phenomenon can be covered up in the sense that it is still quite *undiscovered*. It is neither known nor unknown.[65] Moreover, a phenomenon can be *buried over* [*verschüttet*]. This means that it has at some time been discovered but has deteriorated [verfiel] to the point of getting covered up again. This covering-up can become complete; or rather—and as a rule—what has been discovered earlier may still be visible, though only as a semblance. Yet so much semblance, so much 'Being'.[66] This covering-up as a 'disguising' is both the most frequent and the most dangerous, for here the possibilities of deceiving and misleading are especially stubborn. Within a 'system', perhaps, those structures of Being—and their concepts—which are still available but veiled in their indigenous character, may claim their rights. For when they have been bound together constructively in a system, they present themselves as something 'clear', requiring no further justification, and thus can serve as the point of departure for a process of deduction.

The covering-up itself, whether in the sense of hiddenness, burying-over, or disguise, has in turn two possibilities. There are coverings-up which are accidental; there are also some which are necessary, grounded in what the thing discovered consists in [der Bestandart des Entdeckten]. Whenever a phenomenological concept is drawn from primordial sources, there is a

36

possibility that it may degenerate if communicated in the form of an assertion. It gets understood in an empty way and is thus passed on, losing its indigenous character, and becoming a free-floating thesis. Even in the concrete work of phenomenology itself there lurks the possibility that what has been primordially 'within our grasp' may become hardened so that we can no longer grasp it. And the difficulty of this kind of research lies in making it self-critical in a positive sense.

The way in which Being and its structures are encountered in the mode of phenomenon is one which must first of all be *wrested* from the objects of phenomenology. Thus the very *point of departure* [*Ausgang*] for our analysis requires that it be secured by the proper method, just as much as does our *access* [*Zugang*] to the phenomenon, or our *passage* [*Durchgang*] through whatever is prevalently covering it up. The idea of grasping and explicating phenomena in a way which is 'original' and 'intuitive' ["*originären*" und "*intuitiven*"] is directly opposed to the *naïveté* of a haphazard, 'immediate', and unreflective 'beholding' ["*Schauen*"].

Now that we have delimited our preliminary conception of phenomenology, the terms '*phenomenal*' and '*phenomenological*' can also be fixed in their signification. That which is given and explicable in the way the phenomenon is encountered is called 'phenomenal'; this is what we have in mind when we talk about "phenomenal structures". Everything which belongs to the species of exhibiting and explicating and which goes to make up the way of conceiving demanded by this research, is called 'phenomenological'.

Because phenomena, as understood phenomenologically, are never anything but what goes to make up Being, while Being is in every case the Being of some entity, we must first bring forward the entities themselves if it is our aim that Being should be laid bare; and we must do this in the right way. These entities must likewise show themselves with the kind of access which genuinely belongs to them. And in this way the ordinary conception of phenomenon

becomes phenomenologically relevant. If our analysis is to be authentic, its aim is such that the prior task of assuring ourselves 'phenomenologically' of that entity which is to serve as our example, has already been prescribed as our point of departure.

With regard to its subject-matter, phenomenology is the science of the Being of entities—ontology. In explaining the tasks of ontology we found it necessary that there should be a fundamental ontology taking as its theme that entity which is ontologico-ontically distinctive, Dasein, in order to confront the cardinal problem—the question of the meaning of Being in general. Our investigation itself will show that the meaning of phenomenological description as a method lies in *interpretation*. The λόγος of the phenomenology of Dasein has the character of a ἑρμηνεύειν, through which the authentic meaning of Being, and also those basic structures of Being which Dasein itself possesses, are *made known* to Dasein's understanding of Being. The phenomenology of Dasein is a *hermeneutic* in the primordial signification of this word, where it designates this business of interpreting. But to the extent that by uncovering the meaning of Being and the basic structures of Dasein in general we may exhibit the horizon for any further ontological study of those entities which do not have the character of Dasein, this hermeneutic also becomes a 'hermeneutic' in the sense of working out the conditions on which the possibility of any ontological investigation depends. And finally, to the extent that Dasein, as an entity with the possibility of existence, has ontological priority over every other entity, "hermeneutic", as an interpretation of Dasein's Being, has the third and specific sense of an analytic of the existentiality of existence; and this is the sense which is philosophically *primary*. Then so far as this hermeneutic works out Dasein's historicality ontologically as the ontical condition for the possibility of historiology, it contains the roots of what can be called 'hermeneutic' only in a derivative sense: the methodology of those humane sciences which are historiological in character.

Being, as the basic theme of philosophy, is no class or genus of entities, yet it pertains to every entity. Its 'universality' is to be sought higher up. Being and the structure of Being lie beyond every entity and every possible character which an entity may possess. *Being is the transcendens pure and simple.*[67] And the transcendence of Dasein's Being is distinctive in that it implies the possibility and the necessity of the most radical *individuation*. Every disclosure of Being as the *transcendens* is *transcendental* knowledge. *Phenomenological truth (the disclosedness of Being) is veritas transcendentalis.*

Ontology and phenomenology are not two distinct philosophical disciplines among others. These terms characterize philosophy itself with regard to its object and its way of treating that object. Philosophy is universal phenomenological ontology, and takes its departure from the hermeneutic of Dasein, which, as an analytic of *existence*, has made fast the guiding-line for all philosophical inquiry at the point where it *arises* and to which it *returns*.

The following investigation would not have been possible if the ground had not been prepared by Edmund Husserl, with whose *Logische Untersuchungen* phenomenology first emerged. Our comments on the preliminary conception of phenomenology have shown that what is essential in it does not lie in its *actuality* as a philosophical 'movement' ["Richtung"]. Higher than actuality stands *possibility*. We can understand phenomenology only by seizing upon it as a possibility.

With regard to the awkwardness and 'inelegance' of expression in the analyses to come, we may remark that it is one thing to give a report in which we tell about *entities*, but another to grasp entities in their *Being*. For the latter task we lack not only most of the words but, above all, the 'grammar'. If we may allude to some earlier researches on the analysis of Being, incomparable on their own level, we may compare the ontological sections of Plato's *Parmenides* or the fourth chapter of the seventh book of Aristotle's *Metaphysics* with a narrative section from Thucydides; we can then see the altogether unprecedented character of those formulations which were imposed upon the Greeks by their philosophers. And where our powers are essentially weaker, and where moreover the area of Being to be disclosed is ontologically far more difficult than that which was presented to the Greeks, the harshness of our expression will be enhanced, and so will the minuteness of detail with which our concepts are formed.

8. DESIGN OF THE TREATISE

The question of the meaning of Being is the most universal and the emptiest of questions, but at the same time it is possible to individualize it very precisely for any particular Dasein. If we are to arrive at the basic concept of 'Being' and to outline the ontological conceptions which it requires and the variations which it necessarily undergoes, we need a clue which is concrete. We shall proceed towards the concept of Being by way of an Interpretation of a certain special entity, Dasein, in which we shall arrive at the horizon for the understanding of Being and for the possibility of interpreting it; the universality of the concept of Being is not belied by the relatively 'special' character of our investigation. But this very entity, Dasein, is in itself 'historical', so that its ownmost ontological elucidation necessarily becomes an 'historiological' Interpretation.

Accordingly our treatment of the question of Being branches out into two distinct tasks, and our treatise will thus have two parts:

Part One: the Interpretation of Dasein in terms of temporality, and the explication of time as the transcendental horizon for the question of Being.

Part Two: basic features of a phenomenological destruction of the history of ontology, with the problematic of Temporality as our clue.

Part One has *three divisions*

1. the preparatory fundamental analysis of Dasein;
2. Dasein and temporality;
3. time and Being.[68]

40   Part Two likewise has *three divisions:*

1. Kant's doctrine of schematism and time, as a preliminary stage in a problematic of Temporality;

2. the ontological foundation of Descartes' '*cogito sum*', and how the medieval ontology has been taken over into the problematic of the '*res cogitans*';

3. Aristotle's essay on time, as providing a way of discriminating the phenomenal basis and the limits of ancient ontology.

NOTES

1. '. . . *als thematische Frage wirklicher Untersuchung*'. When Heidegger speaks of a question as 'thematisch', he thinks of it as one which is taken seriously and studied in a systematic manner. While we shall often translate this adjective by its cognate, 'thematic', we may sometimes find it convenient to choose more flexible expressions involving the word 'theme'. (Heidegger gives a fuller discussion on H. 363.)

2. ' "... was einer am Seienden erfasst" '. The word 'Seiendes', which Heidegger uses in his paraphrase, is one of the most important words in the book. The substantive 'das Seiende' is derived from the participle 'seiend' (see note 1, p. 19), and means literally 'that which is'; 'ein Seiendes' means 'something which is'. There is much to be said for translating 'Seiendes' by the noun 'being' or 'beings' (for it is often used in a collective sense). We feel, however, that it is smoother and less confusing to write 'entity' or 'entities'. We are well aware that in recent British and American philosophy the term 'entity' has been used more generally to apply to almost anything whatsoever, no matter what its ontological status. In this translation, however, it will mean simply 'something which *is*'. An alternative translation of the Latin quotation is given by the English Dominican Fathers, *Summa Theologica*, Thomas Baker, London, 1915: 'For that which, before aught else, falls under apprehension, is *being*, the notion of which is included in all things whatsoever a man apprehends.'

3. '. . . in jedem Verhalten zu Seiendem, in jedem Sich-zu-sich-selbst-verhalten . . .' The verb 'verhalten' can refer to any kind of behaviour or way of conducting oneself, even to the way in which one relates oneself to something else, or to the way one refrains or holds oneself back. We shall translate it in various ways.

4. 'Sie macht offenbar, dass in jedem Verhalten und Sein zu Seiendem als Seiendem a priori ein Rätsel liegt.' The phrase 'Sein zu Seiendem' is typical of many similar expressions in which the substantive 'Sein' is followed by the preposition 'zu'. In such expressions we shall usually translate 'zu' as 'towards': for example, 'Being-towards-death', 'Being towards Others', 'Being towards entities within-the-world'.

5. ' "die geheimen Urteile der gemeinen Vernunft" '.

6. '. . . dann bedarf solches Fragen der angemessenen Durchsichtigkeit'. The adjective 'durchsichtig' is one of Heidegger's favourite expressions, and means simply 'transparent', 'perspicuous', something that one can 'see through'. We shall ordinarily translate it by 'transparent'. See H. 146 for further discussion.

7. '. . . in seinem Dass- und Sosein'.

8. '. . . das eigentlich Intendierte . . .' The adverb 'eigentlich' occurs very often in this work. It may be used informally where one might write 'really' or 'on its part', or in a much stronger sense, where something like 'genuinely' or 'authentically' would be more appropriate. It is not always possible to tell which meaning Heidegger has in mind. In the contexts which seem relatively informal we shall write 'really'; in the more technical passages we shall write 'authentically', reserving 'genuinely' for 'genuin' or 'echt'. The reader must not confuse this kind of 'authenticity' with the kind, which belongs to an 'authentic text' or an 'authentic account'. See H. 42 for further discussion. In the present passage, the verb 'intendieren' is presumably used in the medieval sense of 'intending', as adapted and modified by Brentano and Husserl.

9. 'zunächst'. This word is of very frequent occurrence in Heidegger, and he will discuss his use of it on H. 370 below. In ordinary German usage the word may mean 'at first', 'to begin with', or 'in the first instance', and we shall often translate it in such ways. The word is, however, cognate with the adjective 'nah' and its superlative 'nächst', which we shall usually translate as 'close' and 'closest' respectively; and Heidegger often uses 'zunächst' in the sense of 'most closely', when he is describing the most 'natural' and 'obvious' experiences which we have at an uncritical and pre-philosophical level. We have ventured to translate this Heideggerian sense of 'zunächst' as 'proximally', but there are many border-line cases where it is not clear whether Heidegger has in mind this special sense or one of the more general usages, and in such cases we have chosen whatever expression seems stylistically preferable.

10. 'Sein liegt im Dass- und Sosein, in Realität, Vorhandenheit, Bestand, Geltung, Dasein, im "es gibt".' On 'Vorhandenheit' ('presence-at-hand') see note 1, p. 48, H. 25. On 'Dasein', see note 1, p. 27.

11. The word 'Dasein' plays so important a role in this work and is already so familiar to the English-speaking reader who has read about Heidegger, that it seems simpler to leave it untranslated except in the relatively rare passages in which Heidegger himself breaks it up with a hyphen ('Da-sein') to show its etymological construction: literally 'Being-there'. Though in traditional German philosophy it may be used quite generally to stand for almost any kind of Being or 'existence' which we can say that something *has* (the 'existence' of God, for example), in everyday usage it tends to be used more narrowly to stand for the kind of Being that belongs to *persons*. Heidegger follows the everyday usage in this respect, but goes somewhat further in that he often uses it to stand for any *person* who has such Being, and who is thus an 'entity' himself. See H. 11 below.

12. 'faktisch'. While this word can often be translated simply as 'in fact' or 'as a matter of fact', it is used both as an adjective and as an adverb and is so characteristic of Heidegger's style that we shall as a rule translate it either as 'factical' or as 'factically', thus preserving its connection with the important noun 'Faktizität' ('facticity'), and keeping it distinct from 'tatsächlich' ('factual') and 'wirklich' ('actual'). See the discussion of 'Tatsächlichkeit' and 'Faktizität' in Sections 12 and 29 below (H. 56, 135).

13. '. . . deren faktischen Bestand man wohl nicht leugnen wird'.

14. 'Wesensverfassung'. 'Verfassung' is the standard word for the 'constitution' of a nation or any political organization, but it is also used for the 'condition' or 'state' in which a person may find himself. Heidegger seldom uses the word in either of these senses; but he does use it in ways which are somewhat analogous. In one sense Dasein's 'Verfassung' is its 'constitution', the way it is constituted, '*sa condition humaine*'. In another sense Dasein may have several 'Verfassungen' as constitutive 'states' or factors which enter into its 'constitution'. We shall, in general, translate 'Verfassung' as 'constitution' or 'constitutive state' according to the context; but in passages where 'constitutive state' would be cumbersome and there is little danger of ambiguity, we shall simply write 'state'. These states, however, must always be thought of as constitutive and essential, not as temporary or transitory stages like the 'state' of one's health or the 'state of the nation'. When Heidegger uses the word 'Konstitution', we shall usually indicate this by capitalizing 'Constitution'.

15. '. . . weil es in der Beantwortung der Frage nicht um eine ableitende Begründung, sondern um aufweisende Grund-Freilegung geht.' Expressions of the form 'es geht . . . um . . .' appear very often

in this work. We shall usually translate them by variants on '. . . is an issue for. . .'.

16. 'In den *historischen Geisteswissenschaften* . . .' Heidegger makes much of the distinction between 'Historie' and 'Geschichte' and the corresponding adjectives 'historisch' and 'geschichtlich'. 'Historie' stands for what Heidegger calls a 'science of history'. (See H. 375, 378.) 'Geschichte' usually stands for the kind of 'history' that actually *happens*. We shall as a rule translate these respectively as 'historiology' and 'history', following similar conventions in handling the two adjectives. See especially Sections 6 and 76 below.

17. '. . . als durchsichtige Anweisungen des Fragens . . .'

18. '. . . sondern die Interpretation des eigentlich geschichtlich Seienden auf seine Geschichtlichkeit'. We shall translate the frequently occurring term 'Geschichtlichkeit' as 'historicality'. Heidegger very occasionally uses the term 'Historizität', as on H. go below, and this will be translated as 'historicity'.

19. While the terms 'ontisch' ('ontical') and 'ontologisch' ('ontological') are not explicitly defined, their meanings will emerge rather clearly. Ontological inquiry is concerned primarily with *Being*; ontical inquiry is concerned primarily with *entities* and the facts about them.

20. '. . . das Ganze eines Begründungszusammenhanges wahrer Sätze . . .' See H. 357 below.

21. 'Zu dieser Seinsverfassung des Daseins gehört aber dann, dass es in seinem Sein zu diesem Sein ein Seinsverhältnis hat.' This passage is ambiguous and might also be read as: '. . . and this implies that Dasein, in its Being towards this Being, has a relationship of Being.'

22. '. . . dass es ontologisch *ist*'. As 'ontologisch' may be either an adjective or an adverb, we might also write: '. . . that it *is* ontologically'. A similar ambiguity occurs in the two following sentences, where we read 'Ontologisch-sein' and 'ontisch-seiend' respectively.

23. '. . . dass es je sein Sein als seiniges zu sein hat . . .'

24. We shall translate 'existenziell' by 'existentiell', and 'existenzial' by 'existential' There seems to be little reason for resorting to the more elaborate neologisms proposed by other writers.

25. '. . . innerhalb der Welt . . .' Heidegger uses at least three expressions which might be translated as 'in the world': 'innerhalb der Welt', 'in der Welt', and the adjective (or adverb) 'innerweltlich'. We shall translate these respectively by 'within the world', 'in the world', and 'within-the-world'.

26. 'Besinnung'. The earliest editions have 'Bestimmung' instead.

27. 'Und zwar soll sie das Seiende in dem zeigen, wie es *zunächst und zumeist* ist, in seiner durchschnit-

tlichen *Alltäglichkeit*.' The phrase 'zunächst und zumeist' is one that occurs many times, though Heidegger does not explain it until Section 71 (H. 370 below), where 'Alltäglichkeit' too gets explained. On 'zunächst' see our note 1, p. 25, H. 6.

28. The ambiguity of the pronominal references in this sentence and the one before it, reflects a similar ambiguity in the German. (The English-speaking reader should be reminded that the kind of philosophical 'anthropology' which Heidegger has in mind is a study of man in the widest sense, and is not to be confused with the empirical sciences of 'physical' and 'cultural' anthropology.)

29. '*Zeitlichkeit*'. While it is tempting to translate the adjective 'zeitlich' and the noun 'Zeitlichkeit' by their most obvious English cognates, 'timely' and 'timeliness', this would be entirely misleading; for 'temporal' and 'temporality' come much closer to what Heidegger has in mind, not only when he is discussing these words in their popular senses (as he does on the following page) but even when he is using them in his own special sense, as in Section 65 below. (See especially H. 326 below, where 'Zeitlichkeit' is defined.) On the other hand, he occasionally uses the noun 'Temporalität' and the adjective 'temporal' in a sense which he will explain later (H. 19). We shall translate these by 'Temporality' and 'Temporal', with initial capitals.

30. 'Dasein *ist* in der Weise, seiend so etwas wie Sein zu verstehen.'

31. 'seine *temporale* Bestimmtheit'. See our note 3, p. 38, H. 17 above.

32. 'weltgeschichtliches Geschehen'. While the verb 'geschehen' ordinarily means to 'happen', and will often be so translated, Heidegger stresses its etymological kinship to 'Geschichte' or 'history'. To bring out this connection, we have coined the verb 'historize', which might be paraphrased as to 'happen in a historical way'; we shall usually translate 'geschehen' this way in contexts where history is being discussed. We trust that the reader will keep in mind that such 'historizing' is characteristic of all historical entities, and is *not* the sort of thing that is done primarily by historians (as 'philosophizing', for instance, is done by philosophers). (On 'world-historical' see H. 381 ff.)

33. 'Das Dasein "ist" seine Vergangenheit in der Weise *seines* Seins, das, roh gesagt, jeweils aus seiner Zukunft her "geschieht".'

34. 'Historizität'. Cf. note 2, p. 31. H. 10 above.

35. 'defizienter Modus'. Heidegger likes to think of certain characteristics as occurring in various ways or 'modes', among which may be included certain ways of 'not occurring' or 'occurring only to an inadequate extent' or, in general, occurring 'deficiently'. It is as if zero and the negative integers

were to be thought of as representing 'deficient modes of being a positive integer'.

36. '. . . das Dasein hat nicht nur die Geneigtheit, an seine Welt, in der es ist, zu verfallen und reluzent aus ihr her sich auszulegen, Dasein verfällt in eins damit auch seinen mehr oder minder ausdrücklich ergriffenen Tradition.' The verb 'verfallen' is one which Heidegger will use many times. Though we shall usually translate it simply as 'fall', it has the connotation of *deteriorating, collapsing*, or *falling down*. Neither our 'fall back upon' nor our 'falls prey to' is quite right: but 'fall upon' and 'fall on to', which are more literal, would be misleading for 'an . . . zu verfallen'; and though 'falls to the lot of' and 'devolves upon' would do well for 'verfällt' with the dative in other contexts, they will not do so well here.

37. In this passage Heidegger juxtaposes a number of words beginning with the prefix 'über-': 'übergibt' ('transmits'); 'überantwortet' ('delivers over'); 'das Überkommene' ('what has come down to us'); 'überlieferten' ('handed down to us').

38. '. . . der durch sie gezeitigten Verdeckungen.' The verb 'zeitigen' will appear frequently in later chapters. See H. 304 and our note ad loc.

39. We follow the later editions in reading '*der Seinssinn des "sum"* '. The earlier editions have an anacoluthic 'den' for 'der'.

40. The noun οὐσία is derived from one of the stems used in conjugating the irregular verb εἶναι, ('to be'); in the Aristotelian tradition it is usually translated as 'substance', though translators of Plato are more likely to write 'essence', 'existence', or 'being'. Heidegger suggests that οὐσία is to be thought of as synonymous with the derivative noun παρουσία ('being-at', 'presence'). As he points out, παρουσία has a close etymological correspondence with the German 'Anwesenheit', which is similarly derived from the stem of a verb meaning 'to be' (Cf. O.H.G. 'wesan') and a prefix of the place or time at which ('an-'). We shall in general translate 'Anwesenheit' as 'presence', and the participle 'anwesend' as some form of the expression 'have presence'.

41. 'die "*Gegenwart*"'. While this noun may, like παρουσία or 'Anwesenheit', mean the *presence* of someone at some place or on some occasion, it more often means the *present*, as distinguished from the past and the future. In its etymological root-structure, however, it means a *waiting-towards*. While Heidegger seems to think of all these meanings as somehow fused, we shall generally translate this noun as 'the Present', reserving 'in the present' for the corresponding adjective 'gegenwärtig'.

42. The phrase ζῷον λόγον ἔχον is traditionally translated as 'rational animal', on the assumption that λόγος refers to the faculty of *reason*. Heidegger,

however, points out that λόγος is derived from the same root as the verb λέγειν ('to talk', 'to hold discourse'); he identifies this in turn with νοεῖν ('to cognize', 'to be aware of', 'to know'), and calls attention to the fact that the same stem is found in the adjective διαλεκτικός ('dialectical'). (See also H. 165 below.) He thus interprets λόγος as 'Rede', which we shall usually translate as 'discourse' or 'talk', depending on the context. See Section 7 B below (H. 32 ff.) and Sections 34 and 35, where 'Rede' will be defined and distinguished both from 'Sprache' ('language') and from 'Gerede' ('idle talk') (H. 160 ff.).

43. '. . . von etwas Vorhandenem in seiner puren Vorhandenheit . . .' The adjective 'vorhanden' means literally 'before the hand', but this signification has long since given way to others. In ordinary German usage it may, for instance, be applied to the stock of goods which a dealer has 'on hand', or to the 'extant' works of an author; and in earlier philosophical writing it could be used, like the word 'Dasein' itself, as a synonym for the Latin '*existentia*'. Heidegger, however, distinguishes quite sharply between 'Dasein' and 'Vorhandenheit', using the latter to designate a kind of Being which belongs to things *other* than Dasein. We shall translate 'vorhanden' as 'present-at-hand', and 'Vorhandenheit' as 'presence-at-hand'. The reader must be careful not to confuse these expressions with our 'presence' ('Anwesenheit') and 'the Present' ('die Gegenwart'), etc., or with a few other verbs and adjectives which we may find it convenient to translate by 'present'.

44. '. . . des reinen "Gegenwärtigens" von etwas'. The verb 'gegenwärtigen', which is derived from the adjective 'gegenwärtig', is not a normal German verb, but was used by Husserl and is used extensively by Heidegger. While we shall translate it by various forms of 'make present', it does not necessarily mean 'making physically present', but often means something like 'bringing vividly to mind'.

45. 'Das Seiende, das sich in ihm für es zeigt und das als das eigentliche Seiende verstanden wird, erhält demnach seine Auslegung in Rücksicht auf—Gegen-wart, d.h. es ist als Anwesenheit (οὐσία) begriffen.' The hyphenation of 'Gegen-wart' calls attention to the structure of this word in a way which cannot be reproduced in English. See note 2, p. 47, H. 25 above. The pronouns 'ihm' and 'es' presumably both refer back to λέγειν, though their reference is ambiguous, as our version suggests.

46. The appeal to the 'Sachen selbst', which Heidegger presents as virtually a slogan for Husserl's phenomenology, is not easy to translate without giving misleading impressions. What Husserl has in mind is the 'things' that words may be found to signify

when their significations are correctly intuited by the right kind of *Anschauung*. (Cf. his *Logische Untersuchungen*, vol. 2, part 1, second edition, Halle, 1913, p. 6.) We have followed Marvin Farber in adopting 'the things themselves'. (Cf. his *The Foundation of Phenomenology*, Cambridge, Mass., 1943, pp. 202–3.) The word 'Sache' will, of course, be translated in other ways also.

47. '. . . was man "Erscheinung" oder gar "blosse Erscheinung" nennt.' Though the noun 'Erscheinung' and the verb 'erscheinen' behave so much like the English 'appearance' and 'appear' that the ensuing discussion presents relatively few difficulties in this respect for the translator, the passage shows some signs of hasty construction, and a few comments may be helpful. We are told several times that 'appearance' and 'phenomenon' are to be sharply distinguished; yet we are also reminded that there is a sense in which they coincide, and even this sense seems to be twofold, though it is not clear that Heidegger is fully aware of this. The whole discussion is based upon two further distinctions: the distinction between 'showing' ('zeigen') and 'announcing' ('melden') and 'bringing forth' ('hervorbringen'), and the distinction between ('*x*') that which 'shows itself' ('das Sichzeigende') or which 'does the announcing' ('das Meldende') or which 'gets brought forth' ('das Hervorgebrachte'), and ('*y*') that which 'announces itself' ('das Sichmeldende') or which does the bringing-forth. Heidegger is thus able to introduce the following senses of 'Erscheinung' or 'appearance':

1a. an observable event *y*, such as a symptom which announces a disease *x* by showing itself, and in or through which *x* announces itself without showing itself;

1b. *y*'s showing-itself;

2. *x*'s announcing-itself in or through *y*;

3a. the 'mere appearance' *y* which *x* may *bring forth* when *x* is of such a kind that its real nature can *never* be made manifest;

3b. the 'mere appearance' which is the *bringing-forth* of a 'mere appearance' in sense 3a. Heidegger makes abundantly clear that sense 2 is the proper sense of 'appearance' and that senses 3a and 3b are the proper senses of 'mere appearance'. On H. 30 and 31 he concedes that sense 1b corresponds to the primordial sense of 'phenomenon'; but his discussion on H. 28 suggests that 1a corresponds to this more accurately, and he reverts to this position towards the end of H. 30.

48. '. . . als welches es die Struktur des Scheins bestimmt.' (The older editions omit the 'es'.)

49. 'Was sich in *der* Weise *nicht* zeigt, wie das Erscheinende, kann auch nie scheinen.' This passage is ambiguous, but presumably 'das Erscheinende' is to be interpreted as the *x* of our note 1, p. 51, not our *y*. The reader should notice that our standardized translation of 'scheinen' as 'seem' is one which here becomes rather misleading, even though these words correspond fairly well in ordinary usage. In distinguishing between 'scheinen' and 'erscheinen', Heidegger seems to be insisting that 'scheinen' can be done only by the *y* which 'shows itself' or 'does the announcing', not by the *x* which 'announces itself' in or through *y*, even though German usage does not differentiate these verbs quite so sharply.

50. '. . . eine ausgezeichnete Begegnisart von etwas.' The noun 'Begegnis' is derived from the verb 'begegnen', which is discussed in note 2, p. 70, H. 44 below.

51. '. . . einen seienden Verweisungsbezug im Seienden selbst . . .' The verb 'verweisen', which we shall translate as 'refer' or 'assign', depending upon the context, will receive further attention in Section 17 below. See also our note 2, p. 97, H. 68 below.

52. Cf. *Critique of Pure Reason²*, 'Transcendental Aesthetic', Section I, p. 34.

53. On λόγος, 'Rede', etc., see note 3, p. 47, H. 25 above.

54. '. . . Vernunft, Urteil, Begriff, Definition, Grund, Verhältnis.'

55. '. . . offenbar machen das, wovon in der Rede "die Rede" ist.'

56. '. . . von dem selbst her, wovon die Rede ist.'

57. The Greek words for 'truth' (ἡ ἀλήθεια, τὸ ἀληθές) are compounded of the privative prefix ἀ- ('not') and the verbal stem -λαθ- ('to escape notice', 'to be concealed'). The truth may thus be looked upon as that which is un-concealed, that which gets discovered or uncovered ('entdeckt').

58. 'Wenn man . . . Wahrheit als das bestimmt, was "eigentlich" dem Urteil zukommt. . . '

59. '. . . das schlicht hinsehende Vernehmen der einfachsten Seinsbestimmungen des Seienden als solchen.'

60. 'Was nicht mehr die Vollzugsform des reinen Sehenlassens hat, sondern je im Aufweisen auf ein anderes rekurriert und so je etwas *als* etwas sehen lässt, das übernimmt mit dieser Synthesisstruktur die Möglichkeit des Verdeckens.'

61. ' . . . ein *mehrfach fundiertes* Phänomen von Wahrheit.' A 'secondary' or 'founded' phenomenon is one which is based upon something else. The notion of 'Fundierung' is one which Heidegger has taken over from Husserl. See our note 1, p. 86, on H. 59 below.

62. Heidegger is here pointing out that the word λόγος is etymologically akin to the verb λέγειν, which has among its numerous meanings those of *laying out, exhibiting, setting forth, recounting, telling a tale, making a statement*. Thus λόγος as λέγειν can be thought of as the faculty of 'reason' ('Vernunft') which makes such activities possible. But λόγος can also mean τὸ λεγόμενον (*that which* is laid out, exhibited, set forth, told); in this sense it is the underlying subject matter (τὸ ὑποκείμενον) to which one addresses oneself and which one discusses ('Ansprechen und Besprechen'); as such it lies 'at the bottom' ('zum Grunde') of what is exhibited or told, and is thus the 'ground' or 'reason' ('Grund') for telling it. But when something is exhibited or told, it is exhibited in its *relatedness* ('in seiner Bezogenheit'); and in this way λόγος as λεγόμενον comes to stand for just such a relation or relationship ('Beziehung und Verhältnis'). The three senses here distinguished correspond to three senses of the Latin '*ratio*', by which λόγος was traditionally translated, though Heidegger explicitly calls attention to only one of these. Notice that 'Beziehung' (which we translate as 'relation') can also be used in some contexts where 'Ansprechen' (our 'addressing oneself') would be equally appropriate. Notice further that 'Verhältnis' (our 'relationship'), which is ordinarily a synonym for 'Beziehung', can, like λόγος and '*ratio*', also refer to the special kind of relationship which one finds in a mathematical proportion. The etymological connection between 'Vernehmen' and 'Vernunft' should also be noted.

63. . . . in direkter Aufweisung und direkter Ausweisung . . .

64. 'Der phänomenologische Begriff von Phänomen meint als das Sichzeigende das Sein des Seienden, seinen Sinn, seine Modifikationen und Derivate.'

65. 'Über seinen Bestand gibt es weder Kenntnis noch Unkenntnis.' The earlier editions have 'Erkenntnis' where the latter ones have 'Unkenntnis'. The word 'Bestand' always presents difficulties in Heidegger; here it permits either of two interpretations, which we have deliberately steered between: 'Whether there *is* any such thing, is neither known nor unknown', and 'What it comprises is something of which we have neither knowledge nor ignorance.'

66. 'Wieviel Schein jedoch, soviel "Sein".'

67. 'Sein und Seinsstruktur liegen über jedes Seiende und jede mögliche seiende Bestimmtheit eines Seienden hinaus. *Sein ist das transcendens schlechthin.*'

68. Part Two and the third division of Part One have never appeared.

Quality of Life: A Phenomenological Perspective on Explanation, Prediction, and Understanding in Nursing Science

Patricia Benner

A Heideggerian phenomenological approach to explanation, prediction, and understanding in the study of health, illness, and disease is presented. The extremes of objectification and subjectivism as barriers to understanding illness and suffering are explored. It is argued that meaning terms are essential when studying practical activity and relational issues, and that a privileged position is not gained by developing structural analyses or power terms that get behind or beyond meaning. Hermeneutics, or interpretive methodology, is a holistic strategy because it seeks to study the person in the situation rather than isolating person variables and situation variables and then trying to put them back together. Paradigm cases, exemplars, and thematic analysis are described as interpretive and presentational strategies.

Nursing is concerned with health promotion and the treatment of illness and disease. Health and illness are lived experiences and are accessed through perceptions, beliefs, skills, practices, and expectations. Illness is the human experience of dysfunction whereas disease is concerned with biochemical and neurophysiological functioning at the cell, tissue, and organ system levels.[1] The problem with being concerned with both the phenomenal world—health and illness, and the biophysiological world—disease, is that these two levels of discourse call for different kinds of explanation and prediction in the western tradition. Here the author departs from strict naturalists who hold that the ultimate level of explanation and prediction lies at the bio-

physiological level and that the phenomenal level is superfluous, an unnecessary trapping of human culture and language. The problem of two levels of discourse, the phenomenological level and the biophysiological level, is made more interesting by the empirical evidence that the phenomenal realms, the experiences of health and illness, are causally related to the disease and recovery processes at the cellular and tissue levels.[2]

Merleau-Ponty[3] states that no strictly bottom-up explanation—that is, explanation from the cellular level up to the lived experience of health and illness—can adequately explain or accurately predict the particular course of an illness, nor can it explain the maintenance of health. We know that laboratory data frequently do not match the illness experience. People do not die or survive strictly according to our best biochemical and physiological accounts. Fur-

Reprinted by permission from Advances in Nursing Science 8(1):1–14. © 1985, Aspen Publishers, Inc.

thermore, the person's understanding of his or her body and illness and experience must be taken into consideration to account for alterations in the disease process at the tissue level. These puzzles leave those who are concerned with both the phenomenal realms of health and illness and the physiological manifestations of disease dissatisfied with the Platonic and Cartesian legacy of a split between the mind and body. Cassell has alluded to the problem succinctly:

> If the mind-body dichotomy results in assigning the body to medicine, and the person is not in that category, then the only remaining place for the person is in the category of the mind. Where the mind is problematic (not identifiable in objective terms), its very reality diminishes for science, and so, too, does that of the person. Therefore, so long as the mind-body dichotomy is accepted, suffering is either subjective and not truly "real"— not within medicine's domain—or identified exclusively with bodily pain. Not only is such an identification misleading and distorting, for it depersonalizes the sick patient, but it is itself a source of suffering.[4(p640)]

The paradox of the subject/object split of Cartesian dualism is that it is either extremely subjectivizing or extremely objectifying. The self is viewed as a possession and attributes are given objectively as possessions by the subject in a purely intentional way. This view cannot take account of the historical, cultural, embodied, situated person. The self of possession[5-7] is a collection of attributes and objective traits that the self freely chooses and has ultimate control over as an autonomous subject. This view of the self overlooks the participative and constitutive side of the person's participation in a social world. The person is involved in a shared history, tradition, and social network that he or she both constitutes and is constituted by. Health and illness cannot be understood by studying a mind that possesses a list of talents, traits, and attributes, nor can they be understood by strictly studying biophysiological states. Health and ill-

ness of the person can only be understood by studying the person in context. This becomes painfully clear, for example, when patients refuse blood transfusions because they would cut patients off from God and their communities.

Dreyfus explains that the traditional problem of mind-body split comes from the Cartesian tradition of:

1. taking the self as an isolable present at hand (an objectively, self-possessed, uninvolved) entity rather than as a public activity; and
2. trying to generalize a problem that arises in special cases into a problem about every case. This second move only seems possible if one forgets the shared practices, ie, passes over the phenomenon of world.[8(p11)]

In the human sciences this means that we take examples of breakdown and assume that what shows up can also account for normal functioning.

The particular problems of explanation and prediction in the phenomenal realms (health and illness) must be solved before adequate holistic explanations and predictions of prevention and recovery from disease (the biophysiological) can be developed. Covering laws or other strictly naturalistic explanatory and predictive formulas will not work for health and illness because human experience is based on participating in linguistic and cultural practices that are not reducible to context-free elements capable of being related by the kind of covering laws described by Hempel.[9] The closest approximation to similar covering laws in human behavior is rule-governed behavior (although the author argues with Dreyfus,[8] human beings are capable of orderly behavior without recourse to following formal rules). For the sake of argument, Toulmin's[10] claim that positivistic scientists have glossed over the difference between *rule-governed behavior* and *law-governed action* may be taken seriously.

Action and Behavior

The first mistake is to overlook the distinction between action and behavior. Behavior is purposive where the action of physical objects just describes motion trajectories. Taylor[11] points out the difference between action and behavior by noting the differences between the mere action of "raising the arm" and voting behavior. What counts as an adequate explanation of the motion or action of an arm-raising trajectory is not a satisfactory account of voting behavior. Toulmin points out:

> The essential mark of rule-conforming behavior lies in the normative force of relevant rules. An agent who recognizes that he is deviating from a rule acknowledges a claim on him to correct his behavior. By contrast if we consider natural phenomena of a purely law-governed kind, no such distinction makes sense. . . . Psychologists . . . have played down the differences between rule-conforming and law-governed phenomena of physics and physiology.[10]

According to Taylor[11,12] and Dreyfus,[13] the rules we can expect to find in understanding health and illness are of the *ceteris paribus* kind. They will focus on sufficient conditions and make statements such as, all other things being equal, one can expect such and such to occur. Such a statement leaves room for transformations in meanings and changes in human concerns.

The analysis of variance model of interaction will not be sufficient to capture the relational quality of the person in the situation. That is, separating person variables and situational variables and then calculating their independent contribution to a singular main effect does not capture the configurational relationships inherent in the situation.[14,15] At issue is the understanding that the existence of or freedom from disease may be a necessary condition for certain behavior, but a sufficient condition would be the presence of disease together with the person's experience of the disease and the environment, which constitute together a teleological antecedent. A purely deterministic, tissue-level explanation or a purely psychological description will not suffice. The existence of the diseased organ is not the cause of the state (its sufficient condition) and therefore not the cause (the necessary condition) of the behavior either. As Taylor points out, "The widespread assumption that, because certain physiological states are *necessary* conditions of behavior, behavior must be accounted for by nonteleological physiological laws involves an illegitimate inference."[12(p25)]

Thus, any rules of behavior in explaining health and illness will be teleological or goal oriented in their nature. We cannot expect the same kind of deterministic laws found in nonteleological explanations and predictions of natural science. According to Taylor, such teleological laws will not be able to meet the assumptions of atomism that demand that the two terms, linked in a law, be identifiable separately from each other. Atomism is based on the

> notion that the ultimate evidence for any laws we frame about the world is in the form of discrete units of information, each of which could be as it is even if all others were different, i.e., each of which is separably identifiable from its connections with any of the others.[12(p11)]

Teleological laws are going to be transactional because the self both constitutes and is constituted by situation, language, culture, and history. Taylor says:

> In this way, teleological explanation is, as has often been remarked, connected with some form of holism, or anti-atomistic doctrine. . . . Whether the stringent atomist requirement can be met by all valid laws, then, is itself an empirical question, which hinges partly on the question whether all teleological explanation—or any other type of explanation which involves holist assumptions—can be done away with. It cannot be decided by epistemological fiat, by a rule to the effect that the evidence for teleological laws must be such that it can be stated by means of non-teleological laws.[12(pp11–15)]

Such an epistemological fiat amounts to "methodolatry." Teleological explanations require the systematic inclusion of meanings and self-interpretations in the study of health, illness, and suffering. Meanings are not relegated to philosophical inquiry[16] but become legitimate aspects for empirical study. As Wolf has observed in medicine:

> The plain fact is that many of the manifestations of the integrative processes in the brain that govern visceral and general behavior of human beings cannot be reduced to numbers: faith and optimism, on the one hand, or surrender and depression on the other, are such processes. Moreover, neither measurements nor numbers will help one to understand the tangible effects of placebos or of confidence in a doctor. Thus, the intensity of crucially important attitudes, values, and expectations cannot be gauged by the quantity of even the character of a stimulus, but depend on who is involved and in what context.
>
> The recent neglect of descriptive behavioral studies of individual human beings may have resulted in part from an understandable preoccupation with and fascination by increasingly sophisticated technology, but perhaps more important have been an unwarrantedly exclusive concern with quantitation and an unnecessary diffidence in approaching problems of replication, verification, and observer bias. . . . In medicine, we are just beginning to learn to relegate our preoccupation with quantitation to its proper place and to also ask configurational questions in more than one dimension.[14(pp5,7–8)]

Phenomenology

Pragmatic activity, human concerns, and meanings call for investigative strategies that do not require the kind of decontextualization of strict operationalism. Systematic strategies of study that can be verified or falsified by others and that capture relational and configurational patterns are required. Hermeneutics is one such strategy.[17–21]

Hermeneutics, which allows for the study of the person in the situation, offers a way of studying the phenomenal realms of health and illness, and overcomes the problems of extreme subjectivity or objectivity. Hermeneutics has been used to understand everyday practices, meanings, and knowledge embedded in skills, stress, and coping.[19,20] Hermeneutics assumes that the study of pragmatic activity, that is, everyday understanding and practices, and the study of relational issues are distinctly different from the study of objects or even biophysiological events on the tissue and cellular level.

Hermeneutics stems from the systematic study of texts and was originally developed as a tool of biblical exegesis, jurisprudence, and more recently, historical research and literary criticism. The particular kind of hermeneutics the author has used is congruent with a particular theoretical stance (Heideggerian phenomenology) taken toward human beings and human experience.[8,18] Three essential tenets of this phenomenology are: (1) human beings are self-interpreting. Their interpretations are not just possessions of the self; they are constitutive of the self; (2) furthermore, to be a human being means that the kind of being is an issue, that is, the person takes a stand on the kind of being he or she is. Finally, (3) the self is not a radically free arbiter of meaning. Though the meanings available to the individual can undergo transformations, they are limited by a particular language, culture, and history. No higher court for the individual exists than meanings or self-interpretations embedded in language, skills, and practices. No laws, structures, or mechanisms offer higher explanatory principles or greater predictive power than self-interpretations in the form of common meanings, personal concerns, and cultural practices shaped by a particular history. The goal is to understand everyday practices and the experiences of health and illness.[19–21]

Heideggerian phenomenology offers a critique and an alternative to a strictly cost-benefit approach to the study of quality of life wherein benefit is defined primarily in economic or mastery terms. Quality of life can be approached from the perspective of quality of being, and does not need to be approached merely from the perspective of doing and achieving. Such a perspective is highly relational and requires research strategies that uncover meaning and relational qualities.

The kind of hermeneutics described here has its roots in Division I of Heidegger's work.[17] Others who use this kind of hermeneutics are Taylor,[11] Kuhn,[22] Geertz,[23] and Garfinkel.[24] The goal is to find exemplars or paradigm cases that embody the meanings of everyday practices. The data are participant observations, field notes, interviews, and unobtrusive samples of behavior and interaction in natural settings. Human behavior is treated as a text analogue and the task is to uncover the meanings in everyday practice in such a way that they are not destroyed, distorted, decontextualized, trivialized, or sentimentalized.[25] When the interpreter has done a good job, participants can recognize and validate the interpretation. Participants will be somewhat annoyed or pleased that the interpreter has given a meaningful account of their experience. This is not a hermeneutics of suspicion, used by Marx or Freud or the mid-career-Heidegger, where the goal is to discover some latent causal explanation in theoretical or power terms, such as class struggle, Oedipal complex, dependency needs, or anxiety over ungroundedness, but to accurately portray lived meanings in their own terms.[26]

This method is particularly useful for understanding the phenomenal world of health and illness. It provides an appropriate access to increasing the understanding of disease as it is shaped by experiences of health and illness. It is not a mentalistic view of disease; therefore it is not a subjectivistic or completely relativistic view.[27,28] For example, this view holds that the pathology of diabetes exists irrespective of self-understanding and even before the scientific discovery of the dysfunction. But once the scientific explanation exists and is transmitted culturally, the illness experience is transformed and impacts the disease itself. It is known that

psychological stress, even in the form of "fear of diabetic coma," can increase the need for insulin. The person's illness experience both constitutes and is constituted by disease. To try to determine the relative contribution of "uninterpreted disease" and "the cultural interpretation of the disease" to the illness experience is to ignore the constitutive relationship.

Hermeneutic phenomenology is holistic in that it seeks to study the person in the situation, rather than isolating person variables and situation variables and then trying to put them back together.[15] The explanations are teleological and include intentional causality but are not limited to a mentalistic view of pure intentionality. This view allows the explanation of disease through practice and history without having to embrace a purely intentionalistic explanation that would, for example, allocate unconscious responsibility for choosing the site of one's cancer through internal and unconscious conflicts ("unconscious intent").

Underlying all interpretation-laden practices and self-understanding that are handed down through language and culture is the notion of "the background." The full-blown notion of background preunderstanding is one of the major distinctions between Heideggerian phenomenology and Husserlian transcendental phenomenology. It is this background that individuals cannot make fully explicit and cannot get completely clear about or clear of; it gives individuals the conditions of their possibility and the conditions for their perceptions, for their actions, and so forth. It is this background that makes human beings different from the artificial intelligence of the computer that always has to build its story up element by element, whereas human beings always come to a situation with a story, a preunderstanding. This position assumes that background meanings, skills, and practices are not completely rationalizable (cannot be made completely explicit), that this background forms the conditions of possibility, and that the background is handed down and not individually derived. Therefore, this position breaks with the tradition of methodological individualism. In fact, the meaning-giving subject is no longer the unit of analysis. Meaning resides not solely within the individual nor solely within the situation but is a transaction between the two so that the individual both constitutes and is constituted by the situation. Therefore, the unit of analysis is the transaction. This position, however, expects not only the unique or idiosyncratic but commonalities and recurring similarities and differences as well. However, unlike rational empiricism, hermeneutics does not look for these recurring similarities and differences in laws, mechanisms, structures, and processes or even in values that are unrelated to meaning. In this view, meaning is expressive and constitutive as well as designative and denotative.[29]

To review, methodological individualism is avoided by finding commonality and therefore teleological explanation and prediction based on background skills, meanings, and practices shared in a people with a common history and common situations.[8] This position abandons two assumptions of naturalism pointed out by Taylor.[29] The first position is that meaning can be seen in terms of representation of an independent reality (based on the 17th century philosophers, Hobbes and Locke). This is particularly a problem in studying highly skilled performance, pragmatic activities, and human concerns because all of these human activities and capacities are highly relational. The differential attention paid to aspects of the situation varies with the situation in ways that cannot be quantified. Moreover, many of the aspects that are recognized cannot be reduced to mental representations. They are based on perceptual recognitional abilities that Polanyi calls connoisseurship and the author terms graded qualitative distinctions.[19] One strategy for attending to meaningful distinctions in a situation is to reduce the distinctions to an array of patterns, with each pattern signifying a different meaning. This is a decided advance over identifying one variable at a time but cannot cope with the variability and nuances in shifting importance and rapidly changing relevance that can be recognized by human beings in a situation. The mental representation theory is analogous to matching templates on situations, but such an approach is slow and not as skilled as the experienced person who, without knowing the particulars or the reasons, attends to subtle differences in patterns and subtle shifts in relative importance of presenting issues.

The second assumption of naturalism (rational empiricism) that hermeneutic phenomenology questions is that theory can be generated from the standpoint of a monological observer who stands outside the situation and has private meanings that are then tested or matched with public activities.[19] The model of the person (both researcher and participant) in hermeneutic phenomenology does not expect that the person can ever gain a privileged transcendental position. Dreyfus made the point that "There can be no stable science of an entity which as meaning giver is the condition of its own objectification. No science can objectify the skills which make it possible. But this only shows we should abandon the Kantian definition of man."[13(p15)] Dreyfus goes on to note:

> According to Foucault the human sciences involve a unique human self-interpretation, which reaches its fullest expression in Kant. They interpret their domain of investigation, man, as a transcendental/empirical double—a meaning giver who constitutes the world and determines what counts as objects, and yet is an object in the world like any other. This conception of man makes human self-interpretation essential to an understanding of human beings while at the same time stipulating that human beings are meaningless objects amenable to the sort of theory characteristic of the natural sciences.[13(p4)]

Dreyfus[13] points out that this "double aspect theory," ie, the attempt to explain human activity from a totally physicalistic language and the attempt to provide a totally intentionalistic account, ensures that the sciences of man would always be "abnormal" (Kuhn's[30] term for science with competing paradigms). Two schools of thought—one interpretive and one materialistic—would perpetually compete with each other, each with an exclusive and conflicting vocabulary that could not accommodate the explanatory vocabulary of the other.

Heideggerian phenomenology overcomes the problems inherent in the Cartesian "transcendental/empirical double," or subject-object split, by starting with a different notion of the person. The person is studied in the situation and pragmatic involved activity is considered as a way of knowing and being. Dreyfus has called this "embodied intelligence."[31] Self-interpretations based on skills and practices and preunderstanding govern health and illness experiences and influence physiological functioning.

Dreyfus argues, and the author's observation of expert nurses illustrates,[19] that in studying pragmatic activities and human concerns, an approach to theorizing that is dependent on identifying decontextualized features *by definition* leaves out the meaning of the situation or situational understanding. As Dreyfus states: "The meaning of the situation plays an essential role in determining what counts as an event, and it is precisely this contextualized meaning that theory must ignore."[13(p11)] People have direct access to meaningful situations by virtue of education and experience. For example, nurses are trained to approach and interpret situations differently from physicians. Nurses approach clinical situations with a working knowledge of physiology and medicine but also with a knowledge about particular physicians' clinical skills, how available they typically are, and what their typical responses are likely to be. This situational understanding about the physician is augmented by an understanding of the particular patient and his or her typical response patterns in one situation, and even the clinical skill likely to be available on the next shift. Once situational contextual knowledge is spelled out, it becomes clearer why a purely structural account is unsatisfactory. This problem of describing human pragmatic activity with structuralism is illustrated in Bourdieu's

criticism of Levi-Strauss's formal structural theoretical account of gift giving:

> It is all a question of style, which means in this case timing and choice of occasion, for the same act—giving, giving in return, offering one's services, paying a visit, etc.—can have completely different meanings at different times.[32(pp5–6)]

It is possible to make a similar comparison about the meaning of a bed bath.[33] The list of decontextualized functions and features of a bed bath could be endless. However, with understanding of the situation, one can judge whether the bed bath is an unnecessary fostering of dependence, an essential tool for making a thorough yet unobtrusive assessment, a means of communicating with a withdrawn patient, or something else. In this case, theoretical access is not more elegant or more efficient than practical expert understanding of the situation. Clinical know-how has been trivialized by the thought that it could completely be captured by formal statements just as the experiences of health, illness, and suffering have been trivialized by analytically separating the mind and body.

Interpretive Research Strategies

Hermeneutics is a systematic approach to interpreting a text. Interview material and observations are turned into text through transcription. The interpretation entails a systematic analysis of the whole text, a systematic analysis of parts of the text, and a comparison of the two interpretations for conflicts and for understanding the whole in relation to the parts, and vice versa. Whole cases can be compared to other whole cases. Usually, this shifting back and forth between the parts and the whole reveals new themes, new issues, and new questions that are generated in the process of understanding the text itself.

The participant offers a depiction of the lived experience and the interpreter seeks commonalities in meanings, situations, practices, and bodily experiences. Interpreters use their distance and perspectives to understand the immediacy of the lived situation but these experience-distant perspectives must take into account the person *in* the situation. The interpreter enters into a dialogue with the text. For example, in proposing a clinical ethnography of an illness trajectory, the author has recommended that the interpreter consider the following experience-distant perspectives as possible starting points for interpretation: (1) the changing experience of the body; (2) changing social relationships as a result of the illness; (3) changing demands and tasks of different stages in the disease process and illness trajectory; (4) predictable responses and effective coping strategies for treatment side effects and sequelae; and (5) the particular—what the illness interrupts, threatens, and means to the individual.[21] Such predictable sources of commonality provide a starting point for the interpretation, but they do not set limits on what can be discovered in the process of allowing the test itself to make claims and raise issues with the interpreter. Three strategies—paradigm cases, exemplars, and thematic analysis—are useful for allowing the particular claims of the text to stand out and for presenting configurational and transactional relationships.

PARADIGM CASES

A whole case may stand out as a paradigm case, a strong instance of a particular pattern of meanings. Such a case is a "marker" so that once a paradigm case is recognized because of its particular clarity or vividness, other more subtle cases with similar global characteristics can be recognized.

Paradigm cases are useful as a recognitional strategy because early in the interpretive effort the interpreter may recognize only that this case is a strong instance of a particular relationship or meaning but may not be able to articulate *why* the case stands out or *what it depicts*. Through asking questions such as: Similar in what respect or different in what respect? How does this case stand out in relation to other cases?, the inter-

preter is able to put into words what this case is depicting. Paradigm cases are also useful as presentation strategies because the pattern of meanings and concerns depicted by the case often cannot be broken down into small units without losing important aspects of the patterns.

EXEMPLARS

Exemplars are also useful as recognitional tools *and* presentation strategies. An exemplar is smaller than a paradigm case, but like a paradigm case is a strong instance of a particularly meaningful transaction, intention, or capacity. An exemplar is a vignette or story of the particular transaction that captures the meaning in the situation so that the reader is able to recognize the same meaningful transaction in another situation where the objective characteristics might be quite different. Both exemplars and paradigm cases are presentation strategies that allow the depiction of the person *in* the situation. They present the context, the intentions of the actors, and the meanings in the situation.

THEMATIC ANALYSIS

A third interpretive strategy is that of thematic analysis. The interpreter identifies common themes in the interviews and extracts sufficient interview excerpts to present evidence to the reader of the theme. A thematic analysis is useful for presenting common meanings. In all three presentation strategies, sufficient interview documentation is provided to allow the reader to participate in the validation of the findings.

All three interpretive strategies (paradigm cases, exemplars, and thematic analysis) work both as discovery and presentation strategies. They all allow for the presentation of context and meanings. In interpretive research, unlike grounded theory,[34,35] the goal is not to extract theoretical terms or concepts at a higher level of abstraction. The goal is to discover meaning terms and to achieve understanding. If attempts are made to decontextualize the meaning, then the phenomenon is changed or rendered meaningless. This is the same point that Kuhn makes about the practical knowledge of the natural scientist that resides in shared exemplars and not strictly in rules and procedures. He writes:

> When I speak of knowledge embedded in shared exemplars, I am not referring to a model of knowing that is less systematic or less analyzable than knowledge embedded in rules, laws, or criteria of identification. Instead, I have in mind a manner of knowing which is misconstrued if reconstructed in terms of rules that are first abstracted from exemplars and thereafter function in their stead.[30(p192)]

The discovery of paradigm cases, exemplars, and recurring themes can be systematically and rigorously validated by experts and by those who are living out the practical knowledge and meanings presented in these interpretive strategies. However, if the method of validation requires decontextualization, as in operationalism, then the relational issues, that is, the concerns, meanings, and practical knowledge conveyed by presenting the person in context, will be lost. The experiences of health, illness, and suffering are trivialized by analytically separating the mind and body, and by using research strategies that systematically exclude the lived meanings of these experiences.

Bias Control Strategies

Multiple stages of interpretation allow for bias control by exposing contradictions, conflicts, or surprises that cannot be accounted for by an earlier or later interpretation. Actions and practices may not necessarily be rational, but it is assumed that they will have understandable, meaningful patterns. Multiple interviews with the same participants also provide a bias control strategy inasmuch as they allow patterns to emerge and prevent the interpreter from emphasizing a non-recurring, idiosyncratic episode, statement, or behavior. Redundancy provides confidence in the interpretation. The interpreter attempts to be "true" to the text and not read in meanings that are not supported by textual evidence. Expert consensual validation is sought for at least a

subset of the data to guard against the importation of meanings not actually supported by the text. The assumption is that the interpretations offered are based on shared cultural meanings and are therefore recognizable by other readers who share the same culture. This is congruent with the Heideggerian assumption that the meaning and organization of a culture precedes individual meaning-giving activity.[17]

The goal of this kind of commentary is to make the commonplace visible and understood. In achieving this goal, the interpreter has the same problem as the anthropologist who returns home. The anthropologist at home runs the risk of overlooking key meanings, not because they are so esoteric or uncommon, but rather because they are so pervasive.[17] The reader of the interpretation actively participates in the validation process. The reader should approach interpretive works with the following five criteria of internal validity outlined by Cherniss:

> First, they should help us to understand the lives of the subjects; we should better comprehend the complex pattern of human experience as a result of these. Second, the themes should maintain the integrity of the original "data." Third, the interpretations should be internally consistent. Fourth, data that support the findings should be presented. Usually, these data will take the form of excerpts from interviews. Finally, the reported conclusions should be consistent with the reader's own experience. In qualitative research, the readers must critically scrutinize the results of the thematic analysis, playing a more active role in the process of "validation" than they normally would.[36(pp278–279)]

Cherniss's third point on internal consistency should not be misconstrued to mean that the interpretation should reveal only internally consistent practices and commitments by participants. Conflicting, inconsistent practices and commitments are common and are often what is uncovered in doing the interpretation. Interpretations are considered internally consistent if the textual data presented match the interpretations offered.

The author is enough of a pragmatist to believe that the final proof of the hermeneutic phenomenology position lies in the knowledge it uncovers. We have to ask what our theory and method screens allow us to see. Do theories lend themselves best to a chart audit to determine the completeness of records, or do they tell the clinician how to promote healing and wellness and understand illness and suffering to promote comfort and cure? Do theories allow for mere categorization of information or do they provide guidelines for interpreting the information? Are predictions so deterministic that they overlook human possibilities, change, and growth?

Science at this point needs to return individuals to the things themselves, the experience of health, illness, suffering, and the wisdom and ignorance embedded in practice. There must be a return to the systematic study of practice and of health, illness, and suffering.[21] The study of practice should offer more than a sociological description of role relationships. The goal should be to find out the wisdom, frustration, puzzles, dilemmas, and knowledge embedded in practice. The study of health and illness should offer a new understanding of the lived body in health and illness. The hermeneutics of early Heidegger offers a promising methodological approach.[17]

The author is not a single paradigm expectant scientist,[26,37] because a single paradigm in the human sciences claims that one single perspective provides the *one* explanatory vantage point and that all other paradigms are inferior or subordinate. One paradigm would provide a totalitarian explanatory system for all human behavior and would assume one privileged position exists from which to view situations, capacities, and problems of human beings. Such a singular paradigm works in the natural sciences because the background practices, skills, and assumptions of the scientists are not issues for them. Decontextualizing practices can be ignored after standardization because the natural scientist searches for objectified and decontextualized elements that can be related by strict laws.[13] But as Dreyfus and Rabinow point out:

> If the human sciences claim to study human activities, then the human sciences, unlike the natural sciences, must take account of those human activities which make possible their own disciplines.
>
> Thus, while in the natural sciences it is always possible and generally desirable that an unchallenged normal science which defines and resolves problems concerning the structure of the physical universe establish itself, in the social sciences such an unchallenged normal science would only indicate that an orthodoxy had established itself, not through scientific achievement, but by ignoring the background and eliminating all competitors.[26(pp163–164)]

Such a totalitarian stance is not only unattractive; it simply does not offer much in the way of explanation, prediction, and understanding because the theories in human sciences must always presuppose common background meanings and practices. For example, Taylor[11] points out that objective political science is dependent on cultural practices that are not immutable but subject to change in a constitutive way. Political theory in an individual-based contract society such as the United States will not work on a background of different cultural interpretations such as the Japanese cultural background of consensus and group orientation. The scientist is always in a culture and cannot completely step outside the particular historical understanding available during his or her period. There can be no value-free or interpretation-free data language. Consequently, deterministic monological theoretical schemes will necessarily be time bound and limited in their predictive and explanatory power. Such deterministic theoretical schemes are a part of the cultural press for extreme rationalization and objectification. Weber,[38] Adorno,[39] Foucault,[40] and Dreyfus and Rabinow[26] have been concerned with this pervasive press for rationalization in the western tradition.

Certainly the strain of objectification is felt in the study of health, illness, suffering, and disease. The very labeling and technologizing of symptoms add to the stress of the "target population" at "high risk."[41] Discovering that one is in a high-risk group increases the risk. But coming to view oneself as a collection of needs, wants, and health risks that must be scientifically met creates a stressful, effortful life style based on the premises of control and balance.[20] Such a formula works well until the limits of control are confronted, which for the person experiencing illness or suffering is frequent.[20] As a nurse scientist, the author does not want to increase the rationalization and objectification of the notion of health and the experience of illness and suffering by the formal models and methods used to study individuals.

Extreme objectification and subjectification cannot capture the lived experiences of health and illness because human beings are never fully object or fully subject; they exist in a network of concerns and relations. If the way of doing science objectifies or oversubjectifies (in the sense of making the health-illness experience an extremely private, idiosyncratic one), then those individuals using these approaches will unwittingly contribute to the stress-related diseases so prevalent in today's society, do little to treat illness and disease, and finally blunt the ability to alleviate suffering. Heideggerian phenomenology generates forms of explanation and prediction that offer understanding and choice, rather than manipulation and control. Nursing requires access to concrete problems and dilemmas associated with health, illness, suffering, and disease and an understanding of the power of human practices, skills, and relationships that engender hope and promote healing.

REFERENCES

1. Kleinman A, Eisenberg L, Good B: Culture, illness, and care: Clinical lessons from anthropologic and cross-cultural research. *Ann Intern Med* 1978; 88:251–258.
2. West JW, Stein MS (eds): *Critical Issues in Behavioral Medicine*. Philadelphia, Lippincott, 1982.
3. Merleau-Ponty M: *Phenomenology of Perception*. London, Routledge and Kegan Paul, 1962.
4. Cassell EJ: The nature of suffering and the goals of medicine. *N Engl J Med* 1982;30:639–645.
5. Sandel M: *Liberalism and the Limits of Justice*. London, Cambridge Univ. Press, 1982.
6. Gilligan C: *In a Different Voice*. Cambridge, Mass, Harvard Univ. Press, 1982.
7. Yankelovich D: *New Rules in American Life: Searching for Self-Fulfillment in a World Turned Upside Down*. New York, Random House, 1981.
8. Dreyfus HL: *Being-in-the-World: A Commentary on Division I of Being and Time*. Cambridge, Mass, MIT Press, to be published.
9. Hempel C: *Aspects of Scientific Explanation*. New York, The Free Press, 1965.
10. Toulmin S: Concepts and the explanation of human behavior, in Mischel S. (ed): *Human Action*. New York, Academic Press, 1969, pp 87–88.
11. Taylor C: Interpretation and the sciences of man, in Rabinow P, Sullivan M (eds): *Interpretive Social Science*. Berkeley, University of California Press, 1979.
12. Taylor C: *Explanation of Behavior*. New York, Humanities Press, 1964.
13. Dreyfus HL: Why the study of human capacities can never be scientific. *Berkeley Cognitive Science Report*, no. 11. Berkeley, University of California, Cognitive Science Program, Institute of Human Learning, 1984.
14. Wolf S: Introduction: The role of the brain in bodily disease, in Werner H, Hoger MA, Strunkard AJ (eds): *Brain, Behavior, and Bodily Disease*. New York, Raven Press, 1981, pp 1–9.
15. Lazarus RS, Launier R: Stress-related transactions between person and environment, in Pervin L, Lewis M (eds): *Perspectives in Interactional Psychology*. New York, Plenum Press, 1978, pp 287–327.
16. Weisman A: *Coping with Cancer*. New York, McGraw-Hill, 1979.
17. Heidegger M: *Being and Time*, Macquarrie J., Robinson E. (trans). New York, Harper & Row, 1962.
18. Heidegger M: *The Basic Problems of Phenomenology*, Hofstadter A (trans). Bloomington, Ind, Indiana Univ. Press, 1982.
19. Benner P: *From Novice to Expert: Excellence and Power in Clinical Nursing Practice*. Menlo Park, Calif, Addison-Wesley, 1984.
20. Benner P: *Stress and Satisfaction on the Job: Work Meanings and Coping of Mid-Career Men*. New York, Praeger Scientific Press, 1984.
21. Benner P: The oncology clinical nurse specialist as expert coach. *Oncology Nurse Forum* 1985; 12(2):40–44.
22. Kuhn TS: *The Essential Tension*. Chicago, University of Chicago Press, 1977.

23. Geertz C: *The Interpretation of Cultures*. New York, Harper & Row, 1973.

24. Garfinkel H: *Studies in Ethnomethodology*. Englewood Cliffs, NJ, Prentice-Hall, 1967.

25. Lazarus RS: The trivialization of distress, in Rosen JC, Solomon LJ (eds): *Vermont Conference on the Primary Prevention of Psychopathology*, vol. 8. Hanover, NH, University Press of New England, to be published.

26. Dreyfus HL, Rabinow P: *Michel Foucault Beyond Structuralism and Hermeneutics*. Chicago, The University of Chicago Press, 1982.

27. Bernstein R: *Beyond Objectivism and Relativism: Science, Hermeneutics, and Praxis*. Philadelphia, University of Pennsylvania Press, 1983.

28. Palmer RE: *Hermeneutics*. Evanston, Northwestern Univ. Press, 1969.

29. Taylor C: *Dawes Hicks Lecture, Theories of Meaning. Proceedings of the British Academy*, London, British Academy, 1982, pp 283–327.

30. Kuhn TS: *The Structure of Scientific Revolutions*, ed 2, enlarged. Chicago, The University of Chicago Press, 1970.

31. Dreyfus HL: *What Computers Can't Do*. New York, Harper & Row, 1979.

32. Bourdieu P: *Outline of a Theory of Practice*. Cambridge, Cambridge Univ. Press, 1977.

33. Benner P: Issues in competence based testing. *Nurs Outlook* 1982;30:303–309.

34. Glaser BG, Strauss AL: *The Discovery of Grounded Theory*. Chicago, Atherton Press, 1967.

35. Glaser BG: *Theoretical Sensitivity*. Mill Valley, Calif, The Sociology Press, 1978.

36. Cherniss C: *Professional Burnout in Human Services Organizations*. New York, Praeger, 1980.

37. Rabinow P, Sullivan WM (eds): Introduction, The interpretive turn: Emergence of an approach, in *Interpretive Social Science*. Berkeley, University of California Press, 1979.

38. Weber M: *The Protestant Ethic and the Spirit of Capitalism*. New York, Scribner, 1958.

39. Adorno T: *Against Epistemology*, Domingo W. (trans). Cambridge, Mass, MIT Press, 1983.

40. Foucault M: *Madness and Civilization: A History of Insanity in the Age of Reason*. Howard R. (trans). New York, Random House, 1973.

41. Horowitz MJ, Dimon N, Holden M, et al: Stressful impact of news of risk for premature heart disease. *Psychosom Med* 1983;45(1):31–40.

A Heideggerian Phenomenologic Perspective on the Concept of the Person

Victoria Wynn Leonard

Nursing research has been the focus of intense debates on epistemological questions in recent years. This author contends that these methodologic debates have at their base the problem of differing conceptions of the person. In this paper, a Heideggerian phenomenological view of the person will be presented and contrasted with the Cartesian view of person implicit in current empirical research strategies. Methodologic implications of the phenomenological view will then be outlined in a discussion of interpretive research methods, or hermeneutics.

Much recent debate in nursing research centers around the relative merits of quantitative and qualitative research methods. Insight into current philosophical thinking affords us an alternative to this endless, currently irresolvable controversy.

The battle lines in this debate were largely drawn by 17th-century science as part of the controversy over how the private mind apprehends the external world using a mechanically driven and unreliable body. In sum, how do we know what we know? How do we know that what we know is "true"? Must we choose between the subjective, relative truth of the private subject and the objective truth of the raw data? A review of recent trends in philosophy suggests that there are other ways of framing the problem that yield fruitful insights into the problem of how we study human beings.

Much of the current thinking in philosophy that attempts to get beyond the debate over objectivism and relativism stems from the work of Martin Heidegger. It was Heidegger's shift from the problems of epistemology to those of ontology—that is, of what it is to be a human being—that radically altered modern debates on the nature of science and of knowing. Nursing would profit from considering this question of what it is to be a person before considering questions of epistemology. Once fundamental ontologic notions are clarified, the at times acrimonious debate concerning methodology will be resolved, for, as Laudan[1] argues, a research tradition includes both methodologic and ontologic commitments, which are inextricably linked.

To illustrate this point, the present article will first discuss briefly the Cartesian view of the person, then a Heideggerian phenomenologic view, and finally the hermeneutic method will be outlined. Hermeneutics is a method for studying human beings that flows out of the Heideggerian view of the person and is consistent with it. It is critical, however, to consider the Heideggerian notion of the person before considering any notions of methodology. To consider a

Reprinted by permission from Advances in Nursing Science 11(4):40–55. © 1989, Aspen Publishers, Inc.

methodology without an ontological commitment to a view of persons is to beg the question. The question is not which methodology is best or even necessarily which method is right for the question being asked, because method acts as a theoretical screen and often determines the kinds of questions that are asked. The questions to be asked are, first, What does it mean to be a person, and then, in light of the answer, How does one ask the research questions, and, finally, How does one answer the questions posed? Too often the researcher quickly seizes on a method without considering the more profoundly important philosophical assumptions that undergird the method or whether those assumptions are consistent with the researcher's own view of what it means to be a human being.

The Modern Cartesian View of the Person

As a consequence of a world view that follows canons of Cartesianism, we in nursing are preoccupied with a notion of the person as an assemblange of traits or variables such as anxiety, control, and self-esteem, which are viewed as context-free elements to be combined according to formal laws that can be discovered through the scientific method, the goal of which is prediction and control. This notion of person flows from an implicit acceptance of 17th-century Cartesian notions of the self, in which the self is viewed as subject, an uninvolved entity passively contemplating the external world of things via representations that are held in the mind. This self *possesses* a body and, by extension, traits or attributes such as anxiety and self-esteem. The self is always seen as subject and the world, or the environment, as object.

This view of the person led inextricably to 300 years of debate over whether knowledge is real (ie, an accurate representation of an external reality) or ideal (ie, a subjective idea or private view of the world that is idiosyncratic and thus can never be fully shared or communicated). Modern versions of this debate continue in nursing today, as in the debates between transcendental phenomenologists and positivist empiricists.

The Heideggerian Phenomenologic View of the Person

Heideggerian phenomenology criticizes both the objective and subjective positions of Cartesianism for asking an epistemologic question (ie, How do we know what we know?) rather than an ontologic question (ie, What does it mean to be a person?). By coming to grips with the ontologic question nurses, particularly those doing research, could move away from an uncritical belief in science and the scientific method (variously referred to as scientism or the received view) to embrace a multiplicity of methods. This variety could include the scientific method when it does not violate phenomenologic notions of what it is to be a person (eg, in cellular level or epidemiologic studies), for phenomenology does not propose the abolition of traditional science but rather its appropriate use. Its use is appropriate in levels of study where participants' meanings and interpretations do not figure, such as a study of the effects of maternal hyperglycemia on idiopathic neonatal hypoglycemia or a study of the rate of prenatal complications in pregnant women employed in jobs requiring strenuous work. Traditional science has accomplished astonishing results in the past two centuries, particularly with regard to disease, but, as Baron points out, "These accomplishments are not great in and of themselves. They derive their significance from what they mean for human beings and what effect they have on suffering and individual capability."[2(p608)] Phenomenologists argue that traditional science is itself a theory screen that constraints our ability to understand human agency (ie, intentionality in human action constituted or shaped by concerns, purposes, goals, and commitments), limits our imaginative ability to generate questions, and, further, limits the answers we can generate for those questions that we do pose.

The view of person presented in this article is derived primarily from the writings of Heidegger.[3] The author is also indebted to the works of Taylor[4,5] and Dreyfus.[6]

In Heideggerian phenomenology, the view of person derives fundamentally from Heidegger's shift away from epistemologic concern with the relationship of the knower to the known toward the more fundamental concern with ontology: What does it mean to be a person?

> The proximal goal of *Being and Time* is to develop a descriptive metaphysics. Heidegger is not interested in fanciful speculation about Being. He is concerned with what Being means to us, and this requires at the outset an understanding of the being of that entity which understands what it is to be, namely, Dasein. Dasein in the course of its everyday activities and practices is characterized as "Being-in-the-world."[7(p69)]

Dasein is the term Heidegger uses to designate "the being to whose being an understanding of beings belongs."[3(p312)] In discussing what it is to *be*, Heidegger used *Dasein* to reflect the kind of beings we are prior to the reflective, conscious ego of the Cartesian tradition. "In German the word 'Dasein' means simply 'existence,' as in man's everyday existence. But it also means, if you take it apart, 'being there.' This conveys that this activity of human beings is an activity of being in the situation in which coping can go on and things can be encountered."[8(p263)]

THE PERSON AS HAVING A WORLD

The first step in this presentation of a phenomenologic view of person centers on the relationship of the person to the world. "World," in the phenomenologic sense, has a fundamentally different meaning from the common understanding of the world as environment, or nature, or the sum total of the "things" in our world. Phenomenologically, world is the meaningful set of relationships, practices, and language that we have by virtue of being born into a culture. For example, the common expression "the world of

science" reflects the set of relationships, questions, skills, and practices related to science. World, as Heidegger describes it,

> comes not afterward but beforehand, in the strict sense of the word. Beforehand: that which is unveiled and understood already in advance in every existent Dasein before any apprehending of this or that being. The world as already unveiled in advance is such that we do not in fact specifically occupy ourselves with it, or apprehend it, but instead it is so self-evident, so much a matter of course, that we are completely oblivious to it.[3(p165)]

World, according to Heidegger, is *a priori*. It is given in our cultural and linguistic practices and in our history. Language, in particular, sets up a world; it both articulates and makes things show up for us. "For Heidegger, a vocabulary, or the kinds of metaphors one uses can name things into being and change the sensibility of age."[9(p274)] Language creates the possibility for particular ways of feeling and of relating that make sense within a culture. World is the shared skills and practices on which we depend for meaning and intelligibility.

> World cannot be described by trying to enumerate the entities within it; in this process world would be passed over, for world is just what is presupposed in every act of knowing an entity. Every entity in the world is grasped as an entity *in terms of* world, which is always already there. The entities which comprise man's physical world are not themselves world but in a world. Only man has a world.[9(pp132–133)]

World is both constituted by and constitutive of the self. This notion of the self as constituted by world is fundamentally different from the Cartesian notion of the self as a possession.[10] The world is constitutive in that the self is raised up in the world and shaped by it in a process that is not the causal interaction of the self and the world as objects, but rather the nonreflective taking up of the meanings, linguistic skills, cultural practices, and family traditions by which we become persons and by which things become evident for us. The self as possession and project is the modern subject: autonomous, disengaged, disembodied, rationally choosing actions on the basis of explicit, cognitively held principles and values. The self as possession has a body and traits or characteristics that belong to it. As Sandel[10] puts it, my traits are *mine* but not *me*. These traits can thus come and go without altering the self in any constitutive way, that is, without becoming part of who the self is and shaping how that self knows itself. As Ricoeur[11] comments, this modern self is a self robbed of the health of sameness. Along with this view goes a view of the self as a radically free, autonomous agent: "the human subject as a sovereign agent of choice, whose ends are chosen rather than given."[10(p22)]

Heidegger argues that the only way in which one can arrive at this view of the self is by passing over the world, by not seeing that it is world that circumscribes our choices and creates our possibilities. The word "thrownness" is sometimes used to express this Heideggerian view of the person as *situated*, as being-in-the-world and therefore, as Benner says, "not a radically free arbiter of meaning."[12(p5)] The Heideggerian view is also a teleological view of the self, inconceivable apart from and prior to its ends and purposes, whereas for the radically free self of Cartesianism, values and purposes are the products of choice, "the possessions of a self given prior to its ends."[10(p176)] Freedom, in the Heideggerian view, is *situated* freedom.[4,5] Thus, while the self constitutes its world, it is also constrained in the possible ways in which it can constitute the world by its language, culture, history, purposes, and values. In other words, world sets up possibilities as to who a person can and cannot become. As Hoy comments, "personal identity is not a matter of ownership."[13]

Taylor[4] argues that part of the attraction of traditional science for the Western world has been that it includes the view of the self as radically free. Such a view of the self, suggests Taylor, is profoundly appealing to westerners because it coincides with our modern notions of freedom and liberation. However, it is this very

modern identity that causes us to overlook the essential inability of 17th-century science to afford us an understanding of human agency.

World is not a purely intentional, cognitive set of beliefs (a definition that depends on the Cartesian notion of the conscious subject). Nor is it the environment-as-object described by science. Rather, because world is constituted by our common language and culture and is requisite in order for anything to be visible to us at all, the subjective-objective Cartesian dualism that necessarily forces us into idealism (subjectivism) or realism (objectivism) can be replaced by understanding the person as being-in-the-world. World is neither held in the mind nor "out there" to be apprehended. While each of us may constitute his or her own world in the sense of taking up in a personal way the common meanings given in our language and culture, we nevertheless have some aspects of world in common with all other members who share our language and culture. For example, the American notion of upward mobility, which is evident in many aspects of our society, only makes sense within a cultural context in which class lines are somewhat fluid and in which at least some opportunities exist for self-improvement. Such a notion would make little sense in a culture where class lines were fixed and opportunities for self-improvement were not available to most people. Moreover, the notion of upward mobility is not a concept we are taught but rather a concept into which we are born and by which we are constituted.

Heidegger argues that the detached, reflective mode of knowing the world that is exemplified by Descartes is dependent on the preexistence of world, in the sense that the meanings given by our language and culture create the possibility for our noticing anything at all. The taken-for-granted, involved skills and practices of what Heidegger calls the ready-to-hand mode are presupposed by the abstract, theoretical, reflective knowledge that Heidegger calls the present-at-hand mode.

World is so all-pervasive as to be overlooked

by persons, and it only appears to us in a conscious way when disruption or breakdown occur. Heidegger gives us the example of the hammer. In using a hammer we do not think of it and its purpose in an abstract, theoretical way but rather in an assumed, taken-for-granted way—until such a time as the hammer breaks or fails to serve the purpose we intend for it. From the recognition of what it *isn't* doing we derive a sense of what a hammer in the assumed, ready-to-hand mode is like. A notion of "hammer" in the present-at-hand, abstract, theoretical mode will give us a notion of a hammer that excludes hammering in the taken-for-granted, lived experience of hammering.

Heidegger's example of the hammer exemplifies the phenomenologic objection to our emphasis in Western culture on the primacy of the abstract, present-at-hand mode: It overlooks the world (ie, the taken-for-granted, lived experience of our everydayness) and, concomitantly, it misses the meaning that is made intelligible through the linguistic and cultural skills and practices given by world.

THE PERSON AS A BEING FOR WHOM THINGS HAVE SIGNIFICANCE AND VALUE

A second essential facet of the person from a phenomenologic perspective is that persons are beings for whom things have significance and value.

> [Dasein] *finds itself* primarily and constantly *in things* because, tending them, distressed by them, it always in some way or other rests in things. Each one of us is what he pursues and cares for. In everyday terms we understand ourselves and our existence by way of the activities we pursue and the things we take care of.[3(p159)]

Dreyfus points out that it is a "basic characteristic of Dasein that things show up as mattering—as threatening, or attractive, or stubborn, or useful, and so forth,"[8(p264)] and this mattering is the background for more reflective desiring or evaluating. Another aspect of Heidegger's account of significance is the way in which our activity is directed in a transparent, taken-for-granted, nonmental way toward the future (the "for-the-sake-of").

Borgman[14] further expands Heidegger's notion of the things we care for and traces the modern fate in the face of technology. Things are inseparable from Heidegger's view of world and from our engagement with them via practices that guard and protect them from technological reduction to means and ends. That is, the practice of preparing a good meal protects the meal from being reduced to a microwaved frozen dinner. Borgman contrasts things with devices in which means are, as much as possible, invisible and anonymous. In the case of the microwaved meal, the preparation of the food is minimized; only the end, the meal, is important. The practices (means) that are essential to things are irrelevant to devices whose sole purpose or end is the facile production of commodities for private consumption. The practices that gather us together in human community and give richness and meaning wither into empty and meaningless rituals in the face of technology. An example of Borgman's thesis is found in some modern parents' attitudes toward child rearing. The whole enterprise is reduced to the efficient production of a perfect "product" that embodies certain external goods: a physically well-formed, well-educated, well-mannered, employable, attractive young adult. The practices that embody the means for child rearing are considered irrelevant to this project or, worse, are disdained. The everyday, practical routines of feeding, bathing, teaching, entertaining, supervising, and cleaning up after small children that gathered parents and children together and formed the substance of family life in the past are now left to parental substitutes.

In the phenomenologic view, persons not only have a world in which things have significance and value but they have qualitatively different concerns based on their culture, language, and individual situations. Taylor[4] suggests that the scientific rejection of "secondary" properties—that is, those properties, qualities, or feelings that cannot be "intersubjectively univocal" or free of interpretation (eg, "I feel blue")—is one of the factors that make traditional scientific methods inappropriate for the human sciences. Such methods give no weight to motives like shame, guilt, or love, which are incapable of being significance-free.

> These are the ones, therefore, where the variables occur between human cultures, that is, between different ways of shaping and interpreting that significance. So that what is a matter of shame or guilt or dignity, of moral goodness, is notoriously different and often hard to understand from culture to culture: whereas the conditions of medical health are far more uniform.[4(p111)]

Because there can be no significance-free account of desires, feelings, and emotions, our understanding of these kinds of terms necessarily moves in a hermeneutic circle: We understand the term "shame" by referring to the situation that is shameful and to the purpose of covering up the shameful act or saving face. The act, the feeling, and the purpose all refer to each other. Nowhere can one step out of the circle to get a significance-free "brute datum" to ground the account.[5]

Thus, to understand a person's behavior or expressions, one has to study the person in context, for it is only there that what a person values and finds significant is visible. Understanding the relational and configurational context allows for a more appropriate interpretation of the significance that things have for a person. For example, anxiety during pregnancy is a variable often considered to be a possible predictor of events in labor and delivery. In the traditional treatment of variables as context-free elements that the researcher attempts to relate in some law-like way, a tool such as the Spielberger State-Trait Anxiety Inventor would be used to obtain an "intersubjectively univocal" measure of anxiety. Problems arise because the meanings of pregnancy and of parenthood vary widely, and thus the meaning of the anxiety varies

widely. Assuming in advance that anxiety is a trait that is not fundamentally shaped by the meaning of the situation can cause the researcher, or the clinician, to miss the essential piece of the situation that is required to understand what is going on.

Certain events may be predicted, but at the cost of sacrificing an understanding of the transactional process going on between the person and her world. For example, pregnancy in older women with established careers and marriages interrupts long-established rhythms of work and love, and anxiety in these women can be interpreted as the realistic anticipatory working-through of the problems and issues that having the infant will bring. This kind of anxiety is potentially desirable and means that the woman is looking ahead and planning realistically for the new situations of motherhood. In other cases, the pregnancy may not be wanted and motherhood not valued. The anxiety of these women focuses on despair and the foreclosing of possibilities and should raise a red flag to the clinician providing prenatal care.

It can be seen, therefore, how an appreciation for the fact that persons are beings for whom things have significance, and that this significance may change with context, can reveal a different kind of understanding. The meaning of a pregnant woman's anxiety matters to the clinician because by understanding the world of the pregnant woman the clinician is better able to determine whether to intervene to help her to see new possibilities in her situation that will have meaning for her, given her world. The woman's world provides the only access to what is possible for her. Her world can be expanded only in relation to existing concerns and possibilities. This point has great significance for nurses practicing in clinical settings.

THE PERSON AS SELF-INTERPRETING

Another critical piece in the Heideggerian phenomenologic view of the person is that being is self-interpreting. However, it is important that "self-interpreting" be understood as being non-theoretical and noncognitive. We are beings who are engaged in and constituted by our interpretive understanding. Contrary to Husserl's belief that these interpretations are a product of the individual consciousness of subjects, Heidegger claims that these interpretations are not generated in individual consciousness as subjects related to objects, but rather are given in our linguistic and cultural traditions and make sense only against a background of significance. For example, Caudill and Weinstein[15] studied Japanese and American babies and found that by the age of four months the babies had become distinctly Japanese or American. Thus human beings are already, at a very early age, interpreting themselves in light of their cultural background: all of those hidden skills and practices and the linguistic meanings that are so all-pervasive as to be unnoticed and yet make the world intelligible for us, create our possibilities and the conditions for our actions. In the phenomenologic view, then, persons can never perceive "brute facts" out there in the world. Nothing can be encountered without reference to our background understanding. Every encounter entails an interpretation based on our background. "What appears from the 'object' is what one allows to appear and what the thematization of the world at work in his understanding will bring to light."[9(p136)]

THE PERSON AS EMBODIED

The phenomenologic notion of person includes a view of the body that is fundamentally different from the Cartesian notion of the body as object of possession. The Cartesian body is merely *res extensa*, "a machine driven by mechanical causality ... extrinsic to the essential self"[16(p30)] and exhibiting no intelligence or power to respond to the world. In the phenomenologic view, rather than having a body, we are embodied. Our common practices are based on shared, embodied, perceptual capacities.[17,18] Our bodies provide the possibility for the concrete actions of self in the world. It is the body that first grasps the world and moves with intention in that meaningful world. Merleau-Ponty[18] calls this bodily intelligence. In Leder's words, "Viewed as intentional, bodily functioning can express affective, cognitional influences in a way perhaps inexplicable within the Cartesian model."[16(p38)] Those researchers and clinicians who have an implicit understanding of the intentional body but frame their research and clinical problems from a Cartesian body position find themselves articulating multicausal notions of disease, but they are incapable of ever explaining satisfactorily the Cartesian mind-body problem: How do the physical and mental relate? "The paradigm of the lived-body, wherein subjectivity is always corporeally expressed, avoids these problems."[16(p39)]

Baron points out that health is the state of "unselfconscious being that illness shatters."[2(p609)] Our everyday lived experience, in which the embodied self is taken for granted, breaks down in illness, and our ready-to-hand understanding of ourselves as embodied doesn't work for us anymore. Thus it is in the state of "breakdown" that we develop insight into the taken-for-granted understanding of health: the unity of self and healthy body. "That the body is not a mere extrinsic machine but our living center from which radiates all existential possibilities is brought home with a vengeance in illness, suffering, and disability."[16(p34)] This viewpoint affords the clinician a new position from which to understand the patient's experience of illness. Rather than viewing the problem as the breakdown of an objective machine, one approaches illness as a rupture in the patient's ability to negotiate the world. It is one's embodiment that is the problem, suggests Baron,[2] not one's body as objective machine.

The present author would argue that Baron's position pertains even more directly to nursing than to medicine. It is nursing, more than medicine, that seeks to help the patient reclaim a sense of embodiment that allows for taken-for-granted, unselfconscious transaction with the world.

The Person in Time

Finally, the Heideggerian phenomenologic notion of the person includes a view of the person or being-in-time that differs radically from more traditional Western notions of time. Our traditional view of linear time is of an endless succession of "nows": "The common conception thinks of the nows as free-floating, relationless, intrinsically patched on to one another and intrinsically successive."[3(p263)] This "snap-shot" view of time presents us with the problem of conceiving continuity or transition. It also gives us a notion of things existing as static, atemporal entities and leads, in the scientific research tradition, to a system of formal laws that are supposed to be atemporal. For example, Sandel's[10] self of possession has traits that may come and go, but they do not fundamentally alter the self.

Temporality, in this view, is the accrual of events: for example, I had anxiety, but then X occurred and I no longer had anxiety. The "I" does not change, in this view, in the sense of having been constituted by anxiety, because it merely possessed the anxiety. In this view, time is not a constituent of human events. In the Heideggerian phenomenologic view, however, temporality is constitutive of being; for example, Heidegger describes the past as having-been-ness:

> The Dasein can as little get rid of its bygoneness as escape its death. In every sense and in every case everything we have been is an essential determination of our existence. Even if in some way, by some manipulation, I may be able to keep my bygoneness far from myself, nevertheless, forgetting, repressing, suppressing are modes in which I myself am my own having-been-ness.[3(p265)]

"Temporality" is thus the term Heidegger uses to describe a notion of time that is prior to, or more original than, our common sense of time as a linear succession of nows. Linear time creates the problem of relating past and future

to the now, but temporality, argues Heidegger, is directional and relational and applies only to being, not to physical objects. "The not-yet and no longer are not patched onto the now as foreign but belong to its very content. Because of this *dimension content*, the *now* has within itself the *character of a transition*."[3(p249)] Rather than being empty or something (like space) to be filled up, time is "*essentially* content: it *exists as* activity, such as concernful dealing and attention."[19(p1184)] Thus the Cartesian self as possession is not constituted by time, and traits or attributes can be studied without considering their order or meaning in relation to each other; they are context-free elements. The being-in-time, on the other hand, cannot be studied except within the context of the having-beenness and being-expectant, or its past and future, by which it is constituted. If these concepts are applied to the previous example of anxiety in pregnancy, the older pregnant woman with career commitments might have a having-beenness that includes insisting on doing things with great precision and care. Her having-beenness also includes much rumination on whether an infant can be left in the care of a nonparent while the parents both return to full-time work. Her being-expectant includes an awareness that her company expects her to return to full-time work as an equally functioning member of the team. Her anxiety in pregnancy, then, can be seen to be constituted by her past and future.

Having outlined the essential aspects of a Heideggerian phenomenologic view of person, this article now turns to the implications of this view for research.

Hermeneutics as a Method Appropriate to the Heideggerian Phenomenological Study of Human Beings

> A being who exists only in self-interpretation cannot be understood absolutely; and one who can only be understood against the background of distinctions of worth cannot be captured by a scien-

tific language which essentially aspires to neutrality. Our personhood cannot be treated scientifically in exactly the same way we approach our organic being. What it is to possess a liver or heart is something I can define quite independently of the space of questions in which I exist for myself, but not what it is to have a self or be a person.[4(pp3–4)]

Appreciating the implications for research of a phenomenologic view of the person involves going beyond the debates over qualitative versus quantitative and objectivism versus relativism. It involves a fundmental shift in orientation away from traditional notions of objectivity as unitizing and generalizing, with the goals of prediction and control. This notion of objectivity strips human actions of their context and assumes the possibility of an Archimedean point from which a foundational knowledge can be discovered on the basis of "judgments which could be anchored in a certainty beyond subjective intuition."[5(p19)] Heideggerian phenomenologists, on the other hand, propose that there is no Archimedean point, no privileged position for "objective" knowing but rather that all knowledge emanates from persons who are already in the world and seeking to understand other persons who are also already in the world. One is thus always within the hermeneutic circle of interpretation. Researcher and research participant are viewed as sharing common practices, skills, interpretations, and everyday practical understanding by virtue of their common culture and language. Also, since human beings are constituted by temporality, all knowledge, in this view, is temporal. Atemporal, ahistorical, transcendent knowledge of human behavior is impossible.

> The human sciences, because they are engaged in temporal investigation, are not designed to arrive at an atemporal causal certainty. Instead, their investigations have as their object the rendering of life and the world continually understandable.[19(p1186)]

Further, since persons are fundamentally self-interpreting beings for whom things have significance, understanding human action always involves an interpretation by the researcher of the interpretations being made by those persons being studied. This interpretive approach is called hermeneutics.

Hermeneutics is an ancient discipline that can be traced back to the early Greeks. Early Greek root words of hermeneutics suggest the idea of bringing to understanding, particularly where this process involves language. That is, something foreign, strange, and separated in time, space, or experience is revealed so as to seem familiar and comprehensible.[9]

In modern times, according to Palmer,[9] hermeneutics has had two separate focuses. The first is the rules, methods, or theory governing the exegesis of linguistic texts. Biblical exegesis, the best-known example, dates from the 17th century. Legal discourse and literary criticism also draw on hermeneutics. The second focus of hermeneutics has been the philosophical exploration of the character and requisite conditions for understanding. In the early 19th century, according to Palmer,[9] Schleiermacher redefined heremeneutics as the study of understanding itself. His work was followed by that of Dilthey, who saw hermeneutics as the core discipline or foundation for all of the humanities and social sciences (ie, those disciplines that interpret expressions of the inner life of human beings).[9]

In the early 20th century, Heidegger's analysis of being suggested that interpretation is a foundational mode of our being. Heidegger's *Being and Time*[20] is referred to as "a hermeneutic of Dasein," an interpretive effort through which light is shed on the meaning of being. Thus the relevance of hermeneutics to the human sciences today derives primarily from Heidegger's writings. Currently the hermeneutic approach is being taken up by researchers in diverse human science fields, including nursing, that are concerned with understanding human beings.

The goals of hermeneutics are to understand everyday skills, practices, and experiences; to find commonalities in meanings, skills, practices, and embodied experiences; and "to find exemplars or paradigm cases that embody the meanings of everyday practices in such a way that they are not destroyed, distorted, decontextualized, trivialized, or sentimentalized."[12(pp5–6)] Paradigm cases and exemplars are strong instances of a particular pattern of meanings; they provide effective strategies for depicting the person in the situation and for preserving meanings and context. Access to everyday lived experience opens up a new understanding of the person and the possibility for overcoming the subject-object split of Cartesianism.

Furthermore, rather than looking for deterministic or mechanistic explanations of causality, hermeneutics seeks to develop understanding that is based on concerns, commitments, practices, and meanings. This understanding is such that it "will focus on sufficient conditions and make statements such as, all other things being equal, one expects such and such to occur. Such a statement leaves room for transformations in meanings and changes in human concerns."[12(p3)]

Hermeneutics as a methodology makes several assumptions derived from the Heideggerian phenomenologic view of the person. First, it is assumed that the researcher, on the basis of common background meanings given by culture and language, has a preliminary understanding of the human action being studied. It is by virtue of our world that we, as researchers, have the questions we have and see the possibilities we see. Thus we approach our interpretive project with some understanding. Through systematic analysis of the whole, we gain new perspectives and depth of understanding. We use this understanding to examine the parts of the whole, and then we reexamine the whole in light of the insight we have gained from the parts. The interpretive process follows this part-whole strategy until the researcher is satisfied with the depth of his or her understanding. Thus the interpretive process has no clear termination.

A second assumption made in hermeneutics is that there is no Archimedean point from which one can have a "privileged," foundational view of the world that is atemporal and ahistorical. The researcher has a world and exists in historical time just as the subject does. In order to have an objectively valid interpretation, one would have to understand from a position outside history, which is impossible in the phenomenologic view. Objectivity, then, is no longer a process of decontextualization or of securing abstract, eternal truths, but rather of finding what can show up in agreement among those of us sharing common cultural meanings.[15] Skills, practices, and meanings are objective in the sense of being shared, and are therefore verifiable with both research participants and external judges. They are not, however, objective in the sense of being ahistorical, atemporal, or acontextual. Taylor[4] argues that plausibility is the ultimate criterion for any hermeneutic explanation. It should be emphasized, though, that whereas individuals may take up common background meanings in a personal way, these personal meanings are neither infinitely variable nor completely relative. They are bounded by the cultural and linguistic meanings that we all share. Thus, while I may aspire to behave heroically during labor and delivery of an infant, it is not within my background meanings to go off and deliver alone and unattended. My options for giving birth are narrowed by my Western cultural tradition and by my own history. Within that bounded set of meanings I must find my possibilities for acting heroically. And because the background meanings that create those possibilities for me are shared, consensual validation of a hermeneutic interpretation of my heroic behavior is possible. Private, idiosyncratic meanings are not the data of hermeneutic inquiry.

In hermeneutics the role of theory is to show up meanings that arise out of the lived experience. Phenomenology mandates a new account of what constitutes adequate theory. No formal theoretical assumptions or predictions are made nor is formal theory (in the sense of an apparatus of formal propositions, causal mechanisms, and structures) to be used as a grid or screen through which data are filtered. Furthermore, the goal of research is not the development of a formal theory, defined as propositional statements that seek to outline the law-like relationships of atomistic elements within a static structure. The theory that results from hermeneutics involves the presentation of meanings, skills, and practices, the practical knowledge that eludes traditional empirical research.

DATA COLLECTION IN A HERMENEUTIC INQUIRY

In hermeneutics the primary source of knowledge is everyday practical activity. Human behavior becomes a text analogue that is studied and interpreted in order to discover its hidden or obscured meaning. This meaning is hidden because it is so pervasive and taken for granted that it goes unnoticed. The data for the text analogues can come from interviews, participant observation, diaries, and samples of human behavior.[12] Since our everyday lived experience is so taken for granted as to go unnoticed, it is often through breakdowns that the researcher achieves flashes of insight into the lived world. However, it is important to note that the taken-for-granted, everyday, lived world can never be made completely explicit.

VALIDITY ISSUES

Content validity is threatened in a hermeneutic study by social desirability and by the ambiguity inherent in language. The problem of social desirability is addressed by including the participants' descriptions of situations. These chronological narratives are then used as text analogues. Multiple interviews may also be helpful in distinguishing recurring patterns from individual incidents. The problem of ambiguity in language can be addressed by having an interview transcribed and interpreted prior to the next interview, by allowing the researcher to present the interpretation to the participant for validation or clarification, and by involving more than one researcher in consensual validation of the interpretation.[15]

Sandelowski[21] offers a framework for evaluating qualitative research in which four factors are considered: truth value, applicability, consistency, and neutrality. Truth value in a qualitative study is found in the accurate description of human experiences as they are lived and perceived by participants in the study. The effects of maturation and experience are irrelevant to a phenomenologic study, because a change over time is assumed and the study observes that change in its historical context. As does Taylor,[5] Sandelowski argues that credibility is the criterion against which the truth value of qualitative research should be evaluated.

Applicability in qualitative research is the equivalent of generalizability in quantitative research. While the sample size in hermeneutic studies is typically small, applicability can be achieved when the results of the study shed light on or "fit into" contexts outside the study situation. In a hermeneutic study the exemplars and paradigm cases may shed light on other situations that have quite dissimilar objective characteristics. The representativeness of the sample is replaced by the representativeness of the recurring themes and patterns identified by the study.

Consistency replaces reliability in a qualitative study. Hermeneutic studies assume that because subjects exist in time, a study can never be replicated exactly, just as history can never be recreated exactly. The consistency of a qualitative study can be established by the presentation of sufficient data from the text analogues to enable the research reader to participate in the consensual validation of the data.

Sandelowski's fourth criterion for evaluating qualitative research is neutrality. In quantitative studies the researcher is assumed to have an objective, disinterested stance with regard to the study. In qualitative research it is assumed that there is no detached, objective position from which to study human beings. The researcher is a self-interpreting being who is already in the world, as is the subject. The imperative in a hermeneutic study is to make sure that the integrity of the text is maintained and that the researcher does not become enmeshed in the study and thus unable to distinguish his or her own responses from what the text is saying.

Interpretive Analysis

Transcribed interviews, observational notes, diaries, and samples of human action are treated as text analogues for interpretive analysis. The data analysis in a hermeneutic study is carried out via three interrelated processes: thematic analysis, analysis of exemplars, and the search for paradigm cases.

In the thematic analysis each case (ie, all interviews, field notes, and so forth) is read several times in order to arrive at a global analysis. When several cases have been read in this way, lines of inquiry are identified from the theoretical background of the study and from themes that emerge consistently in the data. From this analysis an interpretive plan emerges and a coding protocol is developed. Each interview is then coded using that protocol. (As this microanalysis is carried out, additional lines of inquiry may emerge from the data and be added to the coding protocol). All cases are then subjected to additional interpretive analysis. The interpretive effort culminates in the identification of general categories that form the basis of the study's findings.

The second phase of the interpretive process involves the analysis of specific episodes or incidents: All aspects of a particular situation and the participant's responses to it are coded together. The completely coded event encompasses the individual's situation and his or her concerns and practices. From this analysis come exemplars, stories or vignettes that capture the meaning of a situation in such a way that the meaning can then be recognized in another situation that might have very different objective characteristics. An exemplar is thus "a strong instance of a particularly meaningful transaction, intention, or capacity."[12(p19)]

The last phase of interpretive analysis involves the identification of paradigm cases, strong instances of particular patterns of meaning. Paradigm cases embody the rich descriptive information necessary for an understanding of how an individual's actions and interpretations emerge from his or her situational context: the individual's concerns, practices, and background meanings. These patterns of meaning are not reducible to formal theory or to abstract variables used to predict and control. Instead, "family resemblances" are recognized between a paradigm case and a particular clinical situation that one is trying to understand and explain.[22]

> All three interpretive strategies work both as discovery and presentation strategies. They all allow for the presentation of context and meanings. In interpretive research, unlike in grounded theory, the goal is not to extract theoretical terms or concepts at a higher level of abstraction. The goal is to discover meaning and to achieve understanding.[12(p10)]

Presentation of a study's findings involves distilling the data to their most essential terms while still providing the reader with enough evidence to enable him or her to participate in the validation of the findings.[15]

Disputes in hermeneutic interpretation are resolved on the basis of the plausibility of alternative interpretations, and the plausibility of an interpretation cannot be reduced to a priori criteria. As Bernstein comments, "A fundamental ontological motif of modernity has been variations on the theme of fundamental indeterminism. Our being-in-the-world is fundamentally indeterminate. Wisdom requires learning to live with this."[23] Thus, although we must live with a plurality of interpretations of meaning, we can narrow things down. Moreover, living with a plurality of meanings, or indeterminacy, does not mean that we cannot understand each other.

Heideggerian phenomenology offers a view of the person that is profoundly different from more traditional Cartesian notions. It is a view that has much to offer to nurses who are, in their practice, fundamentally concerned with the lived experiences of health and illness. Hermeneutics is a method that assumes the philosophical tenets of Heideggerian phenomenology. It offers nurse researchers the opportunity to understand the meaningfully rich and complex lived world of those human beings for whom nurses care. Both the theory and the method deserve to receive serious attention from nurse researchers.

REFERENCES

1. Laudan L: *Progress and Its Problems: Toward a Theory of Scientific Growth*. London, Routledge & Kegan Paul, 1977.
2. Baron R: An introduction to medical phenomenology: I can't hear you while I'm listening. *Ann Intern Med* 1985;163:606–611.
3. Heidegger M: *The Basic Problems of Phenomenology*, Hofstader A (trans). Bloomington, Ind, Indiana University Press, 1982.
4. Taylor C: *Human Agency and Language*. Cambridge, England, Cambridge University Press, 1985, vol 1.
5. Taylor C: *Human Agency and Language*. Cambridge, England, Cambridge University Press, 1985, vol 2.
6. Dreyfus H: *Being-in-the-World: A Commentary on Division I of Being and Time*. Cambridge, Mass, MIT press, to be published.
7. Guignon C: *Heidegger and the Problem of Knowledge*. Indianapolis, Ind, Hackett Publishing Co, 1983.
8. Dreyfus H: Husserl, Heidegger and modern existentialism, in Magee B (ed): *The Great Philosophers: An Introduction to Western Philosophy*. London, BBC Books, 1987, pp 252–278.
9. Palmer R: *Hermeneutics*. Evanston, Ill, Northwestern University Press, 1969.
10. Sandel M: *Liberalism and the Limits of Justice*. Cambridge, Cambridge University Press, 1982.
11. Ricoeur P: Self-identity and the interpretation of narrative. Read before the Approaches to Interpretation Conference, sponsored by the Department of Philosophy, California State University, Hayward, Calif, May, 1986.
12. Benner P: Quality of life: A phenomenological perspective on explanation, prediction and understanding in nursing science. *Adv Nurs Sci* 1985;8:1–14.
13. Hoy D: Proceedings. Read before the Approaches to Interpretation Conference, sponsored by the Department of Philosophy, California State University, Hayward, Calif, May, 1986.
14. Borgman A: *Technology and the Character of Contemporary Life*. Chicago, University of Chicago Press, 1984.
15. Caudill W, Weinstein H: Maternal care and infant behavior in Japan and America. *Psychiatry* 1969;32:12–43.
16. Leder D: Medicine and paradigms of embodiment. *J Med Philos* 1984;9:29–43.
17. Benner P, Wrubel J: *The Primacy of Caring*. Menlo Park, Calif, Addison-Wesley, 1989.
18. Merleau-Ponty M: *Phenomenology of Perception*, Smith C (trans). London, Routledge & Kegan Paul, 1962.
19. Faulconer J, Williams R: Temporality in human action. *Am Psychol* 1985;40:1179–1188.
20. Heidegger M: *Being and Time*, Macquarrie J, Robinson E (trans). New York, Harper & Row Inc, 1962.
21. Sandelowski M: The problem of rigor in qualitative research. *Adv Nurs Sci* 1986;8:27–37.
22. Chesla C: *Parents' Caring Practices and Coping With Schizophrenic Offspring: An Interpretive Study*, dissertation. School of Nursing, University of California, San Francisco, Calif, 1988.
23. Bernstein R: Interpretation and its discontents. Read before the Approaches to Interpretation Conference, sponsored by the Department of Philosophy, California State University, Hayward, Calif, May, 1986.

Phenomenology of Perception

M. Merleau-Ponty

What is phenomenology? It may seem strange that this question has still to be asked half a century after the first works of Husserl. The fact remains that it has by no means been answered. Phenomenology is the study of essences; and according to it, all problems amount to finding definitions of essences: the essence of perception, or the essence of consciousness, for example. But phenomenology is also a philosophy which puts essences back into existence, and does not expect to arrive at an understanding of man and the world from any starting point other than that of their 'facticity'. It is a transcendental philosophy which places in abeyance the assertions arising out of the natural attitude, the better to understand them; but it is also a philosophy for which the world is always 'already there' before reflection begins—as an inalienable presence; and all its efforts are concentrated upon re-achieving a direct and primitive contact with the world, and endowing that contact with a philosophical status. It is the search for a philosophy which shall be a 'rigorous science', but it also offers an account of space, time and the world as we 'live' them. It tries to give a direct description of our experience as it is, without taking account of its psychological origin and the causal explanations which the scientist, the historian or the sociologist may be able to provide. Yet Husserl in his last works mentions a 'genetic phenomenology',[1] and even a 'constructive phenomenology'.[2] One may try to do away with these contradictions by making a distinction between Husserl's and Heidegger's phenomenologies; yet the whole of *Sein und Zeit* springs from an indication given by Husserl and amounts to no more than an explicit account of the 'natürlicher Weltbegriff' or the 'Lebenswelt' which Husserl, towards the end of his life, identified as the central theme of phenomenology, with the result that the contradiction reappears in Husserl's own philosophy. The reader pressed for time will be inclined to give up the idea of covering a doctrine which says everything, and will wonder whether a philosophy which cannot define its scope deserves all the discussion which has gone on around it, and whether he is not faced rather by a myth or a fashion.

Even if this were the case, there would still be a need to understand the prestige of the myth and the origin of the fashion, and the opinion of the responsible philosopher must be that *phenomenology can be practised and identified as a manner or style of thinking, that it existed as a movement before arriving at complete awareness of itself as a philosophy*. It has been long on the way, and its adherents have discovered it in every quarter, certainly in Hegel and Kierkegaard, but equally in Marx, Nietzsche and Freud. A purely linguistic examination of the texts in question would yield no proof; we find in texts only what we put into them, and if ever any kind of history has suggested the interpretations which should be put on it, it is the history of philosophy. We shall find in ourselves, and nowhere else, the unity and true meaning of phenomenology. It is less a question of counting up quotations than of determining and expressing in concrete form this *phenomenology for ourselves* which has given a number of present-day readers the impression, on reading Husserl or Heidegger, not so much of encountering a new philosophy as of recognizing what they had been waiting for. Phenomenology is accessible only through a phenomenological method. Let us, therefore, try systematically to bring together the celebrated phenomenological themes as they have grown spontaneously together in life. Perhaps we shall then understand why phenomenology has for so long remained at an initial stage, as a problem to be solved and a hope to be realized.

It is a matter of describing, not of explaining or analysing. Husserl's first directive to phenomenology, in its early stages, to be a 'descriptive psychology', or to return to the 'things themselves', is from the start a rejection of science. I am not the outcome or the meeting-point of numerous causal agencies which determine my bodily or psychological make-up. I cannot conceive myself as nothing but a bit of the world, a mere object of biological, psychological or sociological investigation. I cannot shut myself up within the realm of science. All my knowledge of the world, even my scientific knowledge, is gained from my own particular point of view, or from some experience of the world without which the symbols of science would be meaningless. The whole universe of science is built upon the world as directly experienced, and if we want to subject science itself to rigorous scrutiny and arrive at a precise assessment of its meaning and scope, we must begin by reawakening the basic experience of the world of which science is the second-order expression. Science has not and never will have, by

its nature, the same significance *qua* form of being as the world which we perceive, for the simple reason that it is a rationale or explanation of that world. I am, not a 'living creature' nor even a 'man', nor again even 'a consciousness' endowed with all the characteristics which zoology, social anatomy or inductive psychology recognize in these various products of the natural or historical process—I am the absolute source, my existence does not stem from my antecedents, from my physical and social environment; instead it moves out towards them and sustains them, for I alone bring into being for myself (and therefore into being in the only sense that the word can have for me) the tradition which I elect to carry on, or the horizon whose distance from me would be abolished—since that distance is not one of its properties—if I were not there to scan it with my gaze. Scientific points of view, according to which my existence is a moment of the world's, are always both naïve and at the same time dishonest, because they take for granted, without explicitly mentioning it, the other point of view, namely that of consciousness, through which from the outset a world forms itself round me and begins to exist for me. To return to things themselves is to return to that world which precedes knowledge, of which knowledge always *speaks,* and in relation to which every scientific schematization is an abstract and derivative sign-language, as is geography in relation to the countryside in which we have learnt beforehand what a forest, a prairie or a river is.

This move is absolutely distinct from the idealist return to consciousness, and the demand for a pure description excludes equally the procedure of analytical reflection on the one hand, and that of scientific explanation on the other. Descartes and particularly Kant *detached* the subject, or consciousness, by showing that I could not possibly apprehend anything as existing unless I first of all experienced myself as existing in the act of apprehending it. They presented consciousness, the absolute certainty of my existence for myself, as the condition of there being anything at all; and the act of relating as the basis of relatedness. It is true that the act of relating is nothing if divorced from the spectacle of the world in which relations are found; the unity of consciousness in Kant is achieved simultaneously with that of the world. And in Descartes methodical doubt does not deprive us of anything, since the whole world, at least in so far as we experience it, is reinstated in the *Cogito*, enjoying equal certainty, and simply labelled 'thought about . . .'. But the relations between subject and world are not strictly bilateral: if they were, the certainty of the world would, in Descartes, be immediately given with that of the *Cogito*, and Kant would not have talked about his 'Copernican revolution'. Analytical reflection starts from our experience of the world and goes back to the subject as to a condition of possibility distinct from that experience, revealing the all-embracing synthesis as that without which there would be no world. To this extent it ceases to remain part of our experience and offers, in place of an account, a reconstruction. It is understandable, in view of this, that Husserl, having accused Kant of adopting a 'faculty psychologism',[3] should have urged, in place of a noetic analysis which bases the world on the synthesizing activity of the subject, his own '*noematic reflection*' which remains within the object and, instead of begetting it, brings to light its fundamental unity.

The world is there before any possible analysis of mine, and it would be artificial to make it the outcome of a series of syntheses which link, in the first place sensations, then aspects of the object corresponding to different perspectives, when both are nothing but products of analysis, with no sort of prior reality. Analytical reflection believes that it can trace back the course followed by a prior constituting act and arrive, in the 'inner man'—to use Saint Augustine's expression—at a constituting power which has always been identical with that inner self. Thus reflection itself is carried away and transplanted in an impregnable subjectivity, as yet untouched by being and time. But this is very ingenuous, or at least it is an incomplete form of reflection which loses sight of its own beginning. When I begin to reflect my reflection bears upon an unreflective experience; moreover my reflection cannot be unaware of itself as an event; and so it appears to itself in the light of a truly creative act, of a changed structure of consciousness, and yet it has to recognize, as having priority over its own operations, the world which is given to the subject, because the subject is given to himself. The real has to be described, not constructed or formed. Which means that I cannot put perception into the same category as the syntheses represented by judgements, acts or predications. My field of perception is constantly filled with a play of colours, noises and fleeting tactile sensations which I cannot relate precisely to the context of my clearly perceived world, yet which I nevertheless immediately 'place' in the world, without ever confusing them with my daydreams. Equally constantly I weave dreams round things. I imagine people and things whose presence is not incompatible with the context, yet who are not in fact involved in it: they are ahead of reality, in the realm of the imaginary. If the reality of my perception were based solely on the intrinsic coherence of 'representations', it ought to be for ever hesitant and, being wrapped up in my conjectures on probabilities, I ought to be ceaselessly taking apart misleading syntheses, and reinstating in reality stray phenomena which I had excluded in the first place. But this does not happen. The real is a closely woven fabric. It does not await our judgement before incorporating the most surprising phenomena, or before rejecting the most plausible figments of our imagination. Perception is not a science of the world, it is not even an act, a deliberate taking up of a position; it is the background from which all acts stand out, and is presupposed by them. The world is not an object such that I have in my possession the law of its making; it is the natural setting of, and field for, all my thoughts and all my explicit perceptions. Truth does not 'inhabit' only 'the inner man',[4] or more accurately, there is no inner man, man is in the world, and only in the world does he know himself. When I return to myself from an excursion into the realm of dogmatic common sense or of science, I find, not a source of intrinsic truth, but a subject destined to be in the world.

All of which reveals the true meaning of the famous phenomenological reduction. There is probably no question over which Husserl has spent more time—or to which he has more often returned, since the 'problematic of reduction' occupies an important place in his unpublished work. For a long time, and even in recent texts, the reduction is presented as the return to a transcendental consciousness before which the world is spread out and completely transparent, quickened through and through by a series of apperceptions which it is the philosopher's task to reconstitute on the basis of their outcome. Thus my sensation of redness is *perceived as* the manifestation of a certain redness experienced, this in turn as the manifestation of a red surface, which is the manifestation of a piece of red cardboard, and this finally is the manifestation or outline of a red thing, namely this book. We are to understand, then, that it is the apprehension of certain *hylè*, as indicating a phenomenon of a higher degree, the *Sinngebung*, or active meaning-giving operation which may be said to define consciousness, so that the world is nothing but 'world-as-meaning', and the phenomenological reduction is idealistic, in the sense that there is here a transcendental idealism which treats the world as an indivisible unity of value shared by Peter and Paul, in which their perspectives blend. 'Peter's consciousness' and 'Paul's consciousness' are in communication, the perception of the world 'by Peter' is not Peter's doing any more than its perception 'by Paul' is Paul's doing; in each case it is the doing of pre-personal forms of consciousness, whose communication raises no problem, since it is demanded by the very definition of consciousness, meaning or truth. In so far as I am a consciousness, that is, in so far as something has meaning for me, I am neither here nor there, neither Peter nor Paul; I am in no way distinguishable from an 'other' consciousness, since we are immediately in touch with the world and since the world is, by definition, unique, being the system in which all truths cohere. A logically consistent transcendental idealism rids the world of its opacity and its transcendence. The world is precisely that thing of which we form a representation, not as men or as empirical subjects, but in so far as we are all one light and participate in the One without destroying its unity. Analytical reflection knows nothing of the problem of other minds, or of that of the world, because it insists that with the first glimmer of consciousness there appears in me theoretically the power of reaching some universal truth, and that the other person, being equally without thisness, location or body, the Alter and the Ego are one and the same in the true world which is the unifier of minds. There is no difficulty in understanding how *I* can conceive the Other, because the I and consequently the Other are not conceived as part of the woven stuff of phenomena; they have validity rather than existence. There is nothing hidden behind these faces and gestures, no domain to which I have no access, merely a little shadow which owes its very existence to the light. For Husserl, on the contrary, it is well known that there is a problem of other people, and the *alter ego* is a paradox. If the other is truly for himself alone, beyond his being for me, and if we are for each other and not both for God, we must necessarily have some appearance for each other. He must and I must have an outer appearance, and there must be, besides the perspective of the For Oneself—my view of myself and the other's of himself—a perspective of For Others—my view of others and theirs of me. Of course, these two perspectives, in each one of us, cannot be simply juxtaposed, *for in that case it is not I that the other would see, nor he that I should see.* I must be the exterior that I present to others, and the body of the other must be the other himself. This paradox and the dialectic of the Ego and the Alter are possible only provided that the Ego and the Alter Ego are defined by their situation and are not freed from all inherence; that is, provided that philosophy does not culminate in a return to the self, and that I discover by reflection not only my presence to myself, but also the possibility of an 'outside spectator'; that is, again, provided that at the very moment when I experience my existence—at the ultimate extremity of reflection—I fall short of the ultimate density which would place me outside time, and that I discover within myself a kind of internal weakness standing in the way of my being totally individualized: a weakness which exposes me to the gaze of others as a man among men or at least as a consciousness among consciousnesses. Hitherto the *Cogito* depreciated the perception of others, teaching me as it did that the I is accessible only to itself, since it defined *me* as the thought which I have of myself, and which clearly I am alone in having, at least in this ultimate sense. For the 'other' to be more than an empty word, it is necessary that my existence should never be reduced to my bare awareness of existing, but that it should take in also the awareness that *one* may have of it, and thus include my incarnation in some nature and the possibility, at least, of a historical situation. The *Cogito* must reveal me in a situation, and it is on this condition alone that transcendental subjectivity can, as Husserl puts it,[5] *be* an intersubjectivity. As a meditating Ego, I can clearly distinguish from myself the world and things, since I certainly do not exist in the way in which things exist. I must even set aside from myself my body understood as a thing among things, as a collection of physico-chemical processes. But even if the *cogitatio*, which I thus discover, is without location in objective time and space, it is not without place in the phenomenological world. The world, which I distinguished from myself as the totality of things or of processes linked by causal relationships, I rediscover 'in me' as the permanent horizon of all my *cogitationes* and as a dimension in relation to which I am constantly situating myself. The true *Cogito* does not define the subject's existence in terms of the thought he has of

existing, and furthermore does not convert the indubitability of the world into the indubitability of thought about the world, nor finally does it replace the world itself by the world as meaning. On the contrary it recognizes my thought itself as an inalienable fact, and does away with any kind of idealism in revealing me as 'being-in-the-world'.

It is because we are through and through compounded of relationships with the world that for us the only way to become aware of the fact is to suspend the resultant activity, to refuse it our complicity (to look at it *ohne mitzu-machen*, as Husserl often says), or yet again, to put it 'out of play'. Not because we reject the certainties of common sense and a natural attitude to things—they are, on the contrary, the constant theme of philosophy—but because, being the presupposed basis of any thought, they are taken for granted, and go unnoticed, and because in order to arouse them and bring them to view, we have to suspend for a moment our recognition of them. The best formulation of the reduction is probably that given by Eugen Fink, Husserl's assistant, when he spoke of 'wonder' in the face of the world.[6] Reflection does not withdraw from the world towards the unity of consciousness as the world's basis; it steps back to watch the forms of transcendence fly up like sparks from a fire; it slackens the intentional threads which attach us to the world and thus brings them to our notice; it alone is consciousness of the world because it reveals that world as strange and paradoxical. Husserl's transcendental is not Kant's and Husserl accuses Kant's philosophy of being 'worldly', because it *makes use* of our relation to the world, which is the motive force of the transcendental deduction, and makes the world immanent in the subject, instead of *being filled with wonder* at it and conceiving the subject as a process of transcendence towards the world. All the misunderstandings with his interpreters, with the existentialist 'dissidents' and finally with himself, have arisen from the fact that in order to see the world and grasp it as paradoxical, we must break with our familiar acceptance of it and, also, from the fact that from this break we can learn nothing but the unmotivated upsurge of the world. The most important lesson which the reduction teaches us is the impossibility of a complete reduction. This is why Husserl is constantly re-examining the possibility of the reduction. If we were absolute mind, the reduction would present no problem. But since, on the contrary, we are in the world, since indeed our reflections are carried out in the temporal flux on to which we are trying to seize (since they *sich einströmen*, as Husserl says), there is no thought which embraces all our thought. The philosopher, as the unpublished works declare, is a perpetual beginner, which means that he takes for granted nothing that men, learned or otherwise, believe they know. It means also that philosophy itself must not take itself for granted, in so far as it may have managed to say something true; that it is an ever-renewed experiment in making its own beginning; that it consists wholly in the description of this beginning, and finally, that radical reflection amounts to a consciousness of its own dependence on an unreflective life which is its initial situation, unchanging, given once and for all. Far from being, as has been thought, a procedure of idealistic philosophy, phenomenological reduction belongs to existential philosophy: Heidegger's 'being-in-the-world' appears only against the background of the phenomenological reduction.

A misunderstanding of a similar kind confuses the notion of the 'essences' in Husserl. Every reduction, says Husserl, as well as being transcendental is necessarily eidetic. That means that we cannot subject our perception of the world to philosophical scrutiny without ceasing to be identified with that act of positing the world, with that interest in it which delimits us, without drawing back from our commitment which is itself thus made to appear as a spectacle, without passing from the *fact* of our existence to its *nature*, from the Dasein to the Wesen. But it is clear that the essence is here not the end, but a means, that our effective involvement in the world is precisely what has to be understood and made amenable to conceptualization, for it is what polarizes all our conceptual particularizations. The need to proceed by way of essences does not mean that philosophy takes them as its object, but, on the contrary, that our existence is too tightly held in the world to be able to know itself as such at the moment of its involvement, and that it requires the field of ideality in order to become acquainted with and to prevail over its facticity. The Vienna Circle, as is well known, lays it down categorically that we can enter into relations only with meanings. For example, 'consciousness' is not for the Vienna Circle identifiable with what we are. It is a complex meaning which has developed late in time, which should be handled with care, and only after the many meanings which have contributed, throughout the word's semantic development, to the formation of its present one have been made explicit. Logical positivism of this kind is the antithesis of Husserl's thought. Whatever the subtle changes of meaning which have ultimately brought us, as a linguistic acquisition, the word and concept of consciousness, we enjoy direct access to what it designates. For we have the experience of ourselves, of that consciousness which we are, and it is on the basis of this experience that all linguistic connotations are assessed, and precisely through it that language comes to have any meaning at all for us. 'It is that as yet dumb experience . . . which we are concerned to lead to the pure expression of its own meaning.'[7] Husserl's essences are destined to bring back all the living relationships of experience, as the fisherman's net draws up from the depths of the ocean quivering fish and seaweed. Jean Wahl is therefore wrong in saying that 'Husserl separates essences from existence'.[8] The separated essences are those of language. It is the office of language to cause essences to exist in a state of separation which is in fact merely apparent, since through language they still rest upon the ante-predicative life of consciousness. In the silence of primary consciousness can be seen appearing not only what words mean, but also what things mean: the core of primary meaning round which the acts of naming and expression take shape.

Seeking the essence of consciousness will therefore not consist in developing the *Wortbedeutung* of consciousness and escaping from existence into the universe of things said; it will consist in rediscovering my actual presence to myself, the fact of my consciousness which is in the last resort what the word and the concept of consciousness mean. Looking for the world's essence is not looking for what it is as an idea once it has been reduced to a theme of discourse; it is looking for what it is as a fact for us, before any thematization. Sensationalism 'reduces' the world by noticing that after all we never experience anything but states of ourselves. Transcendental idealism too 'reduces' the world since, in so far as it guarantees the world, it does so by regarding it as thought or consciousness of the world, and as the mere correlative of our knowledge, with the result that it becomes immanent in consciousness and the aseity of things is thereby done away with. The eidetic reduction is, on the other hand, the determination to bring the world to light as it is before any falling back on ourselves has occurred, it is the ambition to make reflection emulate the unreflective life of consciousness. I aim at and perceive a world. If I said, as do the sensationalists, that we have here only 'states of consciousness', and if I tried to distinguish my perceptions from my dreams with the aid of 'criteria', I should overlook the phenomenon of the world. For if I am able to talk about 'dreams' and 'reality', to bother my head about the distinction between imaginary and real, and cast doubt upon the 'real', it is because this distinction is already made by me before any analysis; it is because I have an experience of the real as of the imaginary, and the problem then becomes one not of asking how critical thought can provide for itself secondary equivalents of this distinction, but of making explicit our primordial knowledge of the 'real', of describing our per-

ception of the world as that upon which our idea of truth is for ever based. We must not, therefore, wonder whether we really perceive a world, we must instead say: the world is what we perceive. In more general terms we must not wonder whether our self-evident truths are real truths, or whether, through some perversity inherent in our minds, that which is self-evident for us might not be illusory in relation to some truth in itself. For in so far as we talk about illusion, it is because we have identified illusions, and done so solely in the light of some perception which at the same time gave assurance of its own truth. It follows that doubt, or the fear of being mistaken, testifies as soon as it arises to our power of unmasking error, and that it could never finally tear us away from truth. We are in the realm of truth and it is 'the experience of truth' which is self-evident.[9] To seek the essence of perception is to declare that perception is, not presumed true, but defined as access to truth. So, if I now wanted, according to idealistic principles, to base this *de facto* self-evident truth, this irresistible belief, on some absolute self-evident truth, that is, on the absolute clarity which my thoughts have for me; if I tried to find in myself a creative thought which bodied forth the framework of the world or illumined it through and through, I should once more prove unfaithful to my experience of the world, and should be looking for what makes that experience possible instead of looking for what it is. The self-evidence of perception is not adequate thought or apodeictic self-evidence.[10] The world is not what I think, but what I live through. I am open to the world, I have no doubt that I am in communication with it, but I do not possess it; it is inexhaustible. 'There is a world', or rather: 'There is the world'; I can never completely account for this ever-reiterated assertion in my life. This facticity of the world is what constitutes the *Weltlichkeit der Welt*, what causes the world to be the world; just as the facticity of the *cogito* is not an imperfection in itself, but rather what assures me of my existence. The eidetic method is the method of a phenomenological positivism which bases the possible on the real.

We can now consider the notion of intentionality, too often cited as the main discovery of phenomenology, whereas it is understandable only through the reduction. "All consciousness is consciousness of something"; there is nothing new in that. Kant showed, in the *Refutation of Idealism*, that inner perception is impossible without outer perception, that the world, as a collection of connected phenomena, is anticipated in the consciousness of my unity, and is the means whereby I come into being as a consciousness. What distinguishes intentionality from the Kantian relation to a possible object is that the unity of the world, before being posited by knowledge in a specific act of identification, is 'lived' as ready-made or already there. Kant himself shows in the *Critique of Judgement* that there exists a unity of the imagination and the understanding and a unity of subjects *before the object*, and that, in experiencing the beautiful, for example, I am aware of a harmony between sensation and concept, between myself and others, which is itself without any concept. Here the subject is no longer the universal thinker of a system of objects rigorously interrelated, the positing power who subjects the manifold to the law of the understanding, in so far as he is to be able to put together a world—he discovers and enjoys his own nature as spontaneously in harmony with the law of the understanding. But if the subject has a nature, then the hidden art of the imagination must condition the categorial activity. It is no longer merely the aesthetic judgement, but knowledge too which rests upon this art, an art which forms the basis of the unity of consciousness and of consciousnesses.

Husserl takes up again the *Critique of Judgement* when he talks about a teleology of consciousness. It is not a matter of duplicating human consciousness with some absolute thought which, from outside, is imagined as assigning to it its aims. It is a question of recognizing consciousness itself as a project of the world, meant for a world which it neither embraces nor possesses, but towards which it is perpetually directed—and the world as this pre-objective individual whose imperious unity decrees what knowledge shall take as its goal. This is why Husserl distinguishes between intentionality of act, which is that of our judgements and of those occasions when we voluntarily take up a position—the only intentionality discussed in the *Critique of Pure Reason*—and operative intentionality (*fungierende Intentionalität*), or that which produces the natural and antepredicative unity of the world and of our life, being apparent in our desires, our evaluations and in the landscape we see, more clearly than in objective knowledge, and furnishing the text which our knowledge tries to translate into precise language. Our relationship to the world, as it is untiringly enunciated within us, is not a thing which can be any further clarified by analysis; philosophy can only place it once more before our eyes and present it for our ratification.

Through this broadened notion of intentionality, phenomenological 'comprehension' is distinguished from traditional 'intellection', which is confined to 'true and immutable natures', and so phenomenology can become a phenomenology of origins. Whether we are concerned with a thing perceived, a historical event or a doctrine, to 'understand' is to take in the total intention—not only what these things are for representation (the 'properties' of the thing perceived, the mass of 'historical facts', the 'ideas' introduced by the doctrine)—but the unique mode of existing expressed in the properties of the pebble, the glass or the piece of wax, in all the events of a revolution, in all the thoughts of a philosopher. It is a matter, in the case of each civilization, of finding the Idea in the Hegelian sense, that is, not a law of the physico-mathematical type, discoverable by objective thought, but that formula which sums up some unique manner of behaviour towards others, towards Nature, time and death: a certain way of patterning the world which the historian should be capable of seizing upon and making his own. These are the *dimensions* of history. In this context there is not a human word, not a gesture, even one which is the outcome of habit or absent-mindedness, which has not some meaning. For example, I may have been under the impression that I lapsed into silence through weariness, or some minister may have thought he had uttered merely an appropriate platitude, yet my silence or his words immediately take on a significance, because my fatigue or his falling back upon a ready-made formula are not accidental, for they express a certain lack of interest, and hence some degree of adoption of a definite position in relation to the situation.

When an event is considered at close quarters, at the moment when it is lived through, everything seems subject to chance: one man's ambition, some lucky encounter, some local circumstance or other appears to have been decisive. But chance happenings offset each other, and facts in their multiplicity coalesce and show up a certain way of taking a stand in relation to the human situation, reveal in fact an *event* which has its definite outline and about which we can talk. Should the starting-point for the understanding of history be ideology, or politics, or religion, or economics? Should we try to understand a doctrine from its overt content, or from the psychological make-up and the biography of its author? We must seek an understanding from all these angles simultaneously, everything has meaning, and we shall find this same structure of being underlying all relationships. All these views are true provided that they are not isolated, that we delve deeply into history and reach the unique core of existential meaning which emerges in each perspective. It is true, as Marx says, that history does not walk on its head, but it is also true that it does not think with its feet. Or one should say rather that it is neither its 'head' nor its 'feet' that we have to worry about, but its body. All economic and psychological explanations of a doctrine are true, since the thinker never thinks from any starting-point but the one constituted by what

he is. Reflection even on a doctrine will be complete only if it succeeds in linking up with the doctrine's history and the extraneous explanations of it, and in putting back the causes and meaning of the doctrine in an existential structure. There is, as Husserl says, a 'genesis of meaning' (*Sinngenesis*),[11] which alone, in the last resort, teaches us what the doctrine 'means.' Like understanding, criticism must be pursued at all levels, and naturally, it will be insufficient, for the refutation of a doctrine, to relate it to some accidental event in the author's life: its significance goes beyond, and there is no pure accident in existence or in co-existence, since both absorb random events and transmute them into the rational.

Finally, as it is indivisible in the present, history is equally so in its sequences. Considered in the light of its fundamental dimensions, all periods of history appear as manifestations of a single existence, or as episodes in a single drama—without our knowing whether it has an ending. Because we are in the world, we are *condemned to meaning*, and we cannot do or say anything without its acquiring a name in history.

Probably the chief gain from phenomenology is to have united extreme subjectivism and extreme objectivism in its notion of the world or of rationality. Rationality is precisely measured by the experiences in which it is disclosed. To say that there exists rationality is to say that perspectives blend, perceptions confirm each other, a meaning emerges. But it should not be set in a realm apart, transposed into absolute Spirit, or into a world in the realist sense. The phenomenological world is not pure being, but the sense which is revealed where the paths of my various experiences intersect, and also where my own and other people's intersect and engage each other like gears. It is thus inseparable from subjectivity and intersubjectivity, which find their unity when I either take up my past experiences in those of the present, or other people's in my own. For the first time the philosopher's thinking is sufficiently conscious not to anticipate itself and endow its own results with reified form in the world. The philosopher tries to conceive the world, others and himself and their interrelations. But the meditating Ego, the 'impartial spectator' (*uninteressierter Zuschauer*)[12] do not rediscover an already given rationality, they 'establish themselves',[13] and establish it, by an act of initiative which has no guarantee in being, its justification resting entirely on the effective power which it confers on us of taking our own history upon ourselves.

The phenomenological world is not the bringing to explicit expression of a pre-existing being, but the laying down of being. Philosophy is not the reflection of a pre-existing truth, but, like art, the act of bringing truth into being. One may well ask how this creation is *possible*, and if it does not recapture in things a pre-existing Reason. The answer is that the only pre-existent Logos is the world itself, and that the philosophy which brings it into visible existence does not begin by being *possible*; it is actual or real like the world of which it is a part, and no explanatory hypothesis is clearer than the act whereby we take up this unfinished world in an effort to complete and conceive it. Rationality is not a *problem*. There is behind it no unknown quantity which has to be determined by deduction, or, beginning with it, demonstrated inductively. We witness every minute the miracle of related experiences, and yet nobody knows better than we do how this miracle is worked, for we are ourselves this network of relationships. The world and reason are not problematical. We may say, if we wish, that they are mysterious, but their mystery defines them: there can be no question of dispelling it by some 'solution', it is on the hither side of all solutions. True philosophy consists in relearning to look at the world, and in this sense a historical account can give meaning to the world quite as 'deeply' as a philosophical treatise. We take our fate in our hands, we become responsible for our history through reflection, but equally by a decision on which we stake our life, and in both cases what is involved is a violent act which is validated by being performed.

Phenomenology, as a disclosure of the world, rests on itself, or rather provides its own foundation.[14] All knowledge is sustained by a 'ground' of postulates and finally by our communication with the world as primary embodiment of rationality. Philosophy, as radical reflection, dispenses in principle with this resource. As, however, it too is in history, it too exploits the world and constituted reason. It must therefore put to itself the question which it puts to all branches of knowledge, and so duplicate itself infinitely, being, as Husserl says, a dialogue or infinite meditation, and, in so far as it remains faithful to its intention, never knowing where it is going. The unfinished nature of phenomenology and the inchoative atmosphere which has surrounded it are not to be taken as a sign of failure, they were inevitable because phenomenology's task was to reveal the mystery of the world and of reason.[15] If phenomenology was a movement before becoming a doctrine or a philosophical system, this was attributable neither to accident, nor to fraudulent intent. It is as painstaking as the works of Balzac, Proust, Valéry or Cézanne—by reason of the same kind of attentiveness and wonder, the same demand for awareness, the same will to seize the meaning of the world or of history as that meaning comes into being. In this way it merges into the general effort of modern thought.

NOTES

1. *Méditations cariésiennes*, pp. 120 ff.
2. See the unpublished *6th Méditation cartésienne*, edited by Eugen Fink, to which G. Berger has kindly referred us.
3. *Logische Untersuchungen, Prolegomena zur reinen Logik*, p. 93.
4. In te redi; in interiore homine habitat veritas (Saint Augustine).
5. *Die Krisis der europäischen Wissenschaften und die transzendentale Phänomenologie*, III (unpublished).
6. *Die phänomenologische Philosophie Edmund Husserls in der gegenwärtigen Kritik*, pp. 331 and ff.
7. *Méditations cartésiennes*, p. 33.
8. *Réalisme, dialectique et mystère*, l'Arbalète, Autumn, 1942, unpaginated.

9. *Das Erlebnis der Wahrheit (Logische Untersuchungen, Prolegomena zur reinen Logik)* p. 190.
10. There is no apodeictic self-evidence, the *Formale und transzendentale Logik* (p. 142) says in effect.
11. The usual term in the unpublished writings. The idea is already to be found in the *Formale und transzendentale Logik*, pp. 184 and ff.
12. *6th Méditation cartésienne* (unpublished).
13. Ibid.
14. 'Rückbeziehung der Phänomenologie auf sich selbst,' say the unpublished writings.
15. We are indebted for this last expression to G. Gusdorf, who may well have used it in another sense.

The Universality of the Hermeneutical Problem

Hans-Georg Gadamer

Why has the problem of language come to occupy the same central position in current philosophical discussions that the concept of thought, or 'thought thinking itself', held in philosophy a century and a half ago? By answering this question, I shall try to give an answer indirectly to the central question of the modern age—a question posed for us by the existence of modern science. It is the question of how our natural view of the world—the experience of the world that we have as we simply live out our lives—is related to the unassailable and anonymous authority that confronts us in the pronouncements of science. Since the seventeenth century, the real task of philosophy has been to mediate this new employment of man's cognitive and constructive capacities with the totality of our experience of life. This task has found expression in a variety of ways, including our own generation's attempt to bring the topic of language to the center of philosophical concern. Language is the fundamental mode of operation of our being-in-the-world and the all-embracing form of the constitution of the world. Hence we always have in view the pronouncements of the sciences, which are fixed in nonverbal signs. And our task is to reconnect the objective world of technology, which the sciences place at our disposal and discretion, with those fundamental orders of our being that are neither arbitrary nor manipulable by us, but rather simply demand our respect.

I want to elucidate several phenomena in which the universality of this question becomes evident. I have called the point of view involved in this theme 'hermeneutical', a term developed by Heidegger. Heidegger was continuing a perspective stemming originally from Protestant theology and transmitted into our own century by Wilhelm Dilthey.

What is hermeneutics? I would like to start from two experiences of alienation that we encounter in our concrete existence: the experience of alienation of the aesthetic consciousness and the experience of alienation of the historical consciousness. In both cases what I mean can be stated in a few words. The aesthetic consciousness realizes a possibility that as such we can neither deny nor diminish in its value, namely, that we relate ourselves, either negatively or affirmatively, to the quality of an artistic form. This statement means we are related in such a way that the judgment we make decides in the end regarding the expressive power and validity of what we judge. What we reject has nothing to say to us—or we reject it because it has nothing to say to us. This characterizes our relation to art in the broadest sense of the word, a sense that, as Hegel has shown, includes the entire religious world of the ancient Greeks, whose religion of beauty experienced the divine in concrete works of art that man creates in response to the gods. When it loses its original and unquestioned authority, this whole world of experience becomes alienated into an object of aesthetic judgment. At the same time, however, we must admit that the world of artistic tradition—the splendid contemporaneousness that we gain through art with so many human worlds—is more than a mere object of our free acceptance or rejection. Is it not true that when a work of art has seized us it no longer leaves us the freedom to push it away from us once again and to accept or reject it on our own terms? And is it not also true that these artistic creations, which come down through the millennia, were not created for such aesthetic acceptance or rejection? No artist of the religiously vital cultures of the past ever produced his work of art with any other intention than that his creation should be received in terms of what it says and presents and that it should have its place in the world where men live together. The consciousness of art—the aesthetic consciousness—is always secondary to the immediate truth-claim that proceeds from the work of art itself. To this extent, when we judge a work of art on the basis of its aesthetic quality, something that is really much more intimately familiar to us is alienated. This alienation into aesthetic judgment always takes place when we have withdrawn ourselves and are no longer open to the immediate claim of that which grasps us. Thus one point of departure for my reflections in *Truth and Method* was that the aesthetic sovereignty that claims its rights in the experience of art represents an alienation when compared to the authentic experience that confronts us in the form of art itself.

About thirty years ago, this problem cropped up in a particularly distorted form when National Socialist politics of art, as a means to its own ends, tried to criticize formalism by arguing that art is bound to a people. Despite its misuse by the National Socialists, we cannot deny that the idea of art being bound to a people involves a real insight. A genuine artistic creation stands within a particular community, and such a community is always distinguishable from

the cultured society that is informed and terrorized by art criticism.

The second mode of the experience of alienation is the historical consciousness—the noble and slowly perfected art of holding ourselves at a critical distance in dealing with witnesses to past life. Ranke's celebrated description of this idea as the extinguishing of the individual provided a popular formula for the ideal of historical thinking: the historical consciousness has the task of understanding all the witnesses of a past time out of the spirit of that time, of extricating them from the preoccupations of our own present life, and of knowing, without moral smugness, the past as a human phenomenon. In his well-known essay *The Use and Abuse of History*, Nietzsche formulated the contradiction between this historical distancing and the immediate will to shape things that always cleaves to the present. And at the same time he exposed many of the consequences of what he called the 'Alexandrian', weakened form of the will, which is found in modern historical science. We might recall his indictment of the weakness of evaluation that has befallen the modern mind because it has become so accustomed to considering things in ever different and changing lights that it is blinded and incapable of arriving at an opinion of its own regarding the objects it studies. It is unable to determine its own position *vis-à-vis* what confronts it. Nietzsche traces the value-blindness of historical objectivism back to the conflict between the alienated historical world and the life-powers of the present.

To be sure, Nietzsche is an ecstatic witness. But our actual experience of the historical consciousness in the last one hundred years has taught us most emphatically that there are serious difficulties involved in its claim to historical objectivity. Even in those masterworks of historical scholarship that seem to be the very consummation of the extinguishing of the individual demanded by Ranke, it is still an unquestioned principle of our scientific experience that we can classify these works with unfailing accuracy in terms of the political tendencies of the time in which they were written. When we read Mommsen's *History of Rome*, we know who alone could have written it, that is, we can identify the political situation in which this historian organized the voices of the past in a meaningful way. We know it too in the case of Treitschke or of Sybel, to choose only a few prominent names from Prussian historiography. This clearly means, first of all, that the whole reality of historical experience does not find expression in the mastery of historical method. No one disputes the fact that controlling the prejudices of our own present to such an extent that we do not misunderstand the witnesses of the past is a valid aim, but obviously such control does not completely fulfill the task of understanding the past and its transmissions. Indeed, it could very well be that only *insignificant* things in historical scholarship permit us to approximate this ideal of totally extinguishing individuality, while the great productive achievements of scholarship always preserve something of the splendid magic of immediately mirroring the present in the past and the past in the present. Historical science, the second experience from which I begin, expresses only one part of our actual experience—our actual encounter with historical tradition—and it knows only an alienated form of this historical tradition.

We can contrast the hermeneutical consciousness with these examples of alienation as a more comprehensive possibility that we must develop. But, in the case of this hermeneutical consciousness also, our initial task must be to overcome the epistemological truncation by which the traditional 'science of hermeneutics' has been absorbed into the idea of modern science. If we consider Schleiermacher's hermeneutics, for instance, we find his view of this discipline peculiarly restricted by the modern idea of science. Schleiermacher's hermeneutics shows him to be a leading voice of historical romanticism. But at the same time, he kept the concern of the Christian theologian clearly in mind, intending his hermeneutics, as a general doctrine of the art of understanding, to be of value in the special work of interpreting Scripture. Schleiermacher defined hermeneutics as the art of avoiding misunderstanding. To exclude by controlled, methodical consideration whatever is alien and leads to misunderstanding—misunderstanding suggested to us by distance in time, change in linguistic usages, or in the meanings of words and modes of thinking—that is certainly far from an absurd description of the hermeneutical endeavor. But the question also arises as to whether the phenomenon of understanding is defined appropriately when we say that to understand is to avoid misunderstanding. It is not, in fact, the case that every misunderstanding presupposes a 'deep common accord'?

I am trying to call attention here to a common experience. We say, for instance, that understanding and misunderstanding take place between I and thou. But the formulation 'I and thou' already betrays an enormous alienation. There is nothing like an 'I and thou' at all—there is neither the I nor the thou as isolated, substantial realities. I may say 'thou' and I may refer to myself over against a thou, but a common understanding [*Verständigung*] always precedes these situations. We all know that to say 'thou' to someone presupposes a deep common accord [*tiefes Einverständnis*]. Something enduring is already present when this word is spoken. When we try to reach agreement on a matter on which we have different opinions, this deeper factor always comes into play, even if we are seldom aware of it. Now the science of hermeneutics would have us believe that the opinion we have to understand is something alien that seeks to lure us into misunderstanding, and our task is to exclude every element through which a misunderstanding can creep in. We accomplish this task by a controlled procedure of historical training, by historical criticism, and by a controllable method in connection with powers of psychological empathy. It seems to me that this description is valid in one respect, but yet it is only a partial description of a comprehensive life-phenomenon that constitutes the 'we' that we all are. Our task, it seems to me, is to transcend the prejudices that underlie the aesthetic consciousness, the historical consciousness, and the hermeneutical consciousness that has been restricted to a technique for avoiding misunderstandings and to overcome the alienations present in them all.

What is it, then, in these three experiences that seemed to us to have been left out, and what makes us so sensitive to the distinctiveness of these experiences? What is the *aesthetic* consciousness when compared to the fullness of what has already addressed us—what we call 'classical' in art? Is it not always already determined in this way what will be expressive for us and what we will find significant? Whenever we say with an instinctive, even if perhaps erroneous, certainty (but a certainty that is initially valid for our consciousness) 'this is classical; it will endure', what we are speaking of has already preformed our possibility for aesthetic judgment. There are no purely formal criteria that can claim to judge and sanction the formative level simply on the basis of its artistic virtuosity. Rather, our sensitive-spiritual existence is an aesthetic resonance chamber that resonates with the voices that are constantly reaching us, preceding all explicit aesthetic judgment.

The situation is similar with the historical consciousness. Here, too, we must certainly admit that there are innumerable tasks of historical scholarship that have no relation to our own present and to the depths of its historical consciousness. But it seems to me there can be no doubt that the great horizon of the past, out of which our culture and our present live, influences us in everything we want, hope for, or fear in the future. History is only present to us in light of our futurity. Here we have all learned from Heidegger, for he exhibited precisely the primacy of futurity for our possible recollection and retention, and for the whole of our history.

Heidegger worked out this primacy in his doctrine of the productivity of the hermeneutical circle. I have given the following formulation to this insight: It is not so much our judgments as it is our prejudices that constitute our being.

This is a provocative formulation, for I am using it to restore to its rightful place a positive concept of prejudice that was driven out of our linguistic usage by the French and the English Enlightenment. It can be shown that the concept of prejudice did not originally have the meaning we have attached to it. Prejudices are not necessarily unjustified and erroneous, so that they inevitably distort the truth. In fact, the historicity of our existence entails that prejudices, in the literal sense of the word, constitute the initial directedness of our whole ability to experience. Prejudices are biases of our openness to the world. They are simply conditions whereby we experience something—whereby what we encounter says something to us. This formulation certainly does not mean that we are enclosed within a wall of prejudices and only let through the narrow portals those things that can produce a pass saying, 'Nothing new will be said here'. Instead we welcome just that guest who promises something new to our curiosity. But how do we know the guest whom we admit is one who has something *new* to say to us? Is not our expectation and our readiness to hear the new also necessarily determined by the old that has already taken possession of us? The concept of prejudice is closely connected to the concept of authority, and the above image makes it clear that it is in need of hermeneutical rehabilitation. Like every image, however, this one too is misleading. The nature of the hermeneutical experience is not that something is outside and desires admission. Rather, we are possessed by something and precisely by means of it we are opened up for the new, the different, the true. Plato made this clear in his beautiful comparison of bodily foods with spiritual nourishment: while we can refuse the former (e.g. on the advice of a physician), we have always taken the latter into ourselves already.

But now the question arises as to how we can legitimate this hermeneutical conditionedness of our being in the face of modern science, which stands or falls with the principle of being unbiased and prejudiceless. We will certainly not accomplish this legitimation by making prescriptions for science and recommending that it toe the line—quite aside from the fact that such pronouncements always have something comical about them. Science will not do us this favor. It will continue along its own path with an inner necessity beyond its control, and it will produce more and more breathtaking knowledge and controlling power. It can be no other way. It is senseless, for instance, to hinder a genetic researcher because such research threatens to breed a superman. Hence the problem cannot appear as one in which our human consciousness ranges itself over against the world of science and presumes to develop a kind of anti-science. Nevertheless, we cannot avoid the question of whether what we are aware of in such apparently harmless examples as the aesthetic consciousness and the historical consciousness does not represent a problem that is also present in modern natural science and our technological attitude toward the world. If modern science enables us to erect a new world of technological purposes that transforms everything around us, we are not thereby suggesting that the researcher who gained the knowledge decisive for this state of affairs even considered technical applications. The genuine researcher is motivated by a desire for knowledge and by nothing else. And yet, over against the whole of our civilization that is founded on modern science, we must ask repeatedly if something has not been omitted. If the presuppositions of these possibilities for knowing and making remain half in the dark, cannot the result be that the hand applying this knowledge will be destructive?

The problem is really universal. The hermeneutical question, as I have characterized it, is not restricted to the areas from which I began in my own investigations. My only concern there was to secure a theoretical basis that would enable us to deal with the basic factor of contemporary culture, namely, science and its industrial, technological utilization. Statistics provide us with a useful example of how the hermeneutical dimension encompasses the entire procedure of science. It is an extreme exam-

ple, but it shows us that science always stands under definite conditions of methodological abstraction and that the successes of modern sciences rest on the fact that other possibilities for questioning are concealed by abstraction. This fact comes out clearly in the case of statistics, for the anticipatory character of the questions statistics answer make it particularly suitable for propaganda purposes. Indeed, effective propaganda must always try to influence initially the judgment of the person addressed and to restrict his possibilities of judgment. Thus what is established by statistics seems to be a language of facts, but which questions these facts answer and which facts would begin to speak if other questions were asked are hermeneutical questions. Only a hermeneutical inquiry would legitimate the meaning of these facts and thus the consequences that follow from them.

But I am anticipating, and have inadvertently used the phrase, 'which answers to which questions fit the facts'. This phrase is in fact the hermeneutical *Urphänomen:* No assertion is possible that cannot be understood as an answer to a question, and assertions can only be understood in this way. It does not impair the impressive methodology of modern science in the least. Whoever wants to learn a science has to learn to master its methodology. But we also know that methodology as such does not guarantee in any way the productivity of its application. Any experience of life can confirm the fact that there is such a thing as methodological sterility, that is, the application of a method to something not really worth knowing, to something that has not been made an object of investigation on the basis of a genuine question.

The methodological self-consciousness of modern science certainly stands in opposition to this argument. A historian, for example, will say in reply: It is all very nice to talk about the historical tradition in which alone the voices of the past gain their meaning and through which the prejudices that determine the present are inspired. But the situation is completely different in questions of serious historical research. How could one seriously mean, for example, that the clarification of the taxation practices of fifteenth-century cities or of the marital customs of Eskimos somehow first receive their meaning from the consciousness of the present and its anticipations? These are questions of historical knowledge that we take up as tasks quite independently of any relation to the present.

In answering this objection, one can say that the extremity of this point of view would be similar to what we find in certain large industrial research facilities, above all in America and Russia. I mean the so-called random experiment in which one simply covers the material without concern for waste or cost, taking the chance that some day one measurement among the thousands of measurements will finally yield an interesting finding; that is, it will turn out to be the answer to a question from which someone can progress. No doubt modern research in the humanities also works this way to some extent. One thinks, for instance, of the great editions and especially of the ever more perfect indexes. It must remain an open question, of course, whether by such procedures modern historical research increases the chances of actually noticing the interesting fact and thus gaining from it the corresponding enrichment of our knowledge. But even if they do, one might ask: Is this an ideal, that countless research projects (i.e. determinations of the connection of facts) are extracted from a thousand historians, so that the 1,001st historian can find something interesting? Of course I am drawing a caricature of genuine scholarship. But in every caricature there is an element of truth, and this one contains an indirect answer to the question of what it is that really makes the productive scholar. That he has learned the methods? The person who never produces anything new has also done that. It is imagination [*Phantasie*] that is the decisive function of the scholar. Imagination naturally has a hermeneutical function and serves the sense for what is questionable. It serves the ability to expose real, productive questions, something in which, generally speaking, only he who masters all the methods of his science succeeds.

As a student of Plato, I particularly love those scenes in which Socrates gets into a dispute with the Sophist virtuosi and drives them to despair by his questions. Eventually they can endure his questions no longer and claim for themselves the apparently preferable role of the questioner. And what happens? They can think of nothing at all to ask. Nothing at all occurs to them that is worth while going into and trying to answer.

I draw the following inference from this observation. The real power of hermeneutical consciousness is our ability to see what is questionable. Now if what we have before our eyes is not only the artistic tradition of a people, or historical tradition, or the principle of modern science in its hermeneutical preconditions but rather the whole of our experience, then we have succeeded, I think, in joining the experience of science to our own universal and human experience of life. For we have now reached the fundamental level that we can call (with Johannes Lohmann) the 'linguistic constitution of the world'.[1] It presents itself as the consciousness that is effected by history [*wirkungsgeschichtliches Bewusstsein*] and that provides an initial schematization for all our possibilities of knowing. I leave out of account the fact that the scholar—even the natural scientist—is perhaps not completely free of custom and society and from all possible factors in his environment. What I mean is that precisely *within* his scientific experience it is not so much the 'laws of ironclad inference' (Helmholz) that present fruitful ideas to him, but rather unforseen constellations that kindle the spark of scientific inspiration (e.g. Newton's falling apple or some other incidental observation).

The consciousness that is effected by history has its fulfillment in what is linguistic. We can learn from the sensitive student of language that language, in its life and occurence, must not be thought of as merely changing, but rather as something that has a teleology operating within it. This means that the words that are formed, the means of expression that appear in a language in order to say certain things, are not accidentally fixed, since the do not once again fall altogether into disuse. Instead, a definite articulation of the world is built up—a process that works as if guided and one that we can always observe in children who are learning to speak.

We can illustrate this by considering a passage in Aristotle's *Posterior Analytics* that ingeniously describes one definite aspect of language formation.[2] The passage treats what Aristotle calls the *epagoge*, that is, the formation of the universal. How does one arrive at a universal? In philosophy we say: how do we arrive at a general concept, but even words in this sense are obviously general. How does it happen that they are 'words', that is, that they have a general meaning? In his first apperception, a sensuously equipped being finds himself in a surging sea of stimuli, and finally one day he begins, as we say, to know something. Clearly we do not mean that he was previously blind. Rather, when we say 'to know' [*erkennen*] we mean 'to recognize' [*wiedererkennen*], that is, to pick something out [*herauserkennen*] of the stream of images flowing past as being identical. What is picked out in this fashion is clearly retained. But how? When does a child know its mother for the first time? When it sees her for the first time? No. Then when? How does it take place? Can we really say at all that there is a single event in which a first knowing extricates the child from the darkness of not knowing? It seems obvious to me that we cannot. Aristotle has described this wonderfully. He says it is the same as when an army is in flight, driven by panic, until at last someone stops and looks around to see whether the foe is still dangerously close behind. We cannot say that the army stops when one soldier has stopped. But then another stops. The army does not stop by virtue of the fact that two soldiers stop. When does it actually stop, then? Suddenly it stands its ground again. Suddenly it obeys the command once again. A subtle pun is involved in Aristotle's description, for in Greek 'command' means *arche*, that is, *principium*. When is the principle present as a principle? Through what capacity? This question is in fact the question of the occurrence of the universal.

If I have not misunderstood Johannes Lohmann's exposition, precisely this same teleology operates constantly in the life of language. When Lohmann speaks of linguistic tendencies as the real agents of history in which specific forms expand, he knows of course that it occurs in these forms of realization, of 'coming to a stand' [*Zum-Stehen-Kommen*], as the beautiful German word says. What is manifest here, I contend, is the real mode of operation of our whole human experience of the world. Learning to speak is surely a phase of special productivity, and in the course of time we have all transformed the genius of the three-year-old into a poor and meager talent. But in the utilization of the linguistic interpretation of the world that finally comes about, something of the productivity of our beginnings remains alive. We are all acquainted with this, for instance, in the attempt to translate, in practical life or in literature or wherever; that is, we are familiar with the strange, uncomfortable, and tortuous feeling we have as long as we do not have the right word. When we have found the right expression (it need not always be one word), when we are certain that we have it, then it 'stands', then something has come to a 'stand'. Once again we have a halt in the midst of the rush of the foreign language, whose endless variation makes us lose our orientation. What I am describing is the mode of the whole human experience of the world. I call this experience hermeneutical, for the process we are describing is repeated continually throughout our familiar experience. There is always a world already interpreted, already organized in its basic relations, into which experience steps as something new, upsetting what has led our expectations and undergoing reorganization itself in the upheaval. Misunderstanding and strangeness are not the first factors, so that avoiding misunderstanding can be regarded as the specific task of hermeneutics. Just the reverse is the case. Only the support of familiar and common understanding makes possible the venture into the alien, the lifting up of something out of the alien, and thus the broadening and enrichment of our own experience of the world.

This discussion shows how the claim to universality that is appropriate to the hermeneutical dimension is to be understood. Understanding is language-bound. But this assertion does not lead us into any kind of linguistic relativism. It is indeed true that we live within a language, but language is not a system of signals that we send off with the aid of a telegraphic key when we enter the office or transmission station. That is not speaking, for it does not have the infinity of the act that is linguistically creative and world experiencing. While we live wholly within a language, the fact that we do so does not constitute linguistic relativism because there is absolutely no captivity within a language—not even within our native language. We all experience this when we learn a foreign language, especially on journeys insofar as we master the foreign language to some extent. To master the foreign language means precisely that when we engage in speaking it in the foreign land, we do not constantly consult inwardly our own world and its vocabulary. The better we know the language, the less such a side glance at our native language is perceptible, and only because we never know foreign languages well enough do we always have something of this feeling. But it is nevertheless already speaking, even if perhaps a stammering speaking, for stammering is the obstruction of a desire to speak and is thus opened into the infinite realm of possible expression. Any language in which we live is infinite in this sense, and it is completely mistaken to infer that reason is fragmented because there are various languages. Just the opposite is the case. Precisely through our finitude, the particularity of our being, which is evident even in the variety of languages, the infinite dialogue is opened in the direction of the truth that we are.

If this is correct, then the relation of our modern industrial world, founded by science, which we described at the outset, is mirrored above all on the level of language. We live in an epoch in which an increasing leveling of all life-forms is taking place—that is the rationally necessary requirement for maintaining life on our planet. The food problem of mankind, for example, can only be overcome by the surrender of the lavish wastefulness that has covered the earth. Unavoidably, the mechanical, industrial world is expanding within the life of the individual as a sort of sphere of technical perfection. When we hear modern lovers talking to each other, we often wonder if they are communicating with words or with advertising labels and technical terms from the sign language of the modern industrial world. It is inevitable that the leveled life-forms of the industrial age also affect language, and in fact the impoverishment of the vocabulary of language is making enormous progress, thus bringing about an approximation of language to a technical sign-system. Leveling tendencies of this kind are irresistible. Yet in spite of them the simultaneous building up of our own world in language still persists whenever we want to say something to each other. The result is the actual relationship of men to each other. Each one is at first a kind of linguistic circle, and these linguistic circles come into contact with each other, merging more and more. Language occurs once again, in vocabulary and grammar as always, and never without the inner infinity of the dialogue that is in progress between every speaker and his partner. That is the fundamental dimension of hermeneutics. Genuine speaking, which has something to say and hence does not give prearranged signals, but rather seeks words through which one reaches the other person, is the universal human task—but it is a special task for the theologian, to whom is commissioned the saying-further (*Weitersagen*) of a message that stands written.

NOTES

1. Cf. Johannes Lohmann, *Philosophie und Sprachwissenschaft* (Berlin: Duncker & Humbolt, 1963).
2. Aristotle, *Posterior Analytics*, 100a 11–13.

Natural Science and Hermeneutics: The Concept of Nature in Ancient Philosophy

Hans-Georg Gadamer

Words tell a story. The word "nature" has penetrated so deeply into our linguistic consciousness that we do not even realize that we are dealing with a word borrowed from Latin, and that so far as the word "nature" is understood as a concept the Latin word is merely taken over from the Greek which formed the concept of *physis*. Now, words are vehicles for our mental imagination. The multiple meanings they radiate amount to the wealth of our ideas and thoughts. The formation of a concept, however, requires exact delimitation and differentiation in the way that Aristotle established in an immortal example in Book Delta of his *Metaphysics*. Philosophical analysis requires that different strands of meaning be distinguished to cancel the error of equivocation. But language itself is already the first deposit of the formation of a concept in that it enables such differences in meaning to arise in words. Philosophical analysis only takes the last step. In any case it is reasonable to become conscious of the whole inheritance of thought that lives on in language usage, and to utilize as it were the history of a word as an approach to the analysis of a concept.

The word "nature" clearly preserves today the status of a keyword. It resonates with the crisis of industrialized society on our planet, indicting a development which represents the exploitation of nature and which introduces irreversible processes of devastation and other ruinous changes. Both the general problem of environmental protection and the particular problems of nuclear energy and of air and water pollution have slowly penetrated today into general consciousness. This suggests that we should again become more conscious of how we think about nature and that we should no longer regard it simply as a deposit of reserves to be transformed into human goods. Certainly the emotional tone of the concept of nature goes back already to that criticism of culture which found its powerful spokesman in Rousseau in the late eighteenth century. He became so to speak an advocate, proclaiming the innocence of nature against the corruption of human civilization, and at the same time preaching passionately for a liberation from the forces of a rationalistic ideal of civilization and for a return to nature. To illustrate what Rousseau advocated, we need only recall how that epoch's taste for the artful design of gardens, that extension of human architecture into nature, turned to the style of the English park, to the "English garden" which intended to be a bit of nature. The return to nature also became a slogan of the French Revolution and of the emancipation of the bourgeoisie, giving the word at the same time a wide ranging social relevance. One thinks

Reprinted by permission from *Proceedings of the Boston Area Colloquium in Ancient Philosophy*, Vol. 1, pp. 39–52. Translated by Kathleen Wright. © 1986, University Press of America, Inc., Lanham, MD.

of the sans-culottes and in general of the words, crinoline *(Reifrock)* and peruke.[1] "Nature has now awoken amid the clang of arms"—Hölderlin could write.[2]

But what lies behind this formation of the concept of nature, one which we recognize, and which lives on by chance for a Heidelberger in the name of the Philosopher's Way? This name does not designate the special walk of philosophy professors but alludes to the peculiar phenomenon of people who prefer to take their walks alone, to Rousseauists, to give them a name. This was then something new which appeared in fact quite incomprehensible in view of the habits of older times. Behind this intensification of the development of human culture up to the critical turning point in the spirit of Rousseau, at which point the counterforce of nature and the spiritual power of solitude were again affirmed, lies the birth of modern science. Since then the technical and industrial application of modern science has reached its critical limits. Thus for the history of the formation of the modern concept of nature we are referred back to the fundamental fact that became a reality in the seventeenth century, the birth of modern science based on mathematics.

Newton's physics represents its first achievement, the conceptual explication of which we owe above all to Kant. In Kant we find the most rigorous concept of that nature thematised by the sciences. He defines nature as the lawfulness of phenomena in space and time. It is clear that this definition narrows the wide semantic field of the word "nature" as it survives in language and in the human spirit. Kant conferred on the new science of nature the concept [of nature] which was to be binding for it: what is not the object *(Gegenstand)* of a scientific method can not at all be valid as an object *(Objekt)* of the same.[3] This leads to the provocative formulation: it is the understanding which prescribes to nature its laws. Manifestly this so to speak epistemological confinement of the concept of nature could not occur without recognizing a broader circumscription of the concept of na-

ture. Consequently Kant made room conceptually in the *Critique of Judgement*, the third of his critiques, for the idea of nature as the guide-line for teleological judgement. To regard something as a natural organism and not as a machine clearly assumes a priori that we admit the thought of purpose and purposiveness. Only then can we speak of the "behavior" of organisms which do not execute movements impelled by mechanical forces but which adjust their behavior directed by their own purposes. A science of nature may consider this extended concept of nature to be merely an imperfect causal explanation of all natural events, and all that we call morphology to be provisionally valid, a merely descriptive way of understanding what has yet to become accessible to a true scientific explanation. One thinks of physicalism, of the "unity of science movement." In truth even such an extended concept of nature still signifies an enormous narrowing of the semantic field of the word "nature," the wealth and plenitude of which point back to other sources. This is most clear since the Renaissance when the Judeo-Christian concept of the creation of the world fused with the ancient heritage which was passing over into the modern world under the name of, as we say, Plato's "neo-Platonic" thought (and also this means above all those views which can be traced back to Stoic elements). In particular, the concept of the creative power of nature, of nature as *natura naturans*, goes back to what the ancients had prepared. The *logos* to which one is advised to listen in the manner of the Stoics, is at once the world principle, or better, the world breath which blows through everything and which animates the great cosmos where all is related to all by the power of sympathy. "To live in harmony with nature" is the famous formula of Stoic moral teachings in which the concept of *physis* becomes almost something like a sacred word.

With this we arrive back at the original formation of the concept of *physis* which we owe to Plato and Aristotle. I would like first to confirm this again by a discussion of the history of a word. If we ignore the disputed fragments of Philolaus, which in any case were later in the fifth century, we know of no use of the word *physis* in an absolute sense from the period of the Pre-Socratics. The discussion is always of the nature of something. This means basically that there was not yet a concept of *physis* which had found its expression in the abstract use of the word *physis*. The only apparent exception which we know of is Heracleitus' saying: φύσις κρύπτεσθαι φιλεῖ (frag. 123, Diels), "Nature likes to hide."[4] Even if this quotation which is first found in Porphyrios were to be authentically Heracleitean in its complete wording, it is far from providing evidence for the concept of nature which we encounter in Attic philosophy. Rather it still means the nature of something, in particular of something animate. Thus we find that Empodocles speaks of *physis* (frag, 8) as the usual word corresponding to *thanatos*, the word for the end of life, in order explicitly to reject it as an inappropriate mode of expression since neither birth nor death are actual in so far as they have to do with a mere transformation. I only mention this passage in order to demonstrate that while *physis* was at that time a common word, it clearly did not mean "nature" but instead "birth," "begetting," "planting" of a being. In case the saying of Heracleitus is completely authentic, it presumably means something like: "the true beginnings of a being remain in hiding"—apparently in opposition to the refulgence of death. Euponis indicates the same in a fragment (frag. 221, Kaibel) that can almost be translated by Hölderlin's "still greater power adheres to . . . birth . . .[5] In any case Heracleitus' saying remains no proof for the concept of *physis* around the year 500. In addition, all of the phrases which appear with this root stem from the earlier period, in Homer, naturally lend themselves to be understood in the sense of birth, seed, procreation of a being. Plato clearly echoes this. Even where it sounds almost like the title of a book, Socrates immediately understands that wisdom which they call περὶ φύσεως ἱστορίαν (*Phaedo* 96a8) in the sense of "why

something becomes (gignetai)." And when Plato means that which people call φύσει καὶ φύσις as opposed to that which is *psyche*, that is, that which comes from *techne* and *nous* (*Laws* 892b), he means "genesis." Even Aristotle has this in mind when he characterizes *physis*—as opposed to *techne*—without further ado as "genesis." (*Physics* Book 2, 193b12, Book 12)

Thus it becomes all the more urgent to ask what formed the word into a concept, what led up to the new concept of *physis*. We may recall here the self-representation which Plato puts into the mouth of Socrates in his last hour of life when he displays Socrates conversing about the immortality of the soul. Socrates speaks there in the first instance about the "cause of becoming and passing away" in general. He describes his earlier disappointing experiences with the great scientists of his age, who gave all kinds of interesting responses to this question, for example, that putrefaction is the condition for the genesis of life or that the brain rather than the midriff is the place where consciousness awakes or is located. Socrates relates how he remained dissatisfied with all that these contemporary scientists knew. Thus in the end, and especially after even Anaxagoras' book on *nous* proved to be a disappointment, he saw himself directed to another path. This was the path of the *logoi*, the path of the deposit [ὑπόθεσις] of conceptual generalities intended by the meaning and naturally also by the usage of words. Plato named this path dialectic. What this means over against the previous approach to and questioning of the world becomes clear when Socrates refers to the cosmological ideas or better explanations the earlier research had used to replace the mythological answers of the tradition. Atlas shouldering a burden no longer explained the fixed position of the earth in the center. Instead a cushion of water or air or some representation of an equilibrium attempted to answer this question at the very limit of human imagination about the position of the earth in the cosmos.

Against these attempts at explanation, Socrates proposes his natural understanding of the kind of understanding *(sein natürliches Verständnis von Verstehen)* that is given and firmly based on the linguistic communication that plays itself out between human beings, and which is above all illustrated in his own life situation. He wanted to learn to understand the position of the earth in the cosmos in the same way he understood why he had decided, in spite of all offers to take flight, to take upon himself the fulfillment of his execution. This "hermeneutical" turn represents manifestly a whole program of a physics which would understand natural events in the same way that human beings understand their own mode of behavior. Aristotle's physics is the fulfillment of this programmatic challenge. This means, however, that the concept of *physis* which was so formed constituted itself against the background of human planning, choosing, and making. The model of *techne* and of making is the basis for the formation of all of Aristotle's concepts. The schema of four causes through which he understands the essence of *physis* is obviously patterned on the different components of the activity of an artisan. The matter is there, together with the form which the product is to take on. There is the touch of the maker himself and the anticipation of the form which is projected in regard to the product's goodness, its fitness. What unfolds as it were in the process of the artisan's activity is woven together mysteriously in the essence of *physis*. Nature is not a process of manufacturing which first bestows on an already given matter its form and complete actuality in the final result. Rather the living being, the plant, the animal, or whatever, is already nature throughout the whole course of its growth. *Physis* is ὁδὸς εἰς φύσιν.

Plato's use of the concept of *physis* rests on the same understanding, even if with a notable qualification. At least in his mythical description of the construction of the cosmos, Plato conjures up the figure of a divine artisan and allows him to construct the cosmos in view of the order of ideas and numbers. In the eyes of Aristotle, this image of the *Timaeus* makes use of an empty metaphor. Indeed Aritotle's view of the world-whole and of nature is not at all compatible with the idea that this whole is made. It was solely in the dimension of interpretive concepts that we could recognize above the function of the model of making, not in the statements about the essence of nature as such.

Now, even Plato transcends in a certain way this mythical mode of representation when he sees the essence of *physis* in *psyche*, that is, in the principle of self-movement that distinguishes the animate. He uses the concept of "soul" (ψυχή) in its older meaning which corresponds very well even without any mythology to the most natural experiences. The enigmatic something which differentiates the animate body from the dead is really a primitive experience, and yet it is something invisible and thus closely related, ontologically speaking, to such enigmatic things as numerical relation. Certainly to the question of how the perfection of mathematical relations forms itself into the reality in which we live, the *Sophist*, the *Philebus*, and the *Timaeus* respond that it is necessary to assume a cause, a planning and knowing mind, something like a divine demiurge. Thus Plato seems manifestly to be serious that such an order can not arise "of itself." We have, however, learned how little this may be taken literally from the battle fought in the Academy over the true significance of the demiurge in the *Timaeus*. Even in the ultra-conservative *Laws*, the explication of φύσις as ψυχή points in the same direction: the world order is not brought into being by the hand of an artisan external to it. And above all in Book X of the *Laws, psyche* is introduced as the true *physis* expressly as a defence against the "automatic" genesis of the world.[6]

This is precisely Aristotle's point of departure. Because of his anti-Pythagorean feelings and his aversion to all hypostatizing of mathematical relations, he takes the being that moves itself of itself as the core of reality from which to construct his own physics. We learn this not the least from his ingenious creation of the words *entelecheia* and *energeia*, which are striking expressions for his own basic position. It is immediately evident what these concepts intend to say. The *telos*, the being finished and complete, is not imposed externally on matter even if it is the *telos* of perfect regularity such as the Greeks marveled at with astonishment in the movements of the constellations. This alone does not constitute for Aristotle the true perfection of nature; more importantly, nature has its perfection so to speak in itself. Aristotle's "onto-theology" is linked to this [perfection of nature] only in one of its conclusion; an all-moving god of motion guarantees the beginning and endlessness of the ordered motion of the cosmos. For the concept of *physis*, it is sufficient to be clear about the basic fact that *physis* is conceived to be a counter-concept to the attitude of producing and making. The concept of *techne* (and the concepts of *thesis* and *nomos*), to which the concept of *physis* is opposed, is what first compels the formation of the concept of nature, the nature both of the natural and of the social world, and which prepares the conceptual means for research into it in the form of the four causes.

Let us examine the manner in which Plato and Aristotle (who were the first to do so) bring into focus their predecessors. It is self-evident that both bring their own perspective to bear in their accounts of earlier thought. No ancient thinker was interested in his predecessors in the sense in which we ask historical questions. But the perspectives of Plato and Aristotle differ, thereby clarifying each one's position. We see for example in the *Sophist* how far Plato remains true to the logic of the arithmetic model of the Pythagorean world experience. He organizes earlier thinkers under the perspective of unity, duality, and the triadic, or of unity and multiplicity—in their varying possibilities. In the classic passage of the *Sophist* (242c ff.) which offers a first classification of Pre-Socratic "philosophy," he uses this model so to speak as a conceptual scan of understanding. This problem—that numbers are the union of many—is his own and the Pythagorean problem. To think and to make statements also means to form a union out of many. Thus Plato clearly follows his own comprehension of the dialectic of the one and the many when he directs his attention to the Pre-Socratics. To be sure he allows his "speaker" to voice a reservation that is very characteristic of him which is that he does not claim on the basis of a superior concept to survey the imperfections and deficiencies of earlier thought. Rather he perceives vague anticipations of the truth in these wise men of an earlier age, and explains that it is we alone who are incapable of really understanding and recovering them. In truth this points ironically and indirectly to Plato's own clear knowledge of what being *(Sein)* and a being *(Seiendes)* are: to be one and yet also to be many. Aristotle, on the other hand, openly makes it his object to integrate all of the thinking that preceded him into his own based on a superior art of making conceptual distinctions. That means for him that he certainly also accepted within limits the Pythagorean mathematical projection of the world—as the discovery of eidetic structures—and this completely embraces the Platonic assumption of *eidos* and the assumption of a final cause, of *telos*. He saw, however, the deficiencies of this mathematical projection of the world in the fact that the realization of the regularities and perfections of this world order was not put forward by Plato in a valid way—because it was put forward only "mythically." It thereby ignored undeniable evidence which gives precedence to an understanding of "being" *(Sein)* based on beings that are by nature and on that which moves itself of itself.

It is precisely the older Ionian thinkers and their followers who offer support at least indirectly for Aristotle. If there were to be many, then "primary being" (the material or that "out of which") must always include something like that from which movement arises within itself. Now this indeed represents a conceptual recourse to the original meaning of the word *physis* as we have learned above all from Heidegger: the "emerging" into "presence." Confronted by its counterimage, by a being which is made and produced out of *techne, physis* forms itself into an independent concept and conceptual word. From another point of view, the distinction between θέσει, or νόμῳ and φύσει, which arises with the sophists, may also play a role here. Aristotle's recourse to the Ionian origins signifies in any case a true resumption of the project to think "ontologically" what had remained unthought in the form of cosmogony and of the natural processes which developed themselves from out of themselves. One who would replace the "empty metaphor" of the ordering hand of a master-artisan by concepts would not satisfy himself with a vague and indeterminate recognition of intelligence or *nous* as the ultimate cause of the movement of everything. Rather he would be much more compelled to the positive knowledge that nature brings itself about as it were of itself, develops itself out of itself, and arrives at what it is fitted for.

This unwittingly introduces something which seems exactly privileged to distinguish and to demarcate the natural from the artificially made, namely, the concepts of the of-itself *(Von-selbst)* and of the necessity which govern natural events as opposed to artificial production. These are precisely the key concepts, το αὐτόματον and ἡ ἀνάγκη which are attested to in Democritus, the great unknown contemporary of Socrates. We can understand how this Democritean program to explain the world could appear to be to a certain extent the most consistent implementation of the Ionian beginning. We can equally understand the nineteenth century interpretation of the Pre-Socratics. Especially because of that century's new fervor for the evolutionary theory which had asserted itself against the Aristotelian cosmos of unchanging species thanks to the revolution introduced by Darwin, to a great extent the conviction then was that Democritus had been the researcher with truly more future, and that the suppression of the productive characteristics of the new scientific knowledge of the world in the later tradition was to be attributed to the reactionary influence of Attic philosophy.

The precise question which we must examine is the following: how was it possible for the new concept of "nature" established by Plato and Aristotle to prove itself superior to the consistent development of atomic theory? For this purpose we must investigate two things: how Plato and Aristotle relativized the intrusive concepts of necessity and of-itself by so to speak overarching considerations, and how as a consequence a conception of nature could be established from which the thinking of Western humanity could first free itself at the start of modernity, and that not without losses.

Thus our task will be to see the confrontation between the intrinsic consistency of the idea of nature which began with the Ionian enlightenment and which found its development in atomic theory and the new turn to thinking of nature teleologically, and to ask ourselves how Plato and Aristotle were able successfully to develop a perspective superior to the Ionian worldview. Certainly they could not do so without integrating what was relatively right about the latter. Thus, what role do the of-itself and ἀνάγκη play in nature? Is it not necessity that at any given time impels the unfolding of a being from out of itself, and which directs each living being up to what it is fitted for with, as even we say, the force of nature? How can this be integrated as a subordinate consideration into a greater interpretative context? This problem is already encountered in Plato's *Timaeus*, where indeed in a surprising turn the teleological master-hand of the world demiurge appears to be limited by a counter-authority, and indeed by the conditions which lie in the essence of spatial reality and its basic mathematical structure, and which limit all materialization. It was Plato's ingenious inspiration to bring into play for the whole history of the construction of reality what was precisely a mathematical discovery of his time, namely, the existence of five, and only five regular bodies, the so-called Platonic bodies. With stereometry there emerges a kind of meeting halfway *(Entgegenkommen)* of space; in the structure of space not all regularities are possible for bodies, but precisely those five regular bodies are possible, which Plato then with his own instinctive and playful imaginative power associates with the four elements of the Pythagorean and Empedoclean tradition. In this way the idea of necessity is both still interpreted by means of mathematics and admitted into a higher purposeful association. The master artisan's intention to order encounters a kind of good-willed readiness on the part of the pre-given; whether one wants to call this matter or space it is all the same. The later Platonism which builds on Aristotle openly speaks of a preformed matter which the great world master comes upon.

Aristotle's discussion of the same problem in his physics is more radical, that is, it is entirely articulated by conceptual distinctions and without the "empty metaphor" of the demiurge. There is no mythic world master [artisan] who brings nature into its order. The task now is to analyze conceptually the ontological structure of that nature which forms itself and grows into itself. What is decisive is the truth that we always understand even the naturalness of natural events from our own understanding of teleology. This is especially so when we compare the superior order of the course of the stars with the paltry order created by the hand of man in the *polis* and in the human disposition *(Gemüt)*. It may certainly also be enlightening that the factors of "of-itself" and "by necessity" play a role in the great purposeful connections that are not "made" by anyone, but only on a secondary level. In view of the superior regularity of the course of nature the fact that something takes place of itself appears to be as it were an exception over against that which is in itself arranged purposefully or is brought about intentionally. When someone accidentally meets someone else, or is hit by a stone that fell of itself on his head, then we experience the feeling that something which occurred accidentally and "of itself" is as if intended. But one still thinks even then on the basis of a possible intent: "of itself" means the absence of this intent. This is even more true for the concept of necessity.

There is no doubt something which we call necessary. For example, it holds in all purposeful action for the relation between the necessary means to the end. It is fundamental to every decision in action that one must ask oneself what the means are which could lead to the end, and these means must indeed be known and recognized as that which is necessary for the end. Once more this indicates that it is the primacy of the thought of purpose which admits the concept of necessity and allows it a relative significance. An opposite world-view which elevated contingencies and subordinate necessities to the one and only explanatory principle of the world's order would be incomprehensible from the point of view of such a linguistically and anthropologically centered concept of the world. For the latter world-view, it is unimaginable that such overpowering manifestations of order in the cosmos such as the regularity of the course of the stars or the constancy of the preservation of the species in the events of life should be explicable by the episodic efficacy of automatic causes. One must recognize that the atomistic model of the origin of the world offered at that time no true explanation. When it ought to have explained the order of the heavens or of living beings, it had instead taken up the experienced order in an unacknowledged way into its own model of explanation.

We see therefore that the teleological view of nature did not just suppress a fruitful way to begin to explain [nature], but that it was also something understandable for us. It may sound to us more amusing than serious to explain the world such that a stone falls because it wants to be in its very own place together with other stones, or that fire ascends because it wants to unite itself so to speak with the great fiery space in the sphere of the stars. However, such thinking allows a uniform understanding of the whole of the world surrounding us, in the same way as we understand ourselves in our actions. Socrates's challenge to explain the structure of the world just as he ordered his own action by the good and the just that were evident to him is fulfilled here. It is to be sure impossible for us to admit such an ideal of the order of nature extrapolated from the human life world as an explanatory principle which could compete with the mechanics established by Galileo and its technical application. What the beginning of modern science in the seventeenth century signified is evident in science's great victory march through the whole of modernity up to our age. But one must also consider the rupture this brought into the homogeneity of a world understanding that had maintained its canonical status for many centuries thanks to Aristotelian philosophy. Ever since the start of modern experimental sciences we are exposed to that tension which permeates our entire culture and which has made the talk of two worlds possible. The one [world] is the research of nature represented by modern science. It is distinguished by its knowledge of the laws of nature and its mastery of the forces of nature based on such knowledge. The other [world] is the teleological ordering of the world which holds self-evidently in the linguistic picture of the world which we all share. It permits us even after the Copernican turn to speak of sunrise and sunset—and not of the earth's rotation.

This, then, is the result of our glance at the ancient concept of nature. We cannot overlook or at all underestimate the great liberation of the human powers, of the will to research and of the ability to produce creatively. These powers have become conditions for human life which cannot be abandoned in our technical and industrial world. However the lesson we have to extract from this backward glance at the ancients is that the interpretation of the world that has been gained from life experience and that is fundamental to our cultural and linguistic tradition also remains valid alongside the other, and that in the end it constitutes what is superior for human action. As our world is slowly transformed into a factory for human production on a global scale, we are beginning to become conscious of this. We must remember the insurmountable limits that the natural order imposes upon us if we are not to destroy, in the process of improving nature into an artifical world, the foundations of life for ourselves, who are beings of nature.

NOTES*

1. Gadamer's point is that these words remind us of the connection between revolutionary politics and a change in fashion to what is natural. Men who did not wear culottes (sans-culotte), women who did not wear crinoline petticoats, and all who disdained the wearing of wigs used a fashion which went "back to nature" to make a political statement.
2. Friedrich Hölderlin, *Poems and Fragments*, trans. Michael Hamburger (Cambridge: Cambridge University Press, 1980), p. 393.
3. Gadamer is referring here to the distinction Kant makes between phenomena and noumena, and to the fact that not all that can be thought (noumena) can be the object *(Objekt)* of experience and of an experimental science of nature.
4. *Ancilla to the Pre-Socratics*, trans. Kathleen Freeman (Cambridge: Harvard Univ. Press, 1978), p. 33.
5. Hölderlin, p. 411.
6. Gadamer's point here is that Plato's identification of *physis* with *psyche* in the *Laws* qualifies his own thesis of a demiurge, and argues against the thesis of the automatic ("of-itself") genesis of the world proposed by Democritus.

* All notes are by the translator.

SECTION SIX

CRITICAL THEORY AND FEMINIST CRITIQUE

Marylouise Welch

Funded by an endowment in 1923 in Frankfurt, Germany, a group of philosophers established the Institute of Social Research. Initially the institute focused its studies on empirical Marxist questions. But under the leadership of Max Horkheimer (1895–1971) in the 1930s, the focus shifted to social philosophy and the dialectics of everyday reality. With Theodor Adorno (1903–1969) and Herbert Marcuse (1898–1978), the institute changed course, calling for critique of the objective, disconnected observer/researcher and a true critique of culture (Horkheimer, 1972). Horkheimer called for new research using a critical mode that involved a reexamination of society that challenges basic social, political, cultural and economic assumptions which maintain hegemony. For Horkheimer and Marcuse, critical theory never rests with increased knowledge but must maintain a critical attitude toward our culturally constructed values and beliefs.

Herbert Marcuse was a student of both Husserl and Heidegger and was influenced by their notions of understanding. His version of critical social theory fused insights from phenomenology, hermeneutics, humanist Marxism (recognizing the presence of the dialectic in all things) and Freudian psychoanalysis. All of these thinkers influenced each other and maintained their relationships to the institute, even in exile during World War II. Into this intellectual landscape arrived Jurgen Habermas (b. 1929), perhaps the most renowned of this circle. He is currently the most often cited of the critical theorists, and it is his essay that is contained in this volume.

Habermas rejuvenated critical theory in the 1960s and brought philosophy and social science back together. The institute had moved the questions of critical theory from a social science perspective to a more philosophical realm. Habermas wanted critical theory to return to knowledge anchored in social science as originally delineated by Marx, including examination of the power structures that maintain the forces of oppression in the social system. In the excerpt included in this volume, he advocates for a new role for philosophy as it interacts with human sciences as the mediator between expert knowledge and the lifeworld.

When one is first introduced to Habermas, it is important to clarify his use of the terms rational, reason, critique and reflection. He wrote in his first work (Habermas, 1971) that he was trying to return critical theory to the Enlightenment notion that critique can be a practical force with emancipatory potential (Bernstein, 1985). Critical thought is rational discourse. His goal is to bring self-knowledge and self-reflection back to an individual whose perception is clouded by values imposed by society. Self-reflective means to bend back upon the self and in so doing see something from a new perspective. By making the theory self-reflective, he requires people to account for their own conditions of possibility. "Critical" means to penetrate a given context (Habermas, 1971), and for Habermas, critical thought is committed to rationality.

TECHNICAL, PRACTICAL AND EMANCIPATORY KNOWLEDGE

In his early writings, Habermas (1971) placed critical social theory within a framework of scientific knowledge which contained three categories of cognitive interests: technical, practical and emancipatory. Habermas's development of cognitive interests is a quasitranscendental theory that attempts to specify the relationship between knowledge and human interests. Causal explanations in which instrumental knowledge facilitates technical control over objects is technical knowledge. Understanding in the historical-hermeneutic tradition is what is meant by practical knowledge. It is the intersubjective way of knowing, with a goal of mutual understanding. Recognizing the limitations of these two ways of knowing, he describes emancipatory knowledge as fundamental to critical social science. The goal is for universal knowledge that will liberate individuals and communities from the power of distorted communication by creating knowledge which furthers autonomy and responsibility. This liberation involves scientific inquiry into people's lived experiences with reflection and critique that exposes concealed domination of individuals and groups. Building on emancipatory knowledge, a form of communication can occur that creates an open universal egalitarian dialogue (Habermas, 1971). Emancipatory knowledge directs consciousness into a critical mode of reflections and reveals sources of domination.

COMMUNICATIVE ACTION

Since the publication of *Knowledge and Human Interests* (1971), Habermas has engaged in scholarly dialogue, has done extensive revisions and developed a much denser, more complicated and abstract theory of communicative action that is oriented to active emancipation (Bernstein, 1985). In later Habermas (1985), there is a synthesis of science and philosophy. One notes that his polemics against theory belong to the past as he tries to create a theory whose ultimate goal is to identify and reconstruct the universal conditions of possible understandings.

In this theory, he is incorporating the focus on action from sociology with an analysis of social systems. Humans engage in strategic acts and communicative acts. Strategic acts are instrumental actions that are normative, purposive and goal oriented, guided by efficiency and predictability. They are unreflected and occur in our everyday lives, often involving competition with an aim at individual success.

In communicative action there is a framework for common understandings. These understandings are in language, culture, and traditions, and they make up the realm of the lifeworld. For Habermas all human action involves language. Acts are linguistically constituted, so language embeds us in an interpersonal communicative context. Communicative actions aim to achieve emancipation through a process of mutual understandings. To reach this goal the participants need communicative competence. Habermas elaborates extensively about the requirements for communicative competence, but briefly, it requires a few essential conditions. First, communicative competence involves situations in which one enjoys freedom from the constraints of domination (Habermas, 1979). In other words, the people are free to be open and to take risks. To accomplish this, one engages in critical reflection to reveal the sources of oppression. Ideal speech is central to communicative competence (Habermas, 1979). This means that participants have equal opportunities to present their claims about what they hold to be truth as these validity claims are examined and critiqued, and group consensus is achieved. The key to intersubjective understanding and coordination of actions is the agreement among the participants on the validity claims embedded in the speech acts. If this ideal situation is met, then communicative action occurs. This involves self-reflection to locate ideological distortion and true dialogue leading to emancipatory action. Not only does the process need to reveal the power structures and the hidden meanings but it must establish a consensual plan for action and change.

He looked to research to uncover the structures of rationality embedded in everyday life. As the writers included in this chapter demonstrate, there is no one research method for critical scholarship. Habermas never outlined one but has made clear that there are certain conditions which must be met in order for research to be critical. These conditions include the analysis and unveiling of hidden power structures, the commitment of the study to full and equal participation of researcher (who becomes a participant) and the observed, and finally the study must be committed to a mutually agreed upon plan for change. Through the process of dialogue and self-reflection, critical theory invokes consciousness raising about the hidden source of domination and power. This has been in large measure critical theory's appeal to feminists and nurses.

CRITICAL THEORY AND NURSING

Janice Thompson points out to nursing the possibilities for our scientific development in the writings of the continental philosophers and in particular the ideas in Habermas's critical social theory (Thompson, 1985, 1987). Wells offers an example of a study in which Habermas's theory served as the framework for an analysis of discharge planning. She shows how strategic action—behavior that is technical, efficient and fulfills the needs of administration—has eclipsed communicative action in this process for patients. While many feminists agree with parts of critical social theory, and would see the insights that Wells has gained as fruitful, there remains for them a common concern that it lacks a specific focus on gender and some of its theorists call for universals. Campbell and Bunting give an excellent overview of the commonalities and differences between critical theory and feminist theory while advising caution. Any comparison between the two can only be broad and general because both critical and feminist theories are really families of theories with significant intratheoretical variations. Much of feminist scholarship has described the historically oppressive concerns common to all women. Yet, as Harding points out, each woman has a unique response to her situation, and this uniqueness needs to be captured in our research about gender issues.

DISCUSSION GUIDE

1. Does Habermas's critical theory clarify or mystify the basis of male domination and female subordination in modern society?
2. In what proportion and in what respect does critical theory challenge ideological rationalizations of dominance?
3. Can critical theory be used to serve the self-clarification of the struggles of feminists?
4. Describe the possibilities in effective communicative action for women and for nursing science.
5. How does critical social theory relate to feminist knowledge development?
6. What is truth in critical social theory?

REFERENCES

Bernstein, R. (1985). *Habermas and modernity*. Cambridge: MIT Press.

Habermas, J. (1971). *Knowledge and human interest*. Boston: Beacon Press.

Habermas, J. (1979). *Communication and the evolution of society*. Boston: Beacon Press.

Habermas, J. (1985). *The theory of communicative action: Reason and the rationalization of society*. (Vol. 1). Boston: Beacon Press.

Horkheimer, M. (1972). *Critical theory: Selected essays*. New York: Seabury Press.

Thompson, J. (1985). Practical discourse in nursing: Going beyond empiricism and historicism. *Advances in Nursing Science, 7*(4):59–71.

Thompson, J. (1987). Critical scholarship: The critique of domination in nursing. *Advances in Nursing Science, 10*(1), 27–38.

BIBLIOGRAPHY

Ashley, J. A. (1972). *Hospitals, paternalism and the role of the nurse*. New York: Teacher's College Press, Columbia University.

Benhabib, S., & Cornell, D. (Eds.). (1987). *Feminism as critique*. Cambridge: Polity Press.

Bronner, S. E. (1994). *Of critical theory and its theorists*. Cambridge, MA: Blackwell.

Carr, W., & Kemmis, S. (1983). *Becoming critical: Knowing through action research*. Victoria, Australia: Deakin University Press.

Freiere, P. (1972). *Pedagogy of the oppressed*. Harmondsworth: Penguin.

———. (1985). *The politics of education: Culture, power and liberation*. London: Maxmillian.

Greenleaf, N. (1980). The sex segmented occupations: Relevance for nursing. *Advances in Nursing Science, 2*, 23–37.

Habermas, J. (1971). *Knowledge and human interests*. Boston: Beacon Press.

———. (1973). *Theory and practice*. Boston: Beacon Press.

———. (1990). *Moral consciousness and communicative action*. Cambridge: MIT Press.

Lather, P. (1984). Critical theory, curricular transformation and feminist mainstreaming. *Journal of Education, 166*, 1:49–62.

McCarthy, T. (1985). *The critical theory of Jürgen Habermas*. Cambridge: MIT Press.

Meehan, J. (Ed.). (1995). *Feminists read Habermas: Gendering the subject of discourse*. New York: Routledge.

Melosh, B. (1982). *The physician's hand: Work, culture and conflict in American nursing*. Philadelphia: Temple University Press.

Rabinow, P., & Sullivan, W. M. (Eds.). (1987). *Interpretive social science: A second look.* Berkeley: University of California Press.

Street, A. (1992). *Inside nursing: A critical ethnography of clinical nursing practice.* Albany: State University of New York Press.

Thomas, L. W. (1995). A critical feminist perspective of the health belief model: Implications for nursing theory, research, practice and education. *Journal of Professional Nursing, 11,* 4:246–252.

Titchen, A., & Binnie, A. (1994). Action research: A strategy for theory generation and testing. *International Journal of Nursing Studies, 31,* 1:1–12.

Wheeler, C. E., & Chinn, P. L. (1984). *Peace & power: A handbook of feminist process.* Buffalo, NY: Margaretdaughters.

Towards a Theory of Communicative Competence

Jürgen Habermas

In this, the second of two articles outlining a theory of communicative competence, the author questions the ability of Chomsky's account of *linguistic* competence to fulfil the requirements of such a theory. 'Linguistic competence' for Chomsky means the mastery of an abstract system of rules, based on an innate language apparatus. The model by which communication is understood on this account contains three implicit assumptions, here called 'monologism', 'a priorism', and 'elementarism'. The author offers an outline of a theory of communicative competence that is based on the negations of these assumptions. In opposing the first two assumptions he introduces distinctions, respectively, between semantic universals which process experiences and those that make such processing possible, and between semantic universals which precede all socialization and those that are linked to the conditions of potential socialization. Against elementarism, he argues that the semantic content of all possible natural languages does not consist of combinations of a finite number of meaning components. Differences in systems of classification preclude this, and such differences can be seen to infect all respects of intercultural comparison. Using the notion of 'performative utterance', the author elucidates the role of dialogue-constitutive universals as part of the formal apparatus required of a speaker's capacity to communicate. He then notes what would be required of a general semantics based on a theory of communicative competence; and finally points out how this theory might be used for social analysis.

Chomsky[1] starts from two experiences: the creativity of the speaker and the grammaticalness of language. Considering the finite capacity of human consciousness, every natural language must consist of a finite number of elements. Irrespective of this fact, everyone who masters a language can, with the aid of these elements, understand and produce an infinite number of sentences, some of them unpredictably new. Moreover, every competent speaker can decide

ad hoc whether a sequence of linguistic expressions is formed correctly or violates the system of linguistic rules; he can differentiate 'intuitively' between correct and deviating formulations. And with the aid of the same capability he can also partially understand semantically senseless or grammatically garbled sentences and classify them according to degree of grammaticalness. For these two particular achievements the competent speaker must possess a knowledge grossly disproportionate to his empirical information; the competent speaker must know more than he can have learned in his previous contacts with his linguistic environment. Chomsky explains this asymmetry between knowledge and

Reprinted from Inquiry 13:360–375, 1970, by permission of Scandinavian University Press, Oslo, Norway.

experience by postulating (1) an abstract linguistic system which consists of 'generative' rules. I shall not comment on this, but go on directly to introduce three further assumptions that Chomsky makes.

The asymmetry evident when an adult speaker 'knows' more than he can have learned empirically is especially conspicuous in the case of language acquisition in infants.[2] Chomsky therefore assumes (2) that the development of the abstract system of linguistic rules is based upon the interaction of phase-specific stimulus conveyance and organic maturation processes. In other words, the system of linguistic rules is innate. Chomsky further assumes (3) that this innate language apparatus consists of linguistic universals which predetermine the form of all potential natural languages. The difficulties he encountered in his attempts to ascertain this system of rules by means of the usual inductive methods of segmentation and classification led him, finally, to the assumption (4) that the given linguistic sequences are surface structures which result from the transformation of deep structures. The basic assumption of a transformational grammar proves useful, moreover, in explaining grammatical ambiguities in phrase structure.[3]

'Linguistic competence' is Chomsky's name for the mastery of an abstract system of rules, based on an innate language apparatus, regardless of how the latter is in fact used in actual speech. This competence is a monological capability; it is founded in the species-specific equipment of the solitary human organism. For such a capability to be a sufficient linguistic basis for speech, one would have to be able to reconstruct the communication process itself as a 'monological' one. The information model of communication is suitable for this purpose. I consider this model to be monological because it consistently attributes the intersubjectivity of meaning—that is, the mutual sharing of identical meanings—to the fact that sender and receiver—each an entity for itself—are previously equipped with the same programme. It is this

pre-established code that is supposed to make communication possible. Speech, the actual language behaviour, would then have to be explained as the result of an interaction between linguistic competence and certain psychological, as well as sociological, peripheral conditions which restrict the application of the competence. While the system of linguistic rules determines, on the one hand, whether a sequence of expressions is correct or deviant, these restrictive conditions determine, on the other, whether a correctly formed expression is unusual or acceptable in a given situation.[4]

To begin with, I would like to show some of the difficulties inherent in this model. If general linguistics restricts itself to giving a rational reconstruction of the abstract system of linguistic rules which the ideal speaker has in mind, as it were, prior to all communication, and if the theory of language performance analyses solely restrictive extralinguistic conditions for applying linguistic competence, then not only grammar and phonetics but semantics, too, would have to be developed independently of the pragmatic dimension of language performance as an element of a monological ability. In this framework general semantics has two problems in particular to solve. First, it must clarify the apparatus of rules which help us to project lexical units into grammatical deep structures and to maintain constancy of meaning in transformational processes; secondly, it must reduce the lexica of natural languages to a finite number of meaning components, out of which the basically solitary speaker can construct all possible semantic contents. The elementaristic research strategy,[5] which is supposed to reconstruct any lexical unit with the aid of general semantic markers and reduce them in the form of deductively classified marker hierarchies to some few universals, results conclusively from the monological language model. At the same time it is assumed that language possesses an *a priori* meaning-structure. Bierwisch[6] introduces this structure, matching it with the *a priori* phonetic structure:

Phonological markers represent acoustic properties of objects just as little as semantic markers directly represent environmental characteristics. The universal phonological inventory is a hypothesis about distinctions which the human being can exploit linguistically according to the structure of his organism, i.e. the ear, the speech organs, and the nervous systems controlling them. A universal inventory of semantic markers would be, similarly, a hypothesis about the differentiations in regard to his environment, which the human being can achieve with the help of his sense organs, his nervous system, or in general, his apperceptive constitution. In other words, a complete inventory of semantic markers, from which each individual language makes a specific selection, would in the end be an intrinsically exact characterization of the apperceptive apparatus by which the human being analyses his surroundings practically and intellectually.

Bierwisch's commentary elucidates the implicit assumptions for a programme of general semantics. We can summarize these in thesis-form as follows. The *thesis of monologism* assumes that the universal meaning components belong to the basic equipment of the solitary organism of the speaking subject. The thesis is incompatible with the proposition that semantic universals could also be parts of an intersubjectively produced cultural system. The *thesis of a priorism* assumes that the inventory of ultimate meaning elements—as the condition which makes semantic differentiation possible—precedes all experience. The thesis is incompatible with the proposition that universal semantic fields can also reflect the universality of specific scopes of experience. The *thesis of elementarism* assumes, finally, that the semantic content of all possible natural languages consists of combinations of a finite number of meaning components. This thesis is incompatible with the proposition that semantic fields can be formed and shifted in structural association with global views of nature and society (*Weltbilder*).

I believe that the propositions which are incompatible with the theses can be more credibly argued than the theses themselves. Regarding theses (1) and (2): Universal meanings, which arise in all natural languages, neither automatically precede all experience, nor are they necessarily rooted in the cognitive equipment of the human organism prior to all socialization. The universal distribution of meanings, and even of meaning components, is not a sufficient criterion for the a priorism and monologism of general semantics urged by the Chomsky school of linguistics. Some meanings are *a priori* universal in as much as they establish the conditions of potential communication and general schemes of interpretation; others are *a posteriori* universal, in the sense that they represent invariant features of contingent scopes of experience which, however, are common to all cultures. For that reason we differentiate between semantic universals which process experiences and semantic universals which make this processing possible in the first place (i.e. *a posteriori / a priori*). Furthermore, some meanings are intersubjectively universal in the sense that they are fixed on structures which first develop with the cultural level of linguistic communication itself; other meanings are monologically universal in as much as they refer to structures of the solitary human organism prior to all communication. Therefore we differentiate between semantic universals which precede all socialization and semantic universals which are linked to the condition of potential socialization (monological/intersubjective). The combination of these points of view comprise four classes of semantic universals:

Semantic universals

	a priori	a posteriori
Intersubjective	Dialogue-constitutive universal	Cultural universal
Monological	Universal cognitive schemes of interpretation	Universals of perceptive and motivational constitution

A few examples can suffice as illustration.[7] The dialogue-constitutive universals include personal pronouns, interrogative, imperative, and assertive formators, modal formators and the like. In the cognitive schemes of interpretation which have been absorbed in the linguistic system of rules we include causality and substance, space and time—in fact the deictic formators in general which establish the system of possible denotations. The best analysed example of cultural universals is the system of kinship words and, correspondingly, of universals of organic constitution of the system of colour words. Whether we can also assume a general vocabulary of basic drives and emotional tendencies for the motivational equipment is a more difficult question.

As for thesis (3), the *a posteriori* universal meanings surely make quite evident the limits within which an elementaristic meaning-analysis can take place. The institution of family, for instance, which is based on the sexual privilege of the parents, i.e. on the incest barrier between the generations, as well as between brothers and sisters, is indeed universally distributed;[8] a system of kinship relations which is formed around this institutional core is to be found in all cultures. But an intercultural comparison of the kinship vocabulary shows clearly that this same semantic field is differently classified depending on the prevailing status system, i.e. on the specific definition of the age-, sex- and descent-linked primary roles. It is true, as the ethnological classifications themselves indicate, that we can find descriptive systems which allow us to reconstruct any given kinship vocabulary in terms of a small number of semantic markers. But there is no general criterion for the selection between several conventional descriptive systems. If we follow the standpoint of cognitive validity and choose that descriptive system which corresponds to the relevant evaluation criteria of a culture itself, then practically every culture demands its own system. Even in the case of coincident vocabularies for two different cultures, the kinship relations can be interpreted

differently; and in that case, which of the alternative interpretations is cognitively 'valid' depends solely on the acknowledged definition of social roles.[9]

The system of colour expressions is a case similar to that of kinship vocabulary. The neurophysiological sense organization establishes a culturally invariable scope of experience for colour perception. The semantic field 'colour-words' is as universal as that of kin-terms, but again the classification of this field varies; notwithstanding the relatively high degree of congruence, here too we find no universal cognitively valid descriptive system, for the common patterns of interpretation classify the colour spectrum in different intervals and not only within the physically determinable dimensions of hue, luminosity, and saturation.[10]

On the basis of ethno-linguistic evidence, we must conclude that the fields of meaning which depend upon culturally universal institutions or upon organically universal equipment probably do represent semantically equivalent scopes (family, colour), but that, in addition, the interpretation of these scopes already depends upon the sociocultural background.

The dependence of semantic analysis upon the non-exceedable common context of the society[11] to which the speakers belong is connected with a fundamental difficulty of semantic elementarism. The examples of semantic analysis given by Chomsky, Fodor, Katz, and others reduce complex meanings to simple semantic markers. These markers are usually specifications of the following type: physical items versus non-physical, animated versus inanimate, male versus female, old versus young. Such marker-pairs are introduced as disjunctive specifications, which can then be classified hierarchically or divided into new disjunctions; for example, living creatures are divided into human beings versus non-humans (animals, plants); human beings into male and female; male into men (adults) and children (non-adults); men into married and unmarried (bachelor), etc. Thus it is possible to create conceptual hierarchies with meaning components of increasing complexity inserted in their intersections. This procedure depends on the fundamental relations of hyponymy, and incompatibility can be differentiated as antonymy, complementarity, and converseness.[12] The vocabulary of all natural languages is structured along these fundamental relations. That is undisputed. An elementaristic meaning-analysis must assume, however, that there is, in addition, a universally valid list of ultimate, i.e. independent and irreducible, meaning components. It is the fundamental semantic relations holding between these components which, according to such an analysis, determine the fundamental relations between compound meanings. I wish to dispute this assumption.

The empirical evidence of comparative ethno-linguistics indicates that the structures of culturally and historically changing world views (*Weltbilder*) determine both (a) whether a finite number of independent and irreducible meaning components is assumed at all, or whether, instead, a system of basic, mutually interpreting meaning components is to be presupposed; and (b) which meaning components are recognized to be the ultimate ones in a given case or which system of meaning components is to be recognized as basic. The conceptual hierarchies which the semantic analysis of a given common vocabulary discloses change in accordance with the world view, i.e. the global interpretation of nature and society, which is valid in a social system at a particular stage of development. It is apparent that the examples presented by Chomsky and his colleagues are likewise guided by a global pre-understanding, though admittedly one that possesses a certain plausibility for us as sharers of the ontology governing the everyday understanding of enlightened members of our civilization after three hundred years of modern science and the criticism of religion, a hundred years since Darwin, and fifty years since Freud, i.e. after a subjectivization and privatization of belief systems, together with the rationalization of social life which Max Weber has analysed.

Only the briefest consideration suffices to show whether dichotomies like those between physical and non-physical objects, organic and inorganic nature, and human and non-human being, which are basic for us, could have just the same position in the conceptual hierarchy of animistic, mythical, religious, philosophical or scientifically oriented views of the world. But then, if we are right in saying that they could not, the programme of general semantics could only hope to succeed if the categorial frame of reference for a structuralist analysis of *all possible* global interpretations of nature and society could be elicited systematically from the general theory of language itself.

It follows from these considerations that general semantics cannot be adequately developed on the narrow basis of the monological linguistic competence proposed by Chomsky. The general competence of a native speaker does not extend merely to the mastery of an abstract system of linguistic rules, which—preprogrammed by his organic equipment and the processes of stimulated maturation—he introduces into a communication in order to function as sender or receiver during the transfer of information. That is, it is not enough to understand language communication as an application—limited by empirical conditions—of linguistic competence. On the contrary, producing a situation of potential ordinary-language communication is itself part of the general competence of the ideal speaker. In other words, a situation in which speech, i.e. the application of linguistic competence, becomes in principle possible, depends on a structure of intersubjectivity which is in turn linguistic. This structure is generated neither by the monologically mastered system of linguistic rules, nor by the extra-linguistic conditions of its performance. On the contrary, in order to participate in normal discourse the speaker must have at his disposal, in addition to his linguistic competence, basic qualifications of speech and symbolic interaction (role-behaviour), which we may call *communicative* competence. Thus communicative competence means the mastery of an ideal speech situation.[13]

We can elucidate this, in the first instance, by studying the example of a category of verbs to which J. L. Austin ascribed a performatory use.[14] As is well known, verbs like 'promise', 'announce', 'warn', 'report', 'desire', 'determine', etc. can be used to *perform* the acts they respectively designate rather than refer to or describe them. The meaning of a 'performative utterance' includes a reference to (a) an *act* of utterance in a particular and appropriate interaction relationship ('I hereby promise . . .'), (b) the definition of a (suitable) situation which is explicitly determined by the performance of the speech act itself, and (c) the propositional content of the dependent clause. Austin differentiates between the levels of 'saying something' and of 'doing something' (locutionary level *v.* illocutionary level). Being composed of speech acts and dependent clauses of propositional content, utterances in general have, in addition to the meaning of their propositional content, a meaning which is linked to the speech situation as such. This, following Austin, we can call their 'illocutionary force'. When they use performative expressions, the speech acts are linguistic representations of that illocutionary force, i.e. the universal pragmatic power of utterances. Expressions of this kind retain no given pragmatic feature of contingent speech situations; they explain the meaning of certain idealized features of speech situations in general, which the speaker must master if his competence is to be adequate for participating at all in situations of potential speech. A theory of communicative competence can thus be developed in terms of universal pragmatics.[15]

The performatives have been called discourse operators, i.e. formators of the speech situation which belong to a meta-language for the placing of linguistic expressions in speech situations. Perhaps we should say that ordinary language contains elements which enable it to be used as the meta-language of the speech situation as well. The performatives are not the only ele-ments to be included here. Deictic elements represent the other class of universal pragmatics. In a manuscript on 'Pragmatics, Speech Situation and Deixis', Dieter Wunderlich has analysed six elements which serve to verbalize features of the ideal speech situation.[16] I shall mention two examples of deictic elements. Firstly, personal pronouns. The linguistic description can only explain why the sentence

'I apparently am hungry'

deviates from

'He apparently is hungry',

if 'I' is understood not only as one nominal pronoun among many, but as a reflexive specification of a speaker in a particular situation. An analogous consideration pertains, secondly, to deictic expressions of place and time. The deviant status of a sentence such as

'I fear that it is raining here (now)'

would not be linguistically apprehensible if the pragmatic sense of 'here' and 'now' were to be ignored and the words merely understood as some adverbial specifications among others. The choice between definite and indefinite articles, or between different forms of pronominalization, does not express a characteristic of the nouns but, rather, certain pragmatic relationships.

What can we learn from these considerations? If communicative competence meant no more than that the speaker can relate himself reflexively to speech situations and copy speech situations metalinguistically, then the speech situation itself would have to be presupposed in turn and understood as a simple empirical state—at least a non-linguistically determined state. This is a mistaken view. The 'verbalization' of pragmatic features inherent in speech situations simply lifts onto the level of linguistic communication that illocutionary force which is already generated with the structure of speech situations itself. Utterances are never simply sentences. Even if they do not expressly make pragmatic relations their subject, they are, due to their illocutionary force, integrated from the beginning into a form of intersubjectivity of mutual understanding. This structure of potential speech is, in a manner of speaking, itself of a linguistic nature, for the speech situation already contains all of the reflexive relations. These universal pragmatic features can be expressed in explicit discourse with the aid of the linguistic elements mentioned. If this is the case, however, we should assume that these elements do not serve as a subsequent verbalization of a previously coordinated speech situation; on the contrary, they must be the very factors which enable us to generate the structure of potential speech.[17] It is the dialogue-constitutive universals, as we now prefer to say, that establish in the first place the form of intersubjectivity between any competent speakers capable of mutual understanding.[18] It may be added that the structure of potential speech is present in the speech process even if pragmatic relations are not contained in the explicit content of the linguistic communication, i.e., when we omit the dialogue-constitutive universal in explicit speech. In this case understanding is incomplete on the locutionary level. Only when the dialogue-constitutive universals which give a sentence the status of an utterance are substituted by non-linguistic means, e.g. by gestures and context, can an implicit understanding on the illocutionary level be added compensatorily.

Above all, communicative competence relates to an ideal speech situation in the same way that linguistic competence relates to the abstract system of linguistic rules. The dialogue-constitutive universals at the same time generate and describe the form of intersubjectivity which makes mutuality of understanding possible. Communicative competence is defined by the ideal speaker's mastery of the dialogue-constitutive universals, irrespective of actual restrictions under empirical conditions. We shall disregard the question of how far the motivation of actions involved in language-games is linguistically open to public communication. We shall also disregard the question of whether and to what extent a systematically distorted communication actually takes place. Thus the idealization exists in the fact that we suppose an exclusively linguistic organization of speech and interaction. The ideal speech situation can then be analysed according to the functions of pure dialogue-constitutive universals.

(1) The personal pronouns (and their derivatives) form a reference system between potential speakers. The identity of meanings, the foundation of every communication, is based on intersubjectively valid rules. Their validity is intersubjective, in the strict meaning of the word, if at least two speakers understand the meaning of a symbol on the basis of reciprocal recognition. For only in that case is it possible for both speakers to comprehend and identify the meaning from their own position and from that of the other at the same time. Only this interlacing of perspectives makes an intersubjectively valid meaning, and thus identity of meaning, possible. The system of personal pronouns enables every participant to assume incompatible roles simultaneously, namely that of the I and that of the You. Every being who says 'I' to himself asserts himself towards the Other as absolutely different. And yet at the same time he recognizes himself in the latter as another I, and is conscious of the reciprocity of this relationship; every being is potentially his own Other. These dialogue roles of I and You are reproduced on the level of We and You, while He, She, and they describe roles of virtual or potential participation in the dialogue.

(2) The deictic expressions of space and time, as well as articles and demonstrative pronouns, form the reference system of possible denotations. They link the levels of intersubjectivity on which the subjects converse and interact reciprocally with the levels of objects about which the subjects make propositions. This linking of levels is possible because the cognitive content of the deictic expressions is ambiguous; they contain, respectively, two different schematisms of each underlying category (space and time, sub-

stance and causality). We relate articles and demonstrative pronouns to persons just as to things; space and time deixes refer to 'experienced' as well as to measured spaces and times.

(3) Forms of address (vocative), forms of social contact (greeting), of speech introduction and speech conclusion, indirect discourse, questions and answers, are performatory in that they are directed at the act of speaking as such. They determine the structure of potential speech in as much as they explain the pragmatic meaning of speaking itself. Speech is the medium of communication which already presupposes a tacit consensus about what it means to communicate and an awareness of the possibility of misunderstanding, as well as of error and deception.

(4) The further performatory speech acts form a system which finally enables us to mark the basic differentiations which are fundamental for any speech situation.[19]

(a) Being and appearance. Expressions which refer to the truth value of utterances (not of statements) according to the prototype of 'to claim' and 'to dispute' form the dimension of being and appearance (assure, confirm, deny, certify, testify, doubt, question). All speech acts imply an intended consensus on that which really is, as distinct from that which subjectively only appears to be (the propositional content). This presupposes a differentiation between a public world of intersubjectively acknowledged interpretations and a private world of personal feelings and impressions.

(b) Being and essence. Expressions which refer to the self-representation of persons according to the prototype of 'to reveal' and 'to hide' form the dimension of being and essence (expose, present, allude, express, conceal, obscure, betray, symbolize, virtualize, take at one's word, deceive, etc.). In all speech acts the subjects in their speech-act performances unavoidably express their own selves at the same time as they converse with one another on some propositional topic. This presupposes a differentiation between a communication on objects and a meta-communication on the level of intersubjectivity.

(c) What is and what ought to be. Expressions which refer to the normative status of rules according to the prototype of 'to prescribe' and 'to follow' form the dimension of the 'ought' (order, obey, allow, demand, refuse, resist, recommend, advise, warn, oblige, violate, call to account, etc.). All speech exists in a context of actions and intentions. The mutual recognition of the subjects who communicate with one another includes the certainty that they can conduct themselves reciprocally towards one another's expectations, i.e. act according to valid norms. This presupposes the differentiation between valid rules, which are intentionally followed, and regularities of observable events, which can be stated empirically.

If one thus analyses the structure which we generate and describe by means of pure dialogue-constitutive universals, one arrives at a number of symmetrical relations for the ideal speech situation. Pure intersubjectivity is determined by a symmetrical relation between I and You (We and You), I and He (We and They). An unlimited interchangeability of dialogue roles demands that no side be privileged in the performance of these roles: pure intersubjectivity exists only when there is complete symmetry in the distribution of assertion and dispute, revelation and concealment, prescription and conformity, among the partners of communication. As long as these symmetries exist, communication will not be hindered by constraints arising from its own structure.

(1) In the case of unrestrained discussion (in which no prejudiced opinion cannot be taken up or criticized) it is possible to develop strategies for reaching unconstrained consensus; (2) on the basis of mutuality of unimpaired self-representation (which includes the acknowledgment of the self-representation of the Other as well) it is possible to achieve a significant rapport despite the inviolable distance between the partners, and that means communication under conditions of individuation; (3) in the case of

full complementarity of expectations (which excludes unilaterally constraining norms) the claim of universal understanding exists, as well as the necessity of universalized norms. These three symmetries represent, incidentally, a linguistic conceptualization of what are traditionally known as the ideas of truth, freedom, and justice.

A speech situation determined by pure intersubjectivity is an idealization. The mastery of dialogue-constitutive universals does not itself amount to a capacity actually to establish the ideal speech situation. But communicative competence does mean the mastery of the means of construction necessary for the establishment of an ideal speech situation. No matter how the intersubjectivity of mutual understanding may be deformed, the *design* of an ideal speech situation is necessarily implied in the structure of potential speech, since all speech, even of intentional deception, is oriented towards the idea of truth. This idea can only be analysed with regard to a consensus achieved in unrestrained and universal discourse. Insofar as we master the means for the construction of an ideal speech situation, we can conceive the ideas of truth, freedom, and justice, which interpret each other—although of course only as ideas. On the strength of communicative competence alone, however, and independent of the empirical structures of the social system to which we belong, we are quite unable to realize the ideal speech situation; we can only anticipate it.

It should be possible to demonstrate the deformations of pure intersubjectivity, induced by the social structure, on the basis of asymmetries in the performance of dialogue rules. The uneven distribution of dialogue-constitutive universals in standard communication between individuals and social groups indicates the particular form and deformation of the intersubjectivity of mutual understanding which is built into the social structure. But here I am afraid I must leave the matter at that. The considerations I have spoken of can only claim to be a first attempt to grasp communicative competence in terms of linguistic theory. Let me, however, draw two conclusions, the first of which will lead back to the problem of general semantics.

I imagine that the particular form of intersubjectivity of mutual understanding—that is, the particular structure of potential speech—is the basic linguistic framework which also determines the scope and structure of corresponding world views. Then, the classification of semantic fields is predetermined by the question of how far the net of intersubjectivity must be spread in order to stabilize the identity of the individuals, as well as that of the social group in a given culture or subculture at a given time. The structural differences between the animistic, the mythical, the religious, the philosophical, and the scientistic views of life lie clearly in this dimension. The range of those global interpretations of nature and society extend from the case of total identification of the individual and his group with all non-human phenomena, within an all-embracing association of motivated actions, to the case of total reification of all intersubjective relationships within the framework of objectifying sciences. At this time I cannot pursue this topic further. However, one consequence seems to me to be important in our context. If we could succeed in describing deformations of pure intersubjectivity in the dimension in which dialogue-constitutive universals are applied; and if it were possible, moreover, to distinguish also the categorical frameworks of potential views of life in terms of distributions of dialogue-constitutive universals, then general semantics could be developed on the basis of a theory of communicative competence.

The second and final point is how that theory of communicative competence might be employed for social analysis. As already mentioned, the 'idealization' of the concept of the ideal speech situation does not consist simply in the fact that we disregard contingent empirical limitations. It consists rather of the supposition that the motivational base of all actions is organized linguistically, i.e. within the structure of potential speech. By this idealization we imagine the actual motivations of the actor being identical with the linguistically apprehensible intentions of the speakers. This model of pure communicative action is included in the design of pure intersubjectivity. Now we have reason enough to assume, however, that social action is not only—and perhaps not even primarily—controlled by motives which coincide with the intentions of the actor-speaker, but rather by motives excluded from public communication and fixed to a prelinguistic symbol organization. The greater the share of pre-linguistically fixed motivations which cannot be freely converted in public communication, the greater the deviance from the model of pure communicative action. I would propose to make the empirical assumptions, first, that these deviations increase in proportion to the degree of repression which characterizes the institutional system within a given society; and secondly that the degree of repression depends in turn on the developmental stage of the productive forces and on the organization of authority, that is of the institutionalization of political and economic power.

NOTES

1. N. Chomsky, *Aspects of the Theory of Syntax,* M.I.T. Press, Cambridge, Mass. 1965.
2. D. McNeill, 'Developmental Psycholinguistics', in F. Smith and G. A. Miller (Eds.), *The Genesis of Language,* M.I.T. Press, Cambridge, Mass. 1966, pp. 15–84.
3. N. Chomsky, *Language and Mind,* Harcourt, Brace & World, New York 1968.
4. J. Fodor and M. Garret, 'Some Reflections on Competence and Performance', in J. Lyons and R. J. Wales (Eds.), *Psycho-linguistic Papers,* Edinburgh University Press, Edinburgh 1966, pp. 135–63; R. J. Wales and J. C. Marshall, 'The Organization of Linguistic Performance', ibid., pp. 29–80; C. B. Cazden, 'On Individual Differences in Language Competence and Performance', in *Journal of Special Education,* Vol. 1 (1967) No. 2.

5. J. J. Katz and P. M. Postal, *An Integrated Theory of Linguistic Description,* M.I.T. Press, Cambridge, Mass. 1964.
6. M. Bierwisch, 'Strukturalismus', *Kursbuch,* Vol. 5, Frankfurt a.M. 1966, pp. 97f.
7. J. H. Greenberg (Ed.), *Universals of Language,* M.I.T. Press, Cambridge, Mass. 1963, 1966.
8. C. Lévi-Strauss, *Les Structures élémentaires de la Parenté,* Mouton & Co., Paris 1967.
9. A. Romney, 'Cognitive Aspects of English Kinterms', in *American Anthropologist* (1946), pp. 36–170.
10. H. C. Conklin, 'Hanunvó Color Categories', in D. Hymes (Ed.), *Language in Culture and Society,* Harper & Row, New York 1964, pp. 189–92.
11. J. Lyons, *Introduction to Theoretical Linguistics,* Cambridge University Press, London 1969, pp. 419 f. and pp. 470 ff.
12. Lyons, *Introduction,* op. cit., pp. 446 ff.
13. I propose to use this term in a way similar to that in which Chomsky uses 'linguistic competence'. Communicative competence should be related to a system of rules generating an ideal speech situation, not regarding linguistic codes which link language and universal pragmatics with actual role systems. Dell Hymes, among others, makes use of the term 'communicative competence' in a socio-linguistically limited sense. I don't want to follow this convention.
14. J. L. Austin, *How to Do Things with Words,* Clarendon Press, Oxford 1962.
15. J. R. Searle pursues a similar approach with his theory of speech acts: *Speech Acts,* Cambridge University Press, London 1969.
16. Manuscript T.U. Berlin, Sept. 1969.
17. This is why Searle conceives the linguistic rules which govern speech acts as what he calls 'constitutive rules'. 'Constitutive rules do not merely regulate, they create or define new forms of behavior' (op. cit., p. 33). 'The hypothesis of this book is that speaking a language is a matter of performing speech acts according to systems of constitutive rules' (ibid., p. 38).
18. Searle puts the same argument in the following way: 'If I am trying to tell someone something, then . . . as soon as he recognizes that I am trying to tell him something and exactly what it is I am trying to tell him, I have succeeded in telling it to him. Furthermore, unless he recognizes that I am trying to tell him something and what I am trying to tell him, I do not fully succeed in telling it to him . . . In the case of illocutionary acts we succeed in doing what we are trying to do by getting our audience to recognize what we are trying to do. But the "effect" on the hearer is not a belief or response, it consists

simply in the hearer understanding the utterance of the speaker. It is this effect that I have been calling the illocutionary effect. The way the reflexive intention works then . . . is: the speaker *S* intends to produce an illocutionary effect *IE* in the hearer *H* by means of getting *H* to recognize *S*'s intention to produce *IE*' (ibid., p. 47).

19. Austin claims that there are about a thousand performatives in English. The classification proposed by Austin himself is not convincing. Searle, who presents the most penetrating analysis of the structure of the speech act (cf. op. cit., Ch. 3, pp. 22–71) does not give a systematic account of the classification of speech acts. My proposal is intended to have the role of such an account, but the three criteria offered still lack a reasonable explication.

●●●

Practical Discourse in Nursing: Going Beyond Empiricism and Historicism

Janice L. Thompson

This discussion presents a critical appraisal of recent works in *Advances in Nursing Science* that have dealt with metatheoretical concerns. In metatheoretical analysis, such as that presented by Silva and Rothbart, nurses are beginning to focus on the traditions that have guided research. This process should be extended by reviewing historical stages of development in empiricist and postempiricist philosophy. Recent work in postempiricist philosophy is especially important since it can help nursing transcend historicist insights. Continental philosophy goes beyond historicist critique by focusing on practical discourse within a community of investigators. This is a stage of development that can be rationally decisive for the scientific development of nursing.

Metatheoretical concern is the beginning of a new stage of self-consciousness in nursing. The community of nurse-investigators is coming to know itself by looking critically at the way it practices science.

One important sign of intellectual maturity is self-consciousness. This is a developmental state in which humans gradually become aware of themselves. By looking critically at the ways in which reality is framed and the ways in which humans relate to natural objects and other human subjects, individuals gradually come to know something new about themselves. Self-consciousness begins with a passage from naive perceptions of objects as though they were things in themselves (the natural attitude) to a reflective awareness that, far from being things in themselves, objects exist for humans, the knowing subjects. This transition from a naive,

natural attitude to an awareness of self through the object, is a developmental state that is usually associated with maturity and autonomy.[1]

Nursing researchers are experiencing this transition and becoming self-conscious for the first time in the history of nursing. Articles in *Advances in Nursing Science* have indicated a quickened interest in metatheoretical questions.[2-4] This is a heightened awareness of nursing as a community of investigators concerned about the traditions that are guiding nursing research.

As nursing scholarship engages in this metatheoretical discourse, nursing researchers make the transition from the natural attitude to self-consciousness. They leave behind naive perceptions of objects and look more critically at how nursing science constitutes the human world. This is a passage to self-consciousness: a community of investigators coming to know itself by focusing on the traditions that have guided its research.

In one of the most historically perceptive articles appearing in recent nursing literature, Silva and Rothbart[4] have engaged in this type of self-conscious analysis. They have identified trends in philosophy that have influenced nursing theory and research, and they have identified an important dichotomy or division between two schools of thought in postempiricist philosophy of science. This is the debate between the empiricist tradition and historicist critique, a debate between those who adhere to the tenets of logical empiricism and those who place the process of inquiry within a historically situated, tradition-bound research program. Since the 1960s the historicist critique has been advanced in its greatest intensity by thinkers such as Kuhn, Feyerabend, Lakatos, and Lauden.

By focusing the debate in postempiricist philosophy of science in this way and by emphasizing the contribution of Lauden, Silva and Rothbart present a distinctly American view of the situation in contemporary philosophy. The debate in postempiricist philosophy of science has been joined by many more thinkers, who carry the discourse far beyond the insights of Lauden. Specifically, the contribution of recent continental philosophy is one that can add critical insights by extending the work begun by Silva and Rothbart. And this extension, a continued exploration of the debate in postempiricist philosophy of science, can have a positive influence on nursing's self-understanding.

Empiricist Philosophy

Semantic Analysis

In a remarkable study of the postempiricist era, Bernstein[5] has extended the analysis of historicist and empiricist positions. He has explored developments in contemporary empiricism, and his work can be used to understand why empiricism has had such a major impact on nursing theory and research. The history of contemporary empiricism began with early attempts by logical empiricists to ground knowledge claims in a single term by making a word or a concept the primary epistemological unit. In this stage,

researchers were preoccupied with attempts to isolate "logical proper names" and with proper methods of "ostensive definition."[5(p75)]

It might be argued that this stage of development is still present in nursing. Current theoretical discourse in nursing includes a preoccupation with "proper" techniques of concept analysis,[6,7] in which nursing scholars focus on words or concepts as the fundamental unit of any knowledge claim. A great amount of emphasis is placed on semantic analysis and proper techniques for "operationalizing" concepts. These research practices reflect the influence of early empiricism.

The concern with ostensive definition in nursing may reflect an underlying conviction borrowed from early empiricism, the conviction that there must be permanent, ahistorical standards for grounding knowledge in reality. The attempt to isolate logical proper names and to use rigorous methods for ostensive definition is a search for foundations. Empiricists argue that if concepts are defined clearly and distinctly enough and if they are linked to corresponding pieces of reality, they can serve as fundamental epistemological units, as a stable, unchanging foundation for future knowledge claims.

Hypothesis Testing

Early in the 20th century, empiricism saw a shift of focus, and a new emphasis was placed on the proposition, observation statement, or descriptive sentence as the primary epistemological unit for grounding knowledge. Empiricists including Schlick,[8] Hempel,[9] and Neurath[10] were preoccupied with "protocol sentences." These were new attempts to demonstrate that observation statements or hypotheses that were properly confirmed could be the foundation for future knowledge.

This stage of the empiricist tradition has had a profound effect on nursing scholars. Hypothesis testing and the concern over empirical techniques for confirming hypotheses led quickly to the insights of Popper,[11] who argued that scientific method is a rigorous attempt to *falsify* hypotheses, not to confirm them. This stage of the empiricist tradition was a significant sociological event. It created a definition of "proper" scientific method that touched many nurse scholars, especially those involved in the nurse scientist program.

This phase of development is still apparent in nursing. Current theoretical discourse includes an ongoing concern with hypothesis testing. In the 1960s and 1970s, Dickoff and James[12] and Diers[13] formalized a popular view of hypothesis testing in nursing. These authors presented hypothesis testing as a "middle range tier" in a hierarchy of knowledge claims. At the base of this pyramid were concepts and categories "unique to nursing," which were to be isolated in descriptive, exploratory studies, providing a first level foundation for nursing knowledge. At the next level in this hierarchy, observation statements or hypotheses were to be empirically tested. These provided a second-level foundation for future knowledge claims. Finally, succeeding levels in their hierarchy were to be achieved by the generation of "prescriptive" or "situation producing" theory.

The concern with hypothesis testing in nursing again reflects an underlying "foundationalism" borrowed from early empiricists. The metaphor of a pyramid is a very powerful image of foundationalism as it has affected nursing. In this metaphor, hypothesis testing, or the confirmation of observation statements in the clinical contexts of nursing practice, was to provide a second-level foundation for succeeding knowledge claims.

CONCEPTUAL SCHEMES

Nursing moved very rapidly away from its concern with isolated hypothesis testing. By the early 1980s, nursing discourse showed an increased concern with conceptual schemes as the primary unit of epistemological analysis. This shift paralleled similar developments in the empiricist tradition. The empiricist concern with hypothesis testing

set off the search for a criterion of cognitive meaning that would once and for all distinguish empirically meaningful propositions from those that paraded as cognitively meaningful propositions but failed to meet a "rigorous" criterion of empirical meaning. But with the failure of all such attempts and the increasing realization of the futility of the entire project, there was a shift away from isolated propositions, statements and sentences to a focus on the conceptual scheme or framework as the proper unit of epistemological analysis.[5(p75)]

The shift from "isolated" hypothesis testing to a focus on conceptual schemes is a phase that nursing is currently experiencing. The empiricist tradition moved quickly to this stage when it had difficulty distinguishing empirically meaningful propositions from those that "paraded" as cognitively meaningful propositions. This was a struggle with the normative dimensions of science and with values concerning which statements would be accepted as "valid," "legitimate" knowledge claims and which would be rejected as value statements.

In the 1960s, 1970s, and 1980s, several conceptual schemes have developed in nursing,[14–20] and all of them are scholarly attempts to ground knowledge claims within a conceptual and theoretical context. "Metatheoretical" discourse is now being organized around the project of testing various conceptual models in nursing.[21] With this shift in emphasis, nursing investigators are no longer focusing exclusively on isolated propositions; they have taken up the project of empirically testing conceptual schemes.

The movement of nursing to this third stage of development has been heralded as a "progressive" step and has even been characterized as yielding an "optimistic view of the discipline."[3(p1)] It seems important, however, to identify characteristics of this stage as it has been experienced in the empiricist tradition.

This third stage has proved to be highly unstable for a variety of reasons. There are deep difficulties in trying to clarify just what is a conceptual scheme, how we demarcate one conceptual scheme from another and how radical are the differences among various conceptual schemes. But an even more fundamental difficulty concerns what these so-called conceptual schemes are supposed to be *about*. . . . The very idea that there is a distinction between "something" that is known (uncontaminated by different conceptual schemes) and the various schemes for conceiving or knowing it is suspect.[5(p75)]

Theory testing, the third stage of development, has proved to be unstable because of fundamental difficulties with Cartesian and neo-Kantian assumptions. Such assumptions presume that there is a distinction between the subject and object and that phenomena can be distinguished from the conceptual schemes used to "know" them. Investigators involved in "theory testing" recognize rapidly that their research practices serve as a frame of reference orienting their access to phenomena. Thus, for example, nurse researchers using a Rogerian framework recognize that their language, concepts, and methods frame clinical phenomena in a unique manner, influencing the way Rogerians "have access" to human beings.[21,22]

HISTORICAL DEVELOPMENT

With such recognitions, nurse researchers have experienced a beginning awareness of the biases and prejudices inherent in nursing research programs. In other disciplines, our counterparts in the empiricist tradition have quickly moved to a fourth stage of development, the stage directly preceding and leading to historicist awareness.

The fourth stage of development in the philosophy of science in this century is characterized by the increasing realization that when it comes to interesting questions about the rationality of scientific inquiry, we must focus on the conflict of theories, paradigms, research programs and research traditions in their *historical development*. . . . The unit of appraisal becomes the research program, 'a series of theories rather than an isolated theory.' . . . A research program is something which is not static but which develops and changes over time. . . . In scientific development, we have an historical phenomenon that is analogous to that of tradi-

tion, and indeed, competing traditions, which can inform practice and are modified by further practice.[5(p77)]

This fourth stage of development in the postempiricist era is on the horizon for nursing. Works like that of Silva and Rothbart[4] point to a self-consciousness within nursing and an awareness of research programs as *a series* of theories. New discourse about "metaparadigms"[23] in nursing may *cautiously* be viewed as further evidence for this transition. If a metaparadigm may be construed as a series of theories in the sense described here, then nursing may be starting to focus on its own scientific development by becoming conscious of its own historically changing research programs. This is a gradual process of recognizing that nursing research programs are historically changing traditions. Nursing may be about to confront and, hopefully, transcend historicist insights.

Historicist Debate

As Silva and Rothbart[4] demonstrate, historicism has had a profound influence on recent postempiricist philosophy. Thinkers like Lauden,[24] Feyerabend,[25] Kuhn,[26] Lakatos,[27] and Rorty[28] have consistently challenged empiricist presuppositions. They have demonstrated that scientific disputes generally are *not* resolved by an appeal to the canons of deductive logic. Historicists have found that when disagreements arise within a community of investigators, they usually are not resolved by rigidly adhering to methods of observation, verification, confirmation, or falsification. In times of "crisis," scientific development frequently is steered by imaginative, innovative, "abductive" practices. This historicist discovery has challenged late 20th century empiricist notions about an ahistorical, "logically necessary" scientific method.

Frequently, these historicists' insights have been misinterpreted. Some researchers have protested that the view of science presented by historicism is basically irrational. Historicists seem to be describing science as an activity that relies on emotivism or noncognitivism to settle scientific disputes. Lauden[24] mistakenly interprets Kuhn in this way. But this response to historicism is unfortunate since it misses the main point of historicist critique.

Historicism has been struggling with the practical character of scientific rationality. Historicists have been focusing on deliberation and trying to identify the forms of rational persuasion and argumentation that take place in disputes over rival paradigms, theories, or research programs.

> As a result of recent work in philosophy and history of science, an appreciation of the practical character of rationality in science has been emerging. . . . The "practical" character [of rationality] underscores the role of choice, deliberation, conflicting variable opinions and the judgmental quality of rationality. . . . The sharing of criteria by communities of scientists allows for and indeed requires, interpretation, weighing, and the application of these criteria to specific choices and decisions. . . . Scientific argumentation, especially at those moments of "scientific revolution" requires rational persuasion, persuasion which cannot be assimilated to models of deductive proof and inductive generalization.[5(p74)]

Postempiricist philosophy has been struggling to understand this practical dimension of scientific rationality. Historicists, however, have not been able to uncover the "whys" and "hows" of this process. What kind of rationality is it that moves scientific communities in certain directions and not in others? How does rational deliberation proceed within a community of investigators?

Silva and Rothbart[4] have played an incredibly important role in introducing historicist insights to nursing, but their project must be extended by exploring the postempiricist era in philosophy. This exploration can help the community of nursing scholars understand the practical character of scientific rationality in nursing.

Two thinkers in the continental tradition have added important dimensions to postempiricist philosophy. The works of Gadamer[29] and Habermas[30–33] are late attempts to go beyond historicist insights. These continental thinkers have struggled to recover the practical dimension of rationality in science. They have viewed historically changing research programs as traditions and have explored the ways in which tradition, broadly speaking, mediates human understanding.

Tradition in Postempiricist Philosophy

PREUNDERSTANDING

The work of Gadamer has only recently been discovered in American philosophy. As a student of Heidegger,[34] he has carried on work common to continental philosophy. He is therefore relatively unfamiliar to many American scholars who have been more concerned with issues in analytic philosophy. Focusing on experiences such as aesthetic judgment, jurisprudence, historical understanding, and the interpretation of texts, Gadamer has demonstrated that human understanding occurs through the interpretation of tradition; he has argued that the interpretation of tradition is not just an epistemological category, but an ontological one—lying at the center of being.

For Gadamer, tradition is the total background of practices, vocabulary, concepts, and hypotheses that humans bring to a project. Thus, tradition may be characterized as *preunderstanding,* a total background of prejudices and prejudgments that condition the process of understanding. For those in German philosophy, tradition contains the following forms of prejudice or prejudgment.[35(p10)]

1. *Vorhabe* (fore-having)—The totality of practices which "have us" or make us who we are, and thus determine what we find intelligible. In any science this is the "disciplinary matrix" a student acquires in becoming a scientist which enables him [or her] to determine what are the scientifically relevant facts.

2. *Vorsicht* (fore-sight)—The vocabulary or conceptual scheme we bring to any problem. In the case of our culture this is what, according to the philosophy of the age, counts as real. In science, this is whatever is taken to be relevant dimensions of a problem.
3. *Vorgriff*—A specific hypothesis, which within the overall theory, can be confirmed or disconfirmed by the data.

These characteristics of tradition emphasize not only theoretical biases, but also real social practices or skills acquired in various forms of socialization and apprenticeship. Scientific skills themselves influence the way investigators have access to phenomena. Practical skills influence what investigators find intelligible in a situation and what questions they will ask. Real, concrete social practices, combined with language, theoretical schemes, and hypotheses make up this total background of preunderstanding. This background is the basis for human understanding.

DIALOGUE

With this interpretation of tradition, Gadamer and others in continental philosophy present a view of human inquiry that differs radically from the empiricist position. If all understanding involves some form of prejudice or prejudgment, some empiricists might argue that to gain knowledge, we must "bracket" or overcome this prejudice. For objectivists, this means using the "right method," usually the methods of natural science, to overcome human prejudice. For other empiricists, the point is to test prejudices rather than to remove them. Formalized processes of hypothesis testing that are attempts at confirmation or falsification are the empiricist answer to testing these prejudices.

Gadamer,[29] on the other hand, argues that humans cannot be devoid of prejudices and that prejudices cannot be tested in a straightforward, neutral manner. He does hold, however, that through the interpretation of tradition, humans can discriminate between blind and enabling prejudices.

Gadamer does want to make the all-important distinction between blind prejudices and 'justified prejudices, productive of knowledge. . . . For Gadamer, it is in and through the encounter with what is handed down to us through tradition that we discover which of our prejudices are blind and which are enabling. . . . It is through the *dialogical* encounter with what is at once alien to us, makes a claim upon us and has an affinity with what we are that we can open ourselves to risking and testing our prejudices.[5(p129)]

Thus, the process of human understanding is comparable to the interpretation of tradition. It is a *dialogical* process of discovering inherited "biases" or prejudgments and recognizing some prejudgments as blind and others as genuinely enabling. For Gadamer, this process does not occur through a silent act of self-reflection; it occurs in dialogue, in linguistic experiences.

Gadamer's insights suggest something about the way in which nursing researchers have appropriated the empiricist tradition. Empiricism makes a claim of validity on a community of investigators in dialogical exchange. At first, this claim is made as nursing researchers listen. In graduate and undergraduate education focusing on nursing research, nursing scholars have listened to the authoritative text of the empiricist tradition. Until recently, this tradition has been presented with little critique, and the community of nursing scholars may have listened without questioning the authority of empiricist text.

In this dialogue, listening itself is conditioned by the prejudices of nursing scholars and by all the prejudgments (practices and theories) that have formed them. The community of nursing investigators has most frequently opened itself to the empiricist tradition in paradoxical, contradictory ways. Nurse researchers listen to empiricism with all the preunderstanding of working nurses, a predominantly female labor force in 20th century postindustrialized society. Social practices, language, and conceptual schemes of working class nurses are one layer of prejudice that influences the way nurses listen. But in sometimes contradictory ways, nursing researchers also listen to the empiricist tradition with all of the preunderstanding of aspiring academicians. Social practices, language, and conceptual schemes of upper middle class intellectuals are another layer of prejudice that influences the way nursing scholars listen, what they hear in empiricism, and the questions they ask.

Beyond listening, this dialogue with empiricism also involves interpretation. This is the act of emphasizing some dimensions of empiricist text more than others. Some nursing scholars have chosen to emphasize theoretical dimensions such as concept formation, hypothesis testing, or theory testing, and these choices have been influenced by the prejudices of nursing scholars; that is, by all the conceptual schemes, vocabulary, and research skills acquired in graduate education. These prejudgments may have a parodoxical, contradictory effect on nursing scholars and the interpretation of empiricism. The contradictions of foundationalism in nursing theory development are examples of the paradoxical ways in which nursing has interpreted empiricism.

PHRONESIS

Finally, Gadamer[29] believes that the interpretation of tradition involves the step of application. This process resembles the classical mode of ethicopolitical judgment, *phronesis*. In application, nurse scholars are involved in a distinctive kind of mediation, recognizing something in empiricist text that seems universal and relating it to a particular situation.

> *Phronesis* is a form of reasoning that is concerned with choice and involves deliberation. It deals with that which is variable and about which there can be differing opinions. It is a type of reasoning in which there is a mediation between general principles and a concrete particular situation that requires choice and deliberation. In forming such a judgement, there are no determinate technical rules by which a particular can be subsumed under that which is general or universal. What is required is an interpretation and specification of universals that are appropriate to this particular situation.[5(p54)]

Phronesis is a kind of rationality resembling ethical judgment as it existed before the advent of bourgeois, utilitarian, deontological, or decisionistic ethics in modern times. In this kind of judgment, humans do not use determinate technical rules to subsume a particular problematic concern under a universal principle; instead, something in the tradition that seems universal is at once interpreted or translated and used to understand a particular event or problem.

In applying the empiricist tradition, nursing scholars experience the practical rationality of science; this is a process of deliberation in which values and norms are important. What may seem to be universal in empiricist text depends on the values and norms that nursing scholars have internalized in bourgeois society. Thus, the step of applying empiricist text is itself highly conditioned by the prejudices of nursing scholars.

Nursing researchers frequently apply empiricist text paradoxically. They may deliberate and choose with all the preunderstanding of working class women who use the language and conceptual schemes of a predominantly female labor force. This is a value-laden process of applying empiricism to address the real concerns of nursing labor. But nursing researchers may also apply empiricist text with all the prejudice of aspiring intellectual professionals. This is a value-laden process of applying empiricism to develop "accurate pictures" or "clear views" of clinical reality. This prejudice is closely intertwined with acquiring class privilege in modern professionalized society. Together, these real social layers of prejudice have a powerful, contradictory influence on the ways nurse-researchers *apply* empiricism in particular problem-solving situations.

Gadamer's description of tradition and the ways in which it is appropriated can clarify the scientific development of nursing. These steps of listening, interpreting, and applying empiricist tradition occur in public arenas, in dialogue with others. As nurses appropriate empiricism, the background of preunderstanding, prejudices, and prejudgments may not always be explicit. Nurses may not be aware of the ways in which their conceptual schemes and research skills are forming a layer of prejudice that influences the way they ask questions.

Instead, a community of investigators may accept the empiricist tradition because of its perceived authority and the accumulated weight of evidence, data, reasons, and arguments presented in empiricist science. Later, during times of self-consciousness, a community of investigators may become more critical of empiricist prejudices. This is a time of questioning, a time when the authority of the empiricist tradition may be challenged, a time when nursing scholars recognize some prejudices as enabling and others as blind.

Becoming self-conscious in this way leaves behind blind obedience to the authority of tradition. It leads to recognition that any experience of understanding involves prejudice and that some prejudices may be better than others. This is a point of transition that nursing currently occupies. It is a practical struggle to go beyond empiricist and historicist insights.

Hermeneutics

The point of understanding, in Gadamer's view, is to distinguish which aspects of tradition are enabling and which are not. This is a process of expanding horizons, of moving in the *hermeneutic circle*.

> The process of understanding can never achieve finality. . . . It is always open and anticipatory. We are always understanding and interpreting in light of our anticipatory prejudgments and prejudices, which are themselves changing in history. . . . To understand is to understand *differently*. But this does not mean that our interpretations are arbitrary or distortive. We should always aim . . . at a correct understanding of what the "things themselves" say. But what the "things themselves" say will be different in light of our changing horizons and the different questions we learn to ask.[5(p139)]

For nursing, hermeneutic understanding includes a critical look at the background of prejudice and prejudgment contained in empiricist text. As nursing scholars become more conscious of this horizon of preunderstanding, they judge some dimensions of empiricism to be more enabling than others. Horizons change in this process, prejudices can change, and nurses can learn to ask different questions in new ways.

Gadamer has engaged in his own project of hermeneutic understanding and his own dialogue concerning traditions that inform modern inquiry; he has emerged with strong criticisms of prejudices contained in modern society. And he emphasizes that we are confronted with a world in which there has been a domination of technology based on science, a "false idolatry of the expert," a "scientific mystification of the modern society of specialization," and a "dangerous inner longing to find in science a substitute for lost orientation."[5(p148)] These are powerful criticisms of prejudices that direct nursing scholars and other communities of investigators.

Domination and Authority

Gadamer comes close to addressing the overwhelming presence of modern, distorted, "deforming" prejudices, but he falls short of helping nursing scholars to understand these "blind" prejudgments. The "lacunae" in Gadamer's work comes from his failure to focus on power and domination in modern society. This is a failure to confront real, material, social, and political conditions as sources of domination and authority in contemporary times.

Other investigators in postempiricist philosophy *have* struggled with these questions. Habermas[30-33] has explored conditions that contribute to domination in modern times. He has argued that true dialogue has been suppressed and that the process of rational argumentation and rational persuasion based on *phronesis* has been distorted. And he has recognized widespread, blind obedience to persons in positions of power and to the questions they ask and the answers they provide. The critique of such domination is an important project for intellectuals who are in the process of becoming more self-conscious, "organic" scholars.[35]

In the critique of domination in nursing science questions arise regarding the conditions under which the empiricist tradition has been accepted. Empiricism has been presented as an authoritative foundation for nursing science, and "good reasons" have been given to support its acceptance. But nurses themselves have judged those reasons. It is time now to look critically at how and why nurses have accepted the authority of empiricism. Has this tradition been accepted by relatively blind obedience? Has it been accepted because empiricist science has become the source of power and domination in "specialized" class society or because upper-middle-class masculine voices have defended it? These questions and others like them are important criticisms for nursing scholars who are becoming more self-conscious.

Beyond Empiricist and Historicist Debates

Postempiricist philosophy of science has struggled to go beyond the debate between empiricism and historicism. Thinkers in this era have recognized the importance of historicist discoveries. It has become apparent that there are no permanent, ahistorical algorithms for choosing between rival paradigms. But this discovery has not resulted in a relativized, irrational view of science. In communities of investigators, scientific development is a rational process, and rational dialogue, argumentation, and persuasion determine the directions of future research and practice.

In postempiricist philosophy, an attempt has been made to explore the practical character of this dialogue. It is a process that is similar to the appropriation of tradition. The practical side of scientific rationality includes moments of listening, interpreting, and emphasizing some dimensions of a tradition more than others and then applying whatever seems to be universal in the tradition to concrete, particular situations.

If this process is not blind and if it is truly dialogue, participants come to recognize their own prejudices and, perhaps, to expand these, creating new horizons of preunderstanding. This is a new image of science that has recovered a human emphasis. There is not an objectivistic finality in this image of science, but rather an ongoing dialogue between human beings. In this dialogue, nurses join other investigators in the task of "hammering out" those prejudices that are truly enabling, those that are justified, and those that are productive of knowledge for a more human, humane world.

Works like that of Silva and Rothbart[4] invite nurses to participate in this kind of science. They invite investigators to recognize the human, practical character of rationality in science. These authors have begun a process of reflection, of critical self-appraisal, becoming self-conscious in new, forward looking ways. The transition can be supported by a continued exploration of postempiricist philosophy of science.

Postempiricist philosophy contains an important warning for nurses. "We are fools if we think we can escape prejudices or traditions by an act of will."[5(p167)] Nurses do not choose the empiricist tradition or an alternative to it such as historicism by "wishing." Traditions and prejudices "have us" because they have made a claim to authority. Challenging this authority takes more than an act of will; it takes public discourse.

In public arenas, nurses are engaging in the kind of argumentation that will be rationally decisive for our community of investigators. This is challenging the claims of authority made by scientists in the empiricist tradition, and the challenge may take many forms. It may emerge as:

- feminist critique;
- humanistic criticism of objectivism in science;
- humanistic criticism of domination in science;

- socialist-feminist critique of scientism in the professions; or
- historicist critique of objectivism in science.

Whatever its form, the challenging of empiricism is incredibly important. This is a process of rational deliberation, of choosing prejudices that are most productive of knowledge. The argumentation itself is a sign of intellectual maturity. It is evidence that nurses are coming to self-consciousness, recognizing themselves in the prejudices they endorse. This is an optimistic development, a sign that nursing can engage in the kind of practical discourse that will be rationally decisive for its own scientific development.

REFERENCES

1. Soll I: *An Introduction to Hegel's Metaphysics.* Chicago, University of Chicago Press, 1969.
2. Gortner S: The history and philosophy of nursing science and research. *Adv Nurs Sci* 1983;5(2):1–8.
3. Fawcett J: Hallmarks of success in nursing research. *Adv Nurs Sci* 1984;7(1):1–11.
4. Silva MC, Rothbart D: An analysis of changing trends in philosophies of science on nursing theory development and testing. *Adv Nurs Sci* 1984;6(2):1–11.
5. Bernstein R: *Beyond Objectivism and Relativism: Science, Hermeneutics, and Praxis.* Philadelphia, University of Pennsylvania Press, 1983.
6. Walker L, Avant K: *Strategies for Theory Construction in Nursing.* Norwalk, Conn., Appleton-Century-Crofts, 1983.
7. Chinn P, Jacobs J: *Theory and Nursing: A Systematic Approach.* St Louis, Mosby, 1983.
8. Schlick M: The foundation of knowledge, in Ayer AJ (ed): *Logical Positivism.* Westport, Conn., Greenwood, 1978, pp 209–227.
9. Hempel C: On the standard conception of scientific theories, in *Minnesota Studies in the Philosophy of Science,* vol. 3. Minneapolis, University of Minnesota Press, 1970, pp 142–163.
10. Neurath O: Protocol sentences, in Ayer AJ (ed): *Logical Positivism.* Westport, Conn., Greenwood, 1978, pp 199–208.
11. Popper K: *Conjectures and Refutations: The Growth of Scientific Knowledge.* London, Routledge & Kegan Paul, 1972.
12. Dickoff J, James P: A theory of theories: A position paper. *Nurs Res* 1968;17(3):197–203.
13. Diers D: *Research in Nursing Practice.* Philadelphia, Lippincott, 1979.
14. Rogers M: Nursing: A science of unitary man, in Riehl JP, Roy C (eds): *Conceptual Models For Nursing Practice,* ed 2. New York, Appleton-Century-Crofts, 1980, pp 329–337.
15. Roy C: The Roy adaptation model, in Riehl JP, Roy C (eds): *Conceptual Models For Nursing Practice.* ed 2. New York, Appleton-Century-Crofts, 1980, pp 179–188.
16. King I: *A Theory of Nursing: Systems, Concepts, Process.* New York, Wiley, 1981.
17. Levine M: *Introduction to Clinical Nursing,* ed 2. Philadelphia, F.A. Davis Co., 1973.
18. Orem PE: *Nursing Concepts of Practice.* New York, McGraw-Hill, 1980.
19. Parse R: *Man-Living-Health: A Theory of Nursing.* New York, Wiley, 1981.
20. Paterson JG, Zderad L: *Humanistic Nursing.* New York, Wiley, 1976.
21. Reeder F: Philosophical issues in the Rogerian science of human beings. *Adv Nurs Sci* 1984;6(2):14–23.
22. Wilson L, Fitzpatrick J: Dialectic thinking as a means of understanding systems-in-development: Relevance to Rogers's principles. *Adv Nurs Sci* 1984;6(2):24–41.
23. Fawcett J: *Analysis and Evaluation of Conceptual Models of Nursing.* Norwalk, Conn., Appleton-Century-Crofts, 1983.
24. Lauden L: *Progress and Its Problems: Toward a Theory of Scientific Growth.* London, Routledge & Kegan Paul, 1977.
25. Feyerabend P: *Against Method: Outline For An Anarchistic Theory of Knowledge.* London, Verso/NLB, 1974.
26. Kuhn T: *The Essential Tension: Selected Studies in Scientific Tradition and Change.* Chicago, University of Chicago Press, 1977.
27. Lakatos I: Falsification and the methodology of scientific research programmes, in Lakatos I, Musgrave A: *Criticism and the Growth of Knowledge.* Cambridge, England, Cambridge Univ. Press, 1970, pp 91–195.
28. Rorty R: *Philosophy and the Mirror of Nature.* Princeton, NJ, Princeton Univ. Press, 1979.
29. Gadamer HG: *Truth and Method.* New York, Seabury Press, 1975.
30. Habermas J: *Knowledge and Human Interests.* Boston, Beacon Press, 1971.
31. Habermas J: *Theory and Practice.* Boston, Beacon Press, 1973.
32. Habermas J: *Legitimation Crisis.* Boston, Beacon Press, 1975.

33. Habermas J: *Communication and the Evolution of Society.* Boston, Beacon Press, 1979.
34. Heidegger M: *Being and Time.* London, SCM Press, 1962.
35. Dreyfus H: Holism and hermeneutics. *Rev Metaphysics* 1980;34:3–24.
36. Gramsci A: *Prison Notebooks: Selections,* Hoarc Q, Smith GN (trans). New York, International Publishing Co, 1971.

Critical Theory as a Framework to Enhance Nursing Science

Marilyn A. Ray

The intellectual community of nursing, while continuing its interest in the empiric-analytic and phenomenologic-hermeneutic scientific approaches, is turning to critical science in a quest to gain in-depth understanding of the dynamics of the contemporary human condition in nursing's social and political contexts. With the concern for the social conditions of health and health care reform, the struggle against patriarchal oppression, and the issues of multiculturalism and cultural sensitivity, nursing's interest in the integrality of theory and practice is growing. Critical science has its roots in the philosophic and scientific traditions of Hegel and Marx (Bernstein, 1971, 1978, 1985), Kuhn, Popper, Wittgenstein, Ricoeur and Gadamer (Allen, Benner, & Diekelman, 1986; Bernstein, 1983) and has been refined and reconstructed by Habermas (1981, 1987). This column focuses on the social-philosophic tradition of Habermas as a way of understanding critical science in nursing. The author draws upon the tenets of critical science to outline modes of inquiry to interpret how critical social science can be used to enhance nursing science.

Habermas set a new agenda for critical theory in the twentieth century by detailing a critique of the treatments of modern society by Parsons, Weber, and Marx. He specified a comprehensive approach to the previously competing social paradigms of the *system* (structural-functionalism) and the *lifeworld* (interpretive sociology) by connecting them to formulate the *theory of rational communicative action*. This theory is a systematic synthesis of three non-reducible cognitive interests related to the constitution of knowledge: the *technical,* the *practical,* and the *emancipatory*. Each type of knowledge has its own distinctive corresponding type of discourse in relation to its form of inquiry: functionalist, interpretive, and assertoric respectively (Habermas, 1987; Polkinghorne, 1983). The *technical* cognitive interest is established in the empirical-analytical sciences wherein the form of inquiry requires procedures which confirm or disconfirm empirical hypotheses or theories. The *practical* cognitive interest is highlighted in the phenomenologic-hermeneutic disciplines wherein the aim of inquiry is not knowledge gained from technical control and manipulation but knowledge that clarifies the conditions for communication and intersubjectivity (Bernstein, 1978). Access to understanding the meaning of this knowledge is by reflective interpretation. The *emancipatory* cognitive interest, the approach of a critically oriented science, sets forth the claim that concepts related to control or concepts of meaning and understanding cannot make sense unless there is rational evaluation made by participants in community life (Bernstein, 1985).

Reprinted by permission from Nursing Science Quarterly 5(3):98–101. © 1992, Chestnut House Publications.

The core of critical theory is the notion of emancipating people from conscious or unconscious constraints to facilitate by uncoerced negotiated agreement the making of community life. Though this is the core, the technical and practical are presupposed within the idea of emancipation (Allen, Benner, & Diekelman, 1986). With his concern for the social-political nature of people, Habermas attempted "to articulate and justify critique as a distinctive form of knowledge with its own epistemological integrity" (Bernstein, 1978, p. 205). He argued that an adequate epistemology today must be a social theory. As originally formulated, especially by Marx, critical theory's primary intent centered on political revolutionary action. Habermas' approach, however, took a linguistic turn in relation to theory and practice by focusing on communicative competence in the context of a search for a comprehensive theory of rationality, which is increasingly the focus of different modes of philosophic, social, and political inquiry (Bernstein, 1978). Habermas believes that every group fostering inquiry is located in a context (social and historical) which influences the knowledge produced. This means knowledge is socially constructed through human interaction (Nielsen, 1990). For Habermas, the distinctive form of human interaction is the dialectic of the moral life, where claims to right and wrong are implicit and emergent in all modes of communication (Penman, 1991). All modes of communication rely on the capacity of rationality.

Habermas identifies two processes of rationalization: the *lifeworld* and the *system,* in which the former is concerned with the social, cultural, and personal dimensions, and the latter is concerned with the economic and administrative (political) spheres. Conflicts arise along the seams of the lifeworld and system spheres (Habermas, 1987). Critical science, the theory of communicative action, is intended as a framework for research (preferably interdisciplinary) on shared understanding of "the moments of reason" related to social-economic-political conditions. Although the categories of knowledge and inquiry are interrelated, the focus of investigation shifts away from the technical and practical spheres toward the core phenomenon of the social intersubjectivity of shared understanding with attention to the rational use of language to achieve consensus, where rationality implies a total lack of coercion or manipulation (Brand, 1990; Habermas, 1987). The concept of truth is linked to the idea of rational consensus attained through discourse (Thompson, 1981). Habermas (Bernstein, 1978) notes that all linguistic communication presupposes a background of consensus and is oriented to the idea of truth. This consensus involves four nonreducible validity claims: comprehensibility of the utterance, truth of the content, legitimacy or rightness of the performative content, and veracity of the speaker. Argumentation (practical discourse or reasoned exchange of views with the community of inquirers) itself is the basis for determining whether a consensus is rational or not. Consensus is due simply to the force of the better argument. Consensus, thus, involves a normative dimension wherein the end result of all argumentation involves a form of life in which autonomy (personal freedom) and responsibility are possible.

The fundamental nucleus of investigation in the theory of communicative action is language " . . . 'the ideal speech situation,' in which discourse can fully unfold its potential for rationality" (Brand, 1990, p. 11). Bernstein (1978), however, claims that ideal speech is a fiction, and Bernstein and others (Brand, 1990) criticize Habermas' lack of sufficient attention to the illumination of human agency and motivation (choice and will). These critics specify that being rational requires commitment—rationality not only in itself but for itself. Furthermore, this author notes that little attention is given by Habermas to cultural diversity, language differences, the ethics of accountability, and the ethics of caring, all of which are concerns of nursing. Habermas' work is limited in some nursing situations which might include: (a) the exposure of one to the other in a co-present relationship prior to linguistic interaction; (b) the quality of caring as a human mode of being, with its moral characteristics of commitment, compassion, and justice as the foundation to authentic human interaction; (c) the absence of rational, linguistic communicative interaction (because of unconsciousness or cultural linguistic differences of the other), where feeling, touch, or eye contact may be the modes of communication; and (d) the quality of the relational encounters as a covenantal relationship (bond of trust) as the *promise* of authenticity or answerability to the other. "Other," in these examples, is meant as "individual or collective other." Although Habermas is aware of many of the criticisms, he neglects the inner nature of the individual, the independence of the body and the mind in the body, the ethics of accountability and caring in human encounters, the concern for cultural diversity, and the fact that rational argumentation may not lead to rational action. These shortcomings keep open the intellectual debate, which provides opportunities for generating different ideas and methods of inquiry.

How does critical science, the theory of communicative action, then, relate to nursing? Philosophies and theories of nursing, although not always fully explicit, illuminate many critical theory tenets, such as: theory is inextricably related to practice, and human activity arises within a social context. In addition, other critical science tenets which connect with nursing's interests are: *facilitating emancipation* from oppressive social systems so as to co-create improved conditions for client or community autonomy and responsibility; *bringing to consciousness patriarchal* (male-dominated) *models* in hospitals and universities that support authoritarianism and suppress human caring values; *fostering self-consciousness and an understanding of health* with attention to existing social, political, technologic, and economic conditions; *reforming health care* to include co-equal roles for nursing with other professionals in the delivery of care; *engaging in practical discourse* about health care needs using reasoned communicative action and consensus-building as a means to improving the moral character of community life; and, finally, *studying existing models and theories* to more adequately communicate what is really going on in nursing practice and to more adequately understand the theory-practice link.

Methods which either do or could enhance the connection between critical theory and nursing inquiry are the following: (a) social philosophic-historic methods using critical theory (Allen, 1985, 1986; Allen, Benner, & Diekelman, 1986; Thompson, 1985, 1987); (b) feminist methods (Maguire, 1987; Neil & Watts, 1990; Nielsen, 1990); (c) holistic methods (Schultz, 1987); (d) synthesis of multiple methods (Davidson & Ray, 1991); (e) ethnographic methods (Leininger, 1985); (f) critical-hermeneutic methods (Thompson, 1981); (g) dialectic methods (Moccia, 1986); (h) action research methods (Sussman, 1983); (i) focus group methods (Kingry, Tiedje, & Friedman, 1990); (j) participative research methods (Parker, Gordon, & Brannon, 1992); (k) cooperative methods (Benner, 1991; Newman & Moch, 1991); (l) electronic mass culture and mass media investigational methods (Habermas, 1987; Merelman, 1991); and (m) critical multiplism methods (Coward, 1990). These methods which are at various levels of development in terms of the application of a critical science approach are primarily qualitative in nature utilizing philosophic-historic analysis, or participant observation and interview wherein the researchers and participants are collectively involved in the project to co-identify the quality of the patterns of communicative interaction. Quantitative data can be used, for example, in the synthesis of multiple methods or critical multiplism methods to determine probability levels in causal relationships or evaluative processes. Questionnaires used in focus group or action research methods facilitate initial identification by participants of the foundations of organizational conflict. Video recording captures the intricacies of communicative interactions and adds another dimension to the investigations.

In analyzing the process of interaction (narratives or videotape communications), the researchers and participants examine, through critical reflective interpretation and dialectical processes, the values, ideologies, patterns, rules, characteristics, contradictions, oppositions, tensions, or ethical dilemmas between inner experience as expressed and communicative interactions that form concrete experiences in organizational, community, or nursing situations (social, historical, political, economic, and technological contexts). In the feminist method, attention is given to knowledge that is formulated through patriarchal consciousness (Nielsen, 1990). The primary task of analysis is a depth interpretation where the concept of truth as communicated is linked to the idea of rational consensus that is attained through participant discourse (Thompson, 1981) to co-produce emancipatory direction or solutions to the problems identified.

These research methods, thus, facilitate investigation of the social and cultural conditions including political conditions of nursing and health care by critically interpreting "reasoned moments" and intersubjective communication in social and political contexts. In a sense, the methods underscore a nursing pedagogy-in-action. A critical science approach places the consciousness of nursing directly in relationship with the lifeworld and the administrative system and integrally links theory with practice, and practice with theory. Thus, theory and practice are inseparable. Nursing pedagogy-in-action is a critical nursing science and is the point of reference for continually evaluating the old nursing politics of monopolistic domination and distorted communication including nurses' potential for domination of clients and others. The evaluation is carried out in light of the new nursing politics which is oriented to *self* criticism, to the ethics of responsibility and accountability, and to engagement in authentic, rational communicative interaction. Uniting nursing's prac-

tice activities (ethical communicative interaction) and inquiry illuminates the path for nurses and all participants in shared understanding to restructure health care and enhance or transform existing nursing theory. The emancipatory goal of a more ethically responsible community life that is negotiated through authentic, culturally sensitive communicative interaction is the hope of a critically grounded nursing profession and discipline.

REFERENCES

Allen, D. (1985). Nursing research and social control: Alternative models of science that emphasize understanding and emancipation. *IMAGE: Journal of Nursing Scholarship, 17*(2), 59–64.

Allen, D. (1986). Using philosophical and historical methodologies to understand the concept of health. In P. Chinn (Ed.), *Nursing Research Methodology* (pp. 157–168). Rockville, MD: Aspen.

Allen, D., Benner, P., & Diekelman, N. (1986). Three paradigms for nursing research: Methodological implications. In P. Chinn (Ed.), *Nursing Research Methodology* (pp. 23–38). Rockville, MD: Aspen.

Benner, P. (1991). Experience, narrative and community. *Advances in Nursing Science, 14*(2), 1–21.

Bernstein, R. (1971). *Praxis and action.* Philadelphia: University of Pennsylvania Press.

Bernstein, R. (1978). *The restructuring of social and political theory.* Philadelphia: University of Pennsylvania Press.

Bernstein, R. (1983). *Beyond objectivism and relativism: Science, hermeneutics and praxis.* Philadelphia: University of Pennsylvania Press.

Bernstein, R. (Ed.). (1985). *Habermas and modernity.* Cambridge, MA: MIT Press.

Brand, A. (1990). *The force of reason: An introduction to Habermas' theory of communicative action.* Sydney: Allen and Unwin.

Coward, D. (1990). Critical multiplism: A research strategy for nursing science. *IMAGE: Journal of Nursing Scholarship, 22*(3), 163–167.

Davidson, A., & Ray, M. (1991). Studying the human-environment phenomenon using the science of complexity. *Advances in Nursing Science, 14*(2), 73–87.

Habermas, J. (1981). *The theory of communicative action: Reason and the rationalization of society* (T. McCarthy, Trans.) (Vol. 1). Boston: Beacon.

Habermas, J. (1987). *The theory of communicative action: Lifeworld and system: A critique of functionalist reason* (T. McCarthy, Trans.) (Vol. 2). Boston: Beacon.

Kingry, M., Tiedje, L., & Friedman, L. (1990). Focus groups: A research technique for nursing. *Nursing Research, 39*(2), 124–125.

Leininger, M. (Ed.). (1985). *Qualitative research methods in nursing.* Orlando: Grune & Stratton.

Maguire, P. (1987). *Doing participatory research: A feminist approach.* Amherst, MA: University of Massachusetts, Center for International Education.

Merelman, R. (1991). *Partial visions: Culture and politics in Britain, Canada and the United States.* Madison: University of Wisconsin Press.

Moccia, P. (1986). The dialectic as method. In P. Chinn (Ed.), *Nursing Research Methodology* (pp. 147–156). Rockville, MD: Aspen.

Neil, R., & Watts, R. (1990). *Caring and nursing: Explorations in feminist perspectives.* New York: National League for Nursing.

Newman, M., & Moch, S. (1991). Life patterns of persons with coronary heart disease. *Nursing Science Quarterly, 4,* 161–167.

Nielsen, J. (Ed.). (1990). *Feminist research methods.* Boulder: Westview.

Parker, M., Gordon, S., Brannon, P. (1992). Involving nursing staff in research: A non-traditional approach. *Journal of Nursing Administration, 22*(4), 58–63.

Penman, R. (1991). Goals, games, and moral orders: A paradoxical case in court? *Understanding Face-to-Face Interaction* (pp. 21–42). Hillsdale, NJ: Erlbaum.

Polkinghorne, D. (1983). *Methodology for the human sciences: Systems of inquiry.* Albany: State University of New York Press.

Schultz, P. (1987). Toward holistic inquiry in nursing: A proposal for synthesis of patterns and methods. *Scholarly Inquiry for Nursing Practice: An International Journal, 1*(2), 135–146.

Sussman, G. (1983). Action research: A sociotechnical systems perspective. In G. Morgan (Ed.), *Beyond method: Strategies for social research.* Beverly Hills: Sage.

Thompson, J. (1981). *Critical hermeneutics. A study in the thoughts of Paul Ricoeur and Jurgen Habermas.* Cambridge: Cambridge University Press.

Thompson, J. (1985). Practical discourse in nursing: Going beyond empiricism and historicism. *Advances in Nursing Science, 7*(4), 59–71.

Thompson, J. (1987). Critical scholarship: The critique of domination in nursing. *Advances in Nursing Science, 10*(1), 27–38.

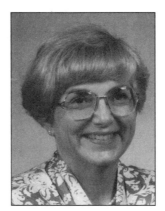

MARILYN A. RAY

The Importance of Critical Theory to Nursing: A Description Using Research Concerning Discharge Decision-Making

Donna L. Wells

Critical theory has emerged as an important research orientation for nursing. It provides for new and broader research questions and offers the potential to extend the knowledge base of nursing. In this paper I describe some applications of Jürgen Habermas's critical theory (1984, 1987) to nursing, using the example of my recently completed doctoral research (Wells, 1994). The theory was employed as a broad perspective for the study in which I investigated the process of decision-making concerning the discharge of elderly patients from the hospital. When data from 31 patient cases were analyzed, the process was found to be determined largely by systemic forces. Habermas's theory was key in understanding the structure of the process as a means-ends, or instrumental one, and in generating ideas for change in the conceptualization of the process of discharge decision-making. Critical theory can advance nursing's understanding of the social organization of everyday practice situations and whether and how they might be reorganized.

Critical theory can orient research to the kinds of questions that relate to prevailing social conditions and the organization of human activity posed in ways that potentially are linked to practical interventions (Morrow, 1994). In the last decade, this perspective has emerged as an important research orientation for nursing (see, for example, Allen, 1987; Hiraki, 1992; McKeever, 1992; Stevens, 1989; Street, 1992; Wells, 1994). Stevens articulated that critical theory provides an archaeology of the sociopolitical and cultural environment, which shapes our practices, our relationships with persons in our care,

and, as Hiraki pointed out, what is accepted as legitimate knowledge. Meleis (1992), in her discussion of nursing theory development, argued that understanding "how individuals experience and respond to health and illness . . . includes making connections and achieving syntheses that go beyond the perception and knowledge of the client and the provider" (the latter focus is characteristic of the phenomenological perspective of some nursing theories) (p. 113). Although admitting a bias toward biobehavioural processes as the central focus in the development of nursing theory, Gortner (1993) acknowledged the potential benefits of critical theory to nursing. Bent (1993) identified another contribution of critical theory to nursing: as a theoretical and research tradition, it can

Reprinted by permission from the Canadian Journal of Nursing Research 27(2): 45–58. © 1995, Canadian Journal of Nursing Research.

help to identify points from which to approach change in the discipline as well as in health care in general.

Critical theory usually refers to the series of ideas that emerged in the 1920s and 1930s in Germany at the University of Frankfurt's Institute of Social Research. But Bronner (1994) has made it clear that, in fact, it began with a number of unorthodox thinkers including Karl Korsch and George Lukacs, who preceded the formation of the Institute. Rabinow and Sullivan (1987) point out that "the great strength of . . . critical theory has been continually to urge that the human sciences cannot be detached from the greater problems of living" (p. 15). Critical theory, throughout its tradition and expounded by Habermas (its current leading representative), has involved analysis and exposure of the sociocultural and political-economic conditions of modern society that can restrict human activity. This knowledge, in turn, is meant to prompt change. The interest of critical theorists thus has been to conjoin theory and critique to achieve praxis, or moral-practical action (Thompson & Held, 1982).

In order to demonstrate how useful Habermas's (1984, 1987) critical theory could be to nursing, I shall describe some of its applications by using the example of my doctoral research (Wells, 1994) about the decision-making process regarding the discharge of elderly patients from hospital. Personal clinical experience and a literature review had suggested to me that conflicting and multiple influences on the process (of a clinical, social, and organizational nature) rendered it complex and, many times, frustrating and adverse for those involved. However, I found no studies focusing directly on elaborating the actual decision-making process, its multiple influences, and the broader context in which the process materializes and unfolds. My research was intended to fill these gaps in knowledge.

The study used the ethnographic research method to (a) describe the process of decision-making regarding the discharge of elderly pa-

tients from hospital, (b) make visible the more local, or immediate, circumstances organizing and giving shape to the everyday process of discharge decision-making, and (c) identify the consequences of the process for the persons involved. The ethnography involved participant observation of the discharge decision-making activities of professionals in a purposively-selected sample of 31 cases of patients 65 or older. These activities of professionals were observed across eight units in a large university hospital and over the patients' total hospital stays, in order to construct an in-depth description and explanation of the process of discharge decision-making. As well, focused interviews were conducted with patients, families, and key professionals involved in the process, in order to test emergent study findings and to fill gaps in the data. Medical-record analysis provided data about patients selected for case study and their clinical trajectory—that is, the course of their disease and its management. This information was important to the analysis of the relationship of the clinical course to discharge decision-making. *The Ethnograph* (Seidel, Kjolseth, & Seymour, 1988) computer software program was used to organize the unstructured data for interpretation, which consisted of identifying themes and patterns and generating the core findings of the study.

Habermas's critical theory was used as the broad framework for the study because it makes possible a discovery of, in Forester's (1985) words, "the institutional contingencies of practical actions" (p. ix), a theme consistent with my research interest. The relation between Habermas's theoretical notions of rationality and social action in modern society, in particular, and the formulation of the study purposes and research questions, is illustrated in the first part of this paper. In the second part, I discuss how Habermas's perspective was also used in the interpretation of the research findings, which revealed that the discharge decision-making process was influenced largely by systemic forces. Habermas's theory offered a way of understanding the structure of the process as a means-ends, or instrumental, one. But the significance of his theoretical ideas goes beyond the interpretation of the empirical findings. Practical insights into ways to achieve change were also generated by way of the theory. An example of these insights is outlined.

The Relation between Habermas's Critical Theory and This Study

Selected elements of Habermas's recent critical theory of society, published in his two-volume *The Theory of Communicative Action* (1984, 1987), broadly oriented the study. His ideas helped to frame the study objectives, beyond a mere description of the process of discharge decision-making for elderly patients, to include a focus on the play of forces underlying the process and the consequences of the process for those involved. In his theory of modern society, Habermas cogently argues that social structure (e.g., the organization of the hospital) is inseparable from social action (e.g., the discharge decision-making activities of practitioners), and that structure can constrain action. As Manicas explains (1987) in his analysis of the concept of social structure, "'structure enters simultaneously into the constitution of the agent and social practices, and exists in the generating moments of this constitution.' It is both medium and product, enabling as well as constraining" (p. 272).

A reading of Habermas's theory suggested that the discharge decision-making process may have come to be structured by a strategic or instrumental (means-ends) mode of reasoning and of human interaction that undergirds our social systems, including health care. Habermas describes a strategic form of social interaction as oriented to "'success,' to the efficient achievement of ends" (Bernstein, 1985, p. 18). Success is measured by the extent to which one's actions actually bring about the intended state of affairs. The mode of rationality supporting strategic ac-

tion is instrumental, directing the choice of means to given—usually material—ends. The modernization of society (e.g., with industrialization and the development of capitalism) and its continuing growth and increasing complexity have necessitated goal-directed action and an instrumental rationality.

One of Habermas's central arguments is that strategic rationality and human action directed to the efficient achievement of ends have come to displace communicative rationality and action. A communicative or discursive form of reasoning directs individuals to question and negotiate issues, to reach mutual understanding (including an understanding of conflict) concerning social needs, interests, and norms. Communicative reasoning works from background assumptions, norms, and values, which represent "cultural resources (including language) usually employed for the organization of everyday life in communication" (Misgeld, 1985, p. 96). Both forms of reasoning have become available to us in modern society as economic and political systems—as well as ways of interpreting the meaning of everyday life events—have become separated from traditional practices, such as those around kinship, and sacred (e.g., religious) forms of authority.

Habermas argues that society's failure to engage strategic and communicative rationality and action in a balanced way is related to systemic imperatives, such as the need for economic growth, administrative efficiency, and scientific and technological progress, which depend on the coordination of human activities using instrumental reasoning. However, what this means, as Misgeld (1985) articulates in his discussion of critical theory and education, is that communicative ways of understanding and interpreting the whys (reasons), wheretos (purposes, ends), and wherefroms (origins, motives) of various human activities are suppressed and not reflected upon. Using the example of the instructional-objectives movement, Misgeld elaborates on the consequences of an instrumental rationalizing attitude toward education:

One does not know when one reads the book [*Objectives for Instruction and Evaluation*] where these units come from or why they must be there other than that they are the best thing to have for the sake of accountability, of improving the efficiency of teaching and of providing guarantees for learning success. (p. 88)

The active reflection of participants (teachers and learners) on the meaning and significance of educational work is bypassed.

The embeddedness of a strategic form of rationality and action in administrative and clinical practices in the hospital may have similar effects. It would mean that patient-related goals are defined according to the exigencies of the organization in order to meet predetermined ends efficiently—for example, in relation to acute medical care and its administrative management, including discharge decision-making, and to education and research in the university hospital. Moreover, reflective kinds of questions concerning the meaning and implications of a means-ends approach—to discharge decision-making, for example—may not be communicatively considered.

Habermas calls the one-sidedness (thus, distortion) that has come to exist in our forms of reasoning and actions *lifeworld colonization*. Associated with this idea is the phenomenon of *cultural impoverishment*, which, he argues, has further contributed to the distorted way of reasoning in modern society. Communicative competence, Habermas argues, has come to take the form only of a specialized discourse or argumentation by expert cultures. As a consequence, increasing distance has been created between these cultures and the broader public. Furthermore, those who are not considered experts may become dependent on those who are for various definitions and decisions about human problems and their solutions.

The phenomenon of growth of professional groups as expert cultures, which has rendered the opinions of nonprofessionals about their health care irrelevant, or at best less important, has been documented in the literature on sociology of medicine (see, e.g., Freidson, 1988). As well, a number of empirical studies have found instances of professional interactions (including those involving nurses) with patients approximating action oriented to success concerning technical interests and preventing the emergence of holistic interpretations (Barrett, 1988; Brown, 1986; Fisher, 1982, 1984a, 1984b; Mishler, 1984; Scambler, 1987; Street, 1992; Waitzkin, 1984, 1989; Waitzkin & Britt, 1989; West, 1983). What this suggests in terms of discharge decision-making for elderly patients is that any significant interaction of a communicative, consensual nature in the definition of their situations may be infrequent, if it occurs at all.

The idea of cultural impoverishment constitutes Habermas's notion of ideology in modern society; that is, with the rise of expert cultures, opportunities for open or critical discourse are veiled. Furthermore, Habermas proposes that professional expertise founded on formal (i.e., scientific and technological) knowledge legitimizes a power relationship of professionals over the public. An imbalance in power results because instrumental rationality systematically displaces communicative rationality. In other words, the goals established by those with power, which may be advanced as a representation of collectively desired goals, cannot be examined, endorsed, or repudiated in a discursive or communicative manner. This is because the institutionalization of scientific, technological, and organizational rationality as the basis for social action makes it increasingly difficult for individuals to distinguish between technical interests on the one hand and practical or moral interests on the other. The concealment of the difference "proves the ideological power of the scientific-technocratic consciousness," Habermas claims (1970, p. 107). As a consequence, the political character of a means-ends or instrumental form of rationality may go unrecognized as a constraint on human activity.

Habermas's conclusion is that although mutual understanding underlies all human action, it does so within the premises of formally regulated or instrumental domains of action. It is not the developments in the economy, administrative systems, science and technology, and expert cultures, per se, that are at issue; it is the subordination of communicative rationality and interaction to instrumental forms of reasoning and action.

In terms of the discharge decision-making process, Habermas's claims remained to be explored because the process and related activities of participants, along with the multiple influences on the process, had not yet been well articulated. Hence, it was still uncertain how the imperatives of the hospital system and of the lifeworld (arriving at shared understandings) were actually interwoven and/or conflicted in this everyday clinical practice situation.

Nevertheless, Habermas's critical perspective was helpful in leading me to ask broad and comprehensive questions about the process of discharge decision-making. Specifically, it directed an inquiry into (a) its basic description (sequences of stages and related activities and discourses of participants), (b) the play of forces underlying the process (reasons, purposes, and ends), (c) the perceptions of those involved (motives, origins), and (d) the consequences of the process for the persons involved (its positive features and pathologies). These questions related to the social context or organization and prevailing conditions of the process. Also, the questions were linked potentially to practical interventions because they were intended to establish the conditions of the process and expose the nature and source of its limits. The study questions thus reflected both the critical and the practical intent of the research consistent with critical theory. As well, they built on personal clinical experience and the research of others.

Habermas's critical theory was more useful than other critical theories (e.g., political economy) because of his central focus on the systemic distortion of communicative action. As well, unlike feminist theory, his theory does not impose a gender constraint in terms of the pop-

ulation that is of research interest. In the hospital, elderly women and men were observed to experience similar problems related to discharge decision-making. Finally, his theory was more relevant than traditional social theories in broadly framing the study purposes and questions. The theoretical schools of functionalism (e.g., structural functionalism) and interpretivism (e.g., phenomenology), for instance, are limited by their view of social reality. In these perspectives, social structure and social action are assumed to serve the purpose of maintaining and/or restoring social order and human action. Description and explanation revolve around "what is" society and "why and how" it tends to hold together. The related inquiry does not entail identification of inherent conflicts and contradictions in social systems and the actions that can constrain human activity. Consequently, there is a quietism about these perspectives; they lack political force. However, it is the explicit task of critical theory to unveil the conditions that limit the full and conscious participation of individuals in society. For nursing, critical theory thus offers a research perspective that may help to uncover the nature of enabling and/or restrictive practices, and thereby create a space for potential change and, ultimately, a better quality of care for patients.

Habermas's Critical Theory and the Findings of This Study

The overarching conclusion, that the decision-making process to discharge elderly patients from hospital was mediated largely by systemic forces, was derived from the three core study findings that emerged during data analysis. The first core result was that the patients' clinical trajectories were not, contrary to what might be expected, a key element in shaping the process. In the majority of cases, decision-making took place without detailed knowledge or understanding of the patients' disease experiences. Characteristically, the patients' clinical outcomes were not manifest until later in the hospitalization; yet, discharge decision-making was tackled early on. For example, in the case study of an 81-year-old woman, the discharge decision-making process presented the following picture:

> Several different decisions were proposed over the course of her hospitalization. Each decision was not intricately linked to her clinical trajectory. Long before the outcome of her disease was known, both home with Home Care and the initiation of nursing home placement were contemplated, and the latter pursued. A Regional Geriatric Program (RGP) consultation was requested during active medical treatment. At the same time, arrangements for Home Care were requested, and plans continued to complete nursing home papers. Finally, the patient did return home with Home Care, but only after a 7-week course of rehabilitation with the RGP. (Wells, 1994, p. 167)

The second central finding explained, in part, why the discharge decision-making process did not follow directly upon the clinical trajectory. Specifically, in all cases studied, the process was shaped, in large part, by a variety of patient-related social factors and organizational or hospital-based parameters, many of which were assumed. The likelihood of discharging the patients was a major concern from the time of admission. The concerns of professionals, and their reasons for discharge decisions, related largely to patient's social situations (e.g., noncompliant health behaviour, social nature of the admission, inadequate social support) and to imperatives of the organization (e.g., fear of recidivism, avoidance of a delay in discharge). As well, the actions and discourses of professionals were oriented strategically, and not communicatively, to accomplish discharge. In the case of a 73-year-old man, (a) discharge decision-making was undertaken early and outside the context of an informed understanding of his actual clinical trajectory, (b) the concerns about and conditions of his discharge were based on various social and organizational factors, many of them unsubstantiated, and (c) the patient and family were approached only when decisions had already been taken at rounds.

The third core result further explained why the discharge decision-making process did not directly result from the patients' clinical trajectories. It was found that professional perceptions of the discharge decision-making process were functional or instrumental in orientation, as opposed to holistic; that is, they were biased toward administrative concerns and those of practitioners, such as bed turnover and the economic viability of the hospital.

In ethnographies, the theoretical approach underpinning a study can be used in the interpretation of the findings (Hammersley, 1992). In this study, Habermas's theory provided a way of understanding the structure of the discharge decision-making process as a means to particular ends (i.e., as strategic or instrumental action). It is systemic forces—mainly institutional imperatives, which are economic or resource related—that shape the discharge decision-making process. The process, accordingly, is characterized by an approach oriented to the successful or efficient achievement of institutional goals—namely, the prompt discharge of patients. The patients' actual clinical trajectories are superseded as a key factor.

Further, in Habermas's terms the discharge decision-making process is instrumentally, or one-sidedly, organized. Systematically distorted communication occurs because communicative action, which is discursive and understanding-oriented, does not materialize in the process. As Habermas's theory indicates, communicative action does not arise, because it is colonized or displaced by a strategic orientation, which also allows professionals to control the process. Contrary to what his theory would suggest, however, the displacement of communicative action does not occur mainly by way of cultural impoverishment (i.e., by the subordination of patients' discourses to the specialized discourses of professionals). Rather, it happens as professionals coordinate the process in a manner oriented toward the prompt discharge of patients on the basis of institutional imperatives. It is the structure of the process that grants professionals decision-making control; this structure is ideological to the extent that it displaces opportunities for a communicative orientation to occur. In this process, ongoing discussions with patients and families were rendered superfluous, and a holistic understanding of patients' discharge situations was not reached.

Habermas argues that the institutionalization of instrumental nationality as the paramount basis of action in our social and political systems undermines communicative action. In so doing, the instrumental structure of action eliminates the evaluation (i.e., self- or critical reflection) of the validity of the instrumental approach itself. In my study, the strategic orientation of the discharge process was unquestioned. Yet, the other study results about the pragmatic and moral consequences of the process indicated that the strategic orientation to discharge decision-making was distressful to patients, families, and professionals. Moreover, too early decision making was, ironically, inefficient for the hospital. In other words, professional and family resources were not always rationally employed in discharge decision-making, there was no apparent effect on patients' length of stay, and the process was unnecessarily complex. Clearly, in terms of nursing knowledge and practice, critical theory can help to illuminate the social-structural basis of an everyday, established practice situation and expose its limitations.

Habermas's communicative-action idea may also represent an intervention strategy for a restructuring of the discharge decision-making process. (A discussion of the serious challenges of this idea of Habermas's is beyond the scope of this paper.) Communicative action, which is marked by a discursive, understanding-oriented attitude concerning social needs, interests, and norms, demands shared, equal participation in decision-making and consensual decision-making. Involvement of all participants in discharge-related issues may bring about a broader and more holistic understanding of patients' clinical situations and discharge requirements, which would in turn foster greater accountability and

lend legitimacy to the process. The process of questioning and negotiating may have the added benefit of participants reflecting on the adequacies and inadequacies of instrumentally oriented practices. Ultimately, a greater balance may be achieved between the legitimate demands of the system (discursively determined) and an acceptable discharge decision-making process. A restructured discharge decision-making process would be valuable to hospital administrators and nurses (as well as other practitioners) trying to meet conflicting goals concerning resource utilization and patient-centred care. Critical theory as a research and theoretical orientation can deepen our understanding of the mechanisms and values that influence our practice. It can be a point of departure from which to examine and restructure our practice in an emancipatory way.

Conclusions

Using the example of my recently completed doctoral research, I have indicated the important contribution that Habermas's critical theory can make to nursing. As White (1988) summarizes, it has been argued that critical theory as designed by Habermas allows for fruitful research concerning forms of social action and pathologies in modern society. It serves to connect practices, such as discharge decision-making, to issues of social organization beyond the perceptions of clients and providers, and thus fulfils a requirement that Meleis (1992) sets out for knowledge development in nursing. Similarly, Street (1992) concludes that knowledge useful to nurses must incorporate ideas about the relationships between practices, the structural elements of the health-care situation, and the larger society. This kind of knowledge can greatly contribute to our understanding of the actual clinical care of patients and to our vision regarding health-care programs and policy.

Habermas's critical theory offers a way in which to achieve change. In Bryan Green's words (1993), "I confess to sharing with critical theorists an intellectual conviction [and a practical commitment] that is political" (p. xiv). Habermas's communicative action model provides a practical vehicle for a restructuring of our everyday practices, which may offset the dominance of a strategic orientation. Hiraki (1992) explains the rationale behind this important theoretical notion of Habermas's: it may be "appropriate for instrumental rationality to inform technical actions that control our natural world. But when instrumental actions affect the social life of people, it exceeds its boundaries" (p. 9). Therefore, decisions about practical life must be made communicatively with the people affected.

REFERENCES

Allen, D. G. (1987). Critical social theory as a model for analyzing ethical issues in family and community health. *Family and Community Health, 10*, 63–72.

Barrett, R. J. (1988). Clinical writing and the documentary construction of schizophrenia. *Culture, Medicine, and Psychiatry, 12*, 265–299.

Bent, K. N. (1993). Perspectives on critical and feminist theory in developing nursing praxis. *Journal of Professional Nursing, 9*, 296–303.

Bernstein, R. J. (Ed.). (1985). *Habermas and modernity.* Cambridge, MA: MIT Press.

Bronner, S. E. (1994). *Of critical theory and its theorists.* Cambridge, MA: Blackwell.

Brown, J. (1986). Professional language: Words that succeed. *Radical Review History, 34*, 33–53.

Fisher, S. (1982). The decision-making context: How doctors and patients communicate. In R. J. DiPietro (Ed.), *Linguistics and the professions* (pp. 51–81). Norwood, NJ: Ablex.

Fisher, S. (1984a). Doctor-patient communication: A social and micro-political performance. *Sociology of Health and Illness, 6*, 1–29.

Fisher, S. (1984b). Institutional authority and the structure of discourse. *Discourse Processes, 7*, 201–224.

Forester, J. (Ed.). (1985). *Critical theory and public life.* Cambridge, MA: MIT Press.

Freidson, E. (1988). *Profession of medicine: A study of the sociology of applied knowledge* (2nd Ed.). Chicago: University of Chicago Press.

Gortner, S. R. (1993). Nursing's syntax revisited: A critique of philosophies said to influence nursing theories. *International Journal of Nursing Studies, 30*, 477–488.

Green, B. S. (1993). *Gerontology and the construction of old age: A study in discourse analysis.* New York: Adline de Gruyter.

Habermas, J. (1970). *Toward a rational society* (J. J. Shapiro, Trans.). Boston: Beacon Press.

Habermas, J. (1984). *The theory of communicative action: Reason and the rationalization of society* (Vol. 1, T. McCarthy, Trans.). Boston: Beacon.

Habermas, J. (1987). *The theory of communicative action: Lifeworld and system: A critique of functionalist reason* (Vol. 2, T. McCarthy, Trans.). Boston: Beacon.

Hammersley, M. (1992). *What's wrong with ethnography?* London: Routledge.

Hiraki, A. (1992). Tradition, rationality, and power in introductory nursing textbooks: A critical hermeneutics study. *Advances in Nursing Science, 14*(3), 1–12.

Manicas, P. I. (1987). *A history and philosophy of the social sciences.* Oxford, UK: Basil Blackwell.

McKeever, P. (1992). *Mothering chronically ill, technology-dependent children: An analysis using critical theory.* Unpublished doctoral dissertation. York University, Toronto.

Meleis, A. I. (1992). Directions for nursing theory development in the 21st century. *Nursing Science Quarterly, 5*, 112–117.

Misgeld, D. (1985). Education and cultural invasion: Critical social theory education as instruction, and the "Pedagogy of the Oppressed." In J. Forester (Ed.), *Critical theory and public life* (pp. 77–118). Cambridge, MA: MIT Press.

Mishler, E. G. (1984). *The discourse of medicine: Dialectics of medical interviews.* Norwood, NJ: Ablex.

Morrow, R. A. (1994). *Critical theory and methodology.* Thousand Oaks, CA: Sage.

Rabinow, P., & Sullivan, W. M. (Eds.). (1987). *Interpretive social science: A second look.* Berkeley, CA: University of California Press.

Scambler, G. (1987). Habermas and the power of medical expertise. In G. Scambler (Ed.), *Sociological theory and medical sociology* (pp. 165–193). London: Tavistock.

Seidel, J. V., Kjolseth, R., & Seymour, E. (1988). *The ethnograph: A user's guide.* Corvallis, OR: Qualis Research Associates.

Stevens, P. E. (1989). A critical social reconceptualization of environment in nursing: Implications for methodology. *Advances in Nursing Science, 11*, 56–68.

Street, A. F. (1992). *Inside nursing: A critical ethnography of clinical nursing practice.* Albany, NY: State University of New York Press.

Thompson, J. B., & Held, D. (Eds.). (1982). *Habermas: Critical debates.* Cambridge, MA: MIT Press.

Waitzkin, H. (1984). Doctor-patient communication: Clinical implications of social scientific research. *Journal of the American Medical Association, 252*, 2441–2447.

Waitzkin, H. (1989). A critical theory of medical discourse: Ideology, social control, and the processing of social context in medical encounters. *Journal of Health and Social Behavior, 30*, 220–239.

Waitzkin, H., & Britt, T. (1989). A critical theory of medical discourse. How patients and health professionals deal with social problems. *International Journal of Health Services, 19*, 577–597.

Wells, D. I. (1994). *On the process of discharge decision-making for elderly patients: A critical ethnography.* Unpublished doctoral dissertation. York University, Toronto.

West, C. (1983). "Ask me no questions . . .": An analysis of queries and replies in physician-patient dialogues. In S. Fisher, & A. D. Todd (Eds.). *The social organization of doctor-patient communication* (pp. 75–106). Washington, DC: Center for Applied Linguistics.

White, S. K. (1988). *The recent work of Jurgen Habermas: Reason, justice & modernity.* New York: Cambridge University Press.

Acknowledgments

This research was generously supported by the Educational Centre for Aging and Health, located at McMaster University, and the Ontario Ministry of Colleges and Universities. The author also wishes to acknowledge the thesis supervision of Dr. Anne Marie Ambert, York University, the research assistance of Ms. Sithy Thaha, and the editorial support of Ms. Barbara Bauer.

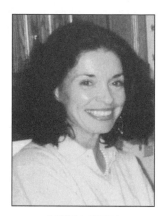

DONNA L. WELLS

The Instability of the Analytical Categories of Feminist Theory

Sandra Harding

Feminist theory began by trying to extend and reinterpret the categories of various theoretical discourses so that women's activities and social relations could become analytically visible within the traditions of intellectual discourse.[1] If women's natures and activities are as fully social as are men's, then our theoretical discourses should reveal women's lives with just as much clarity and detail as we presume the traditional approaches reveal men's lives. We had thought that we could make the categories and concepts of the traditional approaches objective or Archimedean where they were not already.

As we all have come to understand, these attempts revealed that neither women's activities nor gender relations (both inter- and intra-gender relations) can be added to these theoretical discourses without distorting the discourses and our subject matters. The problem here is not a simple one, because liberal political theory and its empiricist epistemology, Marxism, critical theory, psychoanalysis, functionalism, structuralism, deconstructionism, hermeneutics, and the other theoretical frameworks we have explored both do and do not apply to women and to gender relations. On the one hand, we have been able to use aspects or components of each

of these discourses to illuminate our subject matters. We have stretched the intended domains of these theories, reinterpreted their central claims, or borrowed their concepts and categories to make visible women's lives and feminist views of gender relations. After our labors, these theories often do not much resemble what their nonfeminist creators and users had in mind, to put the point mildly. (Think of the many creative uses to which feminists have put Marxist or psychoanalytic concepts and categories; of how subversive these revised theories are of fundamental tendencies in Marxism and Freudianism.) On the other hand, it has never been women's experiences that have provided the grounding for any of the theories from which we borrow. It is not women's experiences that have generated the problems these theories attempt to resolve, nor have women's experiences served as the test of the adequacy of these theories. When we begin inquiries with women's experiences instead of men's, we quickly encounter phenomena (such as emotional labor or the positive aspects of "relational" personality structures) that were made invisible by the concepts and categories of these theories. The recognition of such phenomena undermines the legitimacy of the central analytical structures of these theories, leading us to wonder if we are not continuing to distort women's and men's lives by our extensions and reinterpretations. Moreover, the very fact that we borrow from these theories often has the unfortunate consequence of diverting our energies into endless disputes with the nonfeminist defenders of these theories: we end up speaking not to other women but to patriarchs.

Furthermore, once we understand the destructively mythical character of the essential and universal "man" which was the subject and paradigmatic object of nonfeminist theories, so too do we begin to doubt the usefulness of analysis that has essential, universal woman as its subject or object—as its thinker or the object of its thought. We have come to understand that whatever we have found useful from the perspective of the social experience of Western, bourgeois, heterosexual, white women is especially suspect when we begin our analyses with the social experiences of any other women. The patriarchal theories we try to extend and reinterpret were created to explain not men's experience but only the experience of those men who are Western, bourgeois, white, and heterosexual. Feminist theorists also come primarily from these categories—not through conspiracy but through the historically common pattern that it is people in these categories who have had the time and resources to theorize, and who—among women—can be heard at all. In trying to develop theories that provide the one, true (feminist) story of human experience, feminism risks replicating in theory and public policy the tendency in the patriarchal theories to police thought by assuming that only the problems of *some* women are human problems and that solutions for them are the only reasonable ones. Feminism has played an important role in showing that there are not now and never have been any generic "men" at all—only gendered men and women. Once essential and universal man dissolves, so does his hidden companion, woman. We have, instead, myriads of women living in elaborate historical complexes of class, race, and culture.

I want to talk here about some challenges for theorizing itself at this moment in history, and, in particular, for feminist theorizings. Each has to do with how to use our theories actively to transform ourselves and our social relations, while we and our theories—the agents and visions of reconstruction—are themselves under transformation. Consider, for instance, the way in which we focus on some particular inadequate sexist or earlier feminist analysis and show its shortcomings—often with brilliance and eloquence. In doing so, we speak from the assumptions of some other discourse feminism has adopted or invented. These assumptions always include the belief that we can, in principle, construct or arrive at the perspective from which nature and social life can be seen as they really are. After all, we argue that sexist (or earlier feminist) analyses are wrong, inadequate, or distorting—not that they are equal in scientific or rational grounding to our criticisms.

However, we sometimes claim that theorizing itself is suspiciously patriarchal, for it assumes separations between the knower and the known, subject and object, and the possibility of some powerful transcendental, Archimedean standpoint from which nature and social life fall into what we think is their proper perspective. We fear replicating—to the detriment of women whose experiences have not yet been fully voiced within feminist theory—what we perceive as a patriarchal association between knowledge and power.[2] Our ability to detect androcentrism in traditional analyses has escalated from finding it in the content of knowledge claims to locating it in the forms and goals of traditional knowledge seeking. The voice making *this* proposal is itself super-Archimedean, speaking from some "higher" plane, such that Archimedes' followers in contemporary intellectual life are heard as simply part of the inevitable flux and imperfectly understood flow of human history. (And this is true even when the voice marks its own historical particularity, its femininity.) When it is unreflective, this kind of postmodernism—a kind of absolute relativism—itself takes a definitive stand from yet further outside the political and intellectual needs that guide our day-to-day thinking and social practices. In reaction we wonder how we can not want to say *the way things really are* to "our rulers" as well as to ourselves, in order to voice opposition to the silences and lies emanating from the patriarchal discourses and our own partially brainwashed consciousnesses. On the other hand, there is good reason to agree with a feminist postmodernist suspicion of the relationship between accepted definitions of "reality" and socially legitimated power.

How then are we to construct adequate feminist theory, or even *theories*—whether postmodern or not? Where are we to find the analytical concepts and categories that are free of the patriarchal flaws? What are the analytical categories for the absent, the invisible, the silenced that do not simply replicate in mirror-image fashion the distorting and mystifying categories and projects of the dominant discourses? Again, there are two ways to look at this situation. On the one hand, we can use the liberal powers of reason and the will, shaped by the insights gained through engaging in continuing political struggles, to piece what we see before our eyes in contemporary social life and history into a clear and coherent conceptual form, borrowing from one androcentric discourse here, another one there, patching in between in innovative and often illuminating ways, and revising our theoretical frameworks week by week as we continue to detect yet further androcentrisms in the concepts and categories we are using. We can then worry about the instability of the analytical categories and the lack of a persisting framework from which we continue to build our accounts. (After all, there should be some progress toward a "normal" discourse in our explanations if we are to create a coherent guide to understanding and action.) On the other hand, we can learn how to embrace the instability of the analytical categories; to find in the instability itself the desired theoretical reflection of certain aspects of the political reality in which we live and think; to use these instabilities as a resource for our thinking and practices. No "normal science" for us![3]

I recommend we take the second course, an uncomfortable goal, for the following reason.

The social life that is our object of study and within which our analytical categories are formed and tested is in exuberant transformation.[4] Reason, will power, reconsidering the material—even political struggle—will not slow these changes in ways over which our feminisms should rejoice. It would be a delusion for feminism to arrive at a master theory, at a "normal science" paradigm with conceptual and methodological assumptions that we presume all feminists accept. Feminist analytical categories *should* be unstable—consistent and coherent theories in an unstable and incoherent world are obstacles to both our understanding and our social practices.

We need to learn how to see our theorizing projects as illuminating "riffing" between and over the beats of patriarchal theories, rather than as rewriting the tunes of any particular one (Marxism, psychoanalysis, empiricism, hermeneutics, deconstructionism, to name a few) so that it perfectly expresses *what we think at the moment we want to say*. The problem is that we do not know and should not know just what we want to say about a number of conceptual choices with which we are presented—except that the choices themselves create no-win dilemmas for our feminisms.

In the field in which I have been working—feminist challenges to science and epistemology—this situation makes the present moment an exciting one in which to live and think, but a difficult one in which to conceptualize a definitive overview. That is, the arguments between those of us who are criticizing science and epistemology are unresolvable within the frameworks in which we have been posing them. We need to begin seeing these disputes not as a process of naming issues to be resolved but instead as opportunities to come up with better problems than those with which we started. The destabilization of thought often has advanced understanding more effectively than restabilizations, and the feminist criticisms of science point to a particularly fruitful arena in which the categories of Western thought need destabilization. Though these criticisms began by raising what appeared to be politically contentious but theoretically innocuous questions about discrimination against women in the social structure of science, misuses of technology, and androcentric bias in the social sciences and biology, they have quickly escalated into ones that question the most fundamental assumptions of modern, Western thought. They therefore implicitly challenge the theoretical constructs within which the original questions were formulated and might be answered.

Feminisms are totalizing theories. Because women and gender relations are everywhere, the subject matters of feminist theories are not containable within any single disciplinary framework or any set of them. "The scientific worldview" has also taken itself to be a totalizing theory—anything and everything worth understanding can be explained or interpreted within the assumptions of modern science. Of course there is another world—the world of emotions, feelings, political values, of the individual and collective unconscious, of social and historical particularity explored in novels, drama, poetry, music, and art, and the world within which we all live most of our waking and dreaming hours under constant threat of its increasing reorganization by scientific rationality.[5] One of the projects of feminist theorists is to reveal the relationships between these two worlds—how each shapes and informs the other. In examining feminist criticisms of science, then, we must consider all that science does not, the reasons for these exclusions, how these shape science precisely through their absences—both acknowledged and unacknowledged.

Instead of fidelity to the assumption that coherent theory is a desirable end in itself and the only reliable guide to action, we can take as our standard fidelity to *parameters* of dissonance within and between assumptions of patriarchal discourses. This approach to theorizing captures what some take to be a distinctively women's emphasis on contextual thinking and decision making and on the processes necessary for gaining understanding in a world not of our own making—that is, a world that does not encourage us to fantasize about how we could order reality into the forms we desire.[6] It locates the ways in which a valuably "alienated consciousness," "bifurcated consciousness," "oppositional consciousness" might function at the level of active theory making—as well as at the level of skepticism and rebellion. We need to be able to cherish certain kinds of intellectual, political, and psychic discomforts, to see as inappropriate and even self-defeating certain kinds of clear solutions to the problems we have been posing.

"Bad Science" or "Science as Usual"?

Are sexist assumptions in substantive scientific research the result of "bad science" or simply "science as usual"? The first alternative offers hopes of reforming the kind of science we have; the second appears to deny this possibility.

It is clear that feminist criticisms of the natural and social sciences have identified and described science badly practiced—that is, science distorted by masculine bias in problematics, theories, concepts, methods of inquiry, observations, and interpretations of results of research.[7] There are facts of the matter, these critics claim, but androcentric science cannot locate them. By identifying and eliminating masculine bias through more rigorous adherence to scientific methods, we can get an objective, de-gendered (and in that sense, value-free) picture of nature and social life. Feminist inquiry represents not a substitution of one gender loyalty for the other—one subjectivism for another—but the transcendence of gender which thereby increases objectivity.

In this argument, we use empiricist epistemology because its ends are the same as ours: objective, value-neutral results of research. This feminist empiricism argues that sexism and androcentrism are social biases. Movements for social liberation "make it possible for people to see the world in an enlarged perspective because they remove the covers and blinders that obscure knowledge and observation."[8] Thus the women's movement creates the opportunity for such an enlarged perspective—just as did the bourgeois revolution of the fifteenth to seventeenth centuries, the proletarian revolution of the nineteenth century, and the revolutions overthrowing European and U.S. colonialism in recent decades. Furthermore, the women's movement creates more women scientists and more feminist scientists (men as well as women), who are more likely than nonfeminist men to notice androcentric bias.

Feminist empiricism offers a powerful explanation—though a misleading one—for the greater empirical adequacy of so much of feminist research. It has the virtue of answering the question of how a political movement such as feminism could be contributing to the growth of objective scientific knowledge. In making this argument, however, we avert our eyes from the fact that this appeal to empiricism in fact subverts empiricism in three ways. (1) For empiricism, the social identity of the observer is supposed to be irrelevant to the quality of research results. Feminist empiricism argues that women (or feminists, men and women) as a group are more likely to produce unbiased, objective results of inquiry than are men (or nonfeminists) as a group. (2) We claim that a key origin of androcentric bias lies in the selection of problems for inquiry and in the definition of what is problematic about them. Empiricism insists that its methodological norms are meant to apply only to the context of justification and not to the context of discovery where problematics are identified and defined. Hence we have shown the inadequacy, the impotence, of scientific methods to achieve their goals. (3) We often point out that it is exactly following the logical and sociological norms of inquiry which results in androcentric results of research—appealing to the already existing (Western, bourgeois, homophobic, white, sexist) scientific community for

confirmation of the results of research; generalizing to all humans from observations only of males. Our empiricist criticisms of "bad science" in fact subvert the very understandings of science they are meant to reinforce.

These problems suggest that the most fundamental categories of scientific thought are male biased. Many of the critics of "bad science" also make this second criticism though it undercuts the assumptions of the first.[9] Here they point to historians' descriptions of how sexual politics have shaped science, and science, in turn, has played a significant role in advancing sexual politics. Each has provided a moral and political resource for the other.[10] Furthermore, they show that "pure science"—inquiry immune from the technological and social needs of the larger culture—exists only in the unreflective mental life of some individual scientists and in the rhetoric of science apologists. That is, one does not have to impugn the motives of individual physicists, chemists, or sociologists in order to make a convincing case that the scientific enterprise is structurally and symbolically part and parcel of the value systems of those cultures that maintain it. This argument poses difficulties for us, nonetheless, since if the very concepts of nature, of dispassionate, value-free, objective inquiry, and of transcendental knowledge are androcentric, white, bourgeois, and Western, then no amount of more rigorous adherence to scientific method will eliminate such bias, for the methods themselves reproduce the perspectives generated by these hierarchies and thus distort our understandings.

While these new understandings of the history of science and sexuality expand our understanding immensely, they do not tell us whether a science apparently so inextricably intertwined with the history of sexual politics can be pried loose to serve more inclusive human ends—or whether it is strategically worthwhile to try to do so. Is history destiny? Would the complete elimination of androcentrisms from science leave no science at all? But isn't it important to try to degender science as much as we can in a world where scientific claims are *the* model of knowledge? How can we afford to choose between redeeming science or dismissing it altogether when neither choice is in our best interest?

Successor Science or Postmodernism

The dilemma that arises in criticisms of "bad science" and of "science as usual" reappears at a metalevel in feminist theory's conflicting tendencies toward postmodernism and what I shall call the feminist successor science projects. Feminist empiricism explains (albeit subversively) the achievements of feminist inquiry—of that purported contradiction in terms: a politicized scientific inquiry—by appeal to the familiar empiricist assumptions. In contrast, the feminist standpoint epistemologies articulate an understanding of scientific knowledge seeking that replaces, as successor to, the Enlightenment vision captured by empiricism.[11] Both the standpoint and postmodern tendencies within feminist theory place feminism in an uneasy and ambivalent relationship to patriarchal discourses and projects (just as did feminist empiricism). There are good reasons to think of both as imperfect and converging tendencies toward a postmodernist reality, but there are also good reasons to nourish the tendencies in each which conflict.

The feminist standpoint epistemologies use for feminist ends the Marxist vision in which science can reflect "the way the world is" and contribute to human emancipation. Feminist research claims in the natural and social sciences do appear to be truer to the world, and thus more objective than the sexist claims they replace. They provide an understanding of nature and social life that transcends gender loyalties and does not substitute one gender-loyal understanding for another. Furthermore, these feminist appeals to truth and objectivity trust that reason will play a role in the eventual triumph of feminism, that feminism correctly will be perceived as more than a power politic—though it is that, too. The successor science tendencies

aim to provide more complete, less false, less distorting, less defensive, less perverse, less rationalizing understandings of the natural and social worlds.

This is already a radical project, for the Enlightenment vision explicitly denied that women possessed the reason and powers of dispassionate, objective observation required by scientific thinking. Women could be objects of (masculine) reason and observation but never the subjects, never the reflecting and universalizing human minds. Only men were in fact envisioned as ideal knowers, for only men (of the appropriate class, race, and culture) possessed the innate capacities for socially transcendant observation and reason. The ends and purposes of such a science turned out to be far from emancipatory for anyone.

Marxism reformulated this Enlightenment vision so that the proletariat, guided by Marxist theory and by class struggle, became the ideal knowers, the group capable of using observation and reason to grasp the true form of social relations, including our relations with nature.[12] This Marxist successor to bourgeois science was, like its predecessor, to provide one social group—here, the proletariat—with the knowledge and power to lead the rest of the species toward emancipation. Marxism's epistemology is grounded in a theory of labor rather than a theory of innate (masculine) faculties; so just as not all human faculties are equal in the bourgeois version, here not all labor is equal. It was through struggle in the workplace that the proletariat would generate knowledge. In neither socialist practice nor Marxist theory were any women ever conceptualized as fundamentally defined by their relation to the means of production, regardless of their work force participation. They were never thought of as full-fledged members of the proletariat who could reason and thus know how the world is constructed. Women's distinctive reproductive labor, emotional labor, "mediating" labor thus disappeared within the conceptual framework of Marxist theory, leaving women invisible as a class or social group of agents of knowledge. (Other forms of nonwage or nonindustrial labor similarly disappeared from the center of this conceptual scheme, mystifying the knowing available to slaves and colonized peoples.)

This standpoint tendency in feminist epistemology is grounded in a successor theory of labor or, rather, of distinctively human activity, and seeks to substitute women or feminists (the accounts differ) for the proletariat as the potentially ideal agents of knowledge. Men's (sexists') perceptions of themselves, others, nature, and the relations between all three are characteristically not only partial but also perverse.[13] Men's characteristic social experience, like that of the bourgeoisie, hides from them the politically imposed nature of the social relations they see as natural. Dominant patterns in Western thought justify women's subjugation as necessary for the progress of culture, and men's partial and perverse views as uniquely and admirably human. Women are able to use political struggle and analysis to provide a less partial, less defensive, less perverse understanding of human social relations—including our relations with nature. The standpoint theorists argue that this analysis, not feminist empiricism, accounts for the achievements of feminist theory and research because it is politically engaged theory and research from the perspective of the social experience of the subjugated sex/gender.

The second line of thought, one that can be found within many of these very same writings, expresses a profound skepticism toward the Enlightenment vision of the power of "the" human mind to reflect perfectly a readymade world that is out there for the reflecting. Many feminists share a rejection of the value of the forms of rationality, of dispassionate objectivity, of the Archimedean perspective, which were to be the means to knowledge. Here they are ambivalently related to such other skeptics of modernism as Nietzsche, Wittgenstein, Derrida, Foucault, Lacan, Feyerabend, Rorty, Gadamer, and the discourses of semiotics, psychoanalysis, structuralism, and deconstructionism.[14] What is

striking is how the successor science idea and the postmodern skepticism of science are both embraced by these theorists, though the concepts are diametrically opposed in the nonfeminist discourses.[15]

From the perspective of this postmodern tendency in feminist thinking, the feminist successor science project can appear still too firmly rooted in distinctively masculine modes of being in the world. As one theorist puts the issue, "Perhaps 'reality' can have 'a' structure only from the falsely universalizing perspective of the master. That is, only to the extent that one person or group can dominate the whole, can 'reality' appear to be governed by one set of rules or be constituted by one privileged set of social relations."[16] How can feminism radically redefine the relationship between knowledge and power if it creates yet another epistemology, yet another set of rules for the policing of thought?

However, this postmodern project can appear viciously utopian from the perspective of the successor science tendency.[17] It seems to challenge the legitimacy of trying to describe the way the world is from a distinctively feminist perspective. It can appear of a piece with masculine and bourgeois desire to justify one's activities by denying one's social, embodied location in history; to attempt to transcend one's objective location in politics by appeal to a *mea culpa*, all-understanding, bird's-eye view (the transcendental ego in naturalistic garb) of the frailty of mere humans. That is, in its uneasy affiliation with nonfeminist postmodernism, the feminist postmodernist tendency appears to support an inappropriate relativist stance by the subjugated groups, one that conflicts with feminism's perception that the realities of sexual politics in our world demand engaged political struggle. It appears to support an equally regressive relativism for those mildly estranged members of the subjugating groups with doubts about the legitimacy of their own objective privilege and power (see list above of nonfeminist skeptics of modernism). It is worth keeping in mind that the articulation of relativism as an intellectual position emerges historically only as an attempt to dissolve challenges to the legitimacy of purportedly universal beliefs and ways of life. It is an objective problem, or a solution to a problem, only *from the perspective of the dominating groups.* Reality may indeed appear to have many different structures from the perspectives of our different locations in social relations, but some of those appearances are ideologies in the strong sense of the term: they are not only false and "interested" beliefs but also ones that are used to structure social relations for the rest of us. For subjugated groups, a relativist stance expresses a false consciousness. It accepts the dominant group's insistence that their right to hold distorted views (and, of course, to make policy for all of us on the basis of those views) is intellectually legitimate.

Are not the policing of thought in the service of political power and the retreat to purportedly politically innocent, relativistic, mere interpretations of the world the two sides of the Enlightenment and bourgeois coin to which feminism is opposed? Is it not true—as these theorists all argue in different ways—that men's and women's different kinds of interactions with nature and social life (different "labor") provide women with distinctive and privileged scientific and epistemological standpoints? How can feminism afford to give up a successor science project if it is to empower all women in a world where socially legitimated knowledge and the political power associated with it are firmly lodged in white, Western, bourgeois, compulsorily heterosexual, men's hands? Yet how can we give up our distrust of the historic links between this legitimated knowledge and political power?

One way to see these two tendencies in feminist theory is as converging approaches to a postmodernist world—a world that will not exist until both (conflicting) tendencies achieve their goals. From this perspective, at its best postmodernism envisions epistemology in a world where thought does not need policing. It recognizes the existence today of far less than the ideal speech situation, but disregards (or

fails to acknowledge) the political struggles necessary to bring about change. The standpoint tendency attempts to move us toward that ideal world by legitimating and empowering the "subjugated knowledges" of women, without which that postmodern epistemological situation cannot come into existence. It fails nonetheless to challenge the modernist intimacies between knowledge and power, or the legitimacy of assuming there can be a single, feminist story of reality. Whether or not this is a useful way to see the relationship between the two tendencies, I am arguing that we must resist the temptation to explain away the problems each addresses and to choose one to the exclusion of the other.

The Feminist Standpoint and Other "Others"

Feminist successor science projects stand in an uneasy relation to other emancipatory epistemologies insofar as the former seek to ground a uniquely legitimate and distinctive science and epistemology on the shared characteristics of women's activity. Hilary Rose locates these grounds in the way women's labor unifies mental, manual, and caring labor. Nancy Hartsock focuses on the deeper opposition to the dualities of mental versus manual labor to be found in women's daily, concrete activities both in domestic life and wage labor. Jane Flax identifies the relatively more reciprocal sense of self women bring to all their activities. She suggests that the small gap between men's and women's concepts of self, others, and nature prefigures the possible larger gap between the defensively dualistic knowledge characteristic of male-dominant social orders and the relational and contextual knowledge possible in a future society of "reciprocal selves." Dorothy Smith argues that women's social labor is concrete rather than abstract, that it cannot be articulated to either administrative forms of ruling or the categories of social science, and that it has been socially invisible—combining to create a valuably alienated and bifurcated consciousness in women.[18] How-ever, other emancipatory perspectives claim as resources for their politics and epistemologies similar aspects of their own activity.

On the one hand, of course, feminism is right to identify women and men as classes in opposition at this moment in history. Every-where in the world we find these two classes, and virtually everywhere the men subjugate the women in one way or another.[19] Furthermore, even male feminists receive benefits from an in-stitutionalized sexism they actively struggle to eliminate. Objectively, no individual men can succeed in renouncing sexist privilege any more than individual whites can succeed in renounc-ing racist privilege—the benefits of gender and race accrue regardless of the wishes of the indi-viduals who bear them. Gender, like race and class, is not a voluntarily disposable individual characteristic. After all, fundamentally our fem-inisms address the extraction and transfer of so-cial benefits from women to men *as groups* of humans, on a worldwide scale. Thus the stand-point theorists, in identifying the common as-pects of women's social experience cross-cultur-ally, contribute something important to our work.

On the other hand, the distinctive character-istics of women's activities that Rose, Hartsock, Flax, and Smith identify for our culture are probably to be found also in the labor and social experience of other subjugated groups. There are suggestions in the literature on Native Americans, Africans, and Asians that what femi-nists call feminine versus masculine personali-ties, ontologies, ethics, epistemologies, and worldviews may be what these other liberation movements call non-Western versus Western personalities and worldviews.[20] Thus, should there not also be Native American, African, and Asian sciences and epistemologies, based on the distinctive historical and social experience of these peoples? Would not such successor sci-ences and epistemologies provide similar analy-ses to those of the standpoint theorists? (I set aside the crucial and fatal complication for this

way of thinking—the facts that one-half of these peoples are women and that most women are not Western.) On what grounds would the fem-inist sciences and epistemologies be superior to these others? What is and should be the rela-tionship of the feminist projects to these other emancipatory knowledge-seeking projects?

It is a vast overgeneralization to presume that all Africans, let alone all colonized peoples, share distinctive personalities, ontologies, ethics, epis-temologies, or worldviews. But is it any worse than the presumption that there are commonal-ities to be detected in *all women's* social experi-ences or worldviews? Let us note that we are thinking here about perspectives as inclusive as those referred to in such phrases as the "feudal worldview," the "modern worldview," or the "scientific worldview." Moreover, we women also claim an identity we were taught to de-spise;[21] around the globe we insist on the im-portance of our social experience as *women,* not just as gender-invisible members of class, race, or cultural groups. Similarly, Third World peo-ples claim their colonized social experience as the grounding for a shared identity and as a common source of alternative understandings. Why is it not reasonable to explore how the ex-perience of colonization itself shapes personali-ties and worldviews? How can white Western women insist on the legitimacy of what we think we share with all women and not acknowledge the equal legitimacy of what colonized peoples think they share with each other? In short, we cannot resolve this problem for the feminist standpoint by insisting on the cultural particu-larity of individuals in other cultures while at the same time arguing for the gender similarities of women cross-culturally.

One resolution of this dilemma for the stand-point tendency would be to say that feminist sci-ence and epistemology will be valuable in their own right alongside and as a part of these other possible sciences and epistemologies—not supe-rior to them. With this strategy we have relin-quished the totalizing, "master theory" charac-ter of our theory making which is at least an implicit goal of much feminist theorizing, and we have broken away from the Marxist assumptions that informed the feminist successor science projects. This response to the issue has managed to retain the categories of feminist theory (unstable though they be) and simply set them alongside the categories of the theory making of other subjugated groups. Instead of the "dual systems" theory with which socialist feminists wrestle,[22] this response gives us multisystems theory. Of course, it leaves bifurcated (and perhaps even more finely divided) the identities of all except ruling-class white Western women. There is a fundamental incoherence in this way of thinking about the grounds for feminist approaches to knowledge.

Another solution would be to renounce the goal of unity around shared social experiences in favor of solidarity around those goals that can be shared.[23] From this perspective, each standpoint epistemology—feminist, Third World, gay, working class—names the historical conditions producing the political and conceptual oppositions to be overcome but does not thereby generate universal concepts and political goals. Because gender is also a class and racial category in cultures stratified by class and race as well as by gender, no particular women's experience can uniquely generate the groundings for the visions and politics that will emancipate us from gender hierarchy. A variety of social groups are currently struggling against the hegemony of the Western, white, bourgeois, homophobic androcentric worldview and the politics it both generates and justifies. Our internal racial, sexual, and class struggles, and the differences in our cultural histories which define for us who we are as social beings, prevent our federating around our shared goals. It is history that will resolve or dissolve this problem, not our analytic efforts. Nevertheless, white, Western, bourgeois feminists should attend to the need for a more active theoretical and political struggle against our own racism, classism, and cultural centrism as forces that insure the continued subjugation of women around the world.

Culture versus Nature and Gender versus Sex

Historians and anthropologists show that the way contemporary Western society draws the borders between culture and nature is clearly both modern and culture bound.[24] The culture versus nature dichotomy reappears in complex and ambiguous ways in a number of other oppositions central to modern, Western thinking: reason versus the passions and emotions; objectivity versus subjectivity; mind versus the body and physical matter; abstract versus concrete; public versus private—to name a few. In our culture, and in science, masculinity is identified with culture and femininity with nature in all of these dichotomies. In each case, the latter is perceived as an immensely powerful threat that will rise up and overwhelm the former unless the former exerts severe controls over the latter.

This series of associated dualisms has been one of the primary targets of feminist criticisms of the conceptual scheme of modern science. It is less often recognized, however, how the dualism reappears in feminist thinking about gender, sex, or the sex/gender system. In preceding sections, I have talked about eliminating gender as if the social could be cleanly separated from the biological aspects of our sexual identities, practices, and desires. In feminist discourses, this mode of conceptualizing sexuality is clearly an advance over the biological determinist assumption that gender differences simply follow from sex differences. Since biological determinism is alive and flourishing in sociobiology, endocrinology, ethology, anthropology and, indeed, most nonfeminist discourses, I do not want to devalue the powerful analytical strategy of insisting on a clean separation between the known (and knowable) effects of biology and of culture. Nevertheless, a very different picture of sexual identities, practices, and desires emerges from recent research in biology, history, anthropology, and psychology.[25] Surprisingly, it could also be called biological determinism, though what is determined on this account is the plasticity rather than the rigidity of sexual identity, practice, and desire. Our species is doomed to freedom from biological constraints in these respects, as existentialists would put the issue.

The problem for feminist theory and practice here is twofold. In the first place, we stress that humans are *embodied* creatures—not Cartesian minds that happen to be located in biological matter in motion. Female embodiment is different from male embodiment. Therefore we want to know the implications for social relations and intellectual life of that different embodiment. Menstruation, vaginal penetration, lesbian sexual practices, birthing, nursing, and menopause are bodily experiences men cannot have. Contemporary feminism does not embrace the goal of treating women "just like men" in public policy. So we need to articulate what these differences are. However, we fear that doing so feeds into sexual biological determinism (consider the problems we have had articulating a feminist perspective on premenstrual syndrome and work-related reproductive hazards in ways that do not victimize women). The problem is compounded when it is racial differences between women we want to articulate.[26] How can we choose between maintaining that our biological differences ought to be recognized by public policy and insisting that biology is not destiny for either women or men?

In the second place, we have trouble conceptualizing the fact that the culture versus nature dichotomy and its siblings are not simply figments of thought to be packed up in the attic of outmoded ideas. The tendency toward this kind of dualism is an ideology in the strongest sense of the term, and such tendencies cannot be shucked off by mental hygiene and will power alone. The culture/nature dichotomy structures public policy, institutional and individual social practices, the organization of the disciplines (the social vs. the natural sciences), indeed the very way we see the world around us. Consequently, until our dualistic practices are changed (divisions of social experience into mental vs. manual, into abstract vs. concrete, into emotional vs.

emotion denying), we are forced to think and exist within the very dichotomizing we criticize. Perhaps we can shift the assumption that the natural is hard to change and that the cultural is more easily changed, as we see ecological disasters and medical technologies on the one hand, and the history of sexism, classism, and racism on the other.[27] Nonetheless, we should continue insisting on the distinction between culture and nature, between gender and sex (especially in the face of biological determinist backlash), even as we analytically and experientially notice how inextricably they are intertwined in individuals and in cultures. These dichotomies are empirically false, but we cannot afford to dismiss them as irrelevant as long as they structure our lives and our consciousnesses.

Science as Craft: Anachronism or Resource?

Traditional philosophies of science assume an anachronistic image of the inquirer as a socially isolated genius, selecting problems to pursue, formulating hypotheses, devising methods to test the hypotheses, gathering observations, and interpreting the results of inquiry. The reality of most scientific research today is quite different, for these craft modes of producing scientific knowledge were replaced by industrialized modes in the nineteenth century for the natural sciences, and by the mid-twentieth century for the vast majority of social science research. Consequently, philosophy of science's rules and norms for individual knowledge seekers are irrelevant to the conduct of, and understanding of, most of contemporary science, as a number of science critics have pointed out.[28]

However, it is precisely in areas of inquiry that remain organized in craft ways where the most interesting feminist research has appeared.[29] Perhaps all of the most revolutionary claims have emerged from research situations where individual feminists (or small groups of them) identify a problematic phenomenon, hypothesize a tentative explanation, design and carry out evidence gathering, and then interpret the results of this research. In contrast, when the conception and execution of research are performed by different social groups of persons, as is the case in the vast majority of mainstream natural science and much social science research, the activity of conceptualizing the research is frequently performed by a privileged group and the activity of executing the research by a subjugated group. This situation insures that the conceptualizers will be able to avoid challenges to the adequacy of their concepts, categories, methods, and interpretations of the results of research.

This kind of analysis reinforces the standpoint theorists' argument that a prescriptive theory of knowledge—an epistemology—should be based on a theory of labor or human activity, not on a theory of innate faculties as empiricist epistemology assumes. In fact, the feminist epistemologies mentioned above are all grounded in a distinctive theory of human activity, and in one that gains support from an examination of the preconditions for the emergence of modern science in the fifteenth to seventeenth centuries. Feminists point to the unification of mental, manual, and emotional labor in women's work which provides women with a potentially more comprehensive understanding of nature and social life. As women increasingly are drawn into and seek men's work—from law and policy-making to medicine and scientific inquiry—our labor and social experience violate the traditional distinctions between men's and women's work, thus permitting women's ways of understanding reality to begin to shape public understandings. Similarly, it was a violation of the feudal division of labor that made possible the unity of mental and manual labor necessary to create science's new experimental method.[30]

Traditional philosophy of science's prescriptive image of the scientific inquirer, as craftsman, then, is irrelevant as a model for the activity that occupies the vast majority of scientific workers today. This image instead reflects the practices of the very few scientifically trained workers who are engaged in the construction of new research models. However, since the scientific worldview that feminism criticizes was constructed to explain the activity, results, and goals of the *craft labor* that constituted science in an earlier period, and since contemporary feminist craft inquiry has produced some of the most valuable new conceptualizations, it looks like we need to think more carefully about which aspects of the scientific worldview to reject and retain. Perhaps the mainstream enterprise of today is not scientific at all in the original sense of the term! Can it be that feminism and similarly estranged inquiries are the true offspring of Copernicus, Galileo, and Newton? Can this be true while at the same time these offspring undermine the epistemology that Hume, Locke, Descartes, and Kant developed to explain the birth of modern science? Once again, we are led to what I propose should be regarded as fruitful ambivalence toward the science we have. We should cultivate both "separatist" craft-structured inquiry *and* infuse the industrially structured sciences with feminist values and goals.

These are some of the central conceptual instabilities that emerge in considering the feminist criticism of science. Several of them arise in feminist theorizing more generally. I have been arguing that we cannot resolve these dilemmas in the terms in which we have been posing them and that instead we should learn how to regard the instabilities themselves as valuable resources. If we can learn how to use them, we can match Archimedes' greatest achievement—his inventiveness in creating a new kind of theorizing.

NOTES

1. My thinking about these issues has been greatly improved by the comments of Margaret Andersen and the anonymous reviewers for *Signs: Journal of Women in Culture and Society,* as well as by discussions over the last several years with many of the feminist science critics cited in this paper. I am grateful for support for this research and the larger project of which it is a part provided by the National Science Foundation, a Mina Shaughnessy Fellowship from the Fund for the Improvement of Post-

Secondary Education, University of Delaware Faculty Research Grants, and a Mellon Fellowship at the Wellesley Center for Research on Women. For the larger project, see *The Science Question in Feminism* (Ithaca, N.Y.: Cornell University Press, 1986).

2. See, e.g., Maria C. Lugones and Elizabeth V. Spelman, "Have We Got a Theory for You! Feminist Theory, Cultural Imperialism and the Demand for 'the Women's Voice.'" *Hypatia: A Journal of Feminist Philosophy* (special issue of *Women's Studies International Forum*) 6. no. 6 (1983):573–82; many of the selections in *New French Feminisms,* ed. Elaine Marks and Isabelle de Courtivron (New York: Schocken Books, 1981); Jane Flax, "Gender as a Social Problem: In and For Feminist Theory" *American Studies/Amerika Studien* (June 1986). Donna Haraway, "A Manifesto for Cyborgs: Science, Technology, and Socialist Feminism in the 1980's," *Socialist Review* 80 (1983): 65–107.

3. See Thomas S. Kuhn, *The Structure of Scientific Revolutions* (Chicago: University of Chicago Press, 1970). "Normal science" was Kuhn's term for a "mature science," one where conceptual and methodological assumptions are shared by the inquirers in a field.

4. Perhaps it has always been. But the emergence of "state patriarchy" from the "husband patriarchy" of the first half of the century, the rising of people of color from colonized subjugations, and the on-going shifts in international capitalism all insure that this moment, at any rate, is one of exuberant transformation. See Ann Ferguson, "Patriarchy, Sexual Identity, and the Sexual Revolution." *Signs: Journal of Women in Culture and Society* 7, no. 1 (1981): 158–99, for discussion of the shifts in forms of patriarchy.

5. Milan Kundera, in the article "The Novel and Europe" (*New York Review of Books,* vol. 31, no. 12 [July 19, 1984]), asks if it is an accident that the novel and the hegemony of scientific rationality arose simultaneously.

6. This emphasis is expressed in different ways by Sara Ruddick, "Maternal Thinking," *Feminist Studies* 6, no. 2 (Summer 1980): 342–67; Carol Cilligan, *In a Different Voice: Psychological Theory and Women's Development* (Cambridge, Mass.: Harvard University Press, 1982); Dorothy Smith, "Women's Perspective as a Radical Critique of Sociology," *Sociological Inquiry* 44, no. 1 (1974): 7–13; and "A Sociology for Women," in *The Prism of Sex: Essays in the Sociology of Knowledge,* ed. J. Sherman and E. T. Beck (Madison: University of Wisconsin Press, 1979).

7. See, e.g., the *Signs* review essays in the social sciences, and the papers in Brighton Women and Science Group, *Alice through the Microscope* (London: Virago Press, 1980); Ruth Hubbard, M. S. Henifin, and Barbara Fried, eds., *Biological Woman: The Convenient Myth* (Cambridge, Mass.: Schenkman Publishing Co., 1982); Marian Lowe and Ruth Hubbard, eds., *Woman's Nature Rationalizations of Inequality* (New York: Pergamon Press, 1983); Ethel Tobach and Betty Rosoff, eds., *Genes and Gender I, II, III, IV* (New York: Gordian Press, 1978, 1979, 1981, 1984) (Hubbard and Lowe are the guest editors for vol. 2 in the series, subtitled *Pitfalls in Research on Sex and Gender*); Ruth Bleier, *Science and Gender: A Critique of Biology and Its Theories on Women* (New York: Pergamon Press, 1984).

8. Marcia Millman and Rosabeth Moss Kanter, "Editorial Introduction," in *Another Voice: Feminist Perspectives on Social Life and Social Science* (New York: Anchor Books, 1975), vii.

9. This tension between the two kinds of criticisms is pointed out by Helen Longino and Ruth Doell, "Body, Bias and Behavior: A Comparative Analysis of Reasoning in Two Areas of Biological Science," *Signs* 9, no. 2 (1983): 206–27; and by Donna Haraway, "In the Beginning Was the Word: The Genesis of Biological Theory," *Signs* 6, no. 3 (1981): 469–81. Longino and Doell think "feminists do not have to choose between correcting bad science or rejecting the entire scientific enterprise" (208) and that "only by developing a more comprehensive understanding of the operation of male bias in science, as distinct from its existence, can we move beyond these two perspectives in our search for remedies" (207). Longino and Doell's analysis is helpful indeed in creating this understanding, but since they do not come to grips with the criticisms of "science as usual," my remedy parts from theirs. Haraway does not propose a solution to the dilemma.

10. See, e.g., Elizabeth Fee, "Nineteenth Century Craniology: The Study of the Female Skull," *Bulletin of the History of Medicine* 53, no. 3 (1979): 415–33. Susan Griffin, *Woman and Nature: The Roaring inside Her* (New York: Harper & Row, 1978). Diana Long Hall, "Biology, Sex Hormones and Sexism in the 1920's," *Philosophical Forum* 5 (1973–74): 81–96; Donna Haraway, "Animal Sociology and a Natural Economy of the Body Politic. Parts 1, 2," *Signs* 4, no. 1 (1978): 21–60; Ruth Hubbard, "Have Only Men Evolved?" in Hubbard, Henifin, and Fried, eds. (n. 7 above); L. J. Jordanova, "Natural Facts: A Historical Perspective on Science and Sexuality," in *Nature, Culture and Gender,* ed. Carol MacCormack and Marilyn Strathern (New York: Cambridge University Press, 1980); Carolyn Merchant, *The Death of Nature: Women,*

Ecology and the Scientific Revolution (New York: Harper & Row, 1980); Evelyn Fox Keller, *Reflections on Gender and Science* (New Haven, Conn.: Yale University Press, 1985).

11. Important formulations of the epistemology for a feminist "successor science" have been provided by Jane Flax, "Political Philosophy and the Patriarchal Unconscious: A Psychoanalytic Perspective on Epistemology and Metaphysics," in *Discovering Reality: Feminist Perspectives on Epistemology, Metaphysics, Methodology and Philosophy of Science,* ed. Sandra Harding and Merrill B. Hintikka (Dordrecht: D. Reidel Publishing Co., 1983); Nancy Hartsock, "The Feminist Standpoint: Developing the Ground for a Specifically Feminist Historical Materialism," in Harding and Hintikka, eds., and chap. 10 of *Money, Sex and Power* (Boston: Northeastern University Press, 1983); Hilary Rose, "Hand, Brain and Heart: A Feminist Epistemology for the Natural Sciences," *Signs* 9, no. 1 (1983): 73–90, and "Is a Feminist Science Possible?" (paper presented at MIT, Cambridge, Massachusetts, 1984); D. Smith, "Women's Perspective as a Radical Critique of Sociology," and "A Sociology for Women" (both in n. 6 above).

12. Friedrich Engels, "Socialism: Utopian and Scientific," in *The Marx and Engels Reader,* ed. R. Tucker (New York: W. W. Norton & Co., 1972); George Lukács, "Reification and the Consciousness of the Proletariat," *History and Class Consciousness* (Cambridge, Mass.: MIT Press, 1968).

13. Hartsock, especially, discusses the perversity of the androcentric vision (n. 11 above). I shall subsequently refer to the men vs. women dichotomy since that is the way most of these standpoint theorists put the issue. However, I think these categories are inadequate even for the standpoint projects: it is feminists vs. nonfeminists (sexists) we should be discussing here.

14. Jane Flax discusses this postmodern strain in feminist theory in "Gender as a Social Problem: In and For Feminist Theory" (n. 2 above) and cites these as among the key skeptics of modernism: Friedrich Nietzsche, *On the Genealogy of Morals* (New York: Vintage, 1969), and *Beyond Good and Evil* (New York: Vintage, 1966); Jacques Derrida, *L'écriture et la Différence* (Paris: Editions du Seuil, 1967); Michel Foucault, *The Order of Things* (New York: Vintage, 1973), and *The Archaeology of Knowledge* (New York: Harper & Row, 1972); Jacques Lacan, *Speech and Language in Psychoanalysis* (Baltimore: Johns Hopkins University Press, 1968), and *The Four Fundamental Concepts of Psychoanalysis* (New York: W. W. Norton & Co., 1973); Paul Feyerabend, *Against Method* (New York: Schocken

Books, 1975); Richard Rorty, *Philosophy and the Mirror of Nature* (Princeton, N.J.: Princeton University Press, 1979); Hans-Georg Gadamer, *Philosophical Hermeneutics* (Berkeley: University of California Press, 1976); Ludwig Wittgenstein, *On Certainty* (New York: Harper & Row, 1972), and *Philosophical Investigations* (New York: Macmillan Publishing Co., 1970). See also Jean-François Lyotard, *The Postmodern Condition: A Report on Knowledge,* trans. G. Bennington and B. Massumi (Minneapolis: University of Minnesota Press, 1984).

15. However, different weight is given to one or the other tendency by each theorist. Nevertheless, all are explicitly aware of the tension in their own work between the two kinds of criticisms of modern, Western epistemology. It is another project to explain how each attempts to resolve this tension. See Harding (n. 1 above) for further discussion of these theorists' work.

16. Flax, "Gender as a Social Problem" (n. 2 above), 17.

17. Flax appears to be unaware of this problem. Engels distinguishes utopian and scientific socialisms (n. 12 above).

18. Flax (n. 11 above); Hartsock (both items cited in n. 11 above); Rose (n. 11 above); Smith (n. 6 above).

19. "Virtually everywhere" to give the benefit of the doubt to anthropologists' claims about "egalitarian cultures." See, e.g., Eleanor Leacock, *Myths of Male Dominance* (New York: Monthly Review Press, 1981).

20. Russell Means, "Fighting Words on the Future of the Earth," *Mother Jones* (December 1980): 167; Vernon Dixon, "World Views and Research Methodology," in *African Philosophy: Assumptions and Paradigms for Research on Black Persons,* ed. L. M. King, V. Dixon, and W. W. Nobles (Los Angeles: Fanon Center Publication, Charles R. Drew Postgraduate Medical School, 1976) (but see also Paulin Hountondji, *African Philosophy: Myth and Reality* [Bloomington: Indiana University Press, 1983]): Joseph Needham, "History and Human Values: A Chinese Perspective for World Science and Technology," in *Ideology of/in the Natural Sciences,* ed. Hilary Rose and Steven Rose (Boston: Schenkman Publishing Co., 1979). I have discussed this situation more fully in "The Curious Coincidence of African and Feminine Moralities," in *Women and Moral Theory,* ed. Diana Meyers and Eva Kittay (Totowa, N.J.: Rowman & Allenheld, 1986), and in chap. 7 of Harding (n. 1 above).

21. Michele Cliff, *Claiming an Identity They Taught Me to Despise* (Watertown, Mass.: Persephone Press, 1980).

22. Iris Young, "Beyond the Unhappy Marriage: A Critique of the Dual Systems Theory," in *Women and Revolution,* ed. L. Sargent (Boston: South End Press, 1981).

23. See Bell Hooks, *Feminist Theory from Margin to Center* (Boston: South End Press, 1983), esp. chap. 4; and Haraway, "A Manifesto for Cyborgs" (n. 2 above).

24. See esp. the responses to Sherry Ortner's "Is Female to Male as Nature Is to Culture?" (in *Woman, Culture and Society,* ed. M. Z. Rosaldo and L. Lamphere [Stanford, Calif.: Stanford University Press, 1974]) in MacCormack and Strathern, eds. (n. 10 above).

25. See references cited in nn. 7, 10 above.

26. Inez Smith Reid, "Science, Politics, and Race," *Signs* 1, no. 2 (1975): 397–422.

27. Janice G. Raymond makes this point in "Transsexualism: An Issue of Sex-Role Stereotyping," in Tobach and Rosoff, eds., vol. 2 (n. 7 above).

28. Jerome Ravetz, *Scientific Knowledge and Its Social Problems* (New York: Oxford University Press, 1971); Rose and Rose, eds. (n. 20 above); Rita Arditti, Pat Brennan, Steve Cafrak, eds., *Science and Liberation* (Boston: South End Press, 1980).

29. Hilary Rose in particular has pointed this out in "Hand, Brain and Heart," and in "Is a Feminist Science Possible?" (n. 11 above). Perhaps all new research paradigms must be established through craft activity, as Kuhn argued.

30. Edgar Zilsel, "The Sociological Roots of Science," *American Journal of Sociology* 47, no. 4 (1942): 545–60.

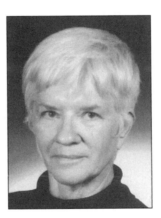

SANDRA HARDING

Voices and Paradigms: Perspectives on Critical and Feminist Theory in Nursing

Jacquelyn C. Campbell • *Sheila Bunting*

Nurse scientists have explored a variety of research methods and a number of philosophic approaches to expand the discipline's ability to describe and investigate nursing's phenomena of interest. This article discusses the similarities and differences in world views, epistemologies, methodologies, and methods of two of these paradigms: critical theory and feminist theory. Attributes of these two stances are contrasted, and the relationship between the methods of analysis and the philosophic point of view are explored. An example of nursing research is given, with discussion of how the approach would differ if the nurse scientist were using critical versus feminist theory as a frame of reference.

Seeking ways to expand the discipline's ability to identify, describe, and research nursing's phenomena of interest, nurse scientists have experimented with a variety of research methods and have explored diverse philosophical approaches. Two such approaches that have intrigued nursing scholars[1,2] and have been compared and sometimes equated with one another are feminist theory and critical theory. Using Harding's[3] descriptive categories of epistemology, methodology, and method, this article will describe the similarities and differences in world views and assumptions of these two theoretic stances. The relationships between the methods of analysis and the philosophical points of view also will be examined, and methods of research that have been used for investigation from each paradigm will be discussed. An example of nursing research, approached separately from each of the two points of view, will be presented, and the differences and similarities in epistemology, methodology, and method will be analyzed.

Differentiating feminist and critical theory approaches is important as a political stance, while recognizing that the two have significant similarities. If feminist theory is considered as a strand or type of critical social theory, this schema again subsumes a femicentric approach to an approach originally developed by men in a period of history when androcentrism dominated academic thought.

Feminist theory, like critical theory, is a family of theories, and the members of that family often disagree on philosophy and strategies. Feminist theories range from those positions that advocate adaptation of the incumbent system to make it more amenable to the progress and promotion of women's interests to those positions of radical separatist feminists.[4,5] For instance, Raymond[6] asserts that feminism means the equality of women with themselves and with all of the women who have fought for women's

Reprinted by permission from Advances in Nursing Science 13(3):1–15. © 1991, Aspen Publishers, Inc.

freedom through the ages. She feels that the issue of women's equality with men obscures the greater liberating potential that women have for empowering each other. Azizah al-Hibri[7] theorizes that prehistoric man turned to production for a sense of power when he realized he was denied the connection to immortality (menstruation and birth) that was inherent in womanhood. Eisler[8] has taken a different but related stance in using "prehistoric" evidence to show that before our aggressive, violent, and domination-oriented culture existed, there was a partnership society based on the characteristics that we now call "feminine," a type of society that can be recreated. Thus the full spectrum of feminist theory takes into account ontologic issues that go beyond the issue of oppression of women, the part of feminist theory that is particularly close to critical theory.

Similarly, critical theory encompasses many different theories and has evolved from a primarily Marxist-based scholarship to a broader emphasis on oppression in general, as well as class oppression. Similar to feminists, some critical theorists have attempted to synthesize and extend other major theories, such as those proposed by Freud, with their premises. Contemporary critical theorists encompass those who emphasize communication (followers of Habermas) and those who emphasize political action through education (followers of Freire), as well as those who espouse a variety of critical theories within other disciplines more specific in their focus. This presence of critical theorists in many different disciplines is another similarity they share with feminist theorists; thus the efforts of nurse scientists to understand and incorporate these paradigms with our own is paralleled in other areas.

The Meaning of "Method"

Controversies among nurse scientists have often focused on the appropriateness of quantitative versus qualitative methods for the conduct of nursing research.[9] Many maintain that human behaviors cannot be isolated and quantified and

that the attempt to do so results in misleading and dehumanizing outcomes rather than in knowledge that is useful for nursing practice. Some suggest, as a compromise, that quantitative and qualitative methods may each serve its own purpose—a "separate but equal" argument—whereas others insist that the two methods can be used at different stages of the same investigation.[10,11] Presently, most nurse researchers consider themselves to belong to one camp or the other, valuing one type of method while acknowledging that the other (less valued) method has its place.

Feminist research has faced questions similar to those nursing has faced concerning the relationships between ideology and method. Can research be quantitative and still be feminist in orientation? Is there a method of inquiry that can be identified as distinctly feminist? Is there a method that could not be considered feminist, regardless of the goals and underlying values of the researcher? Because women's frame of reference has been characterized as relational and contextual,[12,13] qualitative research approaches have been proposed as the only appropriate procedures for investigation of feminist phenomena, both within and outside nursing.[3,9]

Harding[3] states that confusion of the meanings of the terms "method," "methodology," and "epistemology" is at the root of much of the controversies and questions discussed previously. According to Harding, it is not the method used to gather information, but rather the unique purpose of the inquiry, the alternative explanatory hypotheses, and the altered relationships established between researcher and informer (or "subject") that make feminist research distinctive. Her conceptualization will be used to explore the questions posed in this article.

Method vs Methodology vs Epistemology

Harding defines *method* as "a technique for (or way of proceeding in) gathering evidence" and makes the argument that all such techniques can be subsumed under (1) observation, (2) listening to or questioning informants, or (3) examining records (eg, historical documents, existing texts, or medical records).[3(p2)] Each of these concretely described methods has been and can be used in new and creative ways by feminists and by nurses to produce alternative views and explanations of phenomena, but the methods themselves are not bound to a philosophical stance. Consequently they can be used from any world view; thus *the methods do not drive the assumptions.*

Methodology is defined by Harding as "a theory and analysis of how research does or should proceed."[3(p3)] Traditionally, theories of the natural and social sciences have been formulated and applied in ways that assume the masculine viewpoint as the normal viewpoint. It is a critique of methodology when feminists maintain that scientists have chosen study phenomena and explanations for those phenomena from an essentially male point of reference. Examples of feminist methodologies can be found in the discussions of how phenomenological approaches can be modified and used to investigate women's worlds[3] or how Marxist critique can be used to understand the exploitation of women in the plans for care of the community-based elderly.[14] How methods are or should be used are issues of methodology rather than of method in Harding's schema.

An *epistemology* is a theory of knowledge. Epistemology guides methodology, because epistemology concerns the questions of what can be known and who can be a knower. Can subjective truth be thought of as knowledge? Can women be knowers? Epistemology also dictates what criteria beliefs must meet to be considered knowledge and what constitutes justification, or authority against which "truth" is measured (eg, God, common sense, statistical significance, or "scientific proof").[3]

Roots of Critical Theory

Critical theory evolved in Germany during the early 1920s as a response to the technological knowledge being developed by logical positivistic science and its contribution to the oppression of the working classes. The Institute of Social Research was founded in Frankfurt in 1923 and became known as the Frankfurt School. The original group of scholars was interdisciplinary and included Max Horheimer, philosopher and social psychologist; Friedrich Pollack, economist; Theodor Adorno, philosopher and musicologist; Erich Fromm, psychologist; Herbert Marcuse, philosopher; and Leo Lowenthal, popular theorist of culture and literature. They were concerned with the insistence on deterministic objectivism advocated by the natural scientists, who accepted only empirical observations or logical deductions as knowledge.[15] Their goal was a revision of Marxism and its objectivist interpretation of historical materialism. They wanted to integrate a recognition of subjective forms of knowledge into traditional Marxism so that the perceptions and experiences of human beings, as well as "objective" observations, would be considered as having scientific value.

Epistemology of Critical Theory

In keeping with its Marxist roots, the critical theory epistemology from its inception dictated that knowledge should be used for emancipatory political aims. Lukacs,[16] an early critical theorist, believed that the purpose of theory is to analyze the difference between the actual and the possible. He saw reification, the perception that one's productive activity is something alien to one's self, as a major barrier to revolutionary consciousness. Another barrier to consciousness was ideology, belief systems that were presented and treated as facts by the ruling class as a way of controlling workers. Geuss stated that "the heart of the critical theory of society is its criticism of ideology. Ideology is what prevents the agents in the society from correctly perceiving their true situation and real interests."[17(p3)] Thus the goal of critical theory was to nullify the effects of ideology so that the agents' perceptions were freed or "emancipated" to evaluate their true situation. "A critical theory, then, is a reflective theory which gives a kind of knowledge inherently productive of enlightenment and emancipation."[17(p2)]

Because perceptions are greatly influenced by past experiences and culture, critical theory epistemology maintains that standards of truth or evidence are always social and that social life itself is structured by meaning (ie, by rules, conventions, and habits).[1] All meaning and all truth are interpreted within the context of history. History includes the time and other occurrences that contribute to the significance of individual events. Therefore understanding patterns of human behavior involves an understanding of societal structures, such as class structures, which are more important in critical theory epistemology than individual personal meanings. This is a key difference in the epistemologies of critical theory and phenomenology. For the critical theorist, personal meanings are shaped by societal structures and communication processes and are therefore all too often ideologic, historically bound, and distorted.

Methodologic Issues in Critical Theory

To make the epistemological statement that standards of truth are always social (ie, that they are based on negotiation and agreement by a community) would, in Harding's schema, assume certain ensuing methodologies or statements about how research does or should proceed. For instance, agreement about a meaning (or consent to participate) by participants would have to be free from both conscious and unconscious constraints in order to reach the most correct decision. If agreement by participants is coerced, even by hidden ideology, it is not a responsible representative contribution from the community—in effect, not an agreement at all.

The idea of coming to an agreement or negotiation sets the stage for the kind of dialogue that characterizes the interaction between a researcher and the person from whom data is gathered in a critical theory investigation.[18] Because of the emphasis on emancipatory action as an outcome, we believe that an appropriate term

for that other person in the critical theory paradigm is "agent." Obviously this contrasts with the use of the term "subject" in logical positivism and "informant" in naturalistic inquiry.

In the critical theory paradigm, knowledge, or warranted belief, is not discoverable or universal but is created, and its creation and interpretation are grounded in language.[1] This epistemology has implications for the methodology of the study to explore that created knowledge and the language used to communicate it. Either an interview or a text review could be used, with careful attention given to the level of understanding of language as well as to the symbolic and value-laden nature of the words and their meanings to the agent or author. Interviews take the form of dialogue wherein the researcher and agent negotiate and decide together on meanings. Thus, rather than concentrating on the subject's personal meanings, as in phenomenology, the meanings evolve from both the researcher and the agent.

If one's epistemology involves belief that the purpose of knowledge is to release the individual from domination (emancipate) and to further autonomy and responsibility, as is the case in critical theory, then one would expect analysis to be designed to expose hidden power imbalances and enlighten agents about how they ought rationally to act to realize their own best interests.[17-19] Methods, or techniques of gathering information based on this epistemological stance, would include a dialogue similar to that in Freire's *Pedagogy of the Oppressed*.[20] Reflective interviews using "dialogic introspection" were used by McLain[2] to encourage subjects to be aware of the power relationships in collaborative practice situations and to approach the "ideal" open communication advocated by Habermas.[21]

Actually, the most frequent kind of method used by critical theorists has been critical review or "critique." The majority of writings of the critical theorists have been examinations of existing knowledge in various fields using the historical and political context of that knowledge development as background for the "immanent analysis." Adorno[22] described this type of critique as an analysis of the degree of consistency of the interpretations (social opinions) of respondents to questionnaires with the reality of their social structure, a social structure not apparent to the respondents, who are therefore only restating ideology. It was clearly up to the critical theorist to decipher the ideology or determine the "social illusion" in order to juxtapose these subjective findings with objective ones and find a new theory to illuminate the whole.[22(pp254,256)] Even though later critical theorists, such as Habermas and Freire, emphasized the dialogic process toward mutual enlightenment, the assumption can be made that agents (the oppressed) begin the process as less emancipated than the theorists.[20,21] This attitude can result in paternalism, a problem for feminists also.

Characteristics of Feminist Theory

In exploring a world view categorized here as "feminist," we are attempting to describe a frame of reference often associated with women. Yet biologic female sex is neither necessary nor sufficient to be a feminist, as this paradigm could be espoused by either men or women, and many women would find it untenable.

Characteristics of a feminist approach to theory and research identified by Lengermann and Niebrugge-Brantley[23] include a women-centeredness in that (1) women's experiences are the major "object" of investigation, (2) the goal of inquiry is to see the world from the vantage point of a particular group of women, and (3) it is critical and activist in its effort to improve the lot of women and all persons. In addition to these characteristics, dominant threads and patterns that appear and reappear in feminist writing include (1) unity and relatedness of perception, (2) contextual orientation, and (3) emphasis on the subjective.

UNITY AND RELATEDNESS

A feminist world view tends to reject dichotomies and exclusive categories. Women are less comfortable with absolutes than are men,

and they tend to blur the boundaries of their experiences. The personal is political in the minds of women, and they do not make sharp distinctions between work values and personal values or between theory and practice.[24,25] Wheeler and Chinn describe an integration in which "knowing and doing are the same."[26(p7)]

CONTEXTUAL ORIENTATION

It is characteristic of the world view of women that not only do they value personal human relationships, but they also look for and selectively perceive relationships between objects, ideas, and actions. Wheeler and Chinn[26] state that feminist thought is oriented to the power of the whole as opposed to the power of division. Harding and Hintikka[27] point out that women are less likely than men to think in terms of independent discrete units. As an extension of this propensity for context, feminist theory has introduced historicity, materiality, and values as fundamental categories of knowledge.

EMPHASIS ON THE SUBJECTIVE

Women value the lived experience, including the feelings, of themselves and other women. For this they are often accused of being "unscientific" in the logical positivistic sense of science. Women have been known to ignore "hard" data and make decisions on the basis of empirical evidence from their own lives—harking back to the intuitive sense of reality that has provided women with the courage to refute damaging masculine constructions of womanhood throughout history.

CENTRALITY OF GENDER AND IDEALISM

Very consistent throughout feminist theory is the emphasis on gender. Women provide both the object of study, planning, and concern and the subjective framework through which to view the world.[23,26] Critical in the sense of confronting issues and activist in its stance of fighting for a better world for women (and therefore for humanity), feminist theory is idealistic and optimistic in orientation.[23] This quality of idealistic optimism is expressed by Bartky, an existential philosopher, when she describes feminist consciousness as the "apprehension of possibility."[28(p254)] Feminist theorists struggle to communicate their dream, because they have hope for a better future for women and for all. The emphasis is on development, growth, and change—always change for the better—promoted by nonviolent means. Feminist idealism embraces the vision of peace and cessation of racism and class exploitation. Men credited with such feminist attributes by Eisler[8] are Martin Luther King, Jr and Ghandi. Many people believe the time has come to implement the feminist principles of nurturing and conservation to save the earth from ecological devastation.

Epistemology in Feminist Theory

Epistemological issues, or issues regarding adequate theory of knowledge or justification strategy in feminist theory, that derive from the characteristics discussed previously include

- women's experience can be a legitimate source of knowledge—women can be knowers;
- subjective data are valid;
- informants are "experts" on their own lives;
- knowledge is relational and contextual; and
- definitive boundaries between personal and public or personal and political spheres are artificial, as are sharp distinctions between theory and practice.[24–26]

Additional issues addressed by Harding include bias that can exist in the research questions, as well as in the conduct and interpretation of research; thus research questions in the past have addressed questions others wanted answered about women.[3] The questions and the interpretation of the "answers" are very much influenced by the point of view of the person(s) asking the questions. It follows that the researcher's point of view (ie, background, eth-

nic and social class) will greatly affect the analysis and therefore should be included as part of the data. This is part of the "reflexive" research stance that Harding advocates, a stance that also recognizes that all women experience patriarchy differently and that all of the consequent divergent viewpoints are valid.[29] Thus one woman's "emancipation" may not look at all like another woman's. This position better deals with the paternalism previously mentioned and the criticism that the "women's movement" does not represent all women as it was originally formulated.

Methodologic Issues in Feminist Theory

Based on the previous epistemological assumptions, the methodologic conditions include

- research should be based on women's experiences,[3] and the validity of women's perceptions as the "truth" for them should be recognized;
- artificial dichotomies and sharp boundaries are suspect in research involving women and other humans and should be carefully scrutinized;
- the context and relationships of phenomena, such as history and concurrent events, should always be considered in designing, conducting, and interpreting research;
- researchers should recognize that the questions asked are at least as important as the answers obtained ("discovery" and "justification" in Harding's terminology[3]);
- research should address questions women want answered (ie, should be *for* women);
- the researcher's point of view (ie, biases, background, and ethnic and social class) should be described and treated as part of the data, one aspect of ensuring that the researcher is on a plane with the researched;
- research should be nonhierarchical; informants and researchers should be partners;

therefore the term "participant" is an appropriate term for the other person electing to be a part of a research study; and

- interpretations of observations by the researcher should be validated by and shared with the participants so that they may benefit from the research in which they have taken part.

It is these issues of epistemology and methodology and the paradigms from which they spring, not the information-gathering and analytic techniques (ie, methods), that give research investigations the characteristics of feminist research, critical theory, or naturalistic or empirical analytical inquiry.[3]

Differences and Commonalities of Critical and Feminist Theories

Table 32-1 shows some of the similarities and differences in critical and feminist theories. The categories presented are not strictly parallel, and there are subtle variations in language, as well as obvious distinctions. At the ontological level, the beliefs stated are neither mutually exclusive nor necessarily contradictory, but rather are a reflection of the emphasis heard in the collective voices of the two paradigms.

GENDER, CLASS, AND RACE

Although both critical and feminist theories are emancipatory in that they seek to free individuals from conscious and unconscious constraints that interfere with full participation in social interaction,[30] feminist theory is distinguished in that it focuses on women. Feminist theory has the primary goal of presenting a woman-centered patterning of human experience.[23] As pointed out by Fraser,[31] the original critical theorists did not consider gender issues any more than did any of the other androcentric scientific paradigms. Even though contemporary critical theorists are now broadening their approach to include gender issues, gender is not central in critical theory.

Feminists agree with critical theorists that knowledge is socially constructed and that it does not exist outside of the context in which it was created. Both believe that the understanding of patterns of human behavior involves the understanding of both the personal meanings of social structures and the communally agreed upon meanings of those structures. Both agree that social structures can and have resulted in class oppression, but feminists choose division and domination according to gender as the fundamental oppression, although recognizing that

TABLE 32-1. Similarities and differences in feminist and critical theories

Parameter	Feminist Theory	Critical Theory
Ontology (nature of reality, human beings)	Spiritual, physical, relational universe God/dess/nature/humans not separate but intertwined	Reality constructed Human beings capable of rational self-critique
Epistemology (knowledge is:)	Personal is political; affective as important as cognitive Relational, contextual Woman-centered (vs androcentric) Nondichotomous, indivisible	Subjective, rational emphasized Constructed, communal, contextual Emancipatory (vs technical) Disempowered as knowers
Methodology (should to obtain knowledge, do research)	Dialogic if obtaining information from participants Critique of androcentrism and racism Nonhierarchical Validation and sharing with participants	Dialogic if obtaining information from agents Critique of ideology Reveal hidden power imbalances

often it is not the most important oppression for individual women at particular points in time. Feminist theory sees androcentric bias as central, with racism, ethnocentrism, and classism equally problematic but having developed consequent (but within the same historical period) to gender domination.[8] An equally viable stance is that structures of racial domination are central, but this involves a different, although related, paradigm from either critical or feminist theory, with its own epistemology and methodology. In fact, much of contemporary critical theory has moved away from class division as primary and toward a consideration of all forms of oppression together.[30] This is a useful alternative but still different from feminism, which sees Marxist feminism, socialist feminism, and feminism of women of color as different members of the same family.

The recognition of racism as a crucial oppressive mechanism both historically and presently was an important development in both critical and feminist theory and long overdue in both paradigms.[32,33] The addition of the writing and thinking of feminist women of color has immeasurably enriched and radically altered feminist theory. The current scholarly debate on racism, encouraged within feminism with leadership provided by those most fundamentally affected, is not a part of critical theory.

KNOWLEDGE AND UNDERSTANDING

Both feminist and critical theory orientations see historical and contextual influences as important components of information. Both schools of thought endorse subjective perceptions and experiences as knowledge. One of the contrasts between them is an emphasis on rationality in critical theory, whereas in feminist inquiry feelings are also included, respected, valued, and seen as having emancipatory potential. Even Bernstein, a contemporary scholar in the critical tradition who is moving beyond such dualisms in theory, rests his premises on logical arguments, whereas feminist theorists are more likely to use and clearly appeal to emotions in their work and to be criticized for it.[34] Furthermore the epistemologic feminist premise that knowledge cannot be separated into dichotomies and categories generally has not been an emphasis in critical theory.

Another distinction is that critical theory is most interested in knowledge for the emancipation of all humanity or of particular oppressed groups, whereas feminist theory is equally interested in knowledge to improve the condition of any one individual woman. This can be considered an extension of the importance of the personal in feminist thought.

METHODOLOGIES AND METHODS

A related contrast is also based on the importance of the personal and of the individual. Feminist theorists insist on sharing their insights with other women, both their fellow participants in research inquiry and all women. One means of accomplishing this goal is writing research results in language and sources accessible to everyone, as well as in scholarly journals. The original critical theorists wrote for the intellectual world, although some spoke at activist gatherings. They envisioned a world where their level of discourse would be common when class oppression ended, but this is difficult to imagine from the difficulty of the early writings. Even though contemporary critical theorists such as Ryan[33] have made their critique accessible to all, this approach has yet to be widespread or articulated as a critical theory methodology.

In terms of methodology, the feminist condition that researchers and participants should be equal partners would be, and probably should be, critiqued by critical theorists as another example of hidden power imbalances (D Allen, personal communication, 1990). Almost always there are members of the "research team" who have more power than others, and it is equally likely that the researcher(s) will make more of the important decisions about the process than will the participants. The "equal plane" may be a useful ideal, but it is extremely difficult to realize in practice.

At the level of method, both critical and feminist scholars have extensively used critique to analyze prior knowledge and to create new knowledge. Both have been subject to criticism for lack of new theory because of their reliance on critique as method. However, there is much current activity in feminist branches of many disciplines, using dialogic research in many different forms. Critical theory investigations that use dialogue are scarce. In fact, nursing's use of critical theory has generated two of the only investigations found in the literature that use dialogue with observation.[2,35]

The primary means of knowledge generation in critical theory has been a type of record review, or review of previous scientific writings. Habermas describes critical theory as a combination of empirical analytic and hermeneutic methods, with the addition of careful reflection on the nature of the knowledge toward emancipatory enlightenment.[36,37] Thus it would be a mistake to characterize critical theory (or feminist theory) as a qualitative research method or as sharing the assumptions of a "qualitative paradigm." Critical theorists censure logical positivists (and adherents of hermeneutics) for their insistence that their research is the only source of true knowledge. The other two major criticisms of logical positivism in critical theory are the use (rather than the nature) of empirical analytic knowledge primarily for technology and further oppression rather than for emancipation, and the lack of recognition of subject as object. All of these concerns are shared by feminists.

Feminist and Critical Theory Methods in an Investigation

To further illustrate the differences between critical and feminist theory epistemologies and resultant methodologies, we will briefly describe how one of our published investigations would have been differentially shaped by the two world views. The research report "A Test of Two Explanatory Models of Women's Responses to

Battering" describes research that was actually influenced by both critical and feminist theory, but overtly acknowledged neither.[38] In both the critical and feminist theory approaches, the investigator would have clearly stated the political purpose, which was to combat some of the clinical and scientific stigma attached to battered women and to create knowledge emancipatory to women experiencing male violence.

Both the critical and feminist paradigms would have critically examined the theories tested (learned helplessness and grief) in light of the historical origins of these frameworks, and both would have discussed the oppression that has been generated from each framework. Especially pertinent would be the purely behavioral origins, laboratory research tradition, and the uses of learned helplessness. The learned helplessness theory, as applied to battered women, has contributed to their derogatory public image and to the assumption of a pathologic influence on the part of clinicians and researchers. The grief theory, however, has feminist origins, and the image conveyed by the label is more normative. A critical theory orientation would have focused strongly on these linguistic connotations of pathology versus normalcy, whereas a feminist critique of these theoretic origins would have concentrated on the androcentric biases of learned helplessness theory, even though its best known clinical group application has been to women (abused women and, more recently, incest survivors). This application has served to further emphasize presumed "feminine" characteristics and to denigrate the women involved. A feminist analysis would also highlight the inconsistencies in the theory that arise, in part, from inadequate explanations of gender differences in research results.

Critical theory would have emphasized class issues more, in terms of purpose, critique of existing knowledge, data analysis using social class as a variable, and interpretation of findings in terms of class oppression. The individual intrapsychic variables (ie, depression, self-esteem) would probably not have been measured, and more attention would have been paid to the oppressive nature of employment and educational opportunities. A feminist perspective would have been less interested in class and more interested in cultural variations. The feminist perspective would have been more likely to focus on the personal in terms of (1) demonstrating normalcy of response (comparison with other women in problematic relationships both by written report and by discussions with individual women), (2) providing clinical expertise for those emotionally troubled, and (3) explicit recognition that the personal is political.

A further distinction would be in terms of how the dialogue with participants would have been conducted. A critical theorist would be interested in all the women and would leave the dialogue with an increased understanding of their oppression within the relationship and within society. A feminist theorist would give the actual participants the kind of information and support that they sought within the interview process. If they wished to frame their experience in wider political terms, the investigator would discuss these aspects with them, but if they wanted to discuss their experience at a purely personal level, the researcher did nothing to alter that perspective. They would also be given support for whatever course of action they decided on (after having been given safety information), so that the notion of research directed toward emancipation would be performed according to how each woman defined her trajectory, rather than according to the definition of the researcher. Thus the ideal of researcher and participant being on the "same plane" would at least be attempted. If they desired it, women would also be given information about their scores on standardized instruments (measuring depression and self-esteem) as an empowerment strategy. Finally, the results of the study would be mailed to participants who wished to have them, and the investigator would work to publicize the results in media accessible to women (radio and television talk shows). This course of information transmittal would not be considered as important in the critical theory tradition as would scholarly publication.

Thus the research described would have important differences depending on the epistemology and resulting methodology chosen. However, the "bottom line" for both paradigms is creating and using knowledge for emancipation. In the study that was actually performed, normed instruments and sophisticated statistics were used in order to plead the case for the normalcy of battered women in a world where statistics are more persuasive. Empirical evidence is needed to refute oppressive theories that have been developed from empirical evidence, unless the only interest is to convince the already converted.[39] The women in the study also found normed instruments extremely useful in judging for themselves how they were responding in comparison with other women. The combination of in-depth interviews with instrumentation was used to ensure that individual women gained the information they sought from the experience and to provide the kind of context necessary for subjectivity. It was not primarily an attempt at "triangulation" as a methodologic stance. Thus, although the methods did not necessarily reflect the paradigm of the researcher, the actual implementation of the study (methodology) and the epistemology from which the study was conceived reflected the investigator's commitment to emancipation.

• • • • • •

Idealism characterizes both feminists and critical theorists. Both envision a world in which equality enables all individuals to enjoy prosperity and well being, a "transformation of society." Critical theory was rediscovered in this country during the 1960s, when traditional sources of knowledge were being questioned; the same era began the "second wave" of feminism. From that historical reality, which also generated a shared awareness and interest in Marxism, came some of the shared epistemology of the current forms of each. In terms of historical context, there were other eras when class and gender interests joined to struggle against joint oppression (eg, the French Revolution), but women always found that their concerns eventually took a lesser priority, because the acknowledged leaders of each movement were men. Thus the historical context, an important source of knowledge insisted on by both paradigms, indicates the importance of differentiation as well as connections.

Both of these relevant and powerful world views have the potential to shape nursing science so that it is emancipatory as well as knowledge generative.[40] In other disciplines, critical and feminist theorists meet and write in separate forums. Discourse and mutual information shared between the two are needed, and in this respect nursing seems to be ahead of other disciplines. However, there is no need to blur the distinctions between the two. Just as we are making differentiations between logical positivism and naturalistic inquiry, we need to be self-reflectively aware of what these more emancipatory paradigms are and are not and of their differences as well as their common ground.

REFERENCES

1. Allen D, Benner P, Diekelmann NL. Three paradigms for nursing research: Methodological implications. In: Chinn PL, ed. *Nursing Research Methodology: Issues and Implementation*. Rockville, Md: Aspen; 1986.
2. McLain BR. Collaborative practice: A critical theory perspective. *Res Nurs Health*. 1988;11: 391–398.
3. Harding S. Introduction: Is there a feminist model? In: Harding S, ed. *Feminism and Methodology*. Bloomington, Ind: Indiana University Press; 1987.
4. Bunting SM., Campbell JC. Feminism and nursing: Historical perspectives. *ANS*. 1990;12(4): 11–24.
5. Donovan J. *Feminist Theory: The Intellectual Traditions of American Feminism*. New York, NY: Frederick Ungar; 1985.
6. Raymond JG. *A Passion for Friends: Toward a Philosophy of Female Affection*. Boston, Mass: Beacon Press; 1986.
7. al-Hibri A. Capitalism is an advanced stage of patriarchy: But Marxism is not feminism. In: Sargent L., ed. *Women and Revolution: A Discussion of the Unhappy Marriage of Marxism and Feminism*. Boston, Mass: South End; 1981.
8. Eisler R. *The Chalice & the Blade: Our History, Our Future*. San Francisco, Calif: Harper & Row; 1988.
9. Moccia P. A critique of compromise: Beyond the methods debate. *ANS*. 1988;10(4):1–9.
10. Tripp-Reimer T. Combining qualitative and quantitative methodologies. In: Leininger MM, ed. *Qualitative Research Methods in Nursing*. Orlando, Fla: Grune & Stratton; 1985.
11. Porter EJ. The qualitative-quantitative dualism. *Image*. 1989;21(2):98–102.
12. Belenky MF, Clinchy BM, Goldberger NR, Tarule JM. *Women's Ways of Knowing*. New York, NY: Basic Books; 1986.
13. Gilligan C. *In a Different Voice: Psychological Theory and Women's Development*. Cambridge, Mass: Harvard University Press; 1982.
14. Ward D. Gender and cost in caring. Paper presented at the Caring and Nursing Explorations in the Feminist Perspectives Conference, Denver, Colo, October 1988. Sponsored by the School of Nursing, University of Colorado.
15. Ritzer G. *Contemporary Sociological Theory*. 2nd ed. New York, NY: Alfred A. Knopf; 1988.
16. Held D. *Introduction to Critical Theory*. London, England: Hutchinson; 1980.
17. Geuss R. *The Idea of Critical Theory*. Cambridge, Mass: Cambridge University Press; 1981.
18. Lather P. Research as praxis. *Harvard Educ Rev*. 1986;56(3):257–277.
19. Holter IM. Critical theory: A foundation for the development of nursing theories. *Schol Inquiry Nurs Pract*. 1988;2:223–232.
20. Freire P. *Pedagogy of the Oppressed*. New York, NY: Continuum Publishing Co; 1989.
21. Habermas J. *Knowledge and Human Interests*. Boston, Mass: Beacon; 1971.
22. Adorno TW. Subject and object. In: Arato A, Gebhardt E, eds. *The Essential Frankfurt School Reader*. Oxford, England: Basil Blackwell; 1978.
23. Lengermann PM, Niebrugge-Brantley J. Contemporary feminist theory. In: Ritzer G, ed. *Contemporary Sociological Theory*. 2nd ed. New York, NY: Alfred A. Knopf; 1988.
24. de Lauretis T, ed. *Feminist Studies/Critical Studies*. Bloomington, Ind: University of Indiana Press; 1986.
25. Hartsock N. Fundamental feminism: Process and perspective. In: Bunch C, ed. *Building Feminist Theory: Essays from Quest a Feminist Quarterly*. New York, NY: Longman; 1981.
26. Wheeler CE, Chinn PL. *Peace & Power: A Handbook of Feminist Process*. Buffalo, NY: Margaretdaughters; 1984.
27. Harding S, Hintikka MB. *Discovering Reality: Feminist Perspectives on Epistemology, Metaphysics,*

Methodology, and Philosophy of Science. Dordrecht, Holland: Reidel Publishing; 1983.

28. Bartky SL. Toward a phenomenology of feminist consciousness. In: Bishop S, Weinzeweig M, eds. *Philosophy and Women.* Belmont, Calif: Wadsworth; 1979.

29. Harding S. Common causes: Toward a *reflexive* feminist theory. *Women Politics.* 1983;3(4):27–42.

30. Allen D. Nursing research and social control: Alternative models of science that emphasize understanding and emancipation. *Image.* 1985;17(2): 58–74.

31. Fraser N. What's critical about critical theory? In: Benebad S, Cornell D, eds. *Feminism as Critique.* Minneapolis, Minn: University of Minnesota Press; 1987.

32. Hooks B. *Feminist Theory: From Margin to Center.* Boston, Mass: South End Press; 1984.

33. Ryan W. *Equality.* New York, NY: Pantheon Books; 1981.

34. Bernstein R. *Beyond Objectivism and Relativism Science, Hermeneutics, and Praxis.* Philadelphia, Penn: University of Pennsylvania Press; 1983.

35. Hedin BA. A case study of oppressed group behavior in nurses. *Image.* 1986;18(2):53–57.

36. Habermas J. Theory and practice in a scientific society. In: Connerton P, ed. *Critical Sociology.* New York, NY: Penguin; 1976.

37. Adorno TW. Sociology and empirical research. In: Connerton P, ed. *Critical Sociology.* New York, NY: Penguin; 1976.

38. Campbell JC. A test of two explanatory models of women's responses to battering. *Nurs Res.* 1989; 38(1):18–24.

39. Yllo K. Political and methodological debates in wife abuse research. In: Yllo K, Bograd M, eds. *Feminist Perspectives on Wife Abuse.* Newbury Park, Calif: Sage; 1988.

40. Thompson JL. Critical scholarship: The critique of domination in nursing. *ANS.* 1987;10(1):27–38.

SCIENCE AND GENDER

Marylouise Welch

Since the nineteenth century, the natural sciences have commanded an unparalleled position of dominance in our thinking about what we consider to be important knowledge. In some arenas they have replaced religion as the final arbiter of what is truth. As this book has shown, various scholars during the twentieth century began to critique science's unquestioned supremacy. Habermas and the Frankfurt school began some of the critique of science that resonates for feminist theorists. In that critique, the examination of current scientific knowledge, its methods, scope and questions are revealed as socially embedded political practices that are not separable from the knowledge of the producer. Knowledge produced by the sciences is part of the social and political traditions within which its production occurred.

WOMEN IN SCIENTIFIC STUDIES

In the 1970s feminist scholarship began to emerge as other philosophers of science (Feyerabend, 1975) were writing that scientific observation is never value free, never innocent, but always influenced by the interaction of the observed and the observer. In fact, observation is not theory-neutral but rather theory-laden. One example of this emerging critique was the work of Gilligan (1982), which called into question the moral development theories of Kohlberg (1971). She found in her explorations with women facing moral decisions that his hierarchical categories of moral reasoning did not fit the patterns women used to make moral choices. Yet he had developed a hierarchy that he put forth as universal. If you combine with this perspective the concerns of the various avenues of feminist thought, one has a call for a new view of science.

Where to begin to conceptualize science as nonmasculine has permeated the debate on science and gender. It seems daunting when the history of Western thought is a history of male Western thought and therefore, so much of our language, concepts and frameworks are rooted in a male perspective (Bleier, 1986).

Harding (1986) has identified certain salient findings from feminist critiques that are germane to the issue of science and gender. These discoveries include the historical resistance of Western civilization to women's education. One need only examine the history of nursing education for a clear example. Second, scientific findings have been used to support sexist ideology. Scientific theories include many studies of women's biological inability to think in the same manner as men. Because women's brains are physically smaller, and because it was believed that their ovaries and uteri required extra energy to provide for continuation of the species, they were cast as less capable intellectually. Therefore, they were incapable of sophisticated thought, and they were only fit to be mothers (Genova, 1988; Love & Hubbard, 1983). Then there is the concern articulated by Gilligan (1982), which is the total absence of women from the scientific sample, and yet findings are generalized to include all of humanity. Men's values have influenced the selection of scientific questions, methods and interpretations of the findings. These revelations lead to the question, if women had been dominant in science, how would it be different, and if women become more active, how will it be different in the future?

SCIENTIFIC OBSERVATIONS AS VALUE LADEN

Relevant to this line of thinking is the work of Barbara McClintock, who describes her scientific enterprise in different terms from the prevailing voices of the dominant scientific community (Keller, 1983). During McClintock's era she was an outsider to the community of scientists but maintained her own views on how to study maize and genetics.

Keller argues that McClintock's work was devalued because of her observational stance: personal connection with her maize. How could she be objective and establish a neutral theory with such closeness to the object under study? McClintock describes her approach as dwelling amongst the objects (maize) she studies as she shortens the distance between herself (the observer) and the maize (the observed). She maintains a reverence for the maize and seeks to achieve harmony through understanding it. She uses nondomineering, nonhierarchical language. She does not seek to conquer nature but to understand and coexist with it. It is a difficult and lonely position to maintain such an independent stance, but in doing so she was a pioneer calling into question the authority of Western science.

McClintock's independence helped to reveal how, while claiming that science is observing nature in a value-free context, it was failing to acknowledge the extraordinary power of its androcentric bias and assumptions and how they played out politically to determine what is in fact scientific. In describing McClintock's' science and life, Keller (Genova, 1988; Keller, 1983) is describing how science grew from a world full of specific ideological views about gender that has affected the culture of the scientific endeavor. Knowledge is in fact the product of social interaction among members of a community.

In continuing the train of thought of science as historically maintaining an all-male perspective, some authors have raised the issue of who defines what is science? In this anthology, Ginzberg (1989) gives credence to the idea that there have been women scientists throughout history, but due to their powerless positions in society, they were unable to move forward with their work and ideas. They were not a part of the dominant community with the power to determine what constitutes knowledge. One classic writing on this topic is the work of Ehrenreich and English (1973) on witches and midwifery. In this work it is clear that the work of these women in the middle ages was as scientific as anything being done by physicians at universities. Ginzberg believes they were the real empirical scientists of the time. With the advent of obstetrics their oral tradition was steamrolled, some of their knowledge was lost, they were devalued, ridiculed and eventually not allowed to practice. The worst scenario was to vilify them as witches. This historical example makes clear the androcentric value-laden analysis of what constitutes knowledge.

How to recover from this oppressive history and move on with the work of Ehrenreich and English (1973) in restoring the woman's perspective has caused great debate. Feminist theory began by trying to be more rigorous, to use the existing scientific models better in order to become visible within the prevailing scientific discourse. Harding (1987) believes it is impossible to capture accurate knowledge by reinterpreting existing theories that were based on a gender bias view of the world.

However, she also believes that for science to turn its attention now to do exclusively feminist research is not useful. We need to get to a place where scientific endeavors are investigating all humans in order to create useful theories about the nature of our world. It appears that multiple models and research strategies are what is needed. Harding has written extensively about method and feminist research and concluded that there is no one method that is sufficient to capture all of human knowledge (Harding, 1987). What we need to do is find ways to create human science that is inclusive while not totally reducing knowledge to relativity. To be successful, Harding calls for a reflexivity in the scientific process that will put the researcher on the same plane as the object of study, similar to the work of McClintock. Chinn (1998) discusses the effects on the nursing profession of the socially assigned stereotypes of females. If feminist inquiry pushes the scientific community to transcend gender, it will have made a profound contribution to the development of scientific knowledge.

CONCLUSION

As researchers and theoreticians continue to explore the relationship between science and gender, certain common values and beliefs emerge. This is a call for science with a human face where we cooperate with rather than conquer nature, and is a place for scientific inquiry that is not hierarchical, anti-dualistic and allows for difference. It requires a recognition that gender is socially constructed and that all scientific knowledge is grounded in an historical context, which is partial and embodied. The dream of absolute truth is, in the end, only a dream (Keller & Longino 1996).

Nursing has been historically the undervalued part of women's work that has been relegated to art. Its traditions have been oral, invisible, nonhierarchical, suppressed and discredited, and deemed not scientific (Ginzberg, 1989). The feminist critique of gender and science opens a domain of inquiry full of creative opportunity, ripe for nursing's voice and nursing science discoveries.

DISCUSSION GUIDE

1. Describe the three feminist epistemologies: feminist standpoint, feminist empiricism and postmodern feminism.
2. Discuss the role of language as metaphor in gender and science issues. How does McClintock's use of language transform scientific endeavors?

3. Are gender characteristics biologically determined, socially constructed or both?
4. How can nursing use the insights gained from the feminist critique of gender and science to advance nursing science?
5. How does Ginzberg's description of gynocentric science influence the path nursing science should pursue?

REFERENCES

Bleier, R. E. (1986). *Feminist approaches to science*. New York: Pergamon Press.

Chinn, P. L. (1998). Gender and nursing science. In E. C. Polifroni, & M. Welch (Eds.). *Perspectives on philosophy of science in nursing: An historical and contemporary anthology* (pp. 462–468. Philadelphia: Lippincott–Raven.

Ehrenreich, B., & English, D. (1973). *Witches, midwives, and nurses: A history of women healers*. Old Westbury, NY: The Feminist Press.

Feyerabend, P. (1975). *Against method*. London: Verso.

Genova, J. (1988). Women and the mismeasure of thought. *Hypatia, 3* (1):101–117.

Gilligan, C. (1982). *In a different voice*. Cambridge: Harvard University Press.

Ginzberg, R. (1989). Uncovering gynocentric science. In N. Tuma (Ed.), *Feminsim and science*. Bloomington: Indiana University Press.

Harding, S. (1986). *The science question in feminism*. Ithaca: Cornell University Press.

Harding, S. (1987). The method question. *Hypatia, 2* (3):19–35.

Keller, E. F. (1983). *A feeling for the organism: The life and work of Barbara McClintock*. New York: Freeman.

Keller, E. F., & Longino, H. E. (Eds.). (1996). *Feminism and science*. Oxford: Oxford University Press.

Kohlberg, L. (1971). From is to ought: How to commit the naturalistic fallacy and get away with it in the study of moral development. In Mischel (Ed.), *Cognitive development and epistemology*. New York: Academic Press.

Love, M., & Hubbard, R. (Eds.). (1983). *Women's nature: Rationalization of inequality*. New York: Pergamon Press.

BIBLIOGRAPHY

Dickson, G. (1993). The unintended consequences of a male professional ideology for the development of nursing education. *Advances in Nursing Science, 15* (3):67–83.

Harding, S., & Hintikka, M. (Eds.). (1978). *Discovering reality: Feminist perspectives on epistemologies, metaphysics, methodology, and philosophy of science*. Dodrecht, Holland: D. Reidel Publishing Company.

Harding, S. (Ed.). (1987). *Feminism and methodology*. Bloomington: Indiana University Press.

Harding, S. (1991). *Whose science? Whose knowledge? Thinking from women's lives*. Ithaca: Cornell University Press.

Hubbard, R., & Lowe, M. (1979). *Genes and gender*. New York: Gordian Press.

Keller, E. F. (1985). *Reflections on gender and science*. New Haven: Yale University Press.

Rose, H. (1983). Hand, brain and heart: A feminist epistemology for the natural sciences. *Signs: Journal of Women in Culture and Society, 9*:73–90.

Spender, D. (1981). *Men's studies modified: The impact of feminism on the academic disciplines*. Oxford, UK: Pergamon.

Tuana, N. (Ed.). (1989). *Feminism and science*. Bloomington: Indiana University Press.

Gender and Science

Evelyn Fox Keller

I. Introduction

> The requirements of . . . correctness in practical judgements and objectivity in theoretical knowledge . . . belong as it were in their form and their claims to humanity in general, but in their actual historical configuration they are masculine throughout. Supposing that we describe these things, viewed as absolute ideas, by the single word 'objective', we then find that in the history of our race the equation objective = masculine is a valid one (George Simmel, quoted by Horney, 1926, p. 200).

In articulating the commonplace, Simmel steps outside of the convention of academic discourse. The historically pervasive association between masculine and objective, more specifically between masculine and scientific, is a topic which academic critics resist taking seriously. Why is that? Is it not odd that an association so familiar and so deeply entrenched is a topic only for informal discourse, literary allusion, and popular criticism? How is it that formal criticism in the philosophy and sociology of science has failed to see here a topic requiring analysis? The virtual silence of at least the nonfeminist academic community on this subject suggests that the association of masculinity with scientific thought has the status of a myth which either cannot or should not be examined seriously. It has simultaneously the air of being "self-evident" and "nonsensical"—the former by virtue of existing in the realm of common knowledge (i.e., everyone knows it), and the latter by virtue of lying outside the realm of formal knowledge, indeed conflicting with our image of science as emotionally and sexually neutral. Taken seriously, it would suggest that, were more women to engage in science, a different science might emerge. Such an idea, although sometimes expressed by nonscientists, clashes openly with the formal view of science as being uniquely determined by its own logical and empirical methodology.

The survival of mythlike beliefs in our thinking about science, the very archetype of antimyth, ought, it would seem, to invite our curiosity and demand investigation. Unexamined myths, wherever they survive, have a subterranean potency; they affect our thinking in ways we are not aware of, and to the extent that we lack awareness, our capacity to resist their influence is undermined. The presence of the mythical in science seems particularly inappropriate. What is it doing there? From where does it come? And how does it influence our conceptions of science, of objectivity, or, for that matter, of gender?

These are the questions I wish to address, but before doing so it is necessary to clarify and

This article first appeared in Psychoanalysis and Contemporary Thought 1, 3 (1978), published by New York International Universities Press, Inc., New York, NY.

From *Discovering Reality* (pp. 187–205) edited by Sandra Harding and Merrill B. Hintikka. Copyright © 1983. Reprinted with kind permission from Kluwer Academic Publishers.

elaborate the system of beliefs in which science acquires a gender—which amount to a "genderization" of science. Let me make clear at the outset that the issue which requires discussion is *not,* or at least not simply, the relative absence of women in science. While it is true that most scientists have been, and continue to be, men, the make-up of the scientific population hardly accounts, by itself, for the attribution of masculinity to science as an intellectual domain. Most culturally validated intellectual and creative endeavors have, after all, historically been the domain of men. Few of these endeavors, however, bear so unmistakably the connotation of masculine in the very nature of the activity. To both scientists and their public, scientific thought is male thought, in ways that painting and writing—also performed largely by men—have never been. As Simmel observed, objectivity itself is an ideal which has a long history of identification with masculine. The fact that the scientific population is, even now, a population that is overwhelmingly male, is itself a consequence rather than a cause of the attribution of masculinity to scientific thought.[1] What requires discussion is a *belief* rather than a reality, although the ways in which reality is shaped by our beliefs are manifold, and also need articulating.

How does this belief manifest itself? It used to be commonplace to hear scientists, teachers, and parents assert quite baldly that women cannot, should not, be scientists, that they lack the strength, rigor, and clarity of mind for an occupation that properly belongs to men. Now that the women's movement has made offensive such naked assertions, open acknowledgment of the continuing belief in the intrinsic masculinity of scientific thought has become less fashionable. It continues, however, to find daily expression in the language and metaphors we use to describe science. When we dub the objective sciences "hard" as opposed to the softer, i.e., more subjective, branches of knowledge, we implicitly invoke a sexual metaphor, in which "hard" is of course masculine and "soft," feminine. Quite generally, facts are "hard," feelings "soft."

"Feminization" has become synonymous with sentimentalization. A woman thinking scientifically or objectively is thinking "like a man"; conversely, a man pursuing a nonrational, nonscientific argument is arguing "like a woman."

The linguistic rooting of this stereotype is not lost among children, who remain perhaps the most outspoken and least self-conscious about its expression. From strikingly early ages, even in the presence of astereotypic role models, children have learned to identify mathematics and science as male. "Science," my five-year-old son declared, confidently bypassing the fact that his mother was a scientist, "is for men!" The identification between scientific thought and masculinity is so deeply embedded in the culture at large that children have little difficulty internalizing that identification. They grow up not only expecting scientists to be men, but also perceiving scientists as more "masculine" than other male professionals, than, for example, those in the arts. Numerous studies of masculinity and femininity in the professions confirm this observation, with the "harder" sciences as well as the "harder" branches of any profession consistently characterized as more masculine.

In one particularly interesting study of attitudes prevalent among English schoolboys, a somewhat different but critically related dimension of the cultural stereotype emerges. Hudson (1972) observes that scientists are perceived as not only more masculine than are artists, but simultaneously as less sexual. He writes:

> The arts are associated with sexual pleasure, the sciences with sexual restraint. The arts man is seen as having a good-looking, well-dressed wife with whom he enjoys a warm sexual relation; the scientist as having a wife who is dowdy and dull, and in whom he has no physical interest. Yet the scientist is seen as masculine, the arts specialist as slightly feminine (p. 83).

In this passage we see the genderization of science linked with another, also widely perceived image of science as antithetical to Eros. These images are not unrelated, and it is important to bear their juxtaposition in mind as we attempt to understand their sources and functions. What is at issue here is the kind of images and metaphor with which science is surrounded. If we can take the use of metaphor seriously, while managing to keep clearly in mind that it is metaphor and language which are being discussed, then we can attempt to understand the influences they might exert—how the use of language and metaphor can become hardened into a kind of reality. One way is through the internalization of these images by scientists themselves, and I will discuss more explicitly how this can happen later in the paper. As a first step, however, the imagery itself needs to be explored further.

If we agree to pursue the implications of attributing gender to the scientific mind, then we might be led to ask, with what or with whom is the sexual metaphor completed? And, further, what is the nature of the act with which this now desexualized union is consummated? The answer to the first question is immediate. The complement of the scientific mind is, of course, Nature—viewed so ubiquitously as female. "Let us establish a chaste and lawful marriage between Mind and Nature" wrote Bacon (quoted by Leiss, 1972, p. 25), thereby providing the prescription for the birth of the new science. This prescription has endured to the present day—in it are to be found important clues for an understanding of the posture of the virgin groom, of his relation toward his bride, and of the ways in which he defines his mission. The metaphoric marriage of which science is the offspring sets the scientific project squarely in the midst of our unmistakably patriarchal tradition. Small wonder, then, that the goals of science are so persistently described in terms of "conquering" and "mastering" nature. Bacon articulated this more clearly than today's self-consciousness could perhaps permit when he urged: "I am come in very truth leading you to Nature with all her children to bind her to your service and make her your slave" (Farrington, 1951, p. 197).

Much attention has been given recently to the technological abuses of modern science, and in many of these discussions blame is directed toward the distortions of the scientific program intrinsic in its ambition to dominate nature—without, however, offering an adequate explanation of how that ambition comes to be intrinsic to science. Generally such distortions are attributed to technology, or applied science, which is presumed to be clearly distinguishable from pure science. In the latter, the ambition is supposed to be pure knowledge, uncontaminated by fantasies of control. While it is undoubtedly true that the domination of nature is a more central feature of technology, it is impossible to draw a clear line between pure and applied science. History reveals a most complex relation between the two, as complex perhaps as the interrelation between the dual constitutive motives for knowledge—those of transcendence and power. It would be naive to suppose that the connotations of masculinity and conquest affect only the uses to which science is put, and leave untouched its very structure.

Science bears the imprint of its genderization not only in the ways it is used, but in the very description of reality it offers—even in the relation of the scientist to that description. To see this, it is necessary to examine more fully the implications of attributing masculinity to the very nature of scientific thought.

Having divided the world into two parts—the knower (mind) and the knowable (nature)—scientific ideology goes on to prescribe a very specific relation between the two. It prescribes the interactions which can consummate this union, that is, which can lead to knowledge. Not only are mind and nature assigned gender, but in characterizing scientific and objective thought as masculine, the very activity by which the knower can acquire knowledge is also genderized. The relation specified between knower and known is one of distance and separation. It is that between a subject and object radically divided, which is to say no worldly relation. Simply put, nature is objectified. The "chaste and lawful marriage" is consummated through reason rather than feeling, and "observation" rather than "immediate" sensory experience. The modes of intercourse are defined so as to insure emotional and physical inviolability. Concurrent with the division of the world into subject and object is, accordingly, a division of the forms of knowledge into "objective" and "subjective." The scientific mind is set apart from what is to be known, i.e., from nature, and its autonomy is guaranteed (or so it has been traditionally assumed) by setting apart its modes of knowing from those in which that dichotomy is threatened. In this process, the characterization of both the scientific mind and its modes of access to knowledge as masculine is indeed significant. Masculine here connotes, as it so often does, autonomy, separation, and distance. It connotes a radical rejection of any commingling of subject and object, which are, it now appears, quite consistently identified as male and female.

What is the real significance of this system of beliefs, whose structure now reveals a quite intricate admixture of metaphysics, cognitive style, and sexual metaphor? If we reject the position, as I believe we must, that the associations between scientific and masculine are simply "true"—that they reflect a biological difference between male and female brains—then how are we to account for our adherence to them? Whatever intellectual or personality characteristics may be affected by sexual hormones, it has become abundantly clear that our ideas about the differences between the sexes far exceed what can be traced to mere biology; that once formed these ideas take on a life of their own— a life sustained by powerful cultural and psychological forces. Even the brief discussion offered above makes it evident that, in attributing gender to an intellectual posture, in sexualizing a thought process, we inevitably invoke the large world of affect. The task of explaining the associations between masculine and scientific thus becomes, short of reverting to an untenable biological reductionism, the task of understanding the emotional substructure that links our experience of gender with our cognitive experience.

The nature of the problem suggests that, in seeking an explanation of the origins and endurance of this mythology, we look to the processes by which the capacity for scientific thought develops, and the ways in which those processes are intertwined with emotional and sexual development. By so doing, it becomes possible to acquire deeper insight into the structure and perhaps even the functions of the mythology we seek to elucidate. The route I wish to take proceeds along ground laid by psychoanalysts and cognitive psychologists, along a course shaped by the particular questions I have posed. What emerges is a scenario supported by the insights these workers have attained, and held together, it is to be hoped, by its own logical and intuitive coherence.

II. The Development of Objectivity

The crucial insight which underlies much of this discussion—an insight for which we are indebted to both Freud and Piaget—is that the capacity for objectivity, for delineating subject from object, is *not* inborn, although the potential for it into doubt is. Rather, the ability to perceive reality "objectively" is acquired as an inextricable part of the long and painful process by which the child's sense of self is formed. In the deepest sense, it is a function of the child's capacity for distinguishing self from not-self, "me" from "not-me." The consolidation of this capacity is perhaps the major achievement of childhood development.

After half a century's clinical observations of children and adults the developmental picture which emerges is as follows. In the early world of the infant, experiences of thoughts, feelings, events, images, and perceptions are continuous. Boundaries have not yet been drawn to distinguish the child's internal from external environment; nor has order or structure been imposed on either. The external environment, consisting primarily of the mother during this early period, is experienced as an extension of the child. It is only through the assimilation of cumulative experiences of pleasure and pain, of gratification and disappointment, that the child slowly learns to distinguish between self and other, between image and percept, between subject and object. The growing ability to distinguish his or her self from the environment allows for the recognition of a world of external objects—a world subject to ever finer discrimination and delineation. It permits the recognition of an external reality to which the child can relate—at first magically, and ultimately objectively. In the course of time, the inanimate becomes released from the animate, objects from their perspective, and events from wishes; the child becomes capable of objective thought and perception. The process by which this development occurs proceeds through sequential and characteristic stages of cognitive growth, stages which have been extensively documented and described by Piaget and his co-workers.

The background of this development is fraught with intense emotional conflict. The primary object which the infant carves out of the matrix of his/her experiences is an emotional object, namely the mother. And along with the emergence of the mother as a separate being comes the child's painful recognition of his/her own separate existence. Anxiety is unleashed, and longing is born. The child (infant) discovers his dependency and need—and a primitive form of love. Out of the demarcation between self and mother arises a longing to undo that differentiation—an urge to re-establish the original unity. At the same time, there is also growing pleasure in autonomy, which itself comes to feel threatened by the lure of an earlier state. The process of emotional delineation proceeds in fits and starts, propelled and inhibited by conflicting impulses, desires, and fears. The parallel process of cognitive delineation must be negotiated against the background of these conflicts. As objects acquire a separate identity, they remain for a long time tied to the self by a network of magical ties. The disentanglement of self from world, and of thoughts from things, requires relinquishing the magical bonds which

have kept them connected. It requires giving up the belief in the omnipotence—now of the child, now of the mother—that perpetuates those bonds and learning to tolerate the limits and separateness of both. It requires enduring the loss of a wish-dominated existence in exchange for the rewards of living "in reality." In doing so, the child moves from the egocentricity of a self-dominated contiguous world to the recognition of a world outside and independent of himself—a world in which objects can take on a "life" of their own.

The recognition of the independent reality of both self and other is a necessary precondition both for science and for love. It may not, however, be sufficient—for either. Certainly the capacity for love, for empathy, for artistic creativity requires more than a simple dichotomy between subject and object. Autonomy too sharply defined, reality too rigidly defined, cannot encompass the emotional and creative experiences which give life its fullest and richest depth. Autonomy must be conceived of more dynamically and reality more flexibly if they are to allow for the ebb and flow of love and play. Emotional growth does not end with the mere acceptance of one's own separateness; perhaps it is fair to say that it begins there. Out of a condition of emotional and cognitive union with the mother, the child gradually gains enough confidence in the enduring reality of both him/herself and the environment to tolerate their separateness and mutual independence. A sense of self becomes delineated—in opposition, as it were, to the mother. Ultimately, however, both sense of self and of other become sufficiently secure to permit momentary relaxation of the boundary between—without, that is, threatening the loss of either. One has acquired confidence in the enduring survival of both self and other as vitally autonomous. Out of the recognition and acceptance of one's aloneness in the world, it becomes possible to transcend one's isolation, to truly love another.[2]

The final step—of reintroducing ambiguity into one's relation to the world—is a difficult one. It evokes deep anxieties and fears stemming from old conflicts and older desires. The ground of one's selfhood was not easily won, and experiences which appear to threaten the loss of that ground can be seen as acutely dangerous. Milner (1957), in seeking to understand the essence of what makes a drawing "alive," and conversely, the inhibitions which impede artistic expression, has written with rare perspicacity and eloquence about the dangers and anxieties attendant upon opening ourselves to the creative perception so critical for a successful drawing. But unless we can, the world of art is foreclosed to us. Neither love nor art can survive the exclusion of a dialogue between dream and reality, between inside and outside, between subject and object.

Our understanding of psychic autonomy, and along with it, of emotional maturity, owes a great deal to the work of the English psychoanalyst Winnicott. Of particular importance here is Winnicott's concept of the transitional object—an object intermediate between self and other (as, for example, the baby's blanket). It is called a transitional object insofar as it facilitates the transition from the state of magical union with the mother to autonomy, the transition from belief in omnipotence to an acceptance of the limitations of everyday reality. Gradually, it is given up,

> not so much forgotten as relegated to limbo. By this I mean that in health the transitional object does not "go inside" nor does the feeling about it necessarily undergo repression . . . It loses meaning, and this is because the transitional phenomena have become diffused, have become spread out over the whole intermediate territory between "inner psychic reality" and "the external world as perceived by two persons in common," that is to say, over the whole cultural field (Winnicott, 1971, p. 5).

To the diffuse survival of the "creative apperception" he attributes what, "more than anything else, makes the individual feel that life is worth living" (p. 65). Creativity, love, and play are located by Winnicott in the "potential space" between the inner psychic space of "me"

and outer social space of "not-me"—"the neutral area of experience which will not be challenged" (as it was not challenged for the infant)—about which "we will never ask the question: Did you conceive of this or was it presented to you from without" (p. 12).

The inability to tolerate such a potential space leads to psychic distress as surely as the complementary failure to delineate adequately between self and other. "These two groups of people come to us for psychotherapy because in the one case they do not want to spend their lives irrevocably out of touch with the facts of life and in the other because they feel estranged from dream" (p. 67). Both inadequate and excessive delineation between self and other can be seen as defenses, albeit opposite ones, against ongoing anxiety about autonomy.

Emotional maturity, then, implies a sense of reality which is neither cut off from, nor at the mercy of, fantasy; it requires a sufficiently secure sense of autonomy to allow for that vital element of ambiguity at the interface between subject and object. In the words of Loewald (1951), "Perhaps the so-called fully developed, the mature ego is not one that has become fixated at the presumably highest or latest stage of development, having left the others behind it, but is an ego that integrates its reality in such a way that the earlier and deeper levels of ego-reality integration remain alive as dynamic sources of higher organization" (p. 18).

While most of us will recognize the inadequacy of a static conception of autonomy as an emotional ideal, it is easy to fall into the trap of regarding it as an appropriate ideal for cognitive development. That is, cognitive maturity is frequently identified with a posture in which objective reality is perceived and defined as radically divided from the subjective. Our inclination to accept this posture as a model for cognitive maturity is undoubtedly influenced by the definition of objectivity we have inherited from classical science—a definition rooted in the premise that the subject can and should be totally removed from our description of the object. Though that definition has proved unquestionably efficacious in the past, contemporary developments in both philosophy and physics have demonstrated its epistemological inadequacy. They have made it necessary for us to look beyond the classical dichotomy to a more dynamic conception of reality, and a more sophisticated epistemology to support it.

If scientists have exhibited a reluctance to do so, as I think they have, that reluctance should be examined in the light of what we already know about the relation between cognitive and emotional development. Elsewhere (Keller, 1979) I have attempted to show the persistence of demonstrably inappropriate classical ideas even in contemporary physics, where the most dramatic evidence for the failure of classical ideas has come from. There I try to establish some of the consequences of this persistence, and to account for the tenacity of such ideas. In brief, I argue that the adherence to an outmoded, dichotomous conception of objectivity might be viewed as a defense against anxiety about autonomy of exactly the same kind as we find interfering with the capacity for love and creativity. When even physics reveals "transitional phenomena"—phenomena, that is, about which it cannot be determined whether they belong to the observer or the observed—then it becomes essential to question the adequacy of traditional "realist" modes for cognitive maturity as well as for reality. Our very definition of reality requires constant refinement as we continue in the effort to wean our perceptions from our wishes, our fears, and our anxieties; insofar as our conception of cognitive maturity is dictated by our definition of reality, that conception requires corresponding refinement.

III. The Development of Gender

What, the reader may ask, has all this to do with gender? Though the discussion has led us on a sizable detour, the implicit argument which relates it to the genderization of science should already be clear. Before articulating the argument

explicitly, however, we need an account of the development of gender identity and gender identifications in the context of the developmental picture I have presented thus far.

Perhaps the single most important determinant of our conceptions of male and female is provided by our perceptions of and experiences with our parents. While the developmental processes described above are equally relevant for children of both sexes, their implications for the two sexes are bound to differ. The basic and fundamental fact that it is, for most of us, our mothers who provide the emotional context out of which we forget the discrimination between self and other inevitably leads to a skewing of our perceptions of gender. As long as our earliest and most compelling experiences of merging have their origin in the mother-child relation, it appears to be inevitable that that experience will tend to be identified with "mother," while delineation and separation are experienced as a negation of "mother," as "not-mother." In the extrication of self from other, the mother, beginning as the first and most primitive subject, emerges, by a process of effective and affective negation, as the first object.[3] The very processes (both cognitive and emotional) which remind us of that first bond become colored by their association with the woman who is, and forever remains, the archetypal female. Correspondingly, those of delineation and objectification are colored by their origins in the process of separation *from* mother; they become marked, as it were, as "not-mother." The mother becomes an object, and the child a subject, by a process which becomes itself an expression of opposition to and negation of "mother."

While there is an entire world which exists beyond the mother, in the family constellation with which we are most familiar, it is primarily the father (or the father figure) toward whom the child turns for protection from the fear of re-engulfment, from the anxieties and fears of disintegration of a still very fragile ego. It is the father who comes to stand for individuation and differentiation—for objective reality itself; who indeed can represent the "real" world by virtue of being *in* it.

For Freud, reality becomes personified by the father during the oedipal conflict; it is the father who, as the representative of external reality, harshly intrudes on the child's (i.e., boy's) early romance with the mother—offering his protection and future fraternity as the reward for the child's acceptance of the "reality principle." Since Freud, however, it has become increasingly well understood that the rudiments of both gender and reality are established long before the oedipal period, and that reality becomes personified by the father as soon as the early maternal bond comes to be experienced as threatening engulfment, or loss of ego boundaries. A particularly pertinent discussion of this process is presented by Loewald (1951), who writes:

> Against the threatening possibility of remaining in or sinking back into the structureless unity from which the ego emerged, stands the powerful paternal force. . . . While the primary narcissistic identity with the mother forever constitutes the deepest unconscious origin and structural layer of ego and reality, and the motive force for the ego's 'remarkable striving toward unification, synthesis,'—this primary identity is also the source of the deepest dread, which promotes, in identification with the father, the ego's progressive differentiation and structuralization of reality (pp. 15, 17).

Thus it is that, for all of us—male and female alike—our earliest experiences incline us to associate the affective and cognitive posture of objectification with masculine, while all processes which involve a blurring of the boundary between subject and object tend to be associated with the feminine.

The crucial question of course is: What happens to these early associations? While the patterns which give rise to them may be quasi-universal (though strongest, no doubt, in our own form of nuclear family), the conditions which sustain them are not. It is perhaps at this point that specific cultural forces intrude most prominently. In a culture which validates subsequent adult experiences that transcend the subject-ob-ject divide, as we find for example in art, love, and religion, these early identifications can be counteracted—provided, that is, that such experiences are validated as essentially human rather than as "feminine" experience. However, in a culture such as ours, where primary validation is accorded to a science which has been premised on a radical dichotomy between subject and object, and where all other experiences are accorded secondary, "feminine" status, the early identifications can hardly fail to persist. The genderization of science—as an enterprise, as an intellectual domain, as a world view—simultaneously reflects and perpetuates associations made in an earlier, prescientific era. If true, then an adherence to an objectivist epistemology, in which truth is measured by its distance from the subjective, has to be re-examined when it emerges that, by this definition, truth itself has become genderized.

It is important to emphasize, even repeat, that what I have been discussing is a system of beliefs about the meaning of masculine and feminine, rather than any either intrinsic or actual differences between male and female. Children of both sexes learn essentially the same set of ideas about the characteristics of male and female—how they then make use of these ideas in the development of their gender identity as male or female is another question. The relation between the sexual stereotypes we believe in and our actual experience and even observation of gender is a very complex one. It is crucial, however, to make a vigilant effort to distinguish between belief and reality, even, or especially, when the reality which emerges is so influenced by our beliefs. I have not been claiming, for example, that men are by nature more objective, better suited for scientific work, nor that science, even when characterized by an extreme objectivist epistemology, is intrinsically masculine. What I have been discussing are the reasons we might believe all of the above to be true. These beliefs may in fact lead to observed differences between the sexes, though the question of actual differences between men and women in a given culture is ultimately an empirical one. The subsequent issue of how those possible differences might be caused by cultural expectations is yet a separate issue, and requires separate discussion. Without getting into the empirical question of sex differences, about which there is a great deal of debate, it seems reasonable to suggest that we ought to expect that our early beliefs about gender will be subject to some degree of internalization.

To return, then, to the issue of gender development, it is important to recognize that, although children of both sexes must learn equally to distinguish self from other, and have essentially the same need for autonomy, to the extent that boys rest their very sexual identity on an opposition to what is both experienced and defined as feminine, the development of their gender identity is likely to accentuate the process of separation. As boys, they must undergo a twofold "disidentification from mother" (Greenson, 1978)—first for the establishment of a self-identity, and second for the consolidation of a male gender identity. Further impetus is added to this process by the external cultural pressure on the young boy to establish a stereotypic masculinity, now culturally as well as privately connoting independence and autonomy. The cultural definitions of masculine as what can never appear feminine, and of autonomy as what can never be relaxed, conspire to reinforce the child's earliest associations of female with the pleasures and dangers of merging, and male with both the comfort and the loneliness of separateness. The boy's internal anxiety about both self and gender is here echoed by the cultural anxiety; together they can lead to postures of exaggerated and rigidified autonomy and masculinity which can—indeed which may be designed to—defend against that anxiety and the longing which generates it. Many psychoanalysts have come to believe that, because of the boy's need to switch his identification from the mother to the father, his sense of gender identity tends always to be more fragile than the girl's. Her sense of self-identity may, however, be comparatively more vulnerable. It has been suggested that the girl's development of a sense of separateness may be to some degree hampered by her ongoing identification with her mother. Although she too must disentangle herself from the early experience of oneness, she continues to look toward her mother as a model for her gender identity. Whatever vicissitudes her relation to her mother may suffer during subsequent development, a strong identification based on common gender is likely to persist—her need for "disidentification" is not so radical. Cultural forces may further complicate her development of autonomy by stressing dependency and subjectivity as feminine characteristics. To the extent that such traits become internalized, they can be passed on through the generations by leading to an accentuation of the symbiotic bond between mother and daughter (see, e.g., Chodorow, 1974).

It would seem, then, appropriate to suggest that one possible outcome of these processes is that boys may be more inclined toward excessive and girls toward inadequate delineation—growing into men who have difficulty loving and women who retreat from science. What I am suggesting, then, and indeed trying to describe, is a network of interactions between gender development, a belief system which equates objectivity with masculinity, and a set of cultural values which simultaneously elevates what is defined as scientific and what is defined as masculine. The structure of this network is such as to perpetuate and exacerbate distortions in *any* of its parts—including the acquisition of gender identity.

IV. The Development of Scientists

Whatever differences between the sexes such a network might, however, generate—and, as I said earlier, the existence of such differences remains ultimately an empirical question—they are in any case certain to be overshadowed by the inevitably large variations that exist within both the male and female populations. Not all men become scientists, and we must ask whether a science which advertises itself as revealing a reality in which subject and object are unmistakably distinct does not offer special comfort to those who, as individuals (be they male or female), retain particular anxiety about the loss of autonomy. In short, if we can take the argument presented thus far seriously, then we must follow it through yet another step. Would not a characterization of science which appears to gratify particular emotional needs give rise to a self-selection of scientists—a self-selection which would, in turn, lead to a perpetuation of that characterization? Without attempting a detailed discussion of either the appropriateness of the imagery with which science is advertised, or of the personality characteristics which such imagery might select for, it seems reasonable to suggest that such a selection mechanism ought inevitably to operate. The persistence of the characterization of science as masculine, as objectivist, as autonomous of psychological as well as of social and political forces would then be encouraged, through such selection, by the kinds of emotional satisfaction it provides.

If so, the question which then arises is whether, statistically, scientists do indeed tend to be more anxious about their affective as well as cognitive autonomy than nonscientists. Although it is certainly part of the popular image of scientists that they do, the actual measurement of personality differences between scientists and nonscientists has proved to be extremely difficult; it is as difficult, and subject to as much disagreement, as the measurement of personality differences between the sexes. One obvious difficulty arises out of the ambiguity of the term scientist, and the enormous heterogeneity of the scientific population. Apart from the vast differences among individuals, characteristics vary across time, nationality, discipline, and, even, with degree of eminence. The Einsteins of history fail, virtually by definition, to conform to more general patterns either of personality or of intellect. Nevertheless, certain themes, however difficult they may be to pin

down, continually re-emerge with enough prominence to warrant consideration. These are the themes, or stereotypes, on which I have concentrated throughout this paper, and though they can neither exhaustively nor even accurately describe science or scientists as a whole—as stereotypes never can—they do acquire some corroboration from the (admittedly problematic) literature on the "scientific personality." It seems worth noting, therefore, several features which seem to emerge from a number of efforts to describe the personality characteristics which tend to distinguish scientists from nonscientists.

I have already referred to the fact that scientists, particularly physical scientists, score unusually high on "masculinity" tests, meaning only that, on the average, their responses differ greatly from those of women. At the same time, studies (e.g., Roe, 1953, 1956) report that they tend overwhelmingly to have been loners as children, to be low in social interests and skills, indeed to avoid interpersonal contact. McClelland's subsequent studies confirm these impressions. He writes, "And it is a fact, as Anne Roe reports, that young scientists are typically not very interested in girls, date for the first time late in college, marry the first girl they date, and thereafter appear to show a rather low level of heterosexual drive" (1962, p. 321) (by which he presumably means sexual, thereby confirming, incidentally, the popular image of scientists as "asexual" which I discussed earlier). One of McClelland's particularly interesting findings was that 90% of a group of eminent scientists see, in the "mother-son" picture routinely given as part of the Thematic Apperception Test, "the mother and son going their separate ways" (p. 323)—a relatively infrequent response to this picture in the general population. It conforms, however, with the more general observation (emerging from biographical material) of a distant relation to the mother,[4] frequently coupled with "open or covert attitudes of derogation" (Roe, 1956, p. 215).

Though these remarks are admittedly sketchy, and by no means constitute a review of the field, they do suggest a personality profile which seems admirably suited to an occupation seen as simultaneously masculine and asexual. Bacon's image of a "chaste and lawful marriage" becomes remarkably apt insofar as it allows the scientist both autonomy and mastery[5] in his marriage to a bride kept at safe, "objectified" remove.

Conclusion

It is impossible to conclude a discussion of the genderization of science without making some brief comments on its social implications. The linking of scientific and objective with masculine brings in its wake a host of secondary consequences which, however self-evident, may nevertheless need articulating. Not only does our characterization of science thereby become colored by the biases of patriarchy and sexism, but simultaneously our evaluation of masculine and feminine becomes affected by the prestige of science. A circular process of mutual reinforcement is established in which what is called scientific receives extra validation from the cultural preference for what is called masculine, and, conversely, what is called feminine—be it a branch of knowledge, a way of thinking, or woman herself—becomes further devalued by its exclusion from the special social and intellectual value placed on science and the model science provides for all intellectual endeavors. This circularity not only operates on the level of ideology, but is assisted by the ways in which the developmental processes, both for science and for the child, internalize ideological influences. For each, pressures from the other operate, in the ways I have attempted to describe, to create distortions and perpetuate caricatures.

Neither in emphasizing the self-sustaining nature of these beliefs, nor in relating them to early childhood experience, do I wish to suggest that they are inevitable. On the contrary, by examining their dynamics I mean to emphasize the existence of alternative possibilities. The disengagement of our thinking about science from

our notions of what is masculine could lead to a freeing of both from some of the rigidities to which they have been bound, with profound ramifications for both. Not only, for example, might science become more accessible to women, but, far more importantly, our very conception of "objective" could be freed from inappropriate constraints. As we begin to understand the ways in which science itself has been influenced by its unconscious mythology, we can begin to perceive the possibilities for a science not bound by such mythology.

How might such a disengagement come about? To the extent that my analysis rests on the crucial importance of the gender of the primary parent, changing patterns of parenting could be of special importance.[6] But other developments might be of equal importance. Changes in the ethos that sustains our beliefs about science and gender could also come about from the current pressure, largely politically inspired, to re-examine the traditionally assumed neutrality of science, from philosophical exploration of the boundaries or limitations of scientific inquiry, and even, perhaps especially, from events within science itself. Both within and without science, the need to question old dogma has been pressing. Of particular interest among recent developments *within* science is the growing interest among physicists in a process description of reality—a move inspired by, perhaps even necessitated by, quantum mechanics. In these descriptions object reality acquires a dynamic character, akin to the more fluid concept of autonomy emerging from psychoanalysis. Bohr himself perspicaciously provided us with a considerably happier image than Bacon's—one more apt even for the future of physics—when he chose for his coat of arms the yin-yang symbol, over which reads the inscription: *Contraria Sunt Complementa*.

Where, finally, has this analysis taken us? In attempting to explore the significance of the sexual metaphor in our thinking about science, I have offered an explanation of its origins, its functions, and some of its consequences. Necessarily, many questions remain, and it is perhaps appropriate, by way of concluding, to articulate some of them. I have not, for example, more than touched on the social and political dynamics of the genderization of science. This is a crucial dimension which remains in need of further exploration. It has seemed to me, however, that central aspects of this problem belong in the psychological domain, and further, that this is the domain which tends to be least accounted for in most discussions of scientific thought.

Within the particular model of affective and cognitive development I have invoked, much remains to be understood about the interconnections between cognition and affect. Though I have, throughout, assumed an intimate relation between the two, it is evident that a fuller and more detailed conception is necessary.

Finally, the speculations I offer raise numerous questions of historical and psychological fact. I have already indicated some of the relevant empirical questions in the psychology of personality which bear on my analysis. Other questions of a more historical nature ought also to be mentioned. How, e.g., have conceptions of objectivity changed with time, and to what extent have these conceptions been linked with similar sexual metaphors in other prescientific eras, or, for that matter, in other, less technological cultures? Clearly, much remains to be investigated; perhaps the present article can serve to provoke others to help pursue these questions.

NOTES

1. For a further elaboration of this theme, see 'Women in Science: A Social Analysis' (Keller, 1974).
2. See, e.g., Kernberg (1977) for a psychoanalytic discussion of the prerequisites for mature love.
3. To the extent that she personifies nature, she remains, for the scientific mind, the final object as well.
4. These studies are, as is evident, of male scientists. It is noteworthy, however, that studies of the relatively small number of female scientists reveal in women scientists a similar, perhaps even more marked, pattern of distance in relation to the mother. For most, the father proved to be the parent of major emotional

and intellectual importance (see, e.g., Plank and Plank, 1954).

5. Earlier I pointed out how Bacon's marital imagery constitutes an invitation to the "dominance of nature." A fuller discussion of this posture would also require consideration of the role of aggression in the development of object relations and symbolic thought processes—an aspect which has been omitted from the present discussion. Briefly, it can be said that the act of severing subject from object is experienced by the child as an act of violence, and it carries with it forever, on some level, the feeling tone of aggression. For insight into this process we can turn once again to Winnicott, who observes that "it is the destructive drive that creates the quality of externality" (p. 93), that, in the creation and recognition of the object there is always, and inevitably, an implicit act of destruction. Indeed, he says, "it is the destruction of the object that places the object outside the area of the subject's omnipotent control" (p. 90). Its ultimate survival is, of course, crucial for the child's development. "In other words, because of the survival of the object, the subject may now have started to live a life in the world of objects, and so the subject stands to gain immeasurably; but the price has to be pain in acceptance of the ongoing destruction in unconscious fantasy relative to object-relating" (p. 90). It would seem likely that the aggressive force implicit in this act of objectification must make its subsequent appearance in the relation between the scientist and his object, i.e., between science and nature.

6. In this I am joined by Dinnerstein (1976), who has recently written an extraordinarily provocative analysis of the consequences of the fact that it is, and has always been, the mother's "hand that rocks the cradle." Her analysis, though it goes much further and much deeper than the sketch provided here, happily corroborates my own in the places where they overlap. She concludes that the human malaise resulting from the present sexual arrangements can be cured only by dividing the nurturance and care of the infant equally between the mother and the father. Perhaps that is true. I would, however, argue that, at least for the particular consequences I have discussed here, other changes might be of comparable importance.

REFERENCES

Chodorow, N. (1974). 'Family Structure and Feminine Personality,' in *Woman, Culture and Society*, ed. M. Z. Rosaldo & L. Lamphere (Stanford: Stanford University Press), pp. 43–46.

Dinnerstein, D. (1976). *The Mermaid and the Minotaur* (New York: Harper & Row).

Farrington, B. (1951). *Temporus Partus Masculus,* an Untranslated Writing of Francis Bacon. *Centaurus* 1, 193–205.

Greenson, R. (1978). 'Disidentifying from Mother: Its Special Importance for the Boy,' in *Explorations in Psychoanalysis* (New York: International Universities Press, pp. 305–312.

Horney, K. (1926). 'The Flight from Womanhood,' reprinted in *Women and Analysis,* ed. J. Strouse (New York: Dell, 1975), pp. 199–215.

Hudosn, L. (1972). *The Cult of the Fact* (New York: Harper & Row).

Keller, E. F. (1974). 'Women in Science: A Social Analysis,' *Harvard Magazine,* October, pp. 14–19.

Keller, E. F. (1979). 'Cognitive Repression in Contemporary Physics,' *Amer. J. Physics* 47, 718–721.

Keller, E. F. (1980). 'Lewis Carroll: A Study of Mathematical Inhibition.' *J. Amer. Psychoanalytic Assn.* 28, 133–160.

Keller, E. F. (1980). 'Baconian Science: A Hermaphroditic Birth,' *Philosophical Forum* 11.

Keller, E. F. (1979). 'Nature as "Her",' *Proceedings of the Second Sex Conference.* New York University.

Keller, E. F. (1980). 'Feminist Critique of Science: A Forward or Backward Move?' *Fundamenta Scientiae,* Summer, 1980.

Keller, E. F. (1983). 'The Mind's Eye' (with C. R. Grontkowski), this volume.

Kernberg, O. (1977). 'Boundaries and Structure in Love Relations.' *J. Amer. Psychoanal. Assn.* 25, 81–114.

Leiss, W. (1972). *The Domination of Nature* (Boston: Beacon Press, 1974).

Loewald, H. (1951). 'Ego and Reality,' *Internat. J. Psycho-Anal.* 32, 10–18.

McClelland, D. C. (1962). 'On the Dynamics of Creative Physical Scientists,' in *The Ecology of Human Intelligence,* ed. L. Hudson (London: Penguin Books), pp. 309–341.

Milner, M. (1957). *On Not Being Able to Paint* (New York: International Universities Press).

Plank, E. N., & Plank, R. (1954). 'Emotional Components in Arithmetic Leaning as Seen Through Autobiographies.' *The Psychoanalytic Study of the Child* 9, 274–293.

Roe, A. (1953). *The Making of a Scientist* (New York: Dodd, Mead).

Roe, A. (1956). *The Psychology of Occupations* (New York: Wiley).

Winnicott, D. W. (1971). *Playing and Reality* (New York: Basic Books).

Uncovering Gynocentric Science

Ruth Ginzberg

Feminist philosophers of science have produced an exciting array of works in the last several years, from critiques of androcentrism in traditional science to theories about what might constitute feminist science. I suggest here another possibility: that if gynocentric science has existed all along, then the task of identifying a feminist alternative to androcentric science should be a suitable candidate for empirical investigation. Such empirical investigation could provide a solid ground for further theorizing about feminist science at a time when that solid ground is looking rather necessary.

Recent feminist critiques of science have documented a wide variety of forms of androcentrism in traditional Western science (Griffin 1980; Merchant 1980; Bleier 1984; Keller 1985; Harding 1986; Birke 1986; Bleier 1986). There have been some attempts made to define a gynocentric conception of science; Evelyn Fox Keller (1983, 1985) for example, has suggested that we might find clues about gynocentric science by examining the work of women scientists like Barbara McClintock. But many feminist philosophers of science, including Keller, are still at a loss when asked to define what a truly gynocentric alternative might look like. Ruth Bleier articulates the question that many of us struggle with: "[H]ow can we even begin to conceptualize science as non-masculine . . . when most of written civilization—our history, language, conceptual frameworks, literature—has been generated by men?" (Bleier 1986, 15). Some have suggested that we are not yet in a position to identify a fully articulated feminist successor science (Fee 1983; Harding 1986;

Rose 1986). On a Kuhnian model of scientific paradigms, a successor science that would follow the current andro-Eurocentric paradigm could not be fully articulated at this time, partly because of incommensurability and partly because paradigms are never fully articulated even in their own fullest maturity (Kuhn 1970). I would like to toss yet another suggestion into the realm of discourse about feminist science in partial response to Bleier's question: the suggestion that there has been gynocentric science all along, but that we often fail to recognize it as gynocentric *science* because it traditionally has not been awarded the honorific label of 'Science.'

Taking a cue from so many other feminist inquiries, I would like to reexamine women's actual activities in order to discover clues about gynocentric science. My hunch is that if there is such a thing as gynocentric science, it is unlikely that it is just now beginning. I suspect that there is such a thing, and that it has been practiced throughout history—just as other gynocentric traditions have existed throughout history—but that the androcentric record-keepers have failed to notice or record it. In the same way that feminists are beginning to recover some of our artis-

Reprinted with verbal permission from Ruth Ginzberg. This work originally appeared in Hypatia 2(3):89–105, 1987.

tic, political, spiritual and social traditions. I believe that we can now recover some of the scientific traditions of our foresisters by reviewing history with a feminist eye.

For a start, it seems important not to confine our review of history to those activities which have been officially labeled 'Science' until now. As Feyerabend (1975) has argued, 'Science' is—at least in part—a political term. If Feyerabend is correct about this, and I am convinced that he is, then it is imperative that we look beyond the 'official' histories to correct for the political factors working against women. As is typical of oppressed groups, much of women's activity has been outside of the mainstream of Western culture. But that doesn't mean that these activities weren't occurring, or that they weren't valuable, nor does it necessarily mean that they weren't science. It only means that they weren't the subject of favorable attention from the members of the dominant cultures. What I am suggesting is that there are women's activities that haven't been called 'Science' for *political* reasons, even when those activities have been model examples of inquiry leading to knowledge of the natural world. So my partial answer to Bleier's question is that we must look outside of the histories, conceptual frameworks, literature, and possibly even the language, that have been generated by men.

The question, then, becomes that of how to begin. I like Keller's approach as a starting point: She has examined carefully the life and work of a woman scientist who *has* been acknowledged for her scientific work, but who was often seen as a bit "odd" or "incomprehensible." These are hallmarks of the sort of paradigmatic incommensurability described by Kuhn (1970), and should serve as clues about the possible existence of another scientific paradigm. In her biography of Barbara McClintock, Keller (1983, 201) points to such things as "a deep reverence for nature, a capacity for union with that which is to be known," and a sort of holism of approach as being thematic in McClintock's work. There are hints of this sort of theme as well in the work of Rachel Carson, who introduced the concept of ecology to the American public. Anticipating some of the recent, more overtly feminist critiques, Carson wrote in the early 1960's that "The 'control of nature' is a phrase conceived in arrogance, born of the Neanderthal age of biology and philosophy, when it was supposed that nature exists for the convenience of man." Arguing that we were poisoning the entire planet with pesticides in our efforts to 'control' insects rather than learning to live along side them, Carson urged the world to halt "the chemical barrage [which] has been hurled against the fabric of life" (Carson 1964, 261).

In fact some sort of ecology of interconnection is a common theme articulated in feminist conceptions of knowledge (Daly 1978; Rich 1979; Griffin 1980; Merchant 1980; Lorde 1984; Keller 1985; Bleier 1986; Belenky *et al* 1986). In the work of both McClintock and Carson, this epistemology of interconnection is expressed through their careful attention to the dynamics of living systems as pieces of a larger and more awesome natural world which is constantly responding to, and responsive to, itself. As Haunani-Kay Trask has found in her analysis of other work by feminist writers, "their work reverberates with two themes: love (nurturance, care, need, sensitivity, relationship) and power (freedom, expression, creativity, generation, transformation)." These themes are what she had identified as "twin manifestations of the 'life force'" which she names "the feminist Eros" (Trask 1986, 86). We are now in a position to formulate an hypothesis: the hypothesis is that this "feminist Eros" will be an identifying landmark in the epistemology of gynocentric science. Yet while the examination of the work of women who have been recognized as scientists is exciting, it is also unsatisfying; we see only a small fraction of the work that women have done in investigating the world around them from their own perspectives. Following our hypothesis, and Keller's suggestion that a feminist conception of the erotic might yield a fundamentally different conception of science than the one that Plato bequeathed to us, it seems reasonable to suspect that gynocentric science in its natural habitat might already exist, looking somewhat different from androcentric science because of the different conception of the nature and position of the erotic with respect to epistemology (Keller 1985). It is this hitherto unrecognized science that I would like to begin uncovering here.

In searching through women's activities outside of those that have been formally bestowed the label of 'Science,' I have come to suspect that gynocentric science often has been called 'art,' as in the *art* of midwifery, or the *art* of cooking, or the *art* of homemaking. Had these 'arts' been androcentric activities, I have no doubt that they would have been called, respectively obstetrical *science,* food *science,* and family *social science.* Indeed as men have taken an interest in these subjects they have been renamed sciences—and, more importantly, they have been reconceived in the androcentric model of science. There is no question that all of these activities as defined and practiced by women have had important aesthetic, affective, social and erotic dimensions which androcentric science does not acknowledge as Scientific. But that is exactly what our hypothesis predicts for feminist science: that it will be less isolated from other aspects of our lives, less fetishized about individualism, more holistic, more nurturing, more concerned with relations than with objects, perhaps more dialectic, because of the nature and position of the erotic with respect to its epistemology. It might be that the presence of these aesthetic or affective components in gynocentric science underlies some of the reasons that the masculist guardians of Science have not recognized these activities as science, at least not as they were conceived and practiced by women.

Gynocentric Science in Its Natural Habitat

In particular, I would like to suggest that we re-examine midwifery as a paradigm example of gynocentric science. This idea is not originally mine; in 1973 Ehrenreich and English suggested that the "magic" of the 16th Century European witch-healer and midwife "was the science of her time" (Ehrenreich and English 1973, 14). However by no means do I believe that midwifery is the only possible example of gynocentric science. For example, there are good reasons to believe that women's knowledge of food and nutrition historically had to include some fairly sophisticated knowledge of botany and ecosystems, as well as of human nutritional needs. This knowledge undoubtedly was accumulated as women worked in their capacities as the food, nutrition and health experts in a culture that had no pesticides, supermarkets or agricultural extension agents. Food production and preparation were largely women's provinces—and far from being mere social pastimes, they were indispensable to the sustenance of life. Without adequate knowledge of botany and of ecosystems, the life-sustaining gardens maintained primarily by women could have fallen victim to parasites, diseases and the depletion of soil nutrients. The food cultivated for humans would have been eaten by rabbits and deer and the genetic pool of the seed stock could have deteriorated through inbreeding; the concentrated plant populations in women's gardens would have been vulnerable to destruction by parasites and disease. Knowledge about the differences between edible and inedible plants, knowledge about the prevention of spoilage and food poisoning, knowledge about companion planting and crop rotation undoubtedly would have been part of the gynocentric science. One wonders whether food science would have gained the status of a science much sooner (and in a much different way) if women had been defining the sciences.

Pharmacology is another area in which there probably was a substantial tradition of gynocentric science. In his often quoted and equally often ignored remark, Paracelsus—the 'father' of modern pharmacology—attributed his entire knowledge of pharmacology to the wise women of his community. Paracelsus is an enigma in the history of science; modern androcentric historians of science don't know what to make of his mysticism and his holistic approach to the natural world. In the typically androcentric reconstruction of Paracelsus' work, his "Scientific" writings are unbundled from his "Unscientific" writings and packaged separately as Science, though we know that Paracelsus himself objected to this abuse of his own work. Given that he attributed his knowledge of pharmacology to a gynocentric tradition, it might be useful to us to reexamine *all* of what he did say, including that which is often omitted for being "unscientific," perhaps with the idea in mind of gaining clues to what gynocentric science looked like in his time.

But I doubt if gynocentric science is all from eras of long ago. In the twentieth century, for example, the androcentric social sciences have been granted the status of sciences, but the wisdom shared between and among women about the social fabric of their communities is still sneeringly labeled 'gossip.' Recently, however, Belenky *et al* (1986) have suggested that gossip is a paradigm example of what they call "connected knowledge," a way of knowing that their research has found to be highly developed in some women. It would be interesting to investigate the idea that women's traditional vehicles of gossip—garden clubs, sewing circles, coffee klatches, baby showers and backyard fence discussions—actually are part of a gynocentric social science tradition which is oral and dialectic in nature. Another gynocentric field which has emerged in the last century is the field of home economics. Although this field has suffered from the attempts of androcentric educational administrators to turn its academic niche into vocational classes in cooking and sewing for future housewives, home economists undoubtedly have been concerned with home-based *economics*, a branch of economics that studies labor and production in the home. Additionally, there has been a very definite resurgence of gynocentric midwifery in the United States arising out of the women's health movement in the early 1970's. Often working outside of, or in opposition to, the law, lay midwives have organized schools, held conferences, published books and practiced

midwifery in a way quite reminiscent of the midwives of the 16th and 17th centuries—who carried out their work in spite of the threat of the accusation of witchcraft for doing so (Ehrenreich and English 1973; Lang 1972; Arms 1975; Rich 1976; Gaskin 1978).

Women's Knowledge and Gynocentric Science

If I am correct that gynocentric science has existed all along, then there ought to be reasons that it has remained hidden to us, and I think that there are:

First, there is our training, which teaches us that 'science' is work that is done by people who have been awarded the title of Scientist, either by an institution from which they received a degree, or by history. Neither history nor degree-awarding institutions have been willing to award the title of Scientist to those who do not practice traditionally androcentric Western science, so it is to be expected that anyone who is practicing a different sort of science will not be included on the lists of certified Scientists. If we suspect that gynocentric science will be different in kind from androcentric science, even based in a fundamentally different epistemology, then it should be no surprise that gynocentric science would not be recognized as Science, and that gynocentric scientists would not have been labeled Scientists either by institutions or by history.

A second reason that it is easy to overlook gynocentric science is that the work of women has always been invisible in the recorded histories of androcentric Western culture. We are all familiar with the phenomenon of considering women's work to be non-work, as in "She doesn't work; she's a homemaker." Occasionally women scientists such as Marie Curie do make it into the recorded histories of science, but that is because Curie's work was spectacular and individualistic in nature, fitting it well within the model of what men think scientists do. If we are able to make out a case for two distinctly different scientific traditions, an androcentric tradition and a gynocentric tradition, we must not fall into the trap of believing that the practitioners within each of these traditions have been strictly divided along gender lines. Curie's work, though the work of a woman, was part of the androcentric tradition; the work of McClintock, Carson and Paracelsus probably was partially within each of the two traditions, as all three of these scientists seem to have been "claimed" to one extent or another as practitioners of both. Norman Casserley, a man prosecuted by the state of California for practicing midwifery in the early 1970's, probably was working within the gynocentric tradition (Arms 1975). The factors that identify a scientist as a member of one or the other tradition would be based in epistemological basis for inquiry, methodology, problem selection and scientific community—not in gender or sex. But the point is the same: not only women's activities, but all gynocentric activities, have been ignored by the androcentric recorders of history.

The third reason I would like to suggest is that throughout history the gynocentric sciences have been conducted primarily as oral rather than as written traditions. The accumulated wisdom and knowledge of midwives, for example, has been transmitted orally through personal contact and experiential apprenticeships. Midwives have not had professional journals in which they published their findings; they have not had heroes or methodological theoreticians who wrote treatises, nor have they had professional associations which held conferences and published their proceedings, and so on. Since Western androcentric science places such a premium on the written transmission of "results," any activity that has not included a large written component automatically has been excluded from consideration as a science. This undoubtedly is not unrelated to the fact that until very recently in Western history, literacy was much more available to White middle and upper class city-dwelling men than it was to women, the poor, Blacks, Native American tribes, rural families, and so on. Contrary to the usual assump-

tion, which is that illiterate people don't do any science, I would like to propose that they probably do, but that their scientific traditions are oral and dialectic in nature rather than written.

A fourth reason, which is related to the third, is that women's knowledge, and its certification and transmission, may not have been organized hierarchically. The hierarchical organization of androcentric science was exquisitely described by Kuhn (1970) in his description of the socialization of young scientists into a scientific paradigm, and the rise and decline of particular paradigms. What he failed to realize, though Feyerabend (1975) did not, is that the hierarchical organization of both scientific knowledge and scientists is not a *necessary* feature of science, but rather simply a feature of Western science to which we have grown accustomed. While Feyerabend's epistemological anarchy might not provide a good description of the organization of gynocentric knowledge, it does provide the imagination with an alternative to the hierarchical organization of Western scientific knowledge.

A fifth reason, readily visible in the cases of midwifery and 'gossip,' is that there has been a concerted effort to suppress and discredit these bodies of gynocentric knowledge as being erroneous, based in superstition, and connected with harm or evil. More chillingly, history has recorded—although it attempts to forget—a violent campaign of torture and murder in the European witchburnings which was both implicitly and explicitly directed at eradicating various gynocentric traditions (Ehrenreich & English 1973; Daly 1978; Edwards & Waldorf 1984). The influences of force and violence in establishing the Western androcentric scientific tradition as the dominant one should not be underestimated.

Science and Bodily Functions

A look at the gynocentric approach and the androcentric approach to childbirth may provide a case study of one of the longest running disputes between—as Kuhn puts it—competing paradigms. The incommensurability between a gynocentric and an androcentric point of view is clearly visible in the differences between midwives' and scientific doctors' conceptions of childbirth. While medical science views childbirth as an abnormal state of health that has the potential to develop into a serious emergency, midwives have taken a much more holistic view of childbearing than has medical science; childbirth has been viewed as a normal physiological function during which a woman has an increased need for community support. This is not to say that midwives hold the naive view that life- or health-threatening emergencies never arise in the course of childbirth. Occasionally they do. But people also occasionally choke on food, drown in bathtubs, suffer strokes while playing golf and die of heart attacks during sex.

Science Fiction: Consider the following imaginary scenario: Suppose that, recognizing the many possible dangers associated with eating mishaps, the society decided to get much more scientific about the whole process. Federal funds were allocated for setting up elaborate hospital dining halls, and everyone who ate or served food was first urged, then required, to do so under proper medical supervision, "just in case." After all, one could never predict when people might choke on, or have a sudden allergic reaction to, their food. Additionally, experts in the eating sciences had become increasingly concerned about the lack of sterile conditions under which food was typically prepared in the home. Science had already well documented the large numbers of bacterial organisms found in virtually every home kitchen, and its increasing knowledge of the role of bacteria in disease made it obvious that untrained cooks, usually women, in bacteria-laden kitchens could no longer be trusted with the important responsibility of feeding the general population. There was particular concern about the health of children fed in the home. Young children could unknowingly be fed foods to which they might have a violent allergic reaction, and food scien-

tists were alarmed about the numbers of children who were being exposed to the possibility of hives, asthma, lactose intolerance and digestive disturbances during home feeding. It was also suspected that Sudden Infant Death Syndrome and perhaps even some learning disabilities might be linked to unscientific feeding practices. But the dangers of home feeding were not confined to young children. It had long been recognized that eating practices were large factors in adult onset diabetes, heart disease, obesity, anorexia nervosa, diseases of the digestive system, cancer and possibly even drug abuse. At the hospital, each person could be carefully monitored for weight, calorie consumption, vitamin intake, and the percentage of fat and fiber in the diet. Special health problems could be discovered immediately, and each patient's blood and urine could be monitored regularly by the physicians who attended their eating sessions. High risk patients also might have their stomach secretions and peristaltic contractions electronically monitored during each meal at a central nursing station, and a computer controlled alarm would sound if any diner's digestive readings were outside the normal range for the type of meal that was being consumed. Some experts were even starting to suggest that all diners be electronically monitored while they were eating. If there was any indication of a developing eating problem, the patient would probably be admitted to the hospital for intravenous feeding until the problem had cleared up.

Science Reality: This is what androcentric science has done to childbirth.

Human Birth: A Review

As mammals, humans have always given birth to live young. Human pregnancy and childbirth, like eating, always have been biologically successful; that is, they have not been so hazardous or dangerous as to threaten the biological success of the human species. Unlike disease, which threatens the life or the fitness of individuals who suffer from it, pregnancy, childbirth and lactation normally do not threaten the fitness of either mother or child. If pregnancy, childbirth and lactation usually resulted in dead or unfit offspring, or in dead or incapacitated mothers, our species would not have survived. The fact is that the human species not only survives, it thrives with respect to reproduction, particularly when adequate nutrition, shelter and freedom from disease are available to mothers and their offspring. Studies have shown repeatedly that the vast majority of all human pregnancies would end with the birth of a healthy infant to a healthy woman even if she received no prenatal care or advice of any kind from any source (Lang 1972; Guttmacher 1973; Arms 1975; Rich 1976; Oxorn & Foote 1980). With social support, proper nutrition, adequate attention to physical fitness, and the elimination of habits detrimental to health such as smoking, drinking, and drug abuse, some studies have suggested that this figure may approach 95–98% or higher (Lang 1972; Guttmacher 1973; Arms 1975; Gaskin 1978; Edwards & Waldorf 1984). There is documented evidence, for example, that maternal mortality rates were approximately 0.4% in midwife-attended births in the American colonies during the eighteenth century—well before the introduction of modern antibiotics which could cure life-threatening infections (Wertz & Wertz 1979). Midwife-attended home births in Leslie County, KY, one of the poorest rural areas in Appalachia, with the highest birth rate in the country, had a maternal mortality rate of 0.091% from 1925–1955, compared to the national average of 0.34% for white women during the same time period (Arms 1975). This is consistent with the expected levels of health following birth in other species of mammals with typically single gestations. Often touted pseudo-explanations of Western women's difficulties in childbirth simply do not hold up under examination. Evolutionary biology, for example, does not support the idea that Western women could have "evolved" into a species with pelvic structures unsuited for childbirth in the dozen or so generations since androcentric doctors became interested in childbirth. It is possible that women's general levels of physical conditioning and nutrition could have deteriorated over this time period in such a way that the typical Western woman is in poor physical health throughout her childbearing years, but this is entirely environmental, not genetic.

It is also well documented that many of Western women's difficulties in giving birth are the result of the conditions imposed upon them by Western hospitals (Oxorn & Foote 1980; Arms 1975; Mendelsohn 1982). A prime example of this is the condition known as supine hypotensive syndrome. Oxorn & Foote describe the condition this way:

> The clinical picture is one of hypotension when, in the late stages of pregnancy, the woman lies on her back. . . . Other symptoms include nausea, shortness of breath, faintness, pallor, tachycardia, and increased femoral venous pressure. . . . Reduced perfusion of the uterus and placenta leads to fetal hypoxia and changes in the fetal heart rate. (Oxorn & Foote 1980, 115)

This condition may occur to some extent or another in virtually all women who give birth in hospitals, or approximately 97.4% of all births in the United States. This is because hospital births are conducted with the laboring woman ("in the late stages of pregnancy") lying on her back in a bed or on a delivery table. The most common position, known as the lithotomy position, has the woman flat on her back with her legs up in the air in stirrups. Oxorn & Foote list as advantages of this position: more complete asepsis, easier for hospital personnel to monitor the fetal heartbeat without asking the woman to change position, easier for hospital personnel to administer three different kinds of drugs, easier for the doctor to see the birth, good position for the use of forceps and for performing the surgical procedure of episiotomy. As disadvantages they list: risk of supine hypotensive syndrome, sacroiliac or lumbosacral strain, possible thrombosis in the veins of the legs, possible nerve damage, and the danger of aspiration of vomitus (Oxorn & Foote 1980, 114). In contrast, they list the following advantages and disadvantages for women's and midwives' more traditionally preferred squatting position, which is almost never allowed by hospital regulations: Advantages: enlarges the pelvic outlet, enables laboring woman to use her expulsive forces to the greatest advantage, eliminates risk of supine hypotensive syndrome; Disadvantages: difficult "for the accoucher to control the birth and to manage complications," impossible to administer certain types of drugs (Oxorn & Foote 1980, 113).

A feature of the lithotomy position not mentioned by Oxorn & Foote, perhaps because they couldn't decide whether it was an advantage or a disadvantage, is that it increases the amount of symptoms which are taken as indications for performing a cesarean section. The primary fetal indications for cesarean surgery are fetal hypoxia and changes in the fetal heart rate (Oxorn & Foote 1980, 667). These are exactly the fetal conditions that are part of the clinical picture of supine hypotensive syndrome. One would think that since Oxorn & Foote report "the risk of maternal death associated with cesarean section to be 26 times greater than with vaginal delivery" (Oxorn & Foote 1980, 675) the avoidance of cesarean section would be an advantage. However they continually reassure the reader that cesarean section is a fine thing, a tribute to progressive technology. In fact, they advise against the cesarean operation only "when the fetus is dead or in such bad condition that it is unlikely to survive" because "[t]here is no point in submitting the patient to a needless serious operation" (Oxorn & Foote 1980, 669). One cannot help but suspect that physicians who have undergone nearly a decade of training in techniques of medical intervention find it boring and wasteful of their expertise *not* to engage in such interventions whenever possible.

Obviously in this case, when the laboring woman's physiological needs conflict with the convenience or the need for "control" on the part of the hospital staff, it is the woman's physiological needs that are sacrificed. One can hear echoes of Rachel Carson's protest about the "control of nature" and the dangerous effects of that approach in the critiques made by gynocentric investigators about androcentric conceptions of childbirth. Other factors may color androcentric science's research results as well. As Dr. Robert Mendelsohn put it in *Mal(e)practice*, "Doctors know that they can't afford to allow their patients to perceive childbirth as the normal, typically uncomplicated process that it really is. If they did, most women wouldn't need obstetricians" (Mendelsohn 1982, 130). One can almost imagine the same words being written by a dissident physician with respect to eating, in the years following the imaginary scenario in which androcentric science takes control of eating practices. These things are important to keep in mind as we compare gynocentric midwifery with androcentric obstetrical science.

Midwifery and Obstetrics as Competing Scientific Paradigms

Obstetrical science, for the most part, has adopted the view that midwifery is an incomplete, underdeveloped, less successful, and less scientific approach to the same scientific problems that it is attempting to solve. One cannot help but note the similarities between this view of midwifery and the now discredited psychoanalytic and philosophical theories that make out women to be incomplete, underdeveloped, less successful and less rational versions of men. A less biased description might be that midwifery and obstetrical science represent competing scientific paradigms which, like all competing paradigms according to Kuhn (1970), disagree not only about the list of problems to be resolved, but also about the theories, methodologies, and criteria for success that will be used to assess the results achieved.

If gynocentric science is, as I've suggested earlier, "less isolated from other aspects of our lives, less fetishized about individualism, more holistic, more nurturing, more concerned with relations than with objects, perhaps more dialectic, because of the nature and position of the erotic with respect to its epistemology," then these aspects of it should be evident in the work of gynocentric scientists practicing within their paradigm. On the other hand, the androcentric criteria for good science such as abstraction, reductionism, the determination to repress one's feelings to promote 'objectivity' cited by Namenwirth (1986) should be evident in the work of androcentric scientists practicing within their paradigm. Consider these two examples:

Midwifery as Gynocentric Science

. . . I want to stress the importance of good continuous prenatal care. Without the knowledge of excellent health the risks of home birth increase for both mother and child.

To have a healthy pregnancy and good childbirth, certain aspects of existence on the physical, mental, and spiritual plane must be observed and trained to be in harmony with the forces within you, i.e., that of the creation of life.

You should be able to listen closely to everything your body is telling you about what's happening within, how your body feels about what goes into it, what comes out, and just how it feels organically.

As the pregnancy proceeds many things happen and a gradual process of training mind and body takes place.

Food may become a necessary discipline if a diet is not made normally of whole foods. Foods that have been flash grown, processed, refined, nutritionalized and put out as some predigested matter should be avoided.

. . . It's pretty easy to tell if you're doing the above correctly because you will be healthy organically and you can feel that through your entire body.

—*Raven Lang*
Midwife

Obstetrics As Androcentric Science

Once the patient has carefully selected her doctor, she should let him shoulder the full responsibility of her pregnancy and labor, with the comforting knowledge that, no matter what develops, he has had similar cases and her health will be safeguarded by this background of experience.

Most obstetricians prefer to see their patients early in pregnancy, two or three weeks after the first menstrual period is missed. Many women look forward to this first interview with unnecessary dread. Perhaps a friend with previous experience has told them that it is a most embarrassing examination, and such questions! The patient is apt to forget that the doctor has examined literally thousands of women, and in the course of this experience has learned to impersonalize his attitude toward his patients.

At the first visit the obstetrician examines the woman completely from top to toe. It is essential that he determine the exact physical condition of his patient so that he may judge her ability to withstand the strain of pregnancy and labor.

—*Dr. Alan Guttmacher,*
Professor Emeritus of the Department of
Obstetrics and Gynecology at New York's
Mount Sinai Medical School

If incommensurability is to be taken seriously, then we are faced with the ever present problem of theory choice. How are we to evaluate two competing scientific paradigms with respect to their successes at problem solving? "In the first place," wrote Kuhn "the proponents of competing paradigms will often disagree about the list of problems that any candidate for paradigm must resolve. Their standards or their definitions of science are not the same." Going on to explain linguistic incommensurability, he then comes to one of the most compelling observations in *The Structure of Scientific Revolutions:* "In a sense that I am unable to explicate further, the proponents of competing paradigms practice their trades in different worlds" (Kuhn 1970, 150). While the androcentric scientists scratch their heads in perplexed confusion about what Kuhn might possibly mean by this, many feminists smile with the pleasurable sensation of having encountered a clear articulation of the obvious. Many of us are well acquainted with the feeling of dividing our time and attention between two different worlds. Carol Gilligan (1982) has suggested ways in which this plays itself out in ethics; Belenky, Clinchy, Goldberger, and Tarule (1986) have recently done the same for epistemology. There is no reason for us to suspect that we can't do the same thing with respect to science. I don't for a minute want to claim to have demonstrated the existence of a gynocentric science here; what I have tried to do is to articulate an hypothesis that deserves further investigation. My hope is that some empirical investigation will yield fruitful results in this direction, and that these results—in the best of scientific traditions—can feed back into, and interact with, our growing body of theory about the nature of feminist science.

Why Call It 'Science?'

Well, why not?

Women *are* trapped in an androcentric world, as Bleier suggests, one in which language and meaning have been constructed around androcentric goals and enterprises. We've had troubles with language all along. As Marilyn Frye has pointed out, the very terms we use embed in them the connections and distinctions that *men* want to see (Frye 1983, 161). If the term 'science' is to be construed only as a limited range of activities, conducted by properly certified people, under a limited range of circumstances, then perhaps the term 'gynocentric science' is as much a self-contradiction as the term 'military intelligence.' But one of the projects of American feminists has been to claim our right to participate in the making of meaning. We have struggled, for example, to be able to apply the term 'scholarship' to our work, even when much of that work didn't count as scholarship under the old androcentric language rules. For that matter, we've struggled for the right to apply the term 'work' to many of our activities that were once considered not to be work. Feyer-

abend (1975) noticed, even without the benefit of a feminist perspective, that the distinction between science and non-science is political. And as Frye (1983, 105) pointed out, "*definition* is another face of power."

So maybe we are recreating the language a bit by calling midwifery or gossip or cooking 'gynocentric science.' But then, as members of the language-using community, we are entitled. The burden is not on us, but on those who object, to show that this is not a reasonable use of the term 'science.'

Hesitations

Even as I write this, I'm not completely convinced that tugging on the term 'science' to fit gynocentric activities under its umbrella is necessarily the right thing to do. Perhaps, as Marion Namenwirth (1986) suggests, "abstraction, reductionism, the determination to repress one's feelings to promote 'objectivity' have not the same priority to women as they do men." Perhaps, as she doesn't suggest, these qualities are already so tied to the term 'science' that we will choose to dissociate our work from the baggage of the term, and name our gynocentric work something else instead. I find that my own feelings about this waver. On the days when I'm hoping that feminism will make the world better for everybody, I want to tug at the meaning of science to get it to include gynocentric activities. On the days when I'm seeing science as the religion of advanced patriarchy, and philosophy as its theology, I want to withdraw from both entirely. But for those of us who, at least on some days, are struggling to find a feminist conception of science, I offer this suggestion: it's been around us all along. Our task now should be to research it; we need no longer merely fumble about for a theory of what it might be.

REFERENCES

Arms, Suzanne. 1975. *Immaculate deception: A new look at women and childbirth in America*. Boston: Houghton Mifflin.

Belenky, Mary *et al.* 1986. *Women's ways of knowing.* New York: Basic Books.

Birke, Linda. 1986. *Women, feminism and biology: The feminist challenge.* New York: Methuen Press.

Bleier, Ruth. 1984. *Science and gender: A critique of biology and its theories on women.* Elmsford, NY: Pergamon.

———, ed. 1986. *Feminist approaches to science.* Elmsford, NY: Pergamon.

Carson, Rachel. 1964. *Silent spring.* New York: Fawcett Crest.

Daly, Mary. 1978. *Gyn/ecology: The metaethics of radical feminism.* Boston: Beacon Press.

Edwards, Margot and Mary Waldorf. 1984. *Reclaiming birth.* Trumansburg, NY: Crossing Press.

Ehrenreich, Barbara and Deirdre English. 1973. *Witches, midwives, and nurses: A history of women healers.* Old Westbury, NY: The Feminist Press.

Fee, Elizabeth. 1983. Women's nature and scientific objectivity. In *Women's nature: Rationalizations of inequality,* ed. M. Lowe and R. Hubbard, 9–28. Elmsford, NY: Pergamon.

Feyerabend, Paul. 1975. *Against method.* London: Verso.

Frye, Marilyn. 1983. *The politics of reality: Essays in feminist theory.* Trumansburg, NY: Crossing Press.

Gaskin, Ina May. 1978. *Spiritual midwifery.* Summertown, TN: The Book Publishing Company.

Gilligan, Carol. 1982. *In a different voice.* Cambridge, MA: Harvard University Press.

Griffin, Susan. 1980. *Woman and nature: The roaring inside her.* New York: Harper and Row.

Guttmacher, Alan. 1973. *Pregnancy, birth and family planning.* New York: Viking Press.

Harding, Sandra. 1986. *The science question in feminism.* Ithaca, NY: Cornell University Press.

Keller, Evelyn Fox. 1983. *A feeling for the organism: The life and work of Barbara McClintock.* San Francisco: W. H. Freeman.

———. 1985. *Reflections on science and gender.* New Haven, CT: Yale University Press.

Kuhn, Thomas S. 1970. *The structure of scientific revolutions.* Chicago: University of Chicago Press.

Lang, Raven. 1972. *Birth book.* Ben Lomond, CA: Genesis Press.

Lorde, Audre. 1984. *Sister outsider.* Trumansburg, NY: Crossing Press.

Mendelsohn, Robert. 1982. *Mal(e) practice.* Chicago: Contemporary Books.

Merchant, Carolyn. 1980. *The death of nature: Women, ecology and the scientific revolution.* New York: Harper and Row.

Namenwirth, Marion. 1986. Science seen through a feminist prism. In *Feminist approaches to science,* ed. Ruth Bleier. Elmsford, NY: Pergamon.

Oxorn, Harry and William Foote. 1980. *Human labor & birth.* New York: Prentice-Hall.

Rich, Adrienne. 1976. *Of woman born: Motherhood as experience and institution.* New York: Norton.

———. 1979. *On lies, secrets, and silence: Selected prose—1966–78.* New York: Norton.

Rose, Hilary. 1986. Beyond masculinist realities: A feminist epistemology for the sciences. In *Feminist approaches to science,* ed. Ruth Bleier, 57–76. Elmsford, NY: Pergamon.

Stone, Merlin. 1978. *When God was a woman.* New York: Harcourt Brace Jovanovich.

Trask, Haunani-Kay. 1986. *Eros and power.* Philadelphia: University of Pennsylvania Press.

Wertz, Richard and Dorothy Wertz. 1979. *Lying-in: A history of childbirth in America.* New York: Shocken.

After the Neutrality Ideal: Science, Politics, and "Strong Objectivity"

Sandra Harding

There are two kinds of politics with which the new social studies of science have been concerned. One is the older notion of politics as the overt actions and policies intended to advance the interests and agendas of "special interest groups." This kind of politics "intrudes" into "pure science" through consciously chosen and often clearly articulated actions and programs that shape what science gets done, how the results of research are interpreted, and, therefore, scientific and popular images of nature and social relations. This kind of politics is conceptualized as acting *on* the sciences from outside, as "politicizing" science. This is the kind of relationship between politics and science against which the idea of objectivity as neutrality works best.[1]

However, in a sometimes supportive and at other times antagonistic relation to it is a different politics of science. Here power is exercised less visibly, less consciously, and *not on but through* the dominant institutional structures, priorities, practices, and languages of the sciences.[2] Paradoxically, this kind of politics functions through the "depoliticization" of science—through the creation of authoritarian science. As historian Robert Proctor points out:

It is certainly true that, in one important sense, the Nazis sought to politicize the sciences. . . . Yet in an important sense the Nazis might indeed be said to have "depoliticized" science (and many other areas of culture). The Nazis depoliticized science by destroying the possibility of political debate and controversy. Authoritarian science based on the "Führer principle" replaced what had been, in the Weimar period, a vigorous spirit of politicized debate in and around the sciences. The Nazis "depoliticized" problems of vital human interest by reducing these to scientific or medical problems, conceived in the narrow, reductionist sense of these terms. The Nazis depoliticized questions of crime, poverty, and sexual or political deviance by casting them in surgical or otherwise medical (and seemingly apolitical) terms. . . . Politics pursued in the name of science or health provided a powerful weapon in the Nazi ideological arsenal.[3]

The institutionalized, normalized politics of male supremacy, class exploitation, racism, and imperialism, while only occasionally initiated through the kind of violent politics practiced by the Nazis, similarly "depoliticize" Western scientific institutions and practices, thereby shaping our images of the natural and social worlds and legitimating past and future exploitative public policies. In contrast to "intrusive politics," this kind of institutional politics does not force itself into a preexisting "pure" social order and its sciences; it already structures both.

Reprinted by permission from Social Research 59(3):567–587.
© 1992, Social Research.

In this second case, the neutrality ideal provides no resistance to the production of systematically distorted results of research. Even worse, it defends and legitimates the institutions and practices through which the distortions and their exploitative consequences are generated. It certifies as value-neutral, normal, natural, and therefore not political at all the existing scientific policies and practices through which powerful groups can gain the information and explanations that they need to advance their priorities. It functions more through what its normalizing procedures and concepts implicitly prioritize than through explicit directives. This kind of politics requires no "informed consent" by those who exercise it, but only that scientists be "company men," supporting and following the prevailing rules of scientific institutions and their intellectual traditions. This normalizing politics defines the objections of its victims and any criticisms of its institutions, practices, or conceptual world as agitation by special interests that threatens to damage the neutrality of science. Thus, when sciences are already in the service of the mighty, scientific neutrality ensures that "might makes right."

This essay pursues a project begun in other places: to strengthen the notion of objectivity for the natural and social sciences after the demise of the ideal of neutrality.[4] I turn first to the problem of thinking past the epistemological relativism that critics of the neutrality ideal either embrace or commit. Instead, we can begin to discern the possibility of and requirements for a "strong objectivity" by more careful analysis of what is wrong with the neutrality idea. Standpoint epistemologies provide resources for fulfilling these requirements. Finally, I suggest that the usefulness of the notion of truth, like that of epistemological relativism, should be historically relativized; the unnecessary trouble both make in the postneutrality debates originates in their intimate links to the rejected neutrality ideal.

Are Objectivism and Relativism the Only Choices?

The ideal of objectivity as neutrality is widely regarded to have failed not only in history and the social sciences, but also in philosophy and related fields such as jurisprudence.[5] The notion contains a number of elements. In the following passage, Peter Novick describes how it appears in the thinking of historians; but with appropriate adjustments this passage expresses objectivist assumptions more generally:

> The assumptions on which [the ideal of objectivity] rests include a commitment to the reality of the past, and to truth as correspondence to that reality; a sharp separation between knower and known, between fact and value, and, above all, between history and fiction. Historical facts are seen as prior to and independent of interpretation: the value of an interpretation is judged by how well it accounts for the facts; if contradicted by the facts, it must be abandoned. Truth is one, not perspectival. Whatever patterns exist in history are "found," not "made."
>
> The objective historian's role is that of a neutral, or disinterested judge; it must never degenerate into that of advocate or even worse, propagandist. The historian's conclusions are expected to display the standard judicial qualities of balance and evenhandedness. As with the judiciary, these qualities are guarded by the insulation of the historical profession from social pressure or political influence, and by the individual historian avoiding partisanship or bias—not having any investment in arriving at one conclusion rather than another.[6]

What is left of the objectivity ideal when neutrality is abandoned? Fairness, honesty, and an important kind of "detachment," to start. Thomas Haskell, for example, points out that it is absurd to assume—as Novick does—that in giving up the goal of neutrality one must give up the ideal of objectivity:

> The very possibility of historical scholarship as an enterprise distinct from propaganda requires of its practitioners that vital minimum of ascetic self-dis-

cipline that enables a person to do such things as abandon wishful thinking, assimilate bad news, discard pleasing interpretations that cannot pass elementary tests of evidence and logic, and, most important of all, suspend or bracket one's own perceptions long enough to enter sympathetically into the alien and possibly repugnant perspectives of rival thinkers. All of these mental acts—especially coming to grips with a rival's perspective—require *detachment,* an undeniably ascetic capacity to achieve some distance from one's own spontaneous perceptions and convictions, to imagine how the world appears in another's eyes, to experimentally adopt perspectives that do not come naturally—in the last analysis, to develop, as Thomas Nagel would say, a view of the world in which one's own self stands not at the center, but appears merely as one object among many.[7]

Notice that the detachment called for here is not impersonality. The observer is not to act as if s/he were not a social person, or to separate even more from those s/he studies (when it is people or institutions that are the object of study), but, instead, critically to distance from the assumptions that shape *his or her own* "spontaneous perceptions and convictions." Haskell is concerned here with something different from the distorting effects of the intrusion of politics into neutral science. Instead, it is the distorting "politics of the obvious" to which he is drawing attention. Sometimes this can be a matter of idiosyncratic individual assumptions; but these are relatively easily identified by peers who check research designs, sources, and observations. More problematic are the spontaneous perceptions and convictions that are shared by a scientific community and, usually, by the dominant groups in the social order of which the scientists are members by birth and/or achievement. It is reflexivity that is the issue here: self-criticism in the sense of criticism of the widely shared values and interests that constitute one's own institutionally shaped research assumptions.

Haskell's kind of retrieval of the concept of objectivity from its "operationalization" as maximizing neutrality is extremely valuable. How-

ever, to become more than a mere moral and intellectual gesture—to become a competent program that can guide research practices—we need some procedures or strategies to pursue that could systematically lead away from wishful thinking, refusing to come to terms with bad news, refusing "to enter sympathetically into the alien and possibly repugnant perspectives of rival thinkers," etc. Otherwise, it is perfectly clear that only the already marginal groups will be regarded as engaging in these bad habits by those with the most authoritative voices in the social order and our research disciplines. The latter, with no conscious bad intent, will arrive at such judgments by simply following the normalizing procedures of institutions and conceptual schemes legitimated already as value-neutral. Without strategies to maximize this kind of objectivity, these moral exhortations remain only idle gestures.

These "minorities" have additional cause for alarm at the retreat to gestures. In some of the most influential criticisms of objectivism and its assumptions, the effects on historical, sociological, or scientific belief of such macro social structures as the racial order, the class system, imperialism, and the gender order are completely and sometimes even intentionally ignored.[8] In others, the contributions of research and scholarship that begins from the lives of people of color and feminists are devalued and even attacked.[9] Yet the articulation of the perspective from the lives of just such marginalized peoples as racial minorities in the first world, third-world people, women, and the poor has provided some of the most powerful challenges to the adequacy of objectivism. The gestures of mainstream writers to the value of good intentions coupled with their persistent failures to manage to "be fair" to the most "alien and possibly repugnant" competing claims cannot give much hope to those who have persistently lost the most from the conceptual practices of power.[10] Embracing or committing epistemological relativism has the effect of defending the dominant views against their most telling critics. Does relativism itself need to be relativized?

The fall of objectivism and the failure to replace it with a viable alternative program has a double effect for the natural sciences. For one thing, it challenges the procedures in the social studies of science for maximizing the objectivity of the descriptive and prescriptive accounts of the natural sciences that are produced in history, sociology, anthropology, political economy, and philosophy. Have these fields really provided the maximally objective accounts—the least possible partial and distorted ones—of the past practices in the natural sciences? Are the prescriptions for generating future maximally objective accounts likely to advance that goal if they are grounded in accounts of past practices that block our ability to describe, explain, or understand the causes of success and failure in the history of science?

Natural scientists might assume that this is an issue only for the social studies of science. After all, the study of institutions of science, their history and present practices, is not the same as the study of nature. However, the natural sciences can't escape the implications of objectivism's decline so easily. Their choice of procedures to use in identifying and eliminating distorting cultural assumptions from the results of their research are guided by assumptions about which have been the most successful such procedures in the past. The natural sciences do and must assume histories, sociologies, political economies, and philosophies of science whether or not they explicitly articulate such assumptions. Furthermore, this theoretical point is supported by historical evidence since the critics of objectivism also have focused directly on the natural sciences. Following the path of earlier accounts of how bourgeois assumptions have shaped Western sciences, feminist and postcolonial critics recently have pointed to the inadequacy of neutral objectivism to identify the androcentric, Eurocentric, and racist assumptions in many of the most widely accepted scientific claims.[11] The fact that physical nature does not organize itself culturally does not give the natural sciences immu-

nity to these criticisms of how social assumptions and projects inevitably shape the results of human research; what the sciences actually observe is not bare nature but always only nature-as-an-object-of-knowledge—which is always already fully encultured.[12] Thus the natural sciences, too, are confronted with the demise of objectivism and threat of relativism.

Relativizing Relativism

The epistemological relativism that makes unnecessary trouble in the postneutrality discussions is sometimes conflated with sociological relativism. The latter simply describes the obvious fact that different people or cultures have different standards for determining what counts as knowledge; there is no one standard to which they all agree. Sociological relativism simply states a fact that is uncontested by either the epistemological absolutists or relativists, who go on to make further, conflicting, judgments about how to respond to this fact. The absolutists, such as objectivists, say that there is one and only one defensible standard for sorting belief to which—alas—some peoples and societies haven't caught on. The absolutists make a judgment, a prescription, about what standards we all should use in seeking knowledge. The *epistemological* relativists make a different judgment: that each of these (often conflicting) standards that different groups use is equally valid, equally good. There are no defensible grounds for maintaining that any one is better than any other; there can be no one standard for sorting beliefs, they say. My point here is that it is only this epistemological (or judgmental, or cognitive) relativism that is problematic.[13]

It is important to note that relativism is objectivism's twin. While always a theoretical possibility, as a troubling concern it is an historical emergent. On the one hand, it is not a problem justifiable in terms of knowledge projects originating in the lives of marginalized groups. No critics of racism, imperialism, male supremacy, or the class system think that the evidence and arguments they present leave their claims valid only "from their perspective"; they argue for the validity of these claims on objective grounds, not on "perspectivalist" ones. Nor, on the other hand, is there any good reason for an absolutist to be worried about relativism if no one challenges the universal validity of his standards. Relativism appears to have emerged as a disturbing issue only in nineteenth-century Europe, as some anthropologists began to show that the apparently bizarre beliefs and behaviors of "savages" had a rationality of their own, and the rise of socialism and feminism suggested similar possibilities about the working class and women. Many Western anthropologists still defend a relativist stance that simultaneously respects the different rationality of non-Western ways of life, legitimates their own work as reporters of the exotic, and blocks recognition of the authoritarianism of Western standards for science and "progress." Today, disillusioned objectivists are often unable to distinguish between the ethnocentric and relativist stances that they take to be the only alternative to neutrality and that, they insist, are all that feminists, postcolonialists, and other such "special interest groups" can claim, and the systematic procedures for maximizing objectivity that such groups propose. Like its partner, absolutism, relativism can be "relativized." We are not forced to it in rejecting absolutism.[14]

If the demise of the neutrality ideal does not force us to epistemological relativism, perhaps the notion of objectivity can be strengthened as a resource to enable researchers to arrive at less partial and distorting claims.

Objectivism vs. Strong Objectivity

An excessively restricted notion of research methods has ensured that only weak standards of objectivity will be required of research projects. Objectivist methods are designed to identify and eliminate those social and political values and interests that differ between the individuals who constitute a scientific commu-

nity. However, several problems still remain. For one thing, scientific methods in the narrow sense in which research designs designate them—techniques—function only in the "context of justification." That is, they are brought into play only after the "context of discovery": after a problem is identified as a scientific one and a hypothesis and testing procedures are selected.[15] However, it is in the context of discovery that culture-wide assumptions which subsequently are among the most difficult to identify make their way into the research process and shape the claims that result. It is here that problems are identified and designated as scientific ones, concepts selected, and hypotheses formulated. Even the National Academy of Sciences now argues that the notion of scientific methods should be enlarged beyond its familiar meaning of techniques to "include the judgments scientists make about interpretation or reliability of data. They also include the decisions scientists make about which problems to pursue or when to conclude an investigation. Methods involve the ways scientists work with each other and exchange information."[16]

Of course, funding requests (as well as hiring, promotion, and publishing processes) require peer reviews, so one might think that distorting assumptions would tend to be identified here; that a kind of method of discovery—of detecting and eliminating distorting values and interests from the "bold conjectures" that will be tested—is already widely practiced. However, exactly because it is peers who make or contribute importantly to these decisions, it is exactly the assumptions peers share that escape detection here, too.

The same problem appears inside the "context of justification" where it is peers who certify research decisions, processes, and outcomes. Scientific communities that are designed (intentionally or not) to consist only of like-minded individuals lose exactly that economic, political, and cultural diversity that is necessary to enable those who count as peers to detect the dominant culture's values and interests. The main problem here is not that individuals in the community are androcentric, Eurocentric, or economically overprivileged (though that certainly doesn't help), but, instead, that the normalizing, routine conceptual practices of power are exactly those that are least likely to be detected by individuals who are trained not to question the social location and priorities of the institutions and conceptual schemes within which their research occurs. Moreover, even when a conflicting value or interest is detected within such communities, there are no standards or procedures immune to these same criticisms for determining whether the minority or majority claim distorts less. For example, feminist and postcolonial accounts of the history of the natural sciences that are making their way into mainstream publishers' lists are at best regarded by the "natives" of Western science and the social studies of science to be expressing only "special interests" and proposing alternative "ethnosciences"; the dominant views remain the purportedly neutral standard. So objectivism "operationalizes" maximizing objectivity too weakly when its methods can identify only those values and interests that differ within a homogeneous scientific community, and when it has no strategies for gaining causal, critical accounts of the dominant cultural standards.

Furthermore, neutrality operationalizes maximizing objectivity too weakly in another way. Some social values and interests clearly maximize the objectivity of research. As Haskell points out, fairness, honesty, and detachment, which are moral and, indeed, political values and interests, must be activated in order to maximize objectivity. Moreoever, in order to "assimilate bad news," or "to suspend or bracket one's own perceptions long enough to enter sympathetically into the alien and possibly repugnant perspectives of rival thinkers," the material and political conditions must be such that the bad news arrives and the rival thinkers' perspectives are accessible, and that these perspectives are taken seriously as real rivals to the dominant ones. But androcentric, bourgeois, and racist social orders

insure that very little of these necessary material and political conditions will occur. There is little of postcolonial or feminist approaches available in the leading science and social studies of science journals, conference programs, or graduate teaching. Thus, democratizing the social order contributes to maximizing the objectivity of a society's sciences. In short, the most critical—"alien and possibly repugnant"—perspectives, because they conflict with the values and interests that have been conceptualized as neutral, are exactly what get dismissed a priori by objectivists. Thus the sciences are left complicitous with the projects of the most powerful groups in society. The neutrality requirement is not just ineffective at maximizing objectivity; it is an obstacle to it.

These kinds of arguments enable us to begin to see the outlines of a stronger conception of objectivity. Strong objectivity would specify strategies to detect social assumptions that (a) enter research in the identification and conceptualization of scientific problems and the formation of hypotheses about them (the "context of discovery"), (b) tend to be shared by observers designated as legitimate ones, and thus are significantly collective, not individual, values and interests, and (c) tend to structure the institutions and conceptual schemes of disciplines. These systematic procedures would also be capable of (d) distinguishing between those values and interests that block the production of less partial and distorted accounts of nature and social relations ("less false" ones) and those—such as fairness, honesty, detachment, and, we should add, advancing democracy—that provide resources for it. This is the point where standpoint epistemologies can be useful.

Standpoint Epistemologies

Standpoint theories argue that if one wants to detect the values and interests that structure scientific institutions, practices, and conceptual schemes, it is useless to frame one's research questions or to pursue them only within the priorities of these institutions, practices, and conceptual schemes. One must start from *outside* them to gain a causal, critical view of them. One important way to do so is to start thought from marginal lives.

While standpoint theory has been most thoroughly articulated in almost two decades of feminist writings, similar arguments appear in the knowledge and policy claims of postcolonials, people of third-world descent in the first world, lesbians and gays, criticisms of the class system, etc.[17] The convergence of these largely independently developed epistemologies (with their accompanying sociologies, histories, and methodologies of scientific research) creates an additional kind of evidence for any one of them. Here, I can only outline some main tendencies in current thinking about them.

What does it mean to "start thought from marginal lives"? "Marginal lives" are determinate, objective locations in the social structure. Such locations are not just accidently outside the center of power and prestige, but necessarily so. It is the material and symbolic existence of such oppositional margins that keep the center in place: the rich can only be rich if there are others who are economically exploited; masculinity can only be an ideal if it is continuously contrasted with a devalued other: femininity. "Matrix theory," which focuses on the systematic social *relations* between such macrostructuring forces as the class, gender, and race systems, provides an empirically and theoretically more adequate account of these social structures than do the earlier class theories, gender theories, and race theories that did not prioritize the way class, gender, and race construct and maintain each other. The thought that develops from such a starting point emerges from democratic dialogue—the sort characteristic of coalitions—between various marginal communities and, also, the dominant ones.[18] So the standpoint project is, first, to generate scientific problems not from within the debates and puzzles of the research traditions, not from the priorities of funders or dominant policy groups, but from

outside these conceptual frameworks, namely, from the lives of marginalized peoples; and to develop this thought through democratic dialogues between knowledge-producing groups.

These accounts are not fundamentally *about* marginal lives; instead they start off research *from* them; they are about the rest of the local and international social order. The point of identifying these problems is not to generate ethnosciences, but *sciences*—systematic causal accounts of how the natural and social orders are organized such that the everyday lives of marginalized peoples end up in the conditions they do. (From the perspective of standpoint theories, the term "ethnoscience" is more appropriately applied to the dominant sciences that fail to gain the detachment from the conceptual priorities and assumptions of dominant groups that is supposed to be required of sciences.) Moreover, to start from marginal lives is not necessarily to take one's problems in the terms in which they are expressed by marginalized people—and this is as true for researchers who come from such groups as for those who do not. Listening attentively to what bothers them is a crucial assistance in standpoint projects. But the dominant ideology restricts what everyone, including marginalized people, are permitted to see and shapes everyone's consciousnesses. African Americans, too, have argued that African Americans should be satisfied with their lesser places in the social order. Women, like men, have had to learn to think of sexual harassment, not as a matter of "boys will be boys," but as a violation of women's civil rights. Marital rape was a legal and, for most people, conceptual impossibility until recently. Western feminists, like the rest of Westerners, are only beginning to learn how to conceptualize many of our "problems" in anti-Eurocentric terms.

Thus standpoint approaches differ from interpretive ones. Because standpoint theory is persistently misread as a kind of "perspectivalism" that generates relativistic interpretations of nature and social relations, I shall risk repetition here. To start thought from marginal lives is not to take as incorrigible—as the irrefutable grounds for knowledge—what marginal people say or interpretations of their experiences. Listening carefully to what marginalized people say—with fairness, honesty, and detachment—and trying to understand their life worlds are crucial first steps in gaining less partial and distorted accounts of the entire social order; but these could not be the last step. Starting thought from marginal lives is not intended to provide an interpretation of those lives, but instead a causal, critical account of the regularities of the natural and social worlds and their underlying causal tendencies. Thus standpoint theory demands acknowledgment of the sociological relativism that is the fate of all human enterprises including knowledge claims, but rejects epistemological relativism.

To start thought from marginal lives is scientifically and epistemologically preferable for all the reasons historians and social scientists value "stranger," "underclass," and "loser" perspectives on history and social life.[19] What we do enables and limits the kinds of things we can know about ourselves and the world, and if one starts from the activities of those who are necessarily disadvantaged in a particular kind of social order one can come to understand objectively existing features of it that are much harder to detect when one starts thought from the activities of those who benefit most. The "natures" and social conditions of women, the poor, lesbians and gays, and people of color have consistently been regarded as natural and necessary for "human progress" by the dominant groups. Starting thought from these disadvantaged lives enables one to detect the social mechanisms through which power relations are made to appear obviously natural and necessary. The natural sciences have participated in creating and legitimating these distorted accounts, and their institutions and practitioners have benefited from them. Western sciences have played an important role in advancing Western imperialism, and have gained increased prestige from the destruction

of non-Western cultures and their scientific traditions. To examine critically Western sciences from the perspective of this kind of history enables us to detect distorting assumptions structuring it that are shared by most Westerners.

As the history of thought shows, thinkers who are not themselves members of marginalized groups can generate these accounts that maximize strong objectivity. John Stuart Mill was not a woman, though he produced one of the most powerful feminist analyses that begins thinking about social relations between the genders from the perspective of women's lives. Marx and Engels were not members of the proletariat from the perspective of whose lives they began thinking about the class system. Many recent illuminating analyses of the social order have begun from the lives of marginalized people that were very different from the authors' lives. Starting thought from lives other than one's own should not be a controversial idea since it is presumably the goal of a good part of the educational process. Students are expected to be able to understand how the world looked by starting their thought from the objective historical conditions in which lived Aristotle, Galileo, Shakespeare, and other thinkers whose ideas are often "alien and possibly repugnant" to many of these students. What's different here is to expect members of dominant groups to think they can learn anything objectively less false *about themselves* and their conceptual and material universe by thinking about their own, dominant world from the perspective of the objective social conditions of the "have nots" from which (intentionally or not) they benefit. But this is just what is required for the kind of detachment central to maximizing objectivity.

Who Needs Truth?

Finally, we can ask how we should think about the relationship between our best knowledge claims and the nature and social relations that they are intended to describe/interpret. For objectivism, with its ideal of results of research that were socially neutral, truth could appear to be a reasonable way to conceptualize the relationship. The best knowledge claims should be true of the world in the sense of reflecting without distortion the way the world is, of corresponding to a reality that is "out there" and unchanged by human study of it. Claims that satisfied the requirements of knowledge (that constitute "justified true belief") would bear a unique relationship to the world.

Of course there were always obvious contradictions in imagining that the goal of sciences could be to generate true statements since what makes a claim scientific is that it must always be held open to revision on the basis of future possibly disconfirming empirical observations or of revisions in the conceptual frameworks of the sciences. The abandonment in scientific circles of the concept of the crucial experiment in the late nineteenth century reflected that recognition that no empirical observations could "prove" a hypothesis true; (at most) it could only prove it false. However, the last thirty years of the philosophy and history of science have succeeded in undermining dreams of absolute falsification, too. As noted earlier, scientific claims and assumptions form a network, and scientists must choose whether to regard a belief at the analytic center or observational periphery of the network as the one to be revised when refutation of a hypothesis threatens.[20] Historians have pointed out how these choices have been made at different stages in research traditions and for "extrascientific" reasons: young theories must be retained in the face of occasional or even frequent falsifying observations; favored older theories are usually retained until they are forced into retirement by the scientific community's shift in allegiance to an alternative; any theory can always be retained as long as its defenders hold enough institutional power to explain away potential threats to it.[21] Even if the concept of absolute truth could not be used to characterize the results of scientific research, it still could function as an ideal toward which science was moving as long as absolute falsity

could characterize "bold hypotheses" the sciences tested. But once the idea of absolute falsity also becomes indefensible, what could be the use of the concept of truth?

The notion is inextricably linked to objectivism and its absolutist standards.[22] "Less false" claims are all the procedures of the sciences (at best) can generate: the hypothesis passing empirical and theoretical tests is less false than all the alternatives considered. This gap between the best procedures humans have come up with for weighing evidence and the unachievable procedures that a truth standard requires (e.g., testing all possible alternative hypotheses) gives more reason for thinking past objectivism and relativism. Nostalgia for the possibility of certain foundations for our knowledge claims can more easily be left behind us as part of the safety net we no longer need in order to make the best judgments we can about nature and social relations. Who needs truth in science? Only those who are still wedded to the neutrality ideal.

In conclusion, the postneutrality discussions need to turn their backs on epistemological relativism. When they do so they can begin to explore strategies for maximizing objectivity by adopting those methods for detecting systematically distorting assumptions that have proved most powerful in the projects of marginalized groups. This turn to strong objectivity will have benefits for both the natural sciences and the social studies of science.

NOTES

1. See Robert Proctor, *Value-Free Science? Purity and Power in Modern Knowledge* (Cambridge: Harvard University Press, 1991) for a history of the diverse origins and uses of the idea.
2. See the discussion of this second kind of power in, e.g., Joseph Rouse's *Knowledge and Power: Toward a Political Philosophy of Science* (Ithaca, N.Y.: Cornell University Press, 1987).
3. Robert Proctor, *Racial Hygiene: Medicine Under the Nazis* (Cambridge: Harvard University Press, 1988), pp. 290, 293.
4. See *The Science Question in Feminism* (Ithaca, N.Y.: Cornell University Press, 1986); *Whose Science? Whose Knowledge?* (Ithaca, N.Y.: Cornell University

Press, 1991), esp. chs. 5 and 6; my edited collection *The Racial Economy of Science* (Bloomington, Ind.: Indiana University Press, forthcoming 1993); and "Rethinking Standpoint Epistemology" in Linda Alcoff and Elizabeth Potter, eds., *Feminist Epistemologies* (Boston: Routledge, forthcoming).

5. The literature here is huge. For a few particularly striking examples, see Richard Bernstein, *Beyond Objectivism and Relativism* (Philadelphia: University of Pennsylvania Press, 1983); Peter Novick, *That Noble Dream: The "Objectivity Question" and the American Historical Profession* (Cambridge: Cambridge University Press, 1988); Patricia Williams, *The Alchemy of Race and Rights* (Cambridge: Harvard University Press, 1991); chs. 5 and 6 of Evelyn Fox Keller, *Reflections on Gender and Science* (New Haven: Yale University press, 1985); Donna J. Haraway, "Situated Knowledges: The Science Question in Feminism and the Privilege of Partial Perspective," in her *Simians, Cyborgs and Women: The Reinvention of Nature* (New York: Routledge, 1991).

6. Novick, *That Noble Dream*, pp. 1–2.

7. Thomas L. Haskell, "Objectivity Is Not Neutrality: Rhetoric vs. Practice in Peter Novick's *That Noble Dream*," *History and Theory* 29 (1990): 132; citing Thomas Nagel, *The View from Nowhere* (New York: Oxford University Press, 1986), pp. 4–6, 68. See also the important criticisms of Novick's account by Linda Gordon, "AHR Forum: Comments on *That Noble Dream*," *American Historical Review* 96 (June 1991): 683–687.

8. This is the case, for example, for the "strong programme" in the sociology of knowledge and related tendencies in the social studies of science. See, e.g., David Bloor, *Knowledge and Social Imagery* (London: Routledge & Kegan Paul, 1977); Bruno Latour and Steve Woolgar, *Laboratory Life: The Social Construction of Scientific Facts* (Beverly Hills, Calif.: Sage, 1979).

9. Consider, for example, the persistent failure of the social studies of science to come to grips with Joseph Needham's comparative studies of Chinese and Western sciences; see, e.g., *The Grand Titration: Science and Society in East and West* (Toronto: University of Toronto Press, 1970). Or consider Novick and Haskell's trivialization and even demonization of feminist approaches to history. In focusing their discussions of feminist history disproportionately on the Sears case, it is clear that both think it important to jump in and take one side in a discussion within feminist theory that is unfinished and necessarily contentious rather than to try to articulate for their audiences the large concerns that made the Sears case so agonizing for feminists. It is not

that feminists should be immune to criticism—even by scholars who work in other fields such as Novick and Haskell—but that these historians continue gender politics when they assert their right to decide feminist issues rather than trying to understand and explain them.

10. The phrase is Dorothy Smith's; see her *The Conceptual Practices of Power: A Feminist Sociology of Knowledge* (Boston: Northeastern University Press, 1990).

11. The feminist literature is huge. For good review essays and bibliographies, see Londa Schiebinger, "The History and Philosophy of Women in Science: A Review Essay," in Sandra Harding and Jean O'Barr, eds., *Sex and Scientific Inquiry* (Chicago: University of Chicago Press, 1987); A. Wylie, K. Okruhlik, S. Morton, and L. Thielen-Wilson, "Philosophical Feminism: A Bibliographic Guide to Critiques of Science," *New Feminist Research/Nouvelles Recherches Feministes* 18 (June 1990): 2–36. For samples of the postcolonial critiques, see Susantha Goonatilake, *Aborted Discovery: Science and Creativity in the Third World* (London: Zed Books, 1984); Patrick Petitjean, Catherine Jami, Anne Marie Moulin, eds., *Science and Empires: Historical Studies about Scientific Development and European Expansion* (Dordrecht, Holland: Kluwer Academic Publishers, 1992); Ziauddin Sardar, ed., *The Revenge of Athena; Science, Exploitation and the Third World* (London: Mansell Publishing Ltd., 1988).

12. Most people think that the subject matter of the natural sciences is not cultural and therefore that methodological issues raised by the study of people and social institutions are irrelevant to the natural sciences. They disagree on whether, nevertheless, natural-science methods should be the model for the social sciences, but they agree that whatever issues arise for the social sciences because of their distinctive subject matter could not illuminate the natural sciences. In contrast to these disputants, I have argued that nature-as-an-object-of-knowledge is always already encultured for scientists by "conversations" they have with their disciplinary traditions and the surrounding culture, and by the methods they use to interact with nature. Consequently, the natural sciences are usefully conceptualized as a subfield of social research. See *The Science Question* and *Whose Science?*

13. It was Thomas Kuhn's *The Structure of Scientific Revolutions* (Chicago: University of Chicago Press, 1962) that made epistemological relativism a concern in the philosophy of science since, in effect, he showed that all of natural science was located inside social history. At the same time, W. V. O. Quine pointed out that it was always a matter of choice

whether scientists should give up an observational or theoretical claim, or even a logical assumption, when a hypothesis was "falsified by experience": they formed an interconnected network of belief. See his *Word and Object* (Cambridge: MIT Press, 1960). This is not the place to review the subsequent huge literature on epistemological relativism ("relativism," henceforth), but for one interesting recent paper, see S. P. Mohanty, "Us and Them: On the Philosophical Bases of Political Criticism," *Yale Journal of Criticism* 2:2 (1989): 1–31.

14. I have discussed this issue in other places; see, e.g., *Whose Science?*, pp. 153ff.

15. Some may think that discussing these issues in such "rational reconstruction of science" terms is irrelevant to describing, explaining, or understanding what researchers actually do or should be doing. However, since researchers themselves must make assumptions and decisions about how to do research, they, too, have an interest in such "rational reconstructions." It is only distorting and misleading rational reconstructions that should be avoided. The new social studies of science—intentionally or not—provide different rational reconstructions.

16. National Academy of Sciences, *On Being a Scientist* (Washington, D.C.: National Academy of Sciences Press, 1989), pp. 5–6.

17. Central statements of this approach can be found in Smith's *Conceptual Practices of Power* and *The Everyday World as Problematic* (Boston: Northeastern University Press, 1987); Nancy Hartsock, "The Feminist Standpoint: Developing the Ground for a Specifically Feminist Historical Materialism," in S. Harding and M. Hintikka, eds., *Discovering Reality: Feminist Perspectives on Epistemology, Metaphysics, Methodology and Philosophy of Science* (Dordrecht: Reidel Publishing Co., 1983); Hilary Rose, "Hand Brain and Heart: A Feminist Epistemology for the Natural Sciences," *Signs* 9:1 (1983); Alison Jaggar, ch. 11 of *Feminist Politics and Human Nature* (Totowa, N.J.: Roman & Allenheld, 1983). An important recent development of this theory is in chs. 10 and 11 of Patricia Hill Collins, *Black Feminist Thought: Knowledge, Consciousness and the Politics of Empowerment* (New York: Routledge, 1991). Postcolonial standpoint arguments may be found, e.g., in the works cited in note 11.

18. It is women of color who have developed matrix theory and arguments about the importance of gaining knowledge through dialogue between coalition members. See, e.g., Collins, *Black Feminist Thought*.

19. I review many of these in ch. 5 of *Whose Science?*

20. See references in note 13.

21. See my edited collection, *Can Theories Be Refuted? Essays on the Duhem-Quine Thesis* (Dordrecht: Reidel, 1976).

22. The postcolonial science critics are continually amazed at the inability of Westerners to understand that Western sciences, too, are fully housed within distinctively Western religious and cultural meanings. See the earlier citations.

· ·

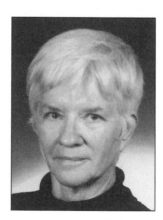

SANDRA HARDING

Reading 36

Gender and Nursing Science

Peggy L. Chinn

Gender is a term that refers to the socialized, acquired traits that render a person's identity as masculine or feminine. It is prescribed for and intended to be associated with a person's biological sex, but abstract or non-human phenomena such as objects, actions, groups, and nature acquire gender associations. As the dictionary notes, use of the term has become confused in recent years:

> Usage Note: Traditionally, *gender* has been used primarily to refer to the grammatical categories of "masculine," "feminine," and "neuter"; but in recent years the word has become well established in its use to refer to sex-based categories, as in phrases such as *gender gap* and the *politics of gender*. This usage is supported by the practice of many anthropologists, who reserve *sex* for reference to biological categories, while using *gender* to refer to social or cultural categories. According to this rule, one would say *The effectiveness of the medication appears to depend on the sex* (not *gender*) *of the patient*, but *In peasant societies, gender* (not *sex*) *roles are likely to be more clearly defined*. This distinction is useful in principle, but it is by no means widely observed, and considerable variation in usage occurs at all levels. (American Heritage Dictionary, Electronic version, 1992)

In this paper, I make the distinction described above, in part because I argue that nursing as a social category has acquired gender traits that are associated with "feminine," regardless of the sex of its individual members.

When I refer to "nursing," or "nursing's perspective," I mean the tradition that is documented as belonging to the profession and discipline of nursing. When I refer to "nurses," I am referring to individuals who alone or collectively hold a viewpoint. I am not assuming the sex of the individual nurse, but I do assume the gender association that is inherent in being a nurse and part of the nursing community.

Gender, as an acquired trait, defines behaviors that are consistent with social norms attributed to being male or female; it also shapes ways of seeing the world. The fact that gender is socially acquired has tremendous implications for a discipline that is predominantly inhabited by women. The discipline itself, like the individuals who comprise the discipline, acquires ways of seeing the world that derive from gendered female experience. Nursing is not neutral. The discipline is so entrenched in its social placement as feminine, that regardless of the sex of its members, it reflects that which is ascribed as being female. Shepherd (1993) stated that the feminine is "the part of us that sees life in context, the interconnectedness of everything, and the consequences of our actions on future generations" (p. 1). This conception of what is feminine is almost identical with typical statements regarding the nature of nursing. Consider the definition of the focus of nursing that Donaldson and Crowley (1978) offered when nursing as a scientific discipline was still in its early stages of development. They stated that the focus of nursing is "the health or wholeness of human beings as they interact within their environments" (p. 113). Smith (1994) commented that while Nightingale set nursing on a path "dedicated to the human-environment relationship and to practices that invite health and healing, the winds of medicine and science have blown us off that course" (p. 57). Smith's comment implies the tension between that which is associated with the feminine (nursing), and that which is associated with the masculine (science and medicine).

Since being female is not typically viewed as an asset in society, moving to a place where the knowledge, actions, and ideas of nurses can be valued is not an easy challenge. I believe, however, that it is time to recognize the strengths that are inherent in nursing perspectives, recognizing that in part this perspective is enriched by a feminine gender association.

Nightingale (1969) established professional nursing with a clear conception of nursing as being concerned with humans in the context of the environment. She also recognized a tension that existed even in the 19th century between nursing's allegiance to medicine, and the feminine concerns for interactions within a context:

> [Nursing] has been limited to signify little more than the administration of medicines and the application of poultices. It ought to signify the proper use of fresh air, light, warmth, cleanliness, quiet, and the proper selection and administration of diet—all at the least expense of vital power to the patient. (Nightingale, 1969, p. 8)

Nightingale's conception sees human health and illness in the context of the environment, and she adamantly ascribed the suffering of illness to the interconnectedness of every aspect of the person's life. Nurses, she believed, could form actions that have significant effects on how people experience illness, and how they recover.

She was unrelenting in her view that women need to be educated in order to serve society well. She envisioned nursing as a women's profession, in part, I think, to assure that the perspectives that she recognized as coming from educated women, would continue to form the philosophic and practical directions for the profession. She wrote *Notes on Nursing* because of her recognition that women's education left them ignorant of their own bodies and lacking in knowledge needed to carry out their responsibilities while caring for the sick. Nightingale passionately believed that women should take their lives as seriously as men do theirs, to prepare themselves for the work they want to do and to do that work wholeheartedly. She saw nursing as a serious occupation, one suited for women to excel and an avenue for women to gain economic independence while making significant contributions to society at large.

In her essay titled *Cassandra*, Nightingale (1979) posed the question: "Why have women passion, intellect, moral activity—these three—and a place in society where no one of the three can be exercised?" (p. 25). In the context of today, and largely because of Nightingale's legacy, women have many more opportunities in society to exercise our passion, intellect, and moral activity. I submit, however, that nurses have not realized our full potential in doing so, and that understanding what it means to exercise our values derived from women's experience could dramatically re-direct the future of nursing and health care. In the discussion that follows, I will set forth a vision of the value of women's perspectives.

Passion

> Women dream till they have no longer the strength to dream. . . . All their plans and visions seem vanished, and they know not where; gone and they cannot recall them. They do not even remember them. And they are left without the food either of reality or of hope. (Nightingale, 1979, p. 49)

Passion, in Nightingale's view, arises from the dream, the yearning for what might be. Nursing's plans, visions, and dreams for health care appear in many forms; accounts in the literature, philosophies written for educational programs or nursing service organizations, proposals for political reform, stories that nurses tell one another, commentaries that detail a longing for what might be. The dreams reflect what is associated with the feminine—yearning for a context or environment that promotes health, healing, and wholeness; recognition of the importance of time spent with another human being nurturing and encouraging growth and healing; valuing a kind of caring that affirms the uniqueness and individuality of every experience; holding and protecting the person's rights, culture, and values (Chinn, 1989).

The reality of what nurses face in practice reflects a system that arises from philosophic viewpoints that have typically eschewed that which is feminine. Nurses are left to dream their dreams, hope for what might be, and ultimately to forsake, even forget, that which could rise to their passion to act. The growing literature in nursing that concerns the values of caring practices, and the necessity for developing knowledge of caring, gives recognition of the value inherent in many of the dreams that nurses dream (Chinn, 1991; Hess, 1996; Rafael, 1996).

Likewise, in the realm of knowledge development, nurses initially adopted methods of traditional science that are imbued with values that are associated with masculine gender—methods that claim objectivity, designed to eliminate any trace of subjectivity. For nurses, pursuing the ideals of science means breaking away from the philosophic values associated with subjectivity—interconnectedness, intuitive grasping of the meaning of a situation, and advocating for the rights and dignity of each individual. As nurses turn to methods of inquiry that are grounded in values of intersubjectivity and meaning, nursing knowledge will increasingly reflect these values (Dahlberg & Drew, 1997; Newman, 1997). Smith (1994) further calls for not only the pursuit of creative empiric approaches to inquiry that can embrace the wholeness of human-envi-

ronment interactions, but also the use of metaphor, poetry, and narrative as means to create understanding and knowledge.

Intellect

> Women often try one branch of intellect after another in their youth . . . But . . . it is impossible to follow up anything systematically. Women often long to enter some man's profession where they would find direction, competition (or rather opportunity of measuring the intellect with others), and above all, time. (Nightingale, 1979, p. 31)

For Nightingale, the single significant barrier to exercising the intellect was the social structure that robbed women of the time to think and to develop intellectual capacities. Today, nurses are burdened with incredible pressures and demands on their time. Many ideas, dreams, or visions that might be brought into reality are stymied for lack of time to develop the idea, to design a plan for implementation, or to explore the resources that might be needed to support and bring the idea to fruition.

Where knowledge development is concerned, time to engage in scholarship and research requires both time and resources, scarce commodities in any setting for nurses. But the ideas and insights that nurses develop in the course of their experiences as nurses—their "intelligence" where their practice is concerned—is one of the vast treasures of the discipline. Recognizing this as a valuable resource is a first step that gained widespread recognition through Benner's (1984) early work focusing on the development of expertise in nursing practice. Drawing on this recognition, nurses who practice and those who teach can now make choices concerning where we place our focus. This does not require abandoning the knowledge of the physical and human sciences, but rather including in our discourses the valuable insights derived from the intelligence of those who practice. This is a gender shift. It requires taking as equally valuable the gendered feminine voices of those who nurse, along with the gendered masculine voices of those who practice traditional science.

Moral Activity

Women dream of a great sphere of steady, not sketchy benevolence, of moral activity, for which they would fain [sic] be trained and fitted, instead of working in the dark, neither knowing nor registering whither their steps lead, whether farther from or nearer to the aim. (Nightingale, 1969, p. 38)

Nightingale viewed moral activity as intimately intertwined with women's passion and intellect. She used the term "high sympathies" in referring to values that embrace concern for the well-being of all of society, not simply concern for one's own well-being and that of one's immediate family and friends. She decried the lack of concern for the hearts and souls of women who yearn to be of use in society. Instead, she observed that women acted on their moral sensibilities in the most sketchy of ways, rarely bringing into full being the social "good" that they envision.

The ethical and moral values that nurses articulate today reflect a collective sense of "moral activity" (Cooper, 1991; Hess, 1996; Liaschenko, 1993; Rafael, 1996). These values are grounded in a foundational moral commitment to remain in a relationship, to treat the relationship with respect and concern. Concern extends to the physical environment and social and political contexts, and how the interactions among people and their contexts shape human health and well-being. In a technological day and age when alienation and isolation seem inevitable, the moral activity of nurses and nursing seems crucial as a means of nurturing human dignity and well-being.

Conclusion

Because of the persisting social and political contexts that confer gender meanings, stereotype individuals and groups with gender associations, and render value judgments based on gender, it is imperative to recognize the powerful influence that gender conveys in terms of how we see the world, how we act in the world, and how we know the world. The ideal, to move beyond gender, is almost unimaginable and can only be envisioned in terms of breaking down gender stereotypes. Again, and in conclusion, I turn to Nightingale, for in her last note in *Notes on Nursing,* she addresses this very issue:

I would earnestly ask my sisters to keep clear of both the jargons now current everywhere (for they *are* equally jargons); of the jargon, namely, about the "rights" of women, which urges women to do all that men do, including the medical and other professions, merely because men do it, and without regard to whether this *is* the best that women can do; and of the jargon which urges women to do nothing that men do, merely because they are women, and should be "recalled to a sense of their duty as women," and because "this is women's work," and "that is men's," and "these are things which women should not do," which is all assertion, and nothing more. . . .

You do not want the effect of your good things to be, "How wonderful for a *woman!*" nor would you be deterred from good things by hearing it said, "Yes, but she ought not to have done this, because it is not suitable for a woman." But you want to do the thing that is good, whether it is "suitable for a woman" or not. (pp. 135–136).

REFERENCES

The American Heritage Dictionary of the English Language. (1992) (Third ed.). Electronic version licensed from InfoSoft International: Houghton Mifflin.

Benner, P. (1984). *From Novice to Expert: Excellence and Power in Clinical Nursing Practice.* Menlo Park, CA: Addison-Wesley.

Chinn, P.L. (1991). *Anthology on caring.* New York: National League for Nursing Press.

Chinn, P.L. (1989). Nursing patterns of knowing and feminist thought. *Nursing Outlook, 10*(2), 71–75.

Cooper, M.C. (1991). Principle-oriented ethics and the ethic of care: A creative tension. *ANS. Advances In Nursing Science, 14*(2), 22–31.

Dahlberg, K., & Drew, N. (1997). A lifeworld paradigm for nursing research. *Journal of Holistic Nursing, 15*(3), 303–317.

Donaldson, S.K., & Crowley, D.M. (1978). The discipline of nursing. *Nursing Outlook, 26,* 113–120.

Hess, J.D. (1996). The ethics of compliance: A dialectic. *ANS. Advances In Nursing Science, 19*(1), 18–27.

Liaschenko, J. (1993). Feminist ethics and cultural ethos: Revisiting a nursing debate. *ANS. Advances In Nursing Science, 15*(4), 71–81.

Newman, M.A. (1997). Experiencing the whole. *ANS. Advances In Nursing Science, 20*(1), 34–39.

Nightingale, F. (1979). *Cassandra.* New York: The Feminist Press.

Nightingale, F. (1969). *Notes on nursing: What it is and what it is not.* New York: Dover Publications, Inc.

Rafael, A.R.F. (1996). Power and caring: A dialectic in nursing. *ANS. Advances In Nursing Science, 19*(1), 3–17.

Shepherd, J. (1993). *Lifting the veil: The feminine face of science.* Boston: Shambhala.

Smith, M.C. (1994). Arriving at a philosophy of nursing: Discovering? Constructing? Evolving? In J.F. Kikuchi, & H. Simmons (Editors), *Developing a Philosophy of Nursing* (pp. 43–60). Thousand Oaks, CA: Sage.

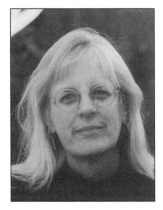

PEGGY CHINN

POSTMODERNISM AND NURSING SCIENCE

Marylouise Welch • E. Carol Polifroni

Throughout this anthology, we have explored fairly standard and commonly accepted themes, concepts and categories within the philosophy of science. The majority of the works cited have presented information from the perspective of the modern period (see time frame in Section 1). However, it is important to be most contemporary in this, the first anthology concerned with philosophy of science in nursing. Thus, attention must be directed to the concept of postmodernism and the postmodernist perspective.

A time frame does not necessarily define a movement, however. In support of the transition to postmodernism, Lister (1991) posits "the way we experience the world is determined by language, or at least by some underlying structure which gives shape to both language and our experience of the world" (p. 208). This notion of some underlying or permeating structure is at the base of a structuralistic philosophy which "replaces a concern for truth or meaning with a concern for underlying structures, with an exploration of how meaning is constructed" (p. 208). However, as the notion of structure is opposed and rejected, whether it be through language, reductionism to a physical science or limitless responsibility, the terms postmodern and poststructuralist arise.

According to Foucault (1972; 1976), a French philosopher who is associated with a postmodern school, postmodernists will not accept a single unified approach to knowledge. Rather, this perspective insists that the view that is used to guide research be congruent with and driven by the question that is asked. This axiom is simple, but paramount for the growth of nursing science. We finish this anthology with writings about a postmodern perspective. Watson describes the postmodern view as a freeing up of thinking to allow for multiple views and analyses of data (1995), multiple causes and effects interacting in a nonlinear manner. Postmodernism does contain some common themes: ideas are temporary, research data is situated in a context, the meaning of reality is transcendent, grand theories are not valid, problems are deconstructed, and findings should be practical (Reed, 1995; Watson, 1995). Reed endorses a modification of modernism by combining critique and communicative reasoning into empirical inquiry. She is proposing a neomodernist framework.

Poststructuralism holds to the general tenets of postmodernism but with some specific values. Basing most of her writing on Foucualt (1972; 1974), Dzurec (1989) describes the important role of politics and power/knowledge in poststructuralist thought. Knowledge does not develop as a result of neutral observations but as a result of power relations. Knowledge is power and rooted in and expressed in politics. For a poststructuralist the aim of science is to reveal the life experiences as they have been dominated and shaped by politics. For Foucault (Rabinow, 1984) politics are a strategy of power with both creative and destructive tendencies. A poststructuralist perspective will help to reveal the issues around power and knowledge in health care for nurses as caregivers and for patients receiving that care.

The concern for truth within postmodernism is replaced with a concern for meaning and utility (Rorty, 1980). The utility of an idea is its practical merit accompanied by the meaning of that practicality to human beings and their search for health and wellness. The postmodern era empowers one to search for this meaning in a multitude of ways without reducing the meaning to empirically verifiable characteristics. Concurrently, the empowerment achieved with postmodernism challenges the scholar to incorporate vigor and principled approaches to the inquiry. One must not fall into a potential abyss of casualness created by the permissiveness and potential empowerment of postmodernism.

The spirit of the postmodernist movement and challenge is reflected in William Butler Yeats' (cited in Watson [1995]) poem "The Second Coming,"

> 'Things fall apart; the center cannot hold; Mere anarchy is loosed upon the world. Surely some revelation is at hand."

Often an intellectual epoch begins with the destruction of something. For example, modern science began with the death of the condemned Galileo. What does the anarchy of the postmodern era herald for the future? It may be nursing's opportunity to harness this intellectual confusion and to truly move the discipline forward.

The readings which follow illustrate the diverse views on both postmodernism and the concerns associated with this era of scientific thought and progress. Watson (1995) lays out the perspectives on postmodernism and challenges the reader by stating "the issue is whether we will take advantage of the fact of change, chaos and ambiguity, deconstruction, and so on, and participate in reconstructing, co-creating a novel and moral direction for knowledge and practice, leading us forward, toward an ever-evolving humanity of possibilities . . ." (p. 63). Reed (1995) states "a post-critical discipline values challenges to the status quo and critiques and exposes oppressive discourses" (p. 82). She believes that the opportunity is before the nursing scholars to do with as they deem appropriate for ongoing knowledge development within the discipline. Reed challenges the reader to use this postcritical perspective to advance our scientific basis for practical aims and purposes; for advancing human science.

CONCLUSION

It is hoped that the reader has gained an understanding of the many perspectives that have and can still influence the development of nursing knowledge. It is important at this point in our disciplinary development to remain open to new views that will enrich our knowledge base and for us to support nurse scientists who are creating new views and methods that will enable us to see/view health-illness in useful perspectives that will improve nursing care. The variety of perspectives that are presented here have been chosen to stimulate the new nursing scholars to think about and ask salient and theoretical questions and to connect these to appropriate philosophical views congruent with the chosen methodology.

The key to any disciplinary development is its definition of knowledge. This anthology has offered multiple definitions from a hypothetico-deductive empirical approach to explanation to a situated, interpretive approach to understanding. It is important for nursing as a discipline to decide what constitutes nursing knowledge and then to identify perspectives that are consonant with that definition. Geertz (1992) describes how the view that we hold determines how we define knowledge. "Who knows the river better, the swimmer or the hydrologist?" (p. 134) It all depends on one's definition of knowledge, and that is derived from one's philosophical stance.

Through the readings of primary sources of philosophers of science and leading nurse theorists this anthology has attempted to generate questions for debate about matters of concern to nursing. Nursing needs more philosophical discussions about which perspective we wish to adopt. If nursing chooses one view, then our discipline would have a clearer focus both internally and to outsiders. However, in reading the positions of the postmodernists it is clear that there are inherent risks to being too comfortable with one perspective. Multiple realities and perspectives are part of any health-illness experience, and nursing may best be served by maintaining an open acceptance of multiple perspectives.

No matter in which direction the discipline may go, it is imperative that any nurse scientist be clear about the philosophical underpinnings of the question and methods that are selected. Nursing literature must begin to insist that theoretic assumptions as well as philosophical ones are clearly identified in all scholarly efforts. So far in nursing we have not settled on a definition of nursing knowledge. Is it essential for nursing to decide on one reality? It is hoped that this anthology has not specifically answered this question but rather it has opened up possibilities for the answer to be found.

DISCUSSION GUIDE

1. Discuss the differences between poststructuralism and postmodernism.
2. How can nursing use the plurality of perspectives in postmodernism to advance its science?
3. What is the value of postmodernism to nursing science?
4. Describe a nursing research question grounded in a neo-postmodern perspective.
5. Is it time to embrace a single perspective? If not now, is this a goal?
6. As one reflects on truth, free will/determinism, explanation, critical social theory, gender, science and phenomenology . . . explore the themes and premises of each. Create a philosophy for yourself which empowers you as a scholar while maintaining the spirit and essence of the chosen perspective.

REFERENCES

Dzurec, L. (1989). The necessity for and evolution of multiple paradigms for nursing research: A poststructuralist perspective. *Advances in Nursing Science, 11*(4), 69–77.

Foucault, M. (1972). *The archaeology of knowledge and the discourse of language.* A.M.S. Smith, trans. New York: Pantheon Books.

Foucault, M. (1976). *The will to know.* Paris: Gallimard.

Geertz, C. (1992). "Local knowledge" and its limits: Some obiter dicta. *Yale Journal of Criticism, 5*(3), 129–135.

Lister, P. (1991). Approaching models of nursing from a postmodernist perspective. *Journal of Advanced Nursing, 16,* 206–212.

Rabinow, P. (ed.). (1984). *The Foucault reader.* New York: Pantheon.

Reed, P. (1995). A treatise on nursing knowledge development for the 21st century: Beyond postmodernism. *Advances in Nursing Science, 17*(3), 70–84.

Rorty, R. (1980). *Philosophy and the mirror of nature.* Oxford: Blackwell.

Watson, J. (1995). Postmodernism and knowledge development in nursing. *Nursing Science Quarterly, 8*(2), 60–64.

BIBLIOGRAPHY

Bernstein, R. (1983). *Beyond objectivism and relativism.* Philadelphia: University of Pennsylvania Press.

Derida, J. (1976). *Of grammatology.* Baltimore: Johns Hopkins University Press.

———. (1982). *Margins of philosophy.* Chicago: University of Chicago Press.

Foucault, M. (1970). *The order of things: An archaeology of the human sciences.* London: Tavistock.

———. (1972). *The archaeology of knowledge and discourse of language.* New York: Pantheon Books.

———. (1973). *The birth of the clinic.* London: Tavistock.

———. (1976). *The will to know.* Paris: Gallimard.

———. (1980). *Power/knowledge.* Brighton, England: Harvester Press.

Kermode, S., & Brown, C. (1996). The postmodernist hoax and its effects on nursing. *International Journal of Nursing Studies, 33*(4), 375–384.

Lather, P. (1991). *Getting smart: Feminist research and pedagogy within the postmodern.* New York: Routledge.

Leitch, V. (1996). *Postmodernism-Local effects, Global flows.* Albany: State University of New York Press.

Lister, P. (1997). The art of nursing in a post-modern context. *Journal of Advanced Nursing, 25,* 38–44.

Lyotard, J. (1979). *The post-modern condition: A report on knowledge.* Minneapolis: University of Minnesota Press.

Mitchell, D. P. (1996). Postmodernism, health and illness. *Journal of Advanced Nursing, 23,* 201–205.

Norris, C. (1993). *The truth about postmodernism.* Oxford: Blackwell.

Polkinghorne, D. (1983). *Methodology for the human sciences: Systems of inquiry.* Albany: State University of New York Press.

Price, K., & Cheek, J. (1996). Exploring the nursing role in pain management from a post-structuralist perspective. *Journal of Advanced Nursing, 24,* 899–904.

Rorty, R. (1989). *Contingency, irony and solidarity.* Cambridge: Cambridge University Press.

Seidman, S. (1994). *Contested knowledge: Social theory in a post-modern era.* Oxford: Blackwell Scientific.

Toulmin, S. (1990). *Cosmopolis: The agenda of modernity.* New York: Free Press.

Turner, B. (Ed.). (1992). *Theories of modernity and postmodernity.* London: Sage.

Vincenza, A. (1994). Chaos theory and some nursing considerations. *Nursing Science Quarterly, 7*(1), 36–42.

Postmodernism and Knowledge Development in Nursing

Jean Watson

Postmodernism as a concept and periodizing point between centuries has been defined as both the beginning and the end of modernity. This article explores some of the dimensions of this moment and movement between centuries and the implications of the postmodern condition on the nursing profession. Amidst the health care reform angst of deconstructing and reconstructing, challenges and opportunities await nursing's evolution into its own postmodern paradigm. Manifestations of such a postmodern paradigm are already reflected in the epistemological shifts of nursing science and knowledge development. Challenges posed for nursing science by this disorientingly free-floating era are brought to light—away from the reaction worldview, past the reciprocal and into the transformative-simultaneous, whereby nursing can emerge within its own unique postmodern discipline.

Postmodern—a response across disciplines to the contemporary crisis of profound uncertainty brought about by crash of modern hope of rationality and technology to solve human dilemmas and quest for a description of "Truth and Reality." (Lather, 1991, p. 20)

Whether reading Derrida (1976), Foucault (1972, 1973), Saussure (1974), Sarup (1988), Smith (1982), Toulmin (1990), Lacan (Benvenuto & Kennedy, 1986), or Lather (1991); whether pondering quantum physics, holograms, literature, music, or art; whether reflecting upon medical or nursing science; whether at a conference in Finland or attending an academic seminar in Sweden, Copenhagen or Colorado; whether in a gallery or coffee bar, there is a prevalent worldwide discourse on postmod-

ernism. From one century to another, there is a struggling to make new meaning, new sense of this modern world which William Butler Yeats captured in 1921, the sense we now share that "things fall apart; the center cannot hold" (Toulmin, 1990, p. 158).

Almost every field of human activity today is engaged in the issues related to postmodern thought, even if it is not labeled as such. Just exactly what is postmodernism is unknown and ambiguous at best. As with any *ism* there is a hesitation to engage in it at that level. However, prominent thinkers suggest postmodern thought is defined by both the beginning and end of modernity (Toulmin, 1990). Indeed, postmodernism has been dubbed the end of the Western mind with its dominance of one reality, primarily the Western worldview, leaving a multiplicity of realities (Tarnas, 1993).

The modern Western mind that stands in contrast to the postmodern has come to convey

Reprinted by permission from Nursing Science Quarterly 8(2):60–64. © 1995, Chestnut House Publications.

positivist reasoning with its neutrality of human values, its concern with control and dominance of one worldview for predicting and sustaining a given reality whereby knowledge = science = reality. Such a modern reality has come to value facts over meaning, has come to value science over church, and physical over nonphysical/metaphysical. Lather (1991) notes that it is considered a periodizing concept and a descriptor for a cultural, aesthetic, philosophical (and the author would add scientific) movement.

One can see the modern-postmodern scientific shift reflected through worldview characteristics referred to in the nursing literature as organismic and mechanistic (Fawcett, 1993). Differing philosophic claims manifest in what Parse (1987) has labeled simultaneity and totality paradigms, informing approaches toward humans and toward health and in what Newman (1992) has identified as the three prevailing paradigms for nursing knowledge development: the particulate-deterministic, the interactive-integrative and the unitary-transformative. These philosophical worldview critiques in nursing, which Fawcett (1993) has named a plethora of paradigms, are reflective of the broader cultural, philosophical transdisciplinary shifts occurring worldwide among the public and academicians alike.

More succinctly, postmodernism/poststructuralism has become "the code name for the crisis of confidence in Western conceptual systems . . . creating a conjunction that shifts our sense of who we are and what is possible" (Lather, 1991, p. 159). Specifically, "the essence of the postmodern argument is that the dualisms which continue to dominate Western thought are inadequate for understanding a world of multiple causes and effects interacting in complex and non-linear ways, all of which are rooted in a limitless array of historical and cultural specificities" (Lather, 1991, p. 21).

The postmodern rise has been most evident in France and throughout Europe during this century, from the *angst* of the existential philosophical movements, to the descriptive, even transcendental phenomenological attempts to grasp the human experience, and beyond, into hermeneutics, critical hermeneutics, interpretative hermeneutics, to feminism, language and semiotics, to deconstruction, to constructivist thinking and onward, toward the disownment of theory, method and dominating systems. The result has been such a decentering of rationality in the predominant reality and worldview that there is a dramatic shift in the understanding of knowledge and science toward an uprising "against all the 'experts' who proposed to speak for or on behalf of others" (Lather, 1991, p. 23). We see a search for ontological and epistemological authenticity (Guba & Lincoln, 1989) whereby "postmodernism as an intellectual movement, challenges the ideas of a single correct approach to knowledge development, of a single truth, and of a single meaning of reality . . . rejecting the ideal that there is one true story about reality" (Uris, 1993, p. 95). Such an ontological and epistemological shift invites and works with context, connections, relations, multiplicity, ambiguity, openness, indeterminacy, patterning, paradox, process, transcendence and mysteries of the human experience of being-in-the-world (Watson, 1992).

Another aspect of the postmodern in contrast to the modern has been most clearly articulated in the field of architecture (Klotz, 1988; Lather, 1991; Toulmin, 1990). Indeed, postmodernism first gained widespread attention through architecture. Toulmin (1990) pointed out that the American architect Venturi argued in the '70s that the age of modern is past and must yield to a new postmodern style. For example, modern architecture is noted to be anonymous, timeless, and indistinguishable—boring, featureless, sterile, and stark—disconnected from its landscape and previous historical referents. Medical facilities in particular during this modern era of the 20th century became distinguishable from hotels or comfortable places to be by adopting the look of "progressive modernity with a clean, efficient, and functional appearance that symbolized the time" (Kingsley, 1988, p. 83). The postmodern style reintroduced elements of beauty, local color, decoration, historical reference, and even fantasy. Such shifts are also now reflected in redesign projects in hospitals and in neighborhoods, whereby sterility, sameness, and functionality are being replaced by emergence of beauty, variety, connection—the use of diverse models of aesthetics toward an integration of the local landscape, color, culture, and even the use of historical archetypal designs, intentionally reconnecting human experiences to human history and myth, across time and space. Postmodern architecture attempts to make places where the soul can live, not just build warehouses in which bodies may dwell (Day, 1990).

While neither "modern" nor "postmodern" has any precise definition, there is general convergence from all parties to the debate that "the modern world committed us to thinking about nature, the human condition, and institutions in a new and 'scientific way' through the use of more 'rational and precise methods' to deal with the problems of human life and society" (Toulmin, 1990, p. 9). Thus, modernity has become a worldview, which some trace back to the French Revolution, to Kant, and even to Descartes' logic and rationality, which, according to Toulmin (1990) was even extended to politics and organization of nation states.

This modern era of course extended directly into the modern medical revolution, which became one of the pinnacles of the world for the 20th century and clearly influenced nursing's modern maturity. Now both fields are grappling with the end of modernity and how to transition from modern, with its assumption of rationality and functionality *in all things,* to the postmodern wherein the modern center no longer holds—things are falling apart.

Shadow Side of Postmodernism: Deconstruction

The falling apart represents what might be considered the down side, or shadow side, of postmodernism. It is commonly associated with what is called deconstruction. The deconstruction of reality, whether through analysis of language, knowledge, or power structures, emerged ironically from the despair of the human condition brought about through modern scientific and technological advances; it was further sparked through the implosion of knowledge, information transfer, and new insights and quests for new meaning of the human condition. All of these forces transformed the human landscape and generated new questions about humanity, nature, and survival. While enlightening insights can be obtained through deconstruction, without critique it can also lead to a void and moral confusion.

Historically, it has been pointed out that the information age and the technologies of electronic communication, which explode the space-time limits of messages and profoundly shape human experience through experiences of multidirectionality and simultaneity, constitute a different kind of human subject and what it means to be human. There is the despatializing of work; there is a language of signifiers that float in relation to referents (Poster, 1987–1988); there is a relativity of time and space which is revealed both in experience and in physics. All have become substitutes for certain forms of social relations, undermining the Cartesian ontology of subject and object (Lather, 1991, p. 21). In this postmodern domain there exist "linguistically transformed representations" (Lather, 1991, p. 21) whereby the unreal is constituted as real, where a virtual reality can recreate a surreal reality.

The formal concept of "deconstruction" (also framed as post-structuralism) gained attention as an avant-garde intellectual movement through the work of Derrida (1976) and Foucault (1972, 1973) in France in the late '60s. The close reading of text for meaning and for power and knowledge relationships became an attempt to discover another picture of reality; to analyze in terms of what is in the text as well as what is not said, or on the margin; to analyze and deconstruct for how knowledge and language function as a form of power and disseminate the effects of power (Sarup, 1988, p. 55). Thus to deconstruct a text is:

> to locate the promising marginal text, to disclose the undecidable moment, to pry it loose with the positive level of the signifier, to reverse the resident hierarchy, only to displace; to dismantle in order to reconstitute what is always already inscribed. (Sarup, 1988, p. 56)

Such efforts toward deconstruction carry over into society and science generally wherein is finally seen that things fall apart and the center can no longer hold, acknowledging that there is *no known solution;* there is no one way of knowing, being, and experiencing reality; recognizing the rationalist model does not fit; people are not here to adapt, to focus on problems to be fixed, but rather to focus on solutions with open possibilities, for what might be. While aspects of deconstruction are liberating, revealing, and giving birth to a new reality, there is the other side. What can also be experienced socially, from such an unraveling of reality, is social and scientific confusion, human and environmental violence, and even moral anarchy, where it is possible to ponder that even humanity cannot hold.

In summary, the other side of the postmodern era's

> openness and indeterminacy is thus the lack of any firm ground for a worldview. Both inner and outer realities have become unfathomably ramified, multidimensional, malleable, and unbounded—bringing a spur to courage and . . . unending relativism and existential finitude. (Tarnas, 1993, p. 398)

As Tarnas points out, with the ascendance of the postmodern mind, the human quest for meaning in the cosmos has devolved upon a hermeneutic enterprise that is disorientingly free-floating: the postmodern exists in a universe whose significance is at once utterly open and without warrantable foundation. Perhaps it is at this point that nursing's transformative paradigm of caring (healing) in the human health experience (Newman, Sime, & Corcoran-Perry, 1991), with its moral foundation and imperative of human caring with respect to human health experience, comes into such powerful light (Fry, 1993; Noddings, 1984; Watson, 1990). It is here, during this latter part of the 20th century, that perhaps the evolution of nursing's modern worldview is shifting from what Fawcett (1993) labeled a *reaction* worldview into the *reciprocal*. As such, the next turn in nursing's development holds great potential for nursing's postmodern paradigm to collapse toward the *transformative-simultaneous*. (See Fawcett, 1993.)

Into the Light of Postmodernism: Reconstruction

Thus, the other side of postmodernism, moving from the reaction worldview, through the reciprocal, and toward the simultaneous, brings with it an aim toward emancipation from oppression, from strict dualism, from domination of rationality, technological controls, and knowledge discourses which have been thrust upon humanity since the rise of modernity. The reconstruction of reality is now being called for, acknowledging that another reality is emerging, in that there is a search for meaning that calls forth personal experience as a truth of its own; that allows for an emergence of beauty, wholeness, and connectedness to replace the emptiness of the initial modern residual associated with the downside of the postmodern condition. The positive side of postmodernism is to acknowledge that this is a historic moment in human evolutionary history as well as nursing's; to realize that the ground of postmodernism and the condition which rises from it is to participate in an explosion of shifting change, complexity, and chaos. What is thus required is nothing less than a radical transformative process of constructing-reconstructing ourselves and our worlds. This reconstruction project for humanity is the light side that counters the down, despairing side of human deconstruction.

So, while we can now acknowledge that the center cannot hold, can we create, recreate, cocreate a new center and a new form of human experience and knowledge which will lead humanity toward emancipation and higher evolution, especially with respect to the art and science of nursing and its caring-healing practices and diverse ways of knowing and being within a wide universe of the human health experience? Or will we submit to further chaos and decline, deconstruction, if not destruction, of humanity and the planet Earth as we know it?

Postmodern Implications for Nursing Knowledge

Is it possible for [nursing science] to be different, that is to forget itself and to become something else—or must it remain a partner in domination and hegemony? (Said, 1989, p. 225)

The postmodern turn in the history of nursing is hallmarked by the fact that the knowledge that has been systematically excluded from the human consciousness now has to be restored and reconnected in order to reconnect with the human condition (Smith, 1982). Some of that knowledge is knowledge of what it means to be human that goes beyond the physicalist, material orientation and fixation of the modern era. Part of that knowledge is an awakening of nursing's moral consciousness and compassion that moves in concentric circles and chains (Noddings, 1984), from self care, to caring for others, to environment, to nature, to caring for and being a part of an evolving universe that people are cocreating.

Nursing, like all other disciplines, must now yield to a postmodern approach, even though it is perhaps yet to be fully redefined. During such redefining during the paradigm shift, even Kuhn (1970) believes that each field of inquiry is called to develop its proper methods, adapted to its special problems and phenomena.

Such postmodern directions are already evident in nursing science knowledge and contemporary nursing theories, even though they may not be labeled as postmodern. (See Newman, 1986, 1992; Newman et al., 1991; Parse, 1981, 1992; Rogers, 1970, 1989; Sarter, 1988; Watson, 1988, 1992). Sarter's (1988) critique of four contemporary nursing theories (Rogers' science of unitary human beings, Newman's health as expanding consciousness, Parse's theory of human becoming, and Watson's theory of transpersonal human caring) revealed shared themes related to what might be considered a redefining of nursing and nursing knowledge from the modern, to the postmodern. This shift in extant nursing science and knowledge matrix is reflected in such shared concepts as evolution of consciousness, self-transcendence, open system, harmony, relativity of space-time, patterning, and holism (Sarter, 1988). Such thinking stands in sharp contrast to previous themes in nursing science associated with concepts such as steady state maintenance, adaptation, linear interactions between humans and the environment, problem-based practice, stress-coping, bio-psycho-social need hierarchy, nursing problem diagnosis, and so on.

The art and science of nursing with its concern with caring-healing and health as a field of study, research, and practice within its own paradigm is realizing that in this postmodern time, science, knowledge, and even images of nursing, health, environment, person become one among many truth games. Thus truth becomes viewed at least as rhetorical as it is procedural (paraphrased from Lather, 1991). The postmodern truth for nursing reconnects with the truth of unfoldment, an expansion and fusing of horizons of meaning, an attending to the authenticity, ethos, and ethic of caring relations, context, continuity, connections, aesthetics, interpretation, and construction. Returning nursing to some of its finest art and artistry from the era of Nightingale is yet to be actualized. This would include acknowledging plasticity and constant change; recognizing all knowledge is constructed as a human endeavor; returning to the context rather than the abstract voice of theory, authority; celebrating ambiguity and pluralism for its openness and possibilities; questioning of all truth statements and assumptions; noting that nothing is fixed, but evolving and fallible—endlessly self-revising and self-reflecting.

The implications for knowledge development in nursing are already reflected in the epistemological shifting from:

- strict rationalist—toward ambiguity, poetic, aesthetic, imaginary;
- analytic, descriptive—toward critical, interpretative hermeneutics, co-constructed meaning;
- phenomena per se—toward lived experience, endlessly deconstructing-reconstructing;
- ontic (fixed) categories, entities—toward the ontologically authentic;
- structure—toward process, patterning, transformation;
- numbers, factual data—toward text, meaning, extracting embedded theory laden in the fact;
- profane—sacred (Watson, 1993).

In summary, as nursing locates itself within the postmodern condition of complexity, with its shadow and light side, and as nursing seeks a dwelling place which is open-ended, ambiguous, dynamically constructed, incessantly questioned, endlessly self-revising, never set, but floating and moving with the river of life:

- Will nurses extract from the margin, uncover, and reconstruct nursing's most ancient and contemporary extant caring-healing-health knowledge and practices?
- Will nurses construct and co-construct ancient and new knowledge of the human health-illness, caring-healing experiences, and thereby move knowledge with its artistry of practice to the center, further clarifying nursing for a new era?
- Will nurses be part of helping nursing to mature and grow up both ontologically and epistemologically, within its own transformative praxis paradigm?

Or will nurses remain as constituted and sustain themselves as highly trained technicians serving a newly "redesigned" medical care system, which has already moved from the modern to the postmodern, with respect to "mindbody-spirit–whole person" medicine as the emerging model for health care reform?

The postmodern challenge is our challenge: the issue is whether we will take advantage of the fact of change, chaos, and ambiguity, deconstruction, and so on, and participate in reconstructing, cocreating a novel and moral direction for knowledge and practice, leading us forward, toward an ever-evolving humanity of possibilities or, will "we go on acting as though nothing ha[s] happened?" (Toulmin, 1990, p. 208).

REFERENCES

Benvenuto, B., & Kennedy, R. (1986). *The works of Jacques Lacan*. London: Free Association Books.

Day, C. (1990). *Places of the soul: Architecture and environmental design as a healing art*. Northamptonshire, England: The Aquarian Press.

Derrida, J. (1976). *On grammatology*. Baltimore: Johns Hopkins University Press.

Fawcett, J. (1993). From a plethora of paradigms to parsimony in worldviews. *Nursing Science Quarterly, 6,* 56–58.

Foucault, M. (1972). *The archaeology of knowledge and the discourse on language* (A.M.S. Smith, Trans.). New York: Pantheon Books.

Foucault, M. (1973). *The birth of the clinic*. (A.M.S. Smith, Trans.). London: Tavistock.

Fry, S. T. (1993). The ethic of care: Nursing's excellence for a troubled world. In D. Gaut (Ed.), *A global agenda for caring* (pp. 175–181). New York: National League for Nursing.

Guba, E., & Lincoln, Y. (1989) *Fourth generation evaluation*. Newbury Park, CA: Sage.

Kingsley, K. (1988). The architecture of nursing. In A. H. Jones (Ed.), *Images of nursing: Perspectives from history, art, and literature*. Philadelphia: University of Pennsylvania Press.

Klotz, H. (1988). *The history of postmodern architecture*. Cambridge: M.I.T. Press.

Kuhn, T. (1970). *The structure of scientific revolutions*. Chicago: University of Chicago Press.

Lather, P. (1991). *Getting smart: Feminist research and pedagogy with/in the postmodern*. New York: Routledge.

Newman, M. A. (1986). *Health as expanding consciousness*. St. Louis: Mosby.

Newman, M. A. (1992). Prevailing paradigms in nursing. *Nursing Outlook, 40*(1), 10–13.

Newman, M. A., Sime, A. M., & Corcoran-Perry, S. A. (1991). The focus of the discipline of nursing. *Advances in Nursing Science 14*(1), 1–6.

Noddings, N. (1984). *Caring: A feminine approach to ethics and moral development.* Berkeley: University of California Press.

Parse, R. R. (1981). *Man-living-health: A theory of nursing.* New York: Wiley.

Parse, R. R. (1987). Nursing science: Major paradigms, theories, and critiques. Philadelphia: Saunders.

Parse, R. R. (1992). Human becoming: Parse's theory of nursing. *Nursing Science Quarterly, 5,* 35–42.

Poster, M. (1987–1988). Foucault, the present and history. *Cultural Critique, 8,* 105–121.

Rogers, M. E. (1970). *An introduction to the theoretical basis of nursing.* Philadelphia: Davis.

Rogers, M. E. (1989). Nursing: A science of unitary human beings. In J. Riehl-Sisca (Ed.), *Conceptual models for nursing practice* (3rd ed.) (pp. 181–188). Englewood Cliffs, NJ: Appleton and Lange.

Said, E. (1989). Representing the colonized: Anthropology's interlocutors. *Critical Inquiry 15,* 205–225.

Sarter, B. (1988). Philosophical sources of nursing theory. *Nursing Science Quarterly, 1,* 52–59.

Sarup, M. (1988). *Post-structuralism and postmodernism.* New York: Harvester Wheatsheaf.

Saussure, F. de, (1974). *Course in general linguistics.* London: Fontana/Collins.

Smith, H. (1982). *Beyond the post-modern mind.* Wheaton, IL: Theosophical Publishing House.

Tarnas, R. (1993). *The passion of the western mind.* New York: Ballantine Books.

Toulmin, S. (1990). *Cosmopolis: The agenda of modernity.* New York: Free Press.

Uris, P. (1993). *Postmodern feminist emancipatory research: A critical analysis of nurses' moral experience of caring in a patriarchal society.* Unpublished doctoral dissertation, University of Colorado, Denver.

Watson, J. (1988). New dimensions of human caring theory. *Nursing Science Quarterly, 1,* 175–181.

Watson, J. (1990). The moral failure of the patriarchy. *Nursing Outlook, 36*(2), 62–66.

Watson, J. (1992). *Postmodern nursing and beyond.* Paper presented at the American Academy of Nursing Annual Meeting, Kansas City.

Watson, J. (1994). Poeticizing as truth through language. In P. Chinn & J. Watson (Eds.), *Art and aesthetics in nursing* (pp. 3–17). New York: National League for Nursing.

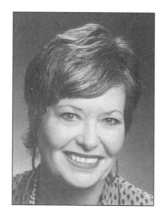

JEAN WATSON

A Treatise on Nursing Knowledge Development for the 21st Century: Beyond Postmodernism

Pamela G. Reed

This article explicates a framework for nursing knowledge development that incorporates both modernist and postmodernist philosophies. The framework derives from an "open philosophy" of science, which links science, philosophy, and practice in development of nursing knowledge. A neomodernist perspective is proposed that upholds modernist values for unified conceptualizations of nursing reality while recognizing the dynamic and value-laden nature of all levels of theory and metatheory. It is proposed that scientific inquiry extend beyond the postmodern critique to identify nursing metanarratives of nursing philosophy and nursing practice that serve as external correctives in the critique process. Philosophic positions related to the science, philosophy, and practice domains are put forth for continued dialogue about future directions for knowledge development in nursing. Key words: *knowledge development, metatheory, philosophy of science, postmodernism*

Among the transitions currently facing nursing is the ending of what someday will be referred to as 20th-century nursing theorizing. For the past several years, nurses have been feeling the ground shift with the reforming of philosophic ideas that launched nursing as a science. Not since the advent of modernism and the birth of modern nursing at the end of the 19th century has nursing science been faced with such a wealth of possibilities for knowledge development. These possibilities have their roots in modernism to be sure, but they also are nurtured by the current dialogue postmodern thought has precipitated.

Postmodernism has engaged nursing in a dialogue to reconcile a basic awareness about the uniqueness and differences in human beings and health, with basic beliefs in universals and values about human phenomena. It is a struggle, as a philosopher characterized that of feminism, to "modify the Enlightenment in the context of late modernity but not to capitulate to the postmodern condition."[1(p195)]

This article presents a framework that will help nursing science bridge modernist and postmodernist philosophies as nursing clarifies contemporary approaches to knowledge development. The framework builds on accomplishments of modernist nursing while exploiting opportunities of the postmodern context and, in this sense, is "neomodernist." The framework reaches beyond postmodern prescriptions for nursing science and proposes a neomodernist perspective on knowledge development that incorporates metanarratives of nursing philosophy and nursing practice into scientific inquiry.

Reprinted by permission from Advances in Nursing Science 17(3):70–84. © 1995, Aspen Publishers, Inc.

Historical Background: Modernism and Postmodernism

From premodern to postmodern times, paths to knowledge have crossed through the Age of Faith, the Age of Reason, to the Culture of Critique. The once dominant religious and metaphysical approach to reasoning about reality was transformed into avenues to truth that separated philosophic "beliefs" from empiric "knowing." Empiricism supplanted the Aristotelian emphasis on rationality that had inspired early modernists. Although modern science enlightened the world and enhanced everyday life, its approach failed to deliver the anticipated empirical base for ultimate meaning and truth about human beings and their world. Also, as philosopher Popper[2] helped scientists realize during the decline of positivism, knowledge development could not be purged of biases, contradictions, and values. Theories, like the fisherman's net, inevitably influenced what data were caught by the scientist. Postmodern thought helped move scientists toward the realization about the embeddedness of research data and the transitory nature of theory.

Postmodernism is a social movement and philosophy that originated among French literary theorists in the 1960s, although postmodern ideas were expressed prior to this time.[3] Postmodernism is a perspective or intellectual style of creating art, of theorizing, of doing science. And it is influencing nursing's approach to knowledge development.

Postmodernism challenges the modernist idea of a single, transcendent meaning of reality and the importance of the search for empirical patterns that correspond to and represent ultimate meaning. Metanarratives, grand or high theories, or other overarching discourses that identify essential truths and propose to re-present reality are not recognized as valid. The "postmodern condition"[4] is a "crisis of confidence in the narratives of truth, science and progress that epitomized modernity"[5(p98)]—a time of paradigms lost. Instead, there is focus on understanding multiple meanings, with the belief that every representation conceals and reveals meanings and that an inextricable link exists between meaning and power.[6] Whereas modernists fragmented the whole to study parts in the attempt to ultimately unify knowledge about the world, postmodernists fragment and dissolve unities, universals, and metanarratives believed to be entangled with values and beliefs that oppress people and fabricate reality. In postmodern thought, problems are not "solved," they are "deconstructed."

Postmodernists generally deny the existence of an essence of human beings, and they have incited ardent debate on the relevance of philosophy for science, given that a central purpose of philosophy is to examine questions about the intrinsic nature of human beings and the world, truth, and knowledge.[7] In postmodern thought, then, there is no autonomous subject to study; the subject is myth. What is studied is what the culture has inscribed on the object of study; in this sense, the focus of study is text. Meaning derives from the relationship between the text and the reader, and the content is not related to an external narrative. There is no transcendent referent for the knowledge builder and no source of meaning about human beings to be discovered and re-presented to others. So, in a phrase, the gods have fled. Any truths that appear to exist have come about not through historical teleologic progress, but as a product of time and chance, contingent on someone redescribing nature in a way that is temporarily useful to the current culture and context.[8,9] Thus, there is an epistemologic shift from concern over the truth of one's findings to concern over the practical significance of the findings.

Framework for Knowledge Development

Postmodernism's iconoclastic and pluralistic attitudes are dislodging nursing from cherished norms about knowledge development that tended to dichotomize essential units of inquiry: research and practice, inductive and deductive reasoning, qualitative and quantitative data. Twenty-first century approaches to developing knowledge will transcend these dichotomies.

Nursing's knowledge development activities have not been daunted by the shifts in philosophic thought, but instead are evolving out of both modernist and postmodernist influences. Nursing is embracing a broadened definition of scholarship that employs various key sources for development of nursing knowledge. These sources derive from the empirical, conceptual, and practice activities of nurses.[10–12] However, consistent with modern science, these domains have been regarded as independent throughout most of 20th-century nursing.

Science, philosophy, and practice have typically represented "orthogonal subspaces" of a discipline; each domain exists in its own dimension and has no image or projection in the plane of the other.[13] The schisms between these subspaces are a problem inherent in knowledge development. Yet despite the orthogonality and despite even the dominance of the scientific over the spiritual or philosophic modes of thought, none has been eliminated. It is as though each subspace represents some irreducible or essential basis of knowledge development. However, the independence between the domains, as enforced by modernists, proved to be an unsatisfactory approach to inquiry.

What instead may be needed for 21st-century nursing theory development is what Polis[13] labeled an "open philosophy," which deliberatively links phenomenon with noumenon and links empirical concepts that can be known through the senses with theoretical concepts of meaning and value that can be known through thought. The postmodern critique of modernism compels nursing to revisit the potential "openness" or linkages between scientific inquiry and the metanarratives of nursing philosophy and nursing practice as a means of both reforming and reaffirming nursing's approaches to knowledge development.

Nursing Science: Modern and Postmodern Influences

A nursing scientist uses valid and reliable systems of inquiry to gain understanding of phenomena of human health and healing processes. The scientist links empirical findings to a conceptual level to create a theoretical story that satisfies certain epistemic criteria, such as predictive accuracy and internal coherence.[14] Nursing science's approach to linking the empirical and theoretical has changed over the history of its science.

Traditional empiricists, of which Nightingale was one, restricted their theorizing to observable processes. Nineteenth-century nursing theorizing did not include much movement up the ladder of abstraction to link empirical and theoretical. Rather than generalizing by abstraction (vertical movement), Nightingale tended to generalize by analogy (horizontal movement). For example, Nightingale's canon about the unhealthful effects of noise on sick people derived from drawing analogies across her observations of disturbing noises, such as rustling dresses, whispered conversations, musical wind instruments, and styles of speaking and reading to patients.[15] Nightingale's theorizing generated empirical generalizations. However, knowledge development by analogy left a gap between the empirical event and theoretical explanation; although this form of knowledge had some predictive power and was used to guide the practitioners of Nightingale's era, it had limited explanatory power.

Prior to and during the half-century hiatus in nursing scientific work between Nightingale and Peplau, a shift in axiology occurred in the scientific community that altered approaches to knowledge development. The shift was precipitated by scientists' growing need to theorize about entities too slow, too small, or otherwise unobservable but inferable from the empirical world, such as gravity or electromagnetism. Hypothetico-deductive logic emerged, whereby vertical links were made between the theoretical and empirical. In this modernist period of science, theory and research were linked through idealized systems of inquiry designed to keep research untainted of values and everyday life and independent of the religious and philosophic roots that once dominated knowledge development.

Peplau's[16] seminal work helped transform nursing from a "science of doing" to a "science of knowing" by reestablishing creative links between theory and research. Her mid-20th century theorizing employed deductive and inductive reasoning, moving up and down the ladder of abstraction to construct nursing knowledge, and produced a nursing practice theory on interpersonal relations.

Today, knowledge is regarded as process and product, as an open system rather than as a fixed set of propositions with truth flowing in top–down fashion, according to Aristotle's ideal of axiomatization.[7] Nursing scientists today are beginning to embrace all three forms of Peirce's[17] system of reasoning—abduction, deduction, and induction—without fragmenting the process. In *abduction* (a term coined by Peirce and similar to retroductive reasoning), the scientist makes a conceptual leap from experience, beliefs, and a preknowledge of patterns to arrive at an educated guess or theory about a phenomenon; the nursing scholar draws from clinical, conceptual, and empirical knowledge to do this. Through *deduction*, the scientist derives empirical events that may occur, given the theory. This deduction is put forth in the form of a hypothesis, research question, grand tour question, or other statement for inquiry. *Induction*, then, refers to the process of subjecting the theoretical ideas to empirical testing. All three forms of reasoning play important roles in knowledge development. Yet postmodernism has introduced some twists to this reasoning process that are relevant to clarifying contemporary approaches to development of nursing knowledge.

First, postmodern thought has sensitized scientists to the primacy of abductive reasoning.

Abduction initiates the reasoning processes[18] and, by definition, introduces values and preunderstandings into science. No data can be free of values and biases.

Second, "empirical testing" is acquiring a broadened definition, whereby the postmodern "empirical" extends beyond the meaning of modernist empiricism. Empirical testing may interface with the practice realm to an extent greater than modernists could tolerate. The "test" of a theory, for example, is not demonstrated primarily (or at all, according to postmodern purists) by correspondence of the empirical with the theoretical but more by the correspondence between the practical and theoretical. The merit of a theory is found in its practical implications and usefulness in solving problems of the discipline.[19,20] Empirical includes the practical.

Third, what qualifies as empirical data has gone beyond empiricism. According to emerging nursing epistemology, acceptable data vary in observability. They include biologic indicators and self-reports, investigator perceptions and informant projections, motor behavior, and personal stories. The modernist distinction between qualitative and quantitative data is blurred for, as is implicit in abduction, no data, whether verbal or numeric symbols, are independent of theory.

Last, scientific work is broader than empirical work. Empirical and nonempirical (or conceptual) knowledge is not hierarchically ordered. Postmodern awareness of the intersubjectivity of knowledge invalidates such ordering and opens the door for valuing contributions to knowledge that are not empirically verifiable in the modernist sense. Nonempirical activities enhance scientific understanding by exposing new and unexpected ideas about a theory or clinical situation in the form of "conceptual innovations."[21] For example, the conceptual innovation from Freudian theory of the "unconscious" revolutionized science and practice of mental health disciplines. Newman's[22] "pattern recognition" and Orem's[23] "self-care" are other conceptual innovations that have attained significance through their meaning in practice as well as their inspiration for theory development.

In the absence of metanarratives about a transcendent truth, postmodernism has further blurred the distinction between the nonempirical and empirical, theory and fact. Theory is regarded as a "forestructure of what form of truth the data will take; theory has priority over what are taken to be facts."[19(p413)] Theory, then, does not represent truth, it creates truth. What Britt[24] stated in reference to the artist and his or her art also applies to the postmodern scientist: Modernists contemplated the meaning of the world and their place in it; postmodernists remake the world as their science demands it.

The Critical Stance: A Call to Armchairs

Given postmodernist influences on the process of knowledge development, the significance of the social critical perspective for science becomes apparent. Data alone do not yield up the theory any more than brushes and paint will produce a painting. Whether qualitative or quantitative, data reside in the researcher's theoretical context. This fact is not a caveat of knowledge development. It is the nature of science, for "when theory does not play a selective role in research, data-gathering activities belong to the realm of journalism."[21(p794)]

Given the subjective and personalized context of theorizing, a critical stance in inquiry helps the scientist develop knowledge that potentially will be more meaningful and useful. More bluntly, some believe that the postmodern critique is a way of salvaging the empiricist tradition.[19,25] The critique serves to keep check on inherent biases and constraints—introduced by the researcher and research focus, the method, theoretical interpretation, and so on—that are not in the best interest of the subject and may oppress or constrain human potential in some way. Neither intuition and empathy nor scientific expertise and statistical significance are

enough to reveal the full meaning of the data. A "call to armchairs"[26] is needed, whereby time is sanctioned for reflection and critique to examine one's assumptions and interpretations through discussion, debate, argument, and compromise with colleagues and participants—all who are affected by the knowledge developed.

Whether science is done using modernist methods, empiric–analytic or historist–hermeneutic, science is incomplete without a critical approach to one's work. Thus, the framework proposed in this article endorses a view put forth by Habermas[27] and other contemporary philosophers[1] that does not advocate the overthrow of modernism, but rather the modification of modernism by integrating the critique and communicative model on reasoning into empirical inquiry. But critique alone is not enough.

Beyond the Critique: A Neomodernist View

The neomodernist framework proposed here extends beyond the critique. The postmodern critique, with its methods of reflexivity and analysis to examine the process and products of the scientist, is not sufficient for knowledge development. Because the one who critiques is part of the culture being critiqued, complicity exists, as critics of postmodernism have explained.[1,28] And the critique cannot serve as its own external corrective; it describes a process but does not provide substance. Thus, it is suggested here that the nursing scientist's critique process be linked to a substantive overarching "ideal" or metanarrative. The metanarrative provides a base for examining knowledge as related to the context of a given discipline.[1] It functions as a "narrative foil"[28] against which scientists critique their work to form and reform knowledge.

Nursing knowledge development need not abandon completely modernist views about high theory or universal ideas. Rather than capitulate entirely to postmodernism, nurses can knowingly involve in their science the realm of perspectives and values, initially put forth by modernist nurses, that distinguish nursing knowledge and the caring application of that knowledge. In adopting a neomodernist view, nursing scientists would draw from the metanarratives of nursing for their critique. Metanarratives of nursing are found in nursing philosophy and nursing practice, as these two domains interface with nursing science in the development of knowledge.

Nursing Philosophy: Metanarratives for Knowledge Development

Philosophy, by definition, goes beyond analysis and critique by assigning values to human experiences.[29] In so doing, philosophy is a source for explicating the metanarratives of a discipline. Nursing philosophy is a statement of foundational and universal assumptions, beliefs, and principles about the nature of knowledge and truth (epistemology) and about the nature of the entities represented in the metaparadigm (ie, nursing practice and human healing processes [ontology]). A variety of philosophic schemes have been identified for understanding the nature of nursing phenomena.

One major scheme derives from philosopher Stephen Pepper's[30] widely recognized 1942 work in which he explicated what he conceived were the major bases of truth about the world. Three of his six worldviews, particularly as modified slightly by Lerner[31] and other developmental psychologists, predominantly have been used by scientists, including nursing scientists,[32] to frame philosophic assumptions of their discipline. Pepper's work predates philosophic schemes identified in nursing, and it likely provided a basis for conceptualizing the nursing worldviews and paradigms.[32-35] These extant nursing schemes, along with Pepper's original worldviews, are useful in organizing basic assumptions about nursing phenomena and in de-

riving a nursing metanarrative from philosophy for knowledge development. The three predominant worldviews are the mechanistic, organismic, and developmental–contextual, the latter previously labeled the "contextual–dialectic" worldview.[36]

Within the *mechanistic* worldview, the metaphor for human beings is the machine, composed of parts that can be measured, controlled, predicted, and added together to understand the whole. The whole is equal to the sum of the parts. Human beings are viewed as inherently at rest. Stability is assumed. Any change that occurs results from external forces and is deterministic and reversible, not developmental. The goal of change is to return to a state of equilibrium and balance. The individual's relationship with the environment is reactive. The unit of study is the part, devoid of context.

Within the *organismic* worldview, the metaphor for human beings is the biologic organism, composed of a complexity of interrelated parts. The parts are understood from the perspective of the whole, and the whole is represented in terms of the biologic organism itself. The environment assumes a more passive role, with the organism viewed as active on the environment. There is interactionism, primarily in the sense that the parts within the person interact and contribute to qualitative, developmental changes. Change is probabilistic and directed toward an end goal.

Within the *developmental–contextual* worldview, the metaphor for human beings is the historic event; that is, the individual is embedded in a context that is dynamic. Change, in both the human being and the environment, is ongoing and irreversible, innovative and developmental. Change occurs not as a result of the person's reaction to or action on the environment, but through a dialectic and interactive relationship with the environment. Change occurs in accord with Werner's[37] "orthogenetic principle" by which living systems develop through patterns of increasing complexity accompanied by increasing organization. Chaos and conflict can provide energy for progressive change. There is no one ideal goal for development that lasts a lifetime; each developmental phase (however defined) is qualitatively different and possesses its own ideals. The whole or basic unit of study is any living structure that manifests developmental patterns of change. Study of the person necessarily involves study of contextual factors.

Various philosophic systems have been put forth by nursing scholars, such as Hall's[33] change and persistence worldviews; Parse's[35] totality and simultaneity paradigms; Newman's[34] particulate–deterministic, interactive–integrative, and unitary–transformative worldviews; and Fawcett's[32] reaction, reciprocal interaction, and simultaneous action worldviews. These schemes reflect Pepper's[30] different depictions of reality and also extend his ideas by constructing worldviews that speak more directly to nursing and its phenomena of concern.

Some nursing scientists have appropriated worldviews from other disciplines, such as medicine and psychology. Medicine has advanced through three paradigms, namely the biomedical, biopsychosocial, and most recently the psychoneuroimmunologic paradigm.[38] Psychology's models of research and practice have evolved across behavioristic, psychodynamic, humanistic, and transpersonal schools of thought.[28,39]

The status quo in nursing seems to be that knowledge developers embrace the diversity of worldviews in critiquing knowledge and clarifying basic beliefs and assumptions about what are relevant and plausible issues of research and practice.[40] While this "plethora of paradigms"[41] available to nurses may be viewed in a positive way, it also may contribute to the potential for fragmentation within the discipline. This concern has been debated.[40,42] In the spirit of postmodernism, nurses must question the status quo and continue to debate the logic of diversity in worldviews underlying nursing knowledge development. From a neomodernist perspective,

this kind of diversity may not be entirely desirable.

Diversity or Fragmentation?

Diversity at the level of the worldview may inhibit clarification of a nursing philosophy[43] and nursing metanarrative for research and critique. The worldviews within each philosophic scheme define and interrelate the nursing metaparadigm concepts in radically different ways. Sanctioning all available worldviews for nursing in one sense reflects the postmodernist retreat from conceptualizing the whole and identifying unifying ideals. In attempting to achieve unity by preserving disparate worldviews, as some advocate,[40] nursing may be sacrificing coherence for diversity.

Does the diversity offer important distinctions in worldviews, each of which has a rightful role in guiding inquiry and critique within a discipline? Or might the diversity in philosophic schemes represent progress in knowledge about the nature of the world, such that some provide for fuller understanding than others? The former position seems less likely. Diversity does not mean that all points of view are equally valid and acceptable for a given context or discipline.[43] Moreover, preserving differences through compromise or coexistence rather than striving to resolve differences in ontology, values, and goals—a purpose of philosophy[44]—blocks dialogue and opportunities to further develop knowledge. Opposing beliefs about the nature of human health and nursing goals can perpetuate even more differences in nursing's epistemic and ethical claims and research funding priorities, "bringing about more confusion in our discipline rather than creating a sense of coherence necessary for its development."[45(p26)]

In addition to the question of the merits of diversity in worldviews for the discipline's progress, there is the more urgent question as to whether entertaining disparate worldviews best serves patients' well-being. Diplomacy and discourse aside, when choices available are between a mechanistic and developmental worldview, or between a paradigm in which the nurse and not the patient possesses the knowledge and authority and a paradigm in which patients are knowledgeable and knowing participants in their own healing process, is not one paradigm more emancipating (for patient and nurse) and more representative of the nature of nursing than the other? The commitment for unity in diversity[42] may not be status quo but may be most appropriate in a postmodern world that tends to fragment focuses of inquiry, human beings, and their world.

To that end, then, the metanarrative of human developmental potential, transformational and self-transcendent capacity for health and healing, and recognition of the developmental histories of persons and their contexts is offered here as an external corrective of choice. It is a metanarrative originating in Lerner's[31] developmental–contextual worldview and congruent with the philosophic ideas expressed in Newman's[34] unitary–transformative paradigm and Parse's[35] simultaneity paradigm.

Given the alternatives, this metanarrative may be the best commitment to be made by the scientist and practitioner, at least at this point in the development of nursing knowledge. In proposing this metanarrative, however, one must acknowledge that inherent in this neomodernist framework is the realization that even metanarratives are temporary and "for the moment."[46] Although metanarratives by definition are more stable than lower levels of theory, their depictions of truth and reality are not fixed and must be open to developmental change themselves, subject in part to influences from the dynamic science and practice dimensions of nursing.

Nursing Practice: A Metanarrative for Knowledge Development

As if anticipating postmodernist values for the reality found in the culture and context of everyday life experiences, nurses have renewed focus on practice as connected to science. Nursing practice is regarded not only as a place of applying knowledge, but also as a place to generate and test ideas for developing knowledge. Early on, Peplau[47] identified practice as the context in which scientific knowledge was transformed into nursing knowledge. Linkages between science and practice help nursing move beyond grand theorizing and operationalize the metanarrative of "responsible participation and consideration of culture and context"[48(pviii)] and the emancipatory potential of nursing knowledge.

From a revisionist perspective of the early nursing theorists such as Peplau[47] and Paterson and Zderad,[49] it can be seen that nursing began moving beyond the reductionist and mechanistic approaches of modernism even before nursing recognition of postpositivism. As a result, nursing practice gave to nursing research a metanarrative that was patient oriented, context sensitive, pattern focused, and participatory. In her practice theory of interpersonal relations, for example, Peplau[47] incorporated practice and theory into her ideas of research. Resembling the hermeneutic circle, Peplau's research process began in practice, spiraled up, drawing in theories—or as she stated, "peeling out theories"—to explain the phenomenon, then returned to practice to examine the new knowledge in light of the experiences and reality of practice.

Paterson and Zderad[49] described a method of "nursology" as the study of nursing practice. They outlined five phases of phenomenologic nursology in which the practitioner role informed the research process: (1) preparing oneself to be an open window, (2) intuiting the rhythm of the other, (3) knowing the other scientifically, (4) synthesizing differences and similarities, and (5) arriving at a conception of the situation that has some universal meaning across many nursing practice situations.

More recently, Newman[50] described research as praxis, meaning an approach to research that takes the form of nursing practice in the researcher's relationship to the participant and in the enactment of values for human transformation through pattern recognition. Similarly, Parse[51] put forth a research methodology based on her "theory of human becoming." One essential step in the research process is "dialogical engagement," which involves establishing a therapeutic presence between researcher and participant.

These and other theorists' models of nursing depict ways in which doing science itself can be linked to the ideals and metanarratives of practice. Guidelines for evaluating the emancipatory potential of the research process and product have been detailed.[52] Nursing practice frameworks are evolving scientific methods that are tailored not only to elicit desired data while protecting research participants' rights, but also to be therapeutic.

THE ESTHETIC ORDER AND NURSING PRACTICE

Postmodernism has stimulated greater awareness among nurses of the culture of practice as a source of ultimate meaning about the object of that practice, human beings' health and healing. Concomitantly, there has been increased interest in research on nursing care processes ranging from nursing care systems to nursing caring behaviors, intuition, nursing presence, and the nurse–patient relationship. Rather than characterize this focus as a return to the mid-20th century focus of research on nurses, it may be more accurately viewed as a focus of inquiry influenced in part by the postmodern emphasis on context. In postmodernism, the ultimate locus of meaning is the culture or context of the object of inquiry.[2] Professional practice is a nursing context. And nursing practice increasingly is being viewed as a legitimate source of knowledge, in part because it is regarded as an esthetic order of nursing, imbued with meaning and beauty.[53]

Amidst the postmodern emphasis on culture and context as something external to the person, nursing must not lose sight of the other context of healing—the patient. The postmodern notion of context must be broadened in nursing to include, if not to emphasize, the pa-

tient as a context of health and healing. Human beings' inner healing nature cannot be dismissed, as postmodernists might have it.[38] Patient as environment was first conceptualized by several nurse theorists (eg, Levine,[54] Orem,[23] Paterson and Zderad,[49] and Neuman[55]) who wrote about the "internal environment" of the person as an inner reality and innate resource for health and development. The significance of an inner healing environment is supported by current worldviews about inner human potential and transformative capacity.[28,30,34,35] A basic assumption of Nightingale was that the natural source of healing resided in the patient.[15] And Rogers[56] wrote emphatically about the coexistence of person and environment, regarding the two as one "person–environment mutual process."

Thus, it is proposed that the esthetic in nursing practice refers not only to the meaningful and beautiful experienced through nursing practice by the nurse, but also, and perhaps more appropriately, to that experienced through nursing practice by the patient. As Kim stated in describing one perspective of esthetics, "Certain aspects of nursing practice may be considered 'art' insofar as they communicate aesthetic ideas to perceivers, especially *clients*."[57(p281)]

This perspective on the esthetics of nursing practice is contrary to the more commonly held view of the esthetic experience residing primarily in the nurse.[56] However, esthetic experience is not found primarily in the type of brushes the painter uses, or the way a musician holds an instrument, or the style of the conductor or poet. Rather, the esthetic is the beauty that is experienced in seeing the painting, hearing the music, and in reading or reciting the poem. Analogously, in nursing, the esthetic is not primarily that experienced by the practitioner; the esthetic is found in the beauty and meaning associated with the patient's experiences of health and healing—the phenomena of concern to nursing. The esthetic is what is desired, meaningful, beautiful—whether it is experienced through the art of a painter, a musician, or a nurse. Given the esthetic order underlying the nurse's art, then, nursing practice is recognized as possessing powerful metanarratives about health and the processes of healing.

NURSING CONCEPTUAL MODELS: ARCHETYPES OF NURSING PRACTICE

The nursing conceptual models are a mechanism of translating the metanarrative of nursing practice for knowledge development. Nursing conceptual models broadly refer to extant conceptual and theoretical systems that describe the nature of nursing practice, patients as human beings, and health. Nursing conceptual models, their biases and preunderstandings notwithstanding,[58] "articulate disciplinary perspectives and underlying philosophical assumptions."[46(p56)] In the modernist era, these models were regarded as ideas to be revered, preserved, unaltered, and used in their entirety. More recently, Whall[59] noted, some are disparaging the conceptual models, reasoning that nursing has matured beyond needing the conceptual models for knowledge development and practice. This reasoning is specious. All levels of theory are needed in generating knowledge for theory-based practice.

The disregard for extant conceptual and theoretical models of nursing may be influenced in part by postmodernists' disinterest in grappling with the wholes that grand-level theories address. In their retreat from dealing with the complexity of a phenomenon, postmodernists fragment objects of inquiry by breaking them into smaller pieces and denying the need to conceptualize the whole.[1] However, from the neomodernist stance proposed in this article, unified conceptualizations of nursing and nursing practice are valued. Nursing conceptual models are more than a modernist artifact; they are archetypes of nursing practice.

Further, these archetypes are dynamic, unlike the archetypes of modernist science. Like the reality they depict, the practice and research contexts in which they are used, the theories they

inspire, and the metaparadigm they represent, nursing conceptual models must be allowed to be open and alterable. As systems of knowledge, they must evolve, lest they move from being extant to becoming extinct. Other conceptual models will likely emerge out of the vestiges of earlier models and the new insights of creative nursing scientists, philosophers, and practitioners who grapple with the whole.

Nursing: A Postcritical Discipline

The neomodernist perspectives on knowledge development presented here build on modernist and postmodern ideas. Characteristic assumptions of postmodernism that all methods and sources of knowledge development are value laden and that the process of constructing and perceiving reality is a dynamic, relational endeavor undergird the framework. It is also recognized that knowledge development is more than science, science more than the empirical, and the empirical more than empiricism. Philosophic and practice dimensions in nursing generate open metanarratives for scientific inquiry that serve as external correctives to the critique of knowledge development. Postmodernism alone can never be a critical theory. As first proposed by Plato, critique of the particulars requires grounding in the universals. Metanarratives provide this grounding and are essential in intellectual pursuits.[2]

Postmodernists have challenged the metanarratives, referring to them as "totalizing discourses" that are fabrications and not representations of reality.[38] Other scholars have explained that science cannot exist in the absence of metanarratives, and they repudiate the notion that there are no legitimated metanarratives.[1,3,5] Language is not so slippery nor meanings so unstable that underlying patterns of individuals and groups cannot be identified. In failing to identify meaningful patterns in the ongoing change of person and environment, science becomes merely history. Thus, nursing, proposed here as a neomodernist science, has identified discourses of nursing philosophy and practice that converge on themes of healing environments, inner human potential, and the developmental–contextual nature of health.

The neomodernist framework proposed here also departs from postmodernism in that the object of inquiry—human processes of health and healing—is regarded as more than a "text" to be deconstructed or disentangled of the discourses that authority figures have inscribed on it.[38] Human beings are more than bodies inscribed by their context. There is text, or meaning, beyond the text that informs and stimulates scientific inquiry. The neomodernist retains a belief in an underlying esthetic order in nursing. This order is revealed through nursing practice processes that enhance healing and development.

Nursing can never return to a pre-postmodern era to regain lost and lofty assumptions about knowledge development and nursing. But nursing still possesses the innovativeness and imagination to continue progressing in the metanarrative Nightingale originally established—empowerment of human beings' natural potential for health and healing.

Nursing, by nature, is a postcritical discipline: Self-reflection, personal autonomy, innate developmental potential, connections between truth and life, emancipatory practice and research, and chaos as opportunity are all valued. These are values and conceptual orientations that distinguish the discipline from others.

Yet within this shared focus, there is a diversity in approaches to knowledge development. As a feminist philosopher recently implied, totality does not have to mean totalitarianism; unity does not mean uniformity.[1] A postcritical discipline values challenges to the status quo and critiques and exposes oppressive discourses. And a postcritical discipline is not timid in committing to an overarching discourse that enables and liberates patients and other persons.

Nursing is a metanarrative that shapes the broader scientific community's understanding of human beings. It is a metanarrative needed in health care reform. And, like all discourse, it warrants ongoing critique. A neomodernist perspective of knowledge development provides for this critique while also fostering the grounding and vision to continue scientific inquiry. An open philosophy that exercises connections between science, philosophy, and practice will help ensure that nursing's metanarratives do not become closed ideologic systems, and it will help ensure that the dialogue on knowledge development continues into the 21st century.

REFERENCES

1. Waugh P. *Postmodernism*. New York, NY: Routledge, Chapman and Hall; 1992.
2. Popper KR. *Conjectures and Refutations: The Growth of Scientific Knowledge*. New York, NY: Harper & Row; 1963.
3. Doherty J, Graham E, Malek M, eds. *Postmodernism and the Social Sciences*. New York, NY: Macmillan; 1992.
4. Lyotard J. *The Postmodern Condition: A Report on Knowledge*. Minneapolis, Minn: University of Minnesota Press; 1979.
5. Burman E. Developmental psychology and the postmodern child. In: Doherty J, Graham E, Malek M, eds. *Postmodernism and the Social Sciences*. New York, NY: Macmillan; 1992.
6. Foucault M. *The Order of Things*. London, England: Tavistock; 1974.
7. Philipse H. Towards a postmodern conception of metaphysics: on the genealogy and successor disciplines of modern philosophy. *Metaphilosophy*. 1994;25:1–44.
8. Rorty R. *Philosophy and the Mirror of Nature*. Oxford, England: Blackwell; 1980.
9. Rorty R. *Contingency, Irony and Solidarity*. Cambridge, NY: Cambridge University Press; 1989.
10. Carper BA. Fundamental patterns of knowing in nursing. *ANS*. 1978;1(1):13–24.
11. Chinn PL, Kramer MK. *Theory and Nursing: A Systematic Approach*. 3rd ed. St. Louis, Mo: Mosby; 1991.
12. Schultz PR, Meleis AI. Nursing epistemology: traditions, insights, questions. *Image J Nurs Schol*. 1989;20:217–221.
13. Polis DF. Paradigms for an open philosophy. *Metaphilosophy*. 1993;24:33–46.

14. Howard GS. Culture tales: a narrative approach to thinking. *Cross-Cultural Psychol Psychother.* 1991;46:187–197.

15. Nightingale F. *Notes on Nursing: What It Is, and What It Is Not.* New York, NY: Dover, 1969.

16. Peplau HE. The art and science of nursing: similarities, differences, and relations. *Nurs Sci Q.* 1988;1:8–15.

17. Peirce CS, Hartshorne C, Weiss P, eds. *Charles Sanders Peirce: Collected Papers.* Cambridge, Mass: Harvard University Press; 1934:5.

18. Staat W. On abduction, deduction, induction and the categories. *Transactions Charles S Peirce Soc.* 1993;29:225–237.

19. Gergen KJ. Exploring the postmodern: perils or potentials? *Am Psychol.* 1994;49:412–417.

20. Laudan L. *Progress and Its Problems: Toward a Theory of Scientific Growth.* Berkeley, Calif: University of California Press; 1977.

21. Kukla A. Nonempirical issues in psychology. *Am Psychol.* 1989;44:785–794.

22. Newman M. *Health as Expanding Consciousness.* 2nd ed. New York, NY: National League for Nursing; 1993.

23. Orem DE. *Nursing: Concepts of Practice.* 4th ed. St. Louis, Mo: Mosby; 1991.

24. Britt D, ed. *Modern Art: Impressionism to Post-Modernism.* Boston, Mass: Little, Brown; 1989.

25. Allen DG. Using philosophical and historical methodologies to understand the concept of health. In: Chinn PL, ed. *Nursing Research Methodology.* Rockville, Md: Aspen Publishers; 1986.

26. Omer H, London P. Metamorphosis in psychotherapy: end of the systems era. *Psychotherapy.* 1988;25:171–180.

27. Habermas J, Lawrence FG, trans. *The Philosophical Discourses of Modernity.* Oxford, England: Polity; 1987.

28. Wilber K. *A Sociable God.* New York, NY: McGraw-Hill; 1983.

29. Sahakian WS. *History of Philosophy.* New York, NY: Barnes & Noble; 1968.

30. Pepper SP. *World Hypotheses: A Study in Evidence.* Berkeley, Calif: University of California Press; 1942.

31. Lerner RM. *Concepts and Theories of Human Development.* 2nd ed. New York, NY: Random House; 1986.

32. Fawcett J. *Analysis and Evaluation of Nursing Theories.* Philadelphia, Pa: F.A. Davis; 1993.

33. Hall BA. The change paradigm in nursing: growth versus persistence. *ANS.* 1981;3(4):1–6.

34. Newman MA. Prevailing paradigms in nursing. *Nurs Outlook.* 1992;40:10–13.

35. Parse RR. *Nursing Science: Major Paradigms, Theories, and Critiques.* Philadelphia, Pa: W.B. Saunders; 1987.

36. Reed PG. Toward a nursing theory of self-transcendence: deductive reformulation using developmental theories. *ANS.* 1991;13:64–77.

37. Werner H. The concept of development from a comparative and organismic point of view. In: Harris DB, ed. *The Concept of Development.* Minneapolis, Minn: University of Minnesota Press; 1957.

38. Fox NJ. *Postmodernism, Sociology, and Health.* Toronto, Canada: University of Toronto Press; 1994.

39. Lundin RW. *Theories and Systems of Psychology.* 2nd ed. Lexington, Mass: Heath; 1979.

40. Barrett EAM. Response: disciplinary perspective: unified or diverse? Diversity reigns. *Nurs Sci Q.* 1992;5:155–157.

41. Fawcett J. From a plethora of paradigms to parsimony in world views. *Nurs Sci Q.* 1993;6:56–58.

42. Northrup DT. Commentary: disciplinary perspective: unified or diverse? A unified perspective within nursing. *Nurs Sci Q.* 1992;5:154–156.

43. Kikuchi JF, Simmons H, eds. *Developing a Philosophy of Nursing.* Thousand Oaks, Calif: Sage; 1994.

44. Moccia P. A critique of compromise: beyond the methods debate. *ANS.* 1988;10(4):1–9.

45. Laurin J. A philosophy of nursing: commentary. In: Kikuchi JF, Simmons H, eds. *Developing a Philosophy of Nursing.* Thousands Oaks. Calif: Sage; 1994.

46. Smith MC. Arriving at a philosophy of nursing: discovering? constructing? evolving? In: Kikuchi JF, Simmons H, eds. *Developing a Philosophy of Nursing.* Thousand Oaks, Calif: Sage; 1994.

47. Peplau HE. Interpersonal relations: a theoretical framework for application in nursing practice. *Nurs Sci Q.* 1992;5(1):13–18.

48. Chinn PL. A window of opportunity. *ANS.* 1994;16(4):viii.

49. Paterson JG, Zderad LT. *Humanistic Nursing.* New York, NY: Wiley; 1976.

50. Newman MA. Newman's theory of health as praxis. *Nurs Sci Q.* 1990;3:37–41.

51. Parse RR. Parse's research methodology with an illustration of the lived experience of hope. *Nurs Sci Q.* 1990;3:9–17.

52. DeMarco R, Campbell J, Wuest J. Feminist critique: searching for meaning in research. *ANS.* 1993; 16(2):26–38.

53. Katims I. Nursing as aesthetic experience and the notion of practice. *Schol Inq Nurs Pract.* 1993; 7:269–278.

54. Levine M. *Introduction to Clinical Nursing.* 2nd ed. Los Angeles, Calif: F.A. Davis; 1973.

55. Neuman B. *The Neuman Systems Model*. 3rd ed. Norwalk, Conn: Appleton-Lange; 1994.

56. Rogers ME. Nursing: a science of unitary man. In: Riehl JP, Roy C, eds. *Conceptual Models for Nursing Practice*. 2nd ed. New York, NY: Appleton-Century-Crofts; 1980.

57. Kim HS. Response to "Nursing as Aesthetic Experience and the Notion of Practice." *Schol Inq Nurs Pract*. 1993;7:279–282.

58. Thompson JL. Practical discourse in nursing: going beyond empiricism and historicism. *ANS*. 1985;7(4):59–71.

59. Whall AL. Let's get rid of all that theory. *Nurs Sci Q*. 1993;6:164–165.

PAMELA G. REED

The Necessity for and Evolution of Multiple Paradigms for Nursing Research: A Poststructuralist Perspective

Laura Cox Dzurec

Viewing a phenomenon from a point beyond its boundaries permits a clearer understanding of it. The evolution of two paradigms, or world views, for nursing research—logical positivism and phenomenology/hermeneutics—is viewed by the author from a perspective beyond either paradigm. That perspective is poststructuralism, a philosophy developed to transcend the limitations of traditional philosophy and to encourage unique thought to develop. Using the ideas of Foucault, a poststructuralist philosopher, the author discusses power/knowledge and discipline as a backdrop for nursing's significant and growing acceptance of multiple paradigms for the conduct of research.

The human sciences, including nursing, have a long tradition of struggling with the problem of identifying an appropriate conceptual framework and methods for the conduct of research. The development of this struggle can be traced through the nursing literature from at least the mid-1960s, when a concern with new approaches to enhancing nursing knowledge became apparent, to the present. A constant factor throughout the struggle has been the presumption of the superiority of one approach over another.

Logical positivism has consistently prevailed as the primary and most highly valued approach to science in nursing, as Reeder[1] demonstrated through analysis of 23 nursing research texts published between 1950 and 1982. Conceptual frameworks other than logical positivism have historically been shunned in influential nursing circles.[2,3] Yet the development of thought that allows other approaches to science, specifically phenomenology/hermeneutics, is emerging. This emergence is reflected, for example, in the devotion of entire journal issues to methodologic concerns (eg, *Adv Nurs Sci* 1986;6[3]), in the publication of research texts devoted entirely to qualitative issues,[4,5] and in the inclusion of qualitative issues in research texts, which have traditionally described science primarily in terms of the techniques of logical positivism.

It is the intent of the author to view this paradigmatic shift in nursing's approach to research from a perspective beyond either of the two dominant research paradigms. Poststructuralist philosophy[6–10] provides such a perspective. Although they admit a need for theoretical structures as frameworks for thinking, research, and theory development, poststructuralists go beyond those frameworks in an effort to evaluate their utility and function in process. This is an

Reprinted by permission from Advances in Nursing Science 11(4):69–77. Inc. © 1989, Aspen Publishers, Inc.

important step for nursing to take as we attempt proactively to identify appropriate directions for research and theory development in nursing.

This article thus provides an overview of significant poststructuralist issues and, from that perspective, outlines the evolution of nursing's use of multiple paradigms for research and theory development. Specifically, the work of Foucault is cited as a foundation for understanding this phenomenon. The evolution of multiple paradigms for nursing research is seen as a necessary outcome of the forces operating within the discipline.

Poststructuralism and Foucault

In general, poststructuralist philosophers hold that life events are accidental, having neither purpose nor direction. While this view may be somewhat shocking initially, the reader is asked to give up, for the moment, previously held ideas about cause and effect, free will, or determinism. The utility of the poststructuralist view will become clear through the process of reevaluating the phenomenon of nursing's paradigmatic shift. Poststructuralists also maintain that while structure (eg, theory and methodology) is useful, it also limits the boundaries of thought. Poststructuralist philosophers thus attempt to view life events in a manner that is free of structure. In so doing they acknowledge that such a stance, in itself, imposes structure. However, no structure can be recognized as the ultimate framework for understanding from a poststructuralist perspective. Given these two general poststructuralist assumptions, it is possible to turn specifically to the observations of Foucault as they were shared with Rabinow[9] in a series of personal interviews.

Foucault's fairly extensive work has focused on power and organization in society. Discourse (ie, human interaction) has represented the basis for his thought. As a poststructuralist, Foucault did not accept a single correct approach to knowledge development. Nor did he accept the authority of a superhuman power or being, such

as one might recognize in some Eastern thought, that directs knowledge development regardless of any human activity so aimed. Foucault simply observed human interactions (events) and recognized them as mechanisms that could be used to discuss, if not finally explain, the human condition. He viewed truth as an outcome of events.

Two particular mechanisms discussed by Foucault are important to attempts to clarify or simplify the process of developing paradigmatic pluralism in nursing. The first of these mechanisms is power/knowledge, and the second is disciplinary instruments. They will be discussed separately.

POWER/KNOWLEDGE

Foucault did not think of power as it is typically viewed but rather saw it as being everywhere. Power is not held; it is an exercise that represents "a strategic situation in a given society."[11(p21)] Power comes from all segments of society and is not localized among a chosen few. Power relations have specific purposes. Certain basic laws or rules are maintained through the network of power relations that pervades society. As Foucault noted, "Power with its prohibitions can only take hold and secure its footing where it is rooted in a whole series of multiple and indefinite power relations that supply the necessary basis for the great negative forms of power."[9(p64)] Therefore, power limits. In this limiting mode, power essentially determines all that can and will be known. It pronounces a rule, and it is maintained at all levels of social hierarchy through the day-to-day interactions of involved individuals.

However, inasmuch as power is a limitation, it is also a productive force. When one acknowledges a rule, one simultaneously acknowledges what the rule forbids. As discourse is produced regarding what is forbidden—what the law will not allow—a new knowledge results. New knowledge is produced as individuals become aware of what the law forbids. With this new knowledge comes a shift in power relations, as more and more people learn about and act upon the newly acquired knowledge.

Because power and knowledge are so intimately involved in this way, Foucault coined the term "power/knowledge." By virtue of its limiting and productive aspects, power/knowledge subtly encourages behavior that is forbidden. As Foucault noted, power "doesn't only weigh on us as a force that says no, but it traverses and produces things. It needs to be considered as a productive network much more than as a negative instance whose function is repression."[9(p61)]

While all people in society are subject to the limiting and productive operations of power/knowledge, not all are consciously aware of those operations. Individual ignorance of the operations of power/knowledge is significant to the maintenance of power, according to Foucault. An important aspect of successful power relations is secrecy, such as that manifest in the techniques used by institutions and organizations to discipline and control society and thereby to maintain their power.

Subtle techniques are used to reward those exemplary individuals who are model citizens and to screen the mechanisms by which power/knowledge operates. These techniques are intended to make power efficient and invisible, while ensuring the visibility of individuals. Thus individual compliance with rules is maintained.

THE INSTRUMENTS OF DISCIPLINE

Foucault noted that the word "discipline" can be defined as either a branch of knowledge or as punishment. From Foucault's perspective, disciplines, including all of the human sciences, are necessarily punitive, as they attempt to maintain power relations and produce knowledge.

Foucault[9] described three specific instruments of discipline used by institutions and organizations in society: examination, normalizing judgment, and hierarchical observation. The three overlap in their functions. Clarification of their roles is important to understanding the development of paradigmatic pluralism in nursing from a poststructuralist perspective.

Examination is used not only to measure levels of knowledge or skill but also to impose diagnostic labels such as "healthy," "schizophrenic," "fit," or "physically incompetent." By examination, the characteristics of one individual are compared with those of a known group. This process also involves normalizing judgment and observation, the other two disciplinary instruments described by Foucault.

Normalizing judgment is a technique that involves the maintenance of acceptable standards. If a person fails to meet expected norms, "little punishments" intended to make an example of the individual's failures and to camouflage power itself are meted out to enforce compliance. Conformity is thus at issue, through which power is maintained.

The third instrument of discipline discussed by Foucault is hierarchical observation. Within society there is a pervasive observational network that allows those at the top of the power structure to view activities in all directions. Observation promotes and maintains the general visibility of the individual, thus supporting the power structure and delimiting power/knowledge. This panopticon is recognizable in closed-circuit television systems in shopping malls, police radar, and even professional meetings, which serve to increase the visibility of individuals and their activities within a discipline.

These three instruments demonstrate the limiting forces of power knowledge. Their function is to maintain the status quo. By recognizing Foucault's[9,11] ideas about power/knowledge and the instruments of discipline, the reader can view the development of multiple paradigms for nursing research from a poststructuralist perspective.

The Tenacity of Logical Positivist Methodology in Nursing

The tenacity of nursing's commitment to logical positivism, which parallels the commitment of all Western human sciences, can be discussed with some degree of understanding when one recognizes that claims to knowledge are also claims to power. A series of "multiple and indefinite power relations"[9(p64)] is apparent in logical positivism as method.

While dominating thought and research in nursing, the logical positivist method also disallowed so-called nonscientific approaches to research and theory development. Most modern nursing contemporaries learned a single way of doing science—logical positivism—without any awareness that this was but one of many possible approaches. (This is true not only of nursing but of the human sciences in general.) It is probably accurate to say that most researchers did not recognize that they were using logical positivist techniques; instead, they believed that they were using *scientific* techniques.

From this narrow vantage point, researchers could and did overcommit to science and its aims. A purpose was born that achieved all but religious status: the advancement of knowledge. It reflected solely the logical positivist method and its inherent assumptions. The fervor with which researchers virtually worshiped logical positivism in the guise of science created power relations that, even as they produced appropriate logical positivist knowledge, simultaneously reinforced the method's grip. Not only were clean, scientific research outcomes assured, but the continuity of the approach was accomplished via the three instruments of discipline (examination, normalizing judgment, and hierarchical observation).

Examinations have been used in nursing to compare individuals' skills and characteristics with those of the larger group of nurses. For example, college entrance examinations are used to screen entrants for graduate and undergraduate programs. In a more direct link to nursing knowledge, objective, multiple-choice, and essay examinations are used in undergraduate classes to ensure that an individual nurse's characteristics match what are considered to be nursing characteristics. Candidacy examinations ensure that doctoral students are prepared to face the rigors of research in a manner appropriate to nursing. In general, the examination can be seen as a mechanism by which a core of nursing knowledge—traditionally couched in logical positivism—has been staunchly maintained.

Those students judged to be unsuccessful in their examinations are subject to normalizing judgment. Failing grades, potential or actual expulsion from programs of study, unsuccessful efforts to publish, and rejection of research grant proposals all are examples of the "little punishments" of normalizing judgment. These punishments are intended, in nursing as in all disciplines, to maintain compliance with acceptable (traditionally logical positivist) standards. By camouflaging power itself and illuminating the individual and his or her efforts, normalizing judgment has served to limit knowledge and power to logical positivist assumptions.

Hierarchical observation occurs at all levels of nursing, from the undergraduate classroom to the postdoctoral seminar and from the hospital to the community. It is visible in the change-of-shift report, in nursing grand rounds, in research and practice conventions. By these mechanisms the activities of nurses are made visible and subjected to further examination and judgment.

Thus, by virtue of the limiting aspects of power/knowledge and the three instruments of discipline, the hold of logical positivism over nursing has been consistently, even if accidentally, maintained. A limiting restraint is not, however, the endpoint of the power of the logical positivist method. Although power/knowledge is limited by disciplinary instruments, those same instruments concomitantly encouraged what was forbidden.

A Productive Outcome of Power/Knowledge: Phenomenology/Hermeneutics

The period beginning in the mid-1960s and stretching to today is perhaps the first in which the power relations in nursing, and in the human sciences in general, have allowed the recognition of logical positivism as a single philosophy of science rather than as science itself. Given this recognition, researchers have begun to identify the specific assumptions of the method as originally delineated by philosophers in the 1930s.[12]

Polkinghorne summarized three primary tenets of the positivist tradition as follows:

> (1) All metaphysics should be rejected and knowledge confined to what has been experienced or can be experienced. (2) The adequacy of knowledge increases as it approximates the forms of explanation achieved by the most advanced sciences. (3) Scientific explanation is limited to only functional and directional laws (Comte) or to only mathematically functional laws (Mach).[12(pp19–20)]

It is fair, both to philosophers of science and to nursing, to say that nurse researchers working within the logical positivist paradigm have subscribed to these three tenets, although they were not always cognizant of the alternatives.

The assumptions of logical positivism have limited study to questions that could be posed in terms of dependent and independent variables. Answers had to be those that conformed to paradigmatic expectations regarding spatiality, temporality, and causality. Unexpected research outcomes were subject to further study so that they too could be understood within the logical positivist frame.[1(pp178–248)]

Viewing the limitations of logical positivist structure from a poststructuralist perspective, one must immediately question why these limitations are necessary. An antistructuralist stance would indicate that logical positivism is simply one among multiple perspectives.

Historically the conceptual system of logical positivism has structured what we have perceived and how we have perceived it in nursing. It has played a central role in the definition of the nursing discipline itself in the definition of nursing practice standards and in the definition of what constitutes acceptable nursing research. But by virtue of the paradoxical effect of power/knowledge as Foucault defined it, the method of logical positivism has been used in increasingly creative ways at the same time that its hold on the scientific community has weakened. Nurse researchers began to identify the limitations imposed by logical positivist assumptions.

The logical positivist method is now being widely questioned as the ultimate approach for the advancement of the discipline of nursing. Another set of "truths" based on other assumptions somehow (fortunately, and probably accidentally) came within the purview of nursing. These truths were the assumptions underlying the phenomenologic/hermeneutic paradigm. In general, this paradigm assumes the potential for multiple experienced realities; a nonspatial, nontemporal, noncausal view of the world; and an irreducible connectedness between the observer and that being observed. The focus of research within the paradigm is everyday, lived experience. Objective inquiry demands that the object of study be viewed in all its fullness and that the integral relationship of subject and object be recognized.

While the utility of these new assumptions was broadly questioned initially, their relevance and utility for nursing have become increasingly apparent to an everwidening body of nurse researchers. The assumptions of phenomenology/hermeneutics lend themselves well to nursing questions about the quality of life, meaning, and lived experience, questions that are irrelevant within the logical positivist framework. The unitary nature of human being and environment that is assumed by this method is consistent with a number of conceptual frameworks for nursing, such as Newman's[13] paradigm of health, Rogers'[14,15] science of unitary human beings, Parse's[16] man-living-health theory, and Paterson and Zderad's[17] humanistic nursing. Parse[18] has labeled the collective view of these nurse researchers "the simultaneity paradigm." The significance of this relatively new paradigm and of the related assumptions of phenomenology/hermeneutics is becoming increasingly clear in nursing.

The new paradigm allows nurse researchers

to understand—that is, to elicit meaning. The aim of research methods used within the paradigm is not to identify modal patterns by which to make normative comparisons of findings. Instead, the aim is to identify idiosyncratic patterns that clarify individuals' personal experiences. While at one time many would have questioned the usefulness of such knowledge, nurse researchers are increasingly recognizing and valuing information about individual uniqueness. Working hypotheses that are useful in discovering further insights about individuals and groups can be developed from such knowledge.

Confusion remains regarding the differentiation of qualitative and quantitative techniques within a single paradigm versus the differentiation of assumptions between paradigms. But this confusion is being openly discussed at professional meetings and by the informed review boards of significant nursing journals. Scholarly work subscribing to non–logical positivist assumptions is increasingly being reviewed by nursing experts as legitimate. Non–logical positivist research is no longer equated with sloppy science. It is now accepted that rigorous scientific research can incorporate either logical positivist methods or other methods.

From Foucault's perspective, nursing's acceptance and use of multiple paradigms for research and theory development were outcomes necessitated by the productive aspects of power/knowledge. Multiple perspectives on nursing research are a "necessary accident." Poststructuralist philosophers would argue that neither logical positivism nor phenomenology/hermeneutics is superior to the other but that the use of either paradigm should be considered in light of the question to be addressed.

This is not a particularly new or shocking observation; however, it is especially significant given the assumptions of poststructuralism. Foucault,[9] like other poststructuralists, wished to obliterate the "hierarchy of appropriateness" that seemed to be inherent in our thinking about relevant frameworks. Nurse researchers

are challenging that hierarchy with the breadth of their current approaches to research and theory development in nursing. Such breadth is essential to the development of the discipline and to the success with which it fulfills its commitments. Moreover, poststructuralist thought encourages us to look beyond what we know to focus on the forces that limit what we can know.

It is vital to nursing's ongoing development that openness to multiple paradigms be maintained. In a recent article, Schlotfeldt noted that the "profession has a commitment to an enhanced research agenda and to identifying the components of the discipline underlying nursing practice."[19(p65)]

Poststructuralist philosophy provides an important and illuminating perspective for this ongoing development. It encourages nurse researchers to focus not only on the content of the questions asked to advance nursing's sanctioned social mission, but on the metaphysical and political assumptions—specifically, those regarding language and power—that structure and limit the content of nursing.

From the poststructuralist perspective, the use of multiple paradigms for the conduct of nursing research is an evolutionary necessity as well as a necessary stance for a responsible discipline. Only from a perspective beyond the limitations of structuring paradigms can nursing hope to become actualized and fully cognizant of what the discipline entails. An awareness of the limitations of a paradigm enables nurse researchers to select research methods that address significant nursing questions. Only through the recognition of multiplicity can nursing hope to advance and fulfill the mission it espouses.

REFERENCES

1. Reeder F: *Nursing research, holism, and philosophies of science: Points of congruence between E Husserl and ME Rogers,* dissertation. New York University, 1984 (University microfilms no 84–21, 466).
2. Knafl KA, Howard MJ: Interpreting, reporting, and evaluating qualitative research. *Res Nurs Health* 1983;7(1):17–24.
3. Tinkle MB, Beaton JL: Toward a new view of sci-

ence: Implications for nursing research. *Adv Nurs Sci* 1983;5(2):27–36.

4. Munhall PL, Oiler CJ: *Nursing Research: A Qualitative Perspective.* New York, Appleton-Century-Crofts, 1986.

5. Parse RR, Coyne AB, Smith MJ: *Nursing Research: Qualitative Methods.* Bowie, Md, Brady Communications Company, 1985.

6. Derrida J: *Margins of Philosophy,* Bass A (trans). Chicago, University of Chicago Press, 1982.

7. Gordon C: Birth of the subject, in Edgley R, Osborne R (eds): *Radical Philosophy Reader.* London, Verso, 1985, pp 69–97.

8. Kristeva J: *Desire in Language: A Semiotic Approach to Literature and Art,* Gora T, Jardine A, Roudiez LS (trans). New York, Columbia University Press, 1980.

9. Rabinow P (ed): *The Foucault Reader.* New York, Pantheon, 1984.

10. Wood DC: An introduction to Derrida, in Edgley R, Osborne R (eds): *Radical Philosophy Reader.* London, Verso, 1985, pp 18–42.

11. Foucault M: *The Will To Know.* Paris: Gallimard, 1976.

12. Polkinghorne D: *Methodology for the Human Sciences: Systems of Inquiry.* Albany, NY, State University of New York Press, 1983.

13. Newman MA: *Health as Expanding Consciousness.* St Louis, Mosby, 1986.

14. Rogers ME: *An Introduction to the Theoretical Basis of Nursing.* Philadelphia, WB Saunders, 1970.

15. Rogers ME: Rogers' science of unitary human beings, in Parse RR (ed): *Nursing Science: Major Paradigms, Theories, and Critiques.* Philadelphia, WB Saunders, 1987, pp 139–146.

16. Parse RR: *Man–Living–Health: A Theory of Nursing.* New York, Wiley, 1981.

17. Paterson J, Zderad LT: *Humanistic Nursing.* New York, Wiley, 1976.

18. Parse RR (ed): *Nursing Science: Major Paradigms, Theories, and Critiques.* Philadelphia, WB Saunders, 1987.

19. Schlotfeldt RM: Defining nursing: A historic controversy. *Nurs Res* 1987;36:64–67.

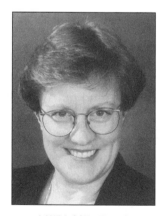

LAURA COX DZUREC

The Dilemma of Nursing Science: Current Quandaries and Lack of Direction

Sheila A. Packard • E. Carol Polifroni

The theme of this paper is the need to address the central question in nursing science. It is hypothesized that in the absence of a central, unifying question, the view of nursing as an applied science, the current research methodological debate, and the social policy statement definition of nursing have hindered nursing's ability to advance the science of nursing. The authors suggest that the terminology of applied science has been wrongfully interpreted as immediate application to nursing practice, that the research methodological debate has occurred because the focus of research efforts is on the means and not the end, and that the policy statement implies a stimulus-response approach to human behavior.

Nursing has been referred to by many as an emerging science. The term, in and of itself, is redundant. As all scholars know, any and all sciences are, by their very nature, evolving and emerging. In fact, growth and emergence are central to the definition of a science. Yet, nurses continue to see this redundancy applied to the acquisition of knowledge in nursing.

What is implied, if not stated, in the idea of emergence is an image of nursing coming into the light or tottering on the brink of scientific discovery. If this is, indeed, indicative of present development and evolution, why is nursing on the edge rather than within the mainstream of science? It is the purpose of this paper to examine factors which influence the conception of nursing as emerging: the notion of applied science, the debate over methodologies, and the social policy statement. Clarity in these areas may be provided through unity in the quest of nursing science.

Nursing as an Applied Science

Nursing is regarded by many as an applied science. This depiction is derived from the fact that theory or theories are judged in part by their immediate applicability to nursing practice. While usefulness may generally be considered an important criterion upon which to base the worth of a theory, the issue is not clear-cut. Questions arise in respect to a common determination of what is really meant by the term "applied science."

Traditionally, an applied science has been seen as the practical application of theories emanating from several disciplines. An example of this might be the applied science of medicine, which, aside from its own unique body of knowledge, utilizes concepts derived from biology, chemistry, and pharmacology among others. When the term is similarly used, something different from practical application of nursing theories is meant. The problem, then, is one of emphasis. In calling nursing an "applied science," one must consider how much nursing knowledge is derived from other fields and how much is self-determined?

Schultz and Meleis (1988) defined nursing epistemology as "the study of the origins of nursing knowledge, its structure and methods, the patterns of knowing of its members, and the criteria for validating its knowledge claims" (p. 217). This definition, in light of the ambiguity attached to the term "applied science," underscores the need for clarification in this area. For a host of reasons (which are beyond the scope of this paper) nursing practice has been governed by paradigms borrowed from other disciplines; among these are psychology, sociology, physics and biology. In addition, much research in nursing has been directed toward testing theory derived from other disciplines, particularly the behavioral sciences.

It would seem imperative, from the standpoint of epistemology, that nursing not confuse the application of theory *per se* with the traditional notion of applied science as a hodgepodge of theories from related fields. In essence, practical usage does not necessitate the incorporation of knowledge from any science other than nursing. While this may not currently be the case, there is hope that the time may come when applied science means the specific utilization of nursing knowledge in nursing practice.

Is nursing only an applied science? Despite much discussion with colleagues, this question remains moot. There are those who would and do argue that the proof positive of any and all nursing theory is its immediate relevancy and therefore applicability to some aspect of nursing practice (Rogers, 1970). The thought here is that the whole point of nursing science is the establishment of a knowledge base upon which to focus decision-making in the provision of care. If this is the only use for nursing theory, then the fate of nursing as *only* an applied science is sealed.

There is, however, the possibility that nursing could and should evolve in part as a pure science; that is, science for its own sake, for the purpose of knowing, as detached from the sole purpose of immediate application. An example in point is theoretical physics, wherein knowledge of the big bang theory or black holes may not be immediately relevant to life on earth in this century. If nursing is defined as an applied science, is there room for discovery of knowledge that may only be relevant in the future? Rogers (in Smith 1988) has stated "Nightingale talked about people; she wasn't just talking about people who were sick. The smallest number of people in this world are the ones who are sick. Our concern is much broader than that handful of people. . . . Practice is how we use knowledge, it is not knowledge itself. . . . I would hate to think that nursing was narrowed to something called intimate personal care. That is a very narrow approach. I don't even know what those words mean" (p. 81).

The point here has to do with the legitimacy of nursing theory which is directed at knowledge about persons whether or not they come into contact with nursing services. Additionally, should relevancy be determined by apparent applicability or is there a place for so-called "pure" or "theoretical" nursing science? If the former is true, then is nursing only an applied science? History demonstrates that some of the most important scientific discoveries come about inadvertently, not as a direct result of specific research aims. More importantly, theory has often preceded application by many years, as in the case of nuclear physics.

In essence then, the term "applied science" as related to nursing is in need of clarification. On

> **"When you don't know the answer, question the question."**
>
> *(Anonymous)*

the one hand, there remains the question of "applying what" (only nursing theories or theories from other disciplines)? And also, there is the question as to whether being an applied science eliminates the potentialities of pure or theoretical science.

The Methods Debate

Recent literature is replete with discussion as to the appropriate methodologies to be used in acquisition of nursing knowledge (Clarke & Yaros, 1988; Duffy, 1987; Moccia, 1988; Norbeck, 1987; Phillips, 1988; and Porter, 1989). As evidenced in the stances taken by various writers, there appears to be growing sentiment that the issue needs to be considered at this juncture in the development of nursing as a science. In the ongoing debate, several camps may be identified: some authors (Clarke & Yaros, 1988; Jayaratne, 1983; Norbeck, 1987) believe that empiricism, if not quantification, is the most appropriate avenue for research endeavors; others (Field & Morse, 1985; Leininger, 1985) maintain that qualitative methodology holds the greatest promise. More recently, writers have advocated triangulation of methods: the use of both qualitative and quantitative approaches within the same study and for the same questions (Duffy, 1987; Gortner & Schultz, 1988; Porter, 1989). However, in response, a number of writers (Moccia, 1988; Phillips, 1988) speak to the overall loss of integrity inherent in triangulation. Finally, there is the stance which favors none of the above but rather the creation of new and different methods ideally suited to the problems faced in nursing research (Moccia, 1988; Parse, 1987; Phillips, 1988). In order to more clearly understand the fundamental issue at stake in the debate, a very brief summary of the points taken by each side is helpful.

ADVOCATES OF QUANTIFICATION

Generally, those who advocate this approach to scientific investigation hold that quantitative methodologies have worked well for other sciences, and have led to understanding of relationships and specific causality. In her article in defense of empiricism Norbeck (1987) contends "it should be a dominant perspective in nursing research because many of the questions that we need to study are consistent with this view. When we plan care for groups of patients, assess the acuity of a unit in the hospital, develop predictive models for at-risk groups or search for causal explanation, we rely on systematically gathered, objective data drawn from relatively large numbers of individuals" (p. 29). Authors favoring the quantitative methods seem to agree that it is not the only way to go about research, but it is important in that statistical data allow us to see what portion of the dependent variable is explained by the identified independent variable(s). Assurances thus may be gained, instrument reliability may be assessed, and generalizability of findings made possible if proper sampling techniques are followed.

ADVOCATES OF QUALITATIVE METHODS

Those who favor qualitative methodologies believe that first-hand experience provides the most meaningful data for nursing science. Qualitative research is considered to be essential in understanding the nature of reality which is dynamic rather than static. It is submitted that since nursing is concerned with the whole human being, an understanding of parts (as is presented in quantitative findings) may be faulty (Rogers 1970). And a richer, fuller appreciation of phenomena is gained through the use of qualitative methodologies. Leininger (1985) encapsulates the views of the proponents of this approach in stating, "the scientific method is far too narrow, reductionistic and controlled to let one know human beings in their totality and help them in times of wellness and illness. Because of this, a cultural movement is slowly taking place in nursing, shifting the focus away from quantitative research methods and paradigms of the scientific mode to qualitative and other alternative research methods" (pp. 2–3).

ADVOCATES OF TRIANGULATION

As a means of resolving divergence between qualitative and quantitative factions, some thinkers support a position which espouses the values of both methodologies, particularly in combination. Gortner and Schultz (1988) believe the emphasis should be on standards of "good" science in nursing regardless of technique. "The very nature of our scientific work, then, asks of us a complex set of perspectives on topics and questions for study through a combination of techniques not seen in other scientific fields. Complex phenomena of interest to nursing are not adequately dealth with by methods that are located within only one perspective or that tend to look solely at one facet" (p. 23). Duffy (1987) contends that while each approach has something unique to offer, a combination or triangulation of approaches increases the likelihood that negative cases will be uncovered. She states, "Triangulation should not be viewed as an end in itself; rather it is a vehicle that, when used appropriately, combines different methods in a variety of ways to produce richer and more insightful analyses of complex phenomena than can be achieved by either method separately" (p. 133). Along these same lines, Porter (1989) puts forth the idea that phenomena could be studied by the concurrent or back and forth use of qualitative and quantitative methods (as in the case of submitting themes from phenomenological investigations to factor analysis). Advocates of triangulation in general seem to believe that it is too early in the development of nursing science to put closure on any type of methodology.

OPPOSERS TO TRIANGULATION

In contrast to the view held by those favoring compromise in and combination of research methods, some authors strongly oppose what Phillips (1988) has called "blended research." Moccia (1988) states that the argument for co-existence closes off important theoretical discussions and alters the focus of nursing science concerns. "The choice between methods has meaning and implications beyond the technical. It is a choice between an open-system and a closed-system view of the world; between knowledge that is legitimately sought and developed for inclusion in nursing science and that which is not legitimate; between definitions of science as a force for change or as a defense of the status quo; and between a nursing practice that hopes to predict and control phenomena and that which attempts to understand and explain them" (p. 3).

Phillips (1988) concurs with this opinion. He contends that method should be congruent with the paradigmatic perspective leading to the identification of the phenomenon under study. Qualitative and quantitative research are derived from different views of reality and are not complementary. It is questionable as to how acausality and causality can be combined in the same research study. He says that triangulation "may reflect the inadequacy of the existing methods for nursing science inquiry" (p. 5).

ADVOCATES OF NEW METHODOLOGIES

Emerging from methods debates is the beginning notion on the part of some thinkers that the controversy on methods, in fact, obscures some salient points with regard to nursing science (Parse, 1987; Phillips, 1988). This is particularly true when the arguments are focused on technique rather than the more fundamental issues in philosophy of science. In her article critiquing compromise, Moccia (1988) questions, "Is science intended to legitimize nursing as a scientific discipline by expanding and refining the ability to predict and prescribe human behavior? Or is it intended to be useful in helping the non-scientific population to understand and explain their experiences in the world? Is there a science to be developed that might combine these polarities" (p. 6)? The sense of some is that while the methods debate takes center stage, the more important aspects of nursing science as a science take place in the wings. Attention perhaps had best be focused on the basic intentions of nursing science along with the concomitant development of new and different methodologies better suited to intentions.

It may be conjectured that the methods debate is healthy and perhaps even inevitable due to forces both within and outside the profession. However, the more important question would seem to be why now? Certainly this issue has arisen in other fields in the past. The controversy is indicative of a deeper, perhaps more philosophical, dispute; namely, the true essence of nursing science.

The Social Policy Statement

Thusfar two factors influencing the development of nursing science have been discussed: the notion of nursing as an applied science and the controversy surrounding methodology. However, a third factor, the *Social Policy Statement* (ANA, 1980) has created difficulties in understanding the position of nursing science at the present time. As Allen (1987) submits, this might not be the case if the statement were merely a public relations document through which nursing is represented to the public. However, the image presented in the policy statement has, with little debate, been accepted by and incorporated into nursing education and practice. As a definition of what nursing is and what nurses do, its impact is pervasive. Choices, including those directly related to nursing research, may emerge from this professional self-image.

The social policy statement defines nursing as "the diagnosis and treatment of human responses to actual or potential health problems" (ANA, 1980, p. 7). It follows that if this is the definition of the nature and scope of nursing practice, nursing science should, to some extent (if not the greatest extent), be aimed at the study of diagnosis and treatment of human responses to actual and potential health problems. This places some significant obstacles in the path of the development of nursing as a science.

Allen (1987) has identified incongruities in the social policy statement centering on the description of person and society. He refers to the view of person in the statement as being, on the one hand, biologically and socially determined while, on the other hand, being both constrained and enabled by biology and socialization. The notion that nurses are primarily concerned with human response implies stimulus. Built into the basic definition of nursing is the cause and effect relationship. Yet, at the same time human behavior may be largely predetermined.

In a similar fashion, the ideas expressed about society in the statement are in conflict. Allen (1987) describes the conflict as the depiction of society as a single organism acting in unison and simultaneously as a group of individuals with different viewpoints and interests.

One is left wondering what nursing is really all about when the essential concepts of person and society are unclear. What is clear, at least, is a quasi-mechanistic view of human beings. But to what are human beings responding? And what is a satisfactory definition of the term health? One can not help but ponder the question, "Would you know health if you saw it?" However, nursing is the diagnosis of the response to health problems and the treatment of the response. The diagnosis is to be determined in actuality and also in potentiality. Nursing science as the foundation of practice is to direct its attention to this arena. What is implied is that nursing, as well as nursing science, is to focus on the response and leave the stimulus to others. If one were to identify a potential health problem or what is meant by the term, would nursing intervention alter or prevent the response? Or is the response inevitable?

Aside from the lack of clarity in the definition statement, the emphasis is placed on diagnosis and treatment, the two activities of the nurse. Is nursing science, in concert with the social policy statement, to study what nurses do as well as the health problems themselves? What about health itself? What about person?

The social policy statement, rather than providing clarity, may well serve to blur the direction of nursing science through a superficial definition of the scope of nursing. As the science struggles for identity, this confusion is added to those previously mentioned in obscuring the direction it must take at the present time.

Toward the Mainstream

The authors have identified three troublesome areas in the development of nursing science: the designation of nursing as an applied science, the controversy over methods, and the ambiguity of the social policy statement. Each in its own right, however, may be seen perhaps more appropriately as a symptom of a larger problem. It is the contention here that the basis of the issue at stake is the lack of a central direction for all of nursing science as evidenced by the absence of an all encompassing question. Each of the areas thusfar addressed point to this need. Confusion in the ranks of scholars as to the nature of nursing science begins with misunderstanding concerning the consensual aim and purpose of nursing science. To that end elaboration on this idea is in order.

Other Disciplines

For the sake of argument and presentation, it is useful to examine the so-called emergence of other recently established disciplines which now refer to themselves as sciences. Education and sociology are examples. Each of these disciplines has played a major part in the education of many nurse scholars.

The essential issue to be addressed in viewing education and sociology is the process of becoming a science. How did these two disciplines make the leap from a general philosophy of learning and a philosophy of social life into their respective scientific modes? The common step taken by both groups was the defining of a fundamental question toward which the fields of education and sociology could be directed. In other words, as will be elaborated, each distinctive science came into being as a science only when the reason for the science (an underlying question in need of an answer) could be identified. It is obvious, then, that efforts directed toward discovery and testing would cease when all laws and principles pertaining to this overriding question were prescribed.

The fundamental question is THE question all scholars in the particular discipline are searching to answer. In other words, once the question is answered, the discipline would have no reason to exist, because all science exists for the purpose of answering the key, fundamental, and essential question. This does not imply that all studies have a singular focus, but rather a unifying focus. The *raison d'être* is to address the fundamental question. However, this is done through the investigation of thousands and thousands of related questions. And, the question is to be answered through every direct and indirect route possible in order to reach the definitive answer.

Sociology is the youngest of the social sciences. The word "sociology" was coined by Comte in his *Positive Philosophy* (1854). He contended that a science of sociology should be based upon systematic observation and classification, not on authority and mere speculation. For this reason, Comte is considered the father of the science of sociology. Spencer (1896) in his work, *Principles of Sociology,* applied the theory of evolution to human society and evolved a grand theory of social evolution. While his premises are no longer accepted, they helped launch sociology into the domain of science.

Essentially, these early founders of the discipline were social philosophers. They developed macro systems of thought, but did neither research, verification, nor measurement of their concepts. They did not collect and classify data nor develop theory with either quantitative or qualitative methodologies. They thought out theory and sought facts to support it. The founders of sociology called for scientific investigation but did little research themselves. Yet, they took the first necessary steps, for the idea of a science of sociology had to precede the building of one.

The true emergence of sociology as a science came about through the work of Durkheim (1895) at the turn of the twentieth century. The crucial step taken by Durkheim was the identification of the aim of sociology. This field of science, he believed, should direct itself toward the study of the relations of the individual to social solidarity. Thus, Durkheim determined that the fundamental question to be answered by the science of sociology was and is: what holds society together? (And, conversely, what breaks society apart?) Each and every investigation in the sociological arena is, in fact, an attempt to more fully answer this immense and distinctive inquiry.

In a similar fashion, the evolution of education as a science was dependent upon the derivation of a basic question, what is thinking and, subsequently, what is learning? Throughout the history of mankind, the question of thinking and learning has been addressed. In ancient times, Confucius, Socrates, and Plato operated on the premise that learning was discovery. In more modern times, Thorndike (1913) believed that learning was based on a stimulus-response continuum. Depending on the particular classification schema, twentieth-century theorists have been divided into several categories of beliefs concerning the theory of learning. Regardless of the classification scheme or specific theory of learning, the fundamental question which is being addressed is the inquiry into what thinking and learning are.

Even though Socrates has been called "the father of education," the fundamental question did not begin with him. He did not raise the question of what learning was, but rather used his method as a means to teach. It was not until the twentieth century that theorists began to question the approach, and raise the central issue of what teaching and learning were all about. What are the concepts and what are the relationships? In the scientific inquiry into learning and thinking, various debates have occurred. Fundamental to each debate is the particular theory of learning the theorists subscribe to and

utilize. But more important and germane to the issue at hand is that each theorist attempts to answer the fundamental question. The science of education is based on the theories of thinking and learning. Without an understanding of what thinking and learning are (the essence of the question), education is only a process and an art.

What may be learned by noting the historical progression of other sciences is the process of emergence. And this emergence in other fields has been contingent upon the articulation of the question rather than the preliminary establishment of theory. As was shown previously, both education and sociology have been able to specify their aims through the identification of an exclusive and simultaneously inclusive question. And each of these sciences is based upon the attempts made to address the question. All research in the discipline is thus, inevitably, directed toward this end in some small part.

The Question and Nursing Science

Are there not parallels which may be drawn between these other sciences and nursing? Nursing science, too, had and has its share of antecedent thinkers. The idea of a science of nursing is well established. Theoreticians have directed attention to concepts relevant to nursing and to the universe of interest to nurses. However, the fundamental question is yet to be elaborated. Disagreement exists as to the focus of nursing science. Recognizing this problem, Peplau (in Smith 1988) has stated, "What is required is an overall rubric that's simple; the focus for the theological profession is the soul and the spirit, and man's relation to God; the focus for medicine is disease, defect and physiological deficits; the focus for law is injustice and grievance; and the focus for architecture is the form and function of buildings. We need a simplified rubric for nursing, and we can't say health because that's a goal, an outcome" (p. 82).

If the central issue of concern to nursing science is indeed human response or the factors involved in health, nursing is not clearly distinguished from the domain of medicine. If the aims are directed toward the phenomenon of caring, how is nursing different from other helping professions? If the purview is the study of nursing care, then it may be argued that the premises are truly tautological.

The problem thus is one of focus. And, this blurring of the aim of nursing science is, at least in part, to blame for such a phenomenon as nurses studying nurses rather than nurses studying issues related to clients. It is also responsible for misunderstandings related to the term "applied science," as well as inconsistencies in the definition of nursing as demonstrated in the social policy statement.

The divergence of opinion with regard to methodology also is, to a large extent, attributable to the unclear direction of nursing science. If you do not know where you are going, how can you best judge the means to get there? All of the philosophical issues raised by this debate are worthy of examination in establishing the focus of nursing science.

Visintainer (1986) uses the analogy of different maps in discussing the relevancy of knowledge. Each type of map (topographical, geological, population density) may represent an aspect of reality, but they share in representing the same spot on earth. To extend that analogy to nursing science, there is the opportunity for development of multiple paradigms, but like various maps they must all be centered on the same location. Certainly, sociologists coming from a Marxist perspective do not examine the same concepts as those espousing a structural-functionalist framework. However, both groups attempt to answer the same central question. It is the ends, rather than the means, that are of paramount importance at this time. Understanding the ends will inevitably clarify the means.

Concepts such as "person" and "health" cannot be immediately defined and put aside. The philosophy of science as it pertains to nursing will hopefully continue to examine, debate, and further elucidate the meaning of such terms. Rather, a central question is required which, by

its very nature, will direct the endeavors of the science as well as its philosophical development. In this regard nursing may be further along than is readily apparent. Sarter (1988) analyzed the philosophical roots of four contemporary nursing theorists, Rogers, Newman, Parse, and Watson. She discussed a pattern which emerged in common across all theorists: the evolutionary is described as the evolution of human consciousness; the way this evolution is characterized varies, but the term applied to it is self-transcending; implications of this view of evolution are seen in the definitions of health; health is this evolution; human beings are seen as open systems; the interaction between person and the world is dynamic, conscious, and essential; the theme of harmony is seen either within the person or between person and world; space and time are non-linear, fluid and relative; space-time forms a matrix in which past and future merge into present; and holism both epistemological and metaphysical is also commonly recognized.

What remains is the identification of THE central question in the science of nursing which directs attention and draws in the ideas of thinkers in nursing. Only by taking this step will the science no longer be described as emerging, but rather as a recognizable and specific branch of scientific endeavor. If the question cannot be determined, nurses then should emphasize the creativity of the craft, call themselves artists and lay science to rest.

REFERENCES

Allen, D. G. (1987). The social policy statement: A reappraisal. *Advances in Nursing Science, 10*(1), 39–48.

American Nurses' Association. (1980). Nursing: A social policy statement. Kansas City, MO: ANA.

Clarke, P. N., & Yaros, P. S. (1988). Commentary: Transitions to new methodologies in nursing science. *Nursing Science Quarterly, 3*, 147–151.

Comte, A. (1854). *The positive philosophy.* (H. Martineau, Trans.). New York: D. Appleton.

Duffy, M. E. (1987). Methodological triangulation: A vehicle for merging quantitative and qualitative research methods. *Image: Journal of Nursing Scholarship, 19*, 130–133.

Durkheim, E. (1895). *The rules of the sociological method.* (G. E. Catlin, Trans.). New York: Free Press.

Field, P. A., & Morse, J. (1985). *Nursing research: The application of qualitative approaches.* Rockville, MD: Aspen Systems.

Gortner, S. R., & Schultz, P. R. (1988). Approaches to nursing science methods. *Image: Journal of Nursing Scholarship, 20,* 22–24.

Jayaratne, T. E. (1983). The value of qualitative methodology for feminist research. In G. Bowlest, & R. D. Klein (Eds.), *Theories of woman's studies* (140–161). Boston: Routledge and Kegan.

Leininger, M. M. (1985). *Qualitative research methods in nursing.* Orlando, FL: Grune and Stratton.

Moccia, P. (1988). A critique of compromise: Beyond the methods debate. *Advances in Nursing Science, 10,* 1–9.

Norbeck, J. S. (1987). In defense of empiricism. *Image: Journal of Nursing Scholarship, 19,* 28–30.

Parse, R. R. (1987). *Nursing science: Major paradigms, theories and critiques.* Philadelphia: Saunders.

Phillips, J. R. (1988). Research blenders. *Nursing Science Quarterly, 1,* 4–6.

Porter, E. J. (1989). The qualitative-quantitative dualism. *Image: Journal of Nursing Scholarship, 21,* 98–102.

Rogers, M. E. (1970). *An introduction to the theoretical basis of nursing.* Philadelphia: Davis.

Sarter, B. (1988). Philosophical sources of nursing theory. *Nursing Science Quarterly, 1,* 52–59.

Schultz, P. R., & Meleis, A. I. (1988). Nursing epistemology: Traditions, insights, questions. *Image: Journal of Nursing Scholarship, 20,* 217–221.

Smith, M. J. (1988). Perspectives on nursing science. *Nursing Science Quarterly, 1,* 80–85.

Spencer, H. (1896). *The principles of sociology.* New York: D. Appleton.

Thorndike, E. L. (1913). *The psychology of learning.* New York: Columbia University.

Visintainer, M. A. (1986). The nature of nursing knowledge and theory in nursing. *Image: Journal of Nursing Scholarship, 18,* 32–38.

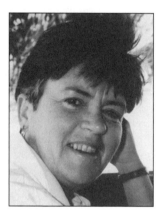

SHEILA A. PACKARD

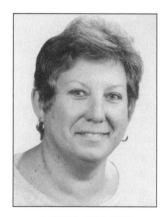

E. CAROL POLIFRONI

Author Index

Note: Page numbers in **boldface** type indicate articles written by contributors; the letter *n* following a page number indicates a footnote. *See also* the separate Subject Index beginning on page 521.

Adorno, T.
　on critical theory, 355, 413, 415
　on rationalization in Western tradition, 312
Aiken, H., on truth, 128, 129
Allen, D.
　on critical theory, 382–384, 387
　on feminist theory, 30, 160, 418
　on positivism, 156
　on scientific approaches for caring, 27
　on social policy statement, 502
　on syntax, 155
　on theory-neutral observations, 62
American Academy of Nursing, on capture of nursing
　　phenomena, 30
American Nurses' Association
　code for practice, 25, 26
　social policy statement, 25, 26, 502–503
　standard of practice, 25
　on values, 25
Anaxagoras, 349
Andersen, M., on feminist theory, 407n1
Aoki, T., on curriculum as lived vs. planned, 52
Aquinas, Thomas
　on adequacy of theory, 102
　Heidegger on, 281
　on truth, 56
Archimedes, objectivity of, 397, 402
Aristotle
　on asymmetry of explanation, 175–176, 178n16
　axiomization ideal of, 481
　on concept establishment, 347
　on determinism, 231
　on explanation, 168
　Heidegger on, 273, 274, 278, 281, 288, 289, 292–294
　on language formation, 345
　logos concept of, 292–294
　on nature, 348–353
　objectivity of, 458
　on truth, 56
　unity of analogy concept of, 274
Arms, S.
　on childbirth traditions, 446
　on gynocentric science, 443, 444

Augustine, St.
　on adequacy of theory, 102
　inner man concept of, 330
Austin, J. L., on communicative competence, 365,
　　370n19
Avenarius, on positivism, 72

Bacon, F.
　on experimentation, 138–139
　as father of philosophy of science, 8
　on gender and science, 429, 437
　on refuting theories, 8
Bain, A., on positivism, 145
Bandura, A. B., self-efficacy theory of, 215
Baron, R.
　on concept of person, 321–322
　on phenomenology, 316
Barrett, R. J., on professional expertise, 390
Bartky, S. L., on feminist theory, 416
Batey, M.
　on science vs. research, 26
　on values of nurse scientist, 27
Beaton, J. L., on universal laws, 65
Beck, L. W., on causality, 172
Becker, M. H.
　on health belief model, 215
　on self-efficacy theory, 216
Belenky, M., on gynocentric science, 441, 443, 449
Belgrave, F. Z., on locus-of-control orientation, 215
Bell Laboratories, crystal lattice work of, 143
Benner, P.
　on caring, 21, 27, 30
　on context, 65
　on critical theory, 382–384
　on expertise, 464
　on explanation, 30, 190
　on freedom, 219
　on Heidegger, 318
　on hermeneutics, 243–244
　on idiosyncratic meaning, 220
　on mechanistic models, 219
　on positivism, 156, 157
　on quality of life, 303–314

Note: The letter *n* following a page number indicates a footnote. *See also* separate Author Index beginning on page 507.